THE WASHINGTON MANUAL®

Rheumatology

Subspecialty Consult

THIRD EDITION

Editors

María C. González-Mayda, MD

Assistant Professor of Medicine
Division of Rheumatology
Washington University School of Medicine
St. Louis, Missouri

Prabha Ranganathan, MD, MSCI

Professor of Medicine
Division of Rheumatology
Washington University School of Medicine
St. Louis, Missouri

Executive Editors

Thomas Ciesielski, MD

Assistant Professor of Medicine
Department of Internal Medicine
Division of General Medicine
Washington University School of Medicine
St. Louis, Missouri

Thomas M. De Fer, MD, FACP

Professor of Medicine
Associate Dean for Medical Student
    Education
Department of Medicine
Washington University School of Medicine
St. Louis, Missouri

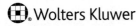 Wolters Kluwer

Philadelphia • Baltimore • New York • London
Buenos Aires • Hong Kong • Sydney • Tokyo

Executive Editor: Sharon Zinner
Development Editor: Thomas Celona
Editorial Coordinator: Tim Rinehart
Marketing Manager: Phyllis Hitner
Production Project Manager: Sadie Buckallew
Design Coordinator: Stephen Druding
Manufacturing Coordinator: Beth Welsh
Prepress Vendor: S4Carlisle Publishing Services

Third edition

9 8 7 6 5 4 3 2

Printed in China

Library of Congress Cataloging-in-Publication Data

Names: González-Mayda, María C., editor.
Title: The Washington manual rheumatology subspecialty consult / [edited by] María C. González-Mayda, Prabha Ranganathan.
Other titles: Rheumatology subspecialty consult
Description: Third edition. | Philadelphia: Wolters Kluwer, 2020. |
  Includes bibliographical references and index.
Identifiers: LCCN 2020005641 | ISBN 9781975113391 (paperback)
Subjects: LCSH: Rheumatism—Diagnosis—Handbooks, manuals, etc. |
  Rheumatism—Treatment—Handbooks, manuals, etc.
Classification: LCC RC927 .W375 2020 | DDC 616.7/23—dc23
LC record available at https://lccn.loc.gov/2020005641

shop.lww.com

CCS0921

Contents

PART I. INTRODUCTION TO THE RHEUMATOLOGY CONSULT

PART II. CORE RHEUMATOLOGIC DISEASES

PART III. SERONEGATIVE SPONDYLOARTHROPATHIES

PART IV. CRYSTALLINE ARTHRITIDES

PART V. VASCULITIDES

PART VI. INFECTION-RELATED DISORDERS

PART VII. OTHER RHEUMATIC DISORDERS

Contributing Authors

Richard D. Brasington, MD
Professor of Medicine
Division of Rheumatology
Washington University School of Medicine
St. Louis, Missouri

Philip Chu, MD
Hospitalist
Division of Hospital Medicine
Washington University School of Medicine
St. Louis, Missouri

Jennifer L. Demertzis, MD
Associate Professor of Radiology
Department of Radiology
Washington University School of Medicine
St. Louis, Missouri

Vladimir Despotovic, MD
Associate Professor of Medicine
Department of Pulmonary and Critical Care
  Medicine
Washington University School of Medicine
St. Louis, Missouri

Colin Diffie, MD
Instructor in Medicine
Division of Rheumatology
Washington University School of Medicine
St. Louis, Missouri

Devon M. DiVito, MD
Fellow
Musculoskeletal Section
Mallinckrodt Institute of Radiology
Washington University School of Medicine
St. Louis, Missouri

Jaime Flores-Ruiz, MD
Resident
Department of Medicine
Washington University School of Medicine
St. Louis, Missouri

Anneliese M. Flynn, MD
Fellow
Division of Rheumatology
Washington University School of Medicine
St. Louis, Missouri

Yuka Furuya, MD
Fellow
Division of Pulmonary and Critical Care
  Medicine
Washington University School of Medicine
St. Louis, Missouri

María C. González-Mayda, MD
Assistant Professor of Medicine
Division of Rheumatology
Washington University School of Medicine
St. Louis, Missouri

Michiko Inaba, MD
Fellow
Division of Rheumatology
Washington University School of Medicine
St. Louis, Missouri

Divya Jayakumar, MD
Fellow
Division of Rheumatology
Washington University School of Medicine
St. Louis, Missouri

Heather A. Jones, MD
Assistant Professor
Division of Dermatology
Washington University School of Medicine
St. Louis, Missouri

Amy M. Joseph, MD
Professor of Medicine
Division of Rheumatology
Washington University School of Medicine
St. Louis, Missouri

Alfred H. J. Kim, MD, PhD
Assistant Professor of Medicine
Division of Rheumatology
Washington University School of Medicine
St. Louis, Missouri

Iris Lee, MD
Fellow
Division of Rheumatology
Washington University School of Medicine
St. Louis, Missouri

Kelvin J. Lee, MD
Fellow
Division of Rheumatology
Washington University School of Medicine
St. Louis, Missouri

Jonathan J. Miner, MD, PhD
Assistant Professor of Medicine
Division of Rheumatology
Washington University School of Medicine
St. Louis, Missouri

Michael A. Paley, MD, PhD
Fellow
Division of Rheumatology
Washington University School of Medicine
St. Louis, Missouri

Deborah L. Parks, MD
Professor of Medicine
Division of Rheumatology
Washington University School of Medicine
St. Louis, Missouri

Prabha Ranganathan, MD, MSCI
Professor of Medicine
Division of Rheumatology
Washington University School of Medicine
St. Louis, Missouri

Christine N. Schafer, MD
Resident
Division of Dermatology
Washington University School of Medicine
St. Louis, Missouri

Deepali Sen, MD
Assistant Professor of Medicine
Division of Rheumatology
Washington University School of Medicine
St. Louis, Missouri

Adrian Shifren, MD
Associate Professor of Medicine
Division of Pulmonary and Critical Care
   Medicine
Washington University School of Medicine
St. Louis, Missouri

Shuang Song, MD, PhD
Fellow
Division of Rheumatology
Washington University School of Medicine
St. Louis, Missouri

Can M. Sungur, MD, PhD
Fellow
Division of Rheumatology
Washington University School of Medicine
St. Louis, Missouri

Wayne M. Yokoyama, MD
Professor of Medicine
Division of Rheumatology
Washington University School of Medicine
St. Louis, Missouri

Roseanne F. Zhao, MD, PhD
Fellow
Division of Rheumatology
Washington University School of Medicine
St. Louis, Missouri

Lisa A. Zickuhr, MD
Instructor in Medicine
Division of Rheumatology
Washington University School of Medicine
St. Louis, Missouri

Chairman's Note

It is a pleasure to present the new edition of *The Washington Manual*® Subspecialty Consult Series: *Rheumatology Subspecialty Consult*. This pocket-size book continues to be an excellent primary reference for medical students, interns, residents, and other practitioners who need ready access to practical clinical information to diagnose and treat patients with a wide variety of autoimmune and rheumatologic disorders. Medical knowledge continues to increase at an astounding rate, which creates a challenge for physicians to keep up with the biomedical discoveries, genomic and immunologic advances, and novel therapeutics that can positively impact patient outcomes. The *Rheumatology Subspecialty Consult* addresses this challenge by concisely and practically providing current scientific information for clinicians to aid them in the diagnosis, investigation, and treatment of autoimmune and rheumatologic diseases.

I want to personally thank the authors, who are house officers, fellows, and attendings at the Washington University School of Medicine and Barnes-Jewish Hospital. Their commitment to patient care and education is unsurpassed, and their efforts and skill in compiling this manual are evident in the quality of the final product. In particular, I would like to acknowledge our editors, Drs. María C. González-Mayda and Prabha Ranganathan, and the executive editors, Drs. Thomas Cielsielski and Tom De Fer, who have worked tirelessly to produce another outstanding edition of this manual. I believe this subspecialty manual will meet its desired goal of providing practical knowledge that can be applied at the bedside and in outpatient settings to improve patient care.

Victoria J. Fraser, MD
Adolphus Busch Professor of Medicine
Chair of the Department of Medicine
Washington University School of Medicine
St. Louis, Missouri

Preface

As we started to plan for the third edition of this manual, it became clear that there have been tremendous advances in rheumatology, especially in new treatments, in the last eight years. Cognizant of this, we have thoroughly revised and updated each chapter and added a few new chapters. We have written this manual as a quick reference guide to rheumatology for the general internist and subspecialist. The target audience also includes medical students, residents, fellows, and other medical professionals who care for patients with rheumatic diseases. This manual is not intended to be exhaustive; rather, it serves as a compendium of rheumatology. The editors would like to thank all the contributing authors for taking time out of their busy schedules to participate in this project. A special thanks to our supportive families for putting up with the long hours we spent editing and proofreading the material. We wish our readers well in their study of rheumatology, a dynamic field that continues to inspire and excite us.

María C. González-Mayda

Prabha Ranganathan

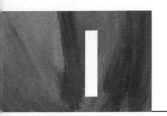

Introduction to the Rheumatology Consult

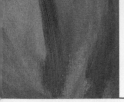

Approach to the Rheumatology Patient

Iris Lee and María C. González-Mayda

GENERAL PRINCIPLES

- Musculoskeletal complaints account for the majority of outpatient visits in the community.
  - Many are self-limited or localized problems that improve with symptomatic treatment.
  - Other conditions (e.g., septic arthritis, crystal-induced arthritis, fractures) require urgent diagnosis and treatment.
- A thorough history and physical examination are necessary to help narrow your diagnosis.
  - Musculoskeletal conditions may be classified according to their symptom presentation—inflammatory versus noninflammatory and articular versus nonarticular.
  - Musculoskeletal problems may also be the initial presentation of diseases such as cancer and endocrinopathies.
- Use specific ancillary tests such as radiographs, labs, and arthrocentesis to help confirm your initial diagnosis.
- Rheumatic diseases mainly involve the musculoskeletal system.
  - Inflammatory disorders are often accompanied by systemic features (fever and weight loss) and other organ involvement (kidney, skin, lung, eye, blood).
  - Because these diseases affect multiple organ systems, they are challenging to diagnose, complicated to treat, and often humbling to study.
- Inpatient consultations usually involve patients with known diagnoses (a patient with lupus admitted with a flare) or with multiple organ system involvement and the suspicion of a systemic rheumatic disease (a patient with respiratory and kidney failure with positive antineutrophil cytoplasmic antibody [ANCA]).

Classification

The following is an approach to patients with musculoskeletal complaints and to common inpatient consults. Regional problems (i.e., nonsystemic musculoskeletal disorders) are discussed in Chapter 8.

Inflammatory versus Noninflammatory

The characteristics of inflammatory and noninflammatory disorders are presented in Table 1-1. These distinctions are useful but not absolute.

- **Inflammatory Disorders**
  - Characterized by systemic symptoms (fever, stiffness, weight loss, fatigue). Joint stiffness is common after prolonged rest (morning stiffness) and improves with activity.
    - Duration of more than 1 hour suggests an inflammatory condition.
    - Noninflammatory conditions may cause stiffness, usually lasting less than 1 hour, and the joint symptoms increase with use and weight bearing.
  - Signs of joint inflammation on physical examination (**erythema, warmth, swelling, pain**)
  - Lab evidence of inflammation (elevated erythrocyte sedimentation rate [ESR], elevated C-reactive protein [CRP], hypoalbuminemia, normochromic normocytic anemia, thrombocytosis). Inflammatory disorders may be **immune mediated** (systemic lupus erythematosus [SLE], rheumatoid arthritis [RA]), **reactive** (reactive arthritis [ReA]), **infectious** (gonococcal [GC] arthritis), or **crystal induced** (gout, pseudogout).

TABLE 1-1	NONINFLAMMATORY VERSUS INFLAMMATORY DISORDERS	
Symptoms	Noninflammatory Disorders (e.g., OA)	Inflammatory Disorders (e.g., RA, lupus)
Morning stiffness	Focal, brief, <1 hour. Typically ≤30 minutes	Significant, prolonged, >1 hour
Constitutional symptoms	Absent	Present
Peak period of discomfort	After prolonged use	After prolonged inactivity
Locking or instability	Implies loose body, internal derangement, or weakness	Uncommon
Symmetry (bilateral)	Occasional	Common

OA, osteoarthritis; RA, rheumatoid arthritis.

- **Noninflammatory Disorders**
  - Characterized by absence of systemic symptoms, **pain without erythema or warmth**, normal lab tests.
  - Osteoarthritis (OA), fibromyalgia, and traumatic conditions are common noninflammatory disorders.

Articular versus Nonarticular
- Pain may originate from:
  - **Articular structures** (synovial membrane, cartilage, intra-articular ligaments, capsule, or juxta-articular bone surfaces).
  - **Periarticular structures** (bursae, tendons, muscle, bone, nerve, skin).
  - **Nonarticular structures** (i.e., cardiac pain referred to the shoulder).
- **Articular Disorders**
  - Cause deep or diffuse pain that worsens with active and passive movement.
  - Physical examination may show deformity, warmth, swelling, effusion, or crepitus.
    - **Arthralgia** refers to joint pain without abnormalities on joint examination.
    - **Arthritis** indicates the presence of abnormality in the joint (warmth, swelling, erythema, tenderness).
    - **Synovitis** (inflammation of the synovial membrane that covers the joint) presents as boggy, tender swelling around the joint. The joint loses its sharp edges on examination. Synovitis is easy to detect in finger and wrist joints.
- **Nonarticular Disorders**
  - Usually have point tenderness and increased pain with active, but not passive, movement.
  - Physical examination does not usually show joint deformity or swelling.

DIAGNOSIS

Clinical Presentation
- The evaluation of musculoskeletal complaints should determine whether the disorder is inflammatory or noninflammatory, whether the joints or the periarticular structures are involved, and the number and pattern of joints involved. The latter is important in the diagnosis.

- Number and pattern of joints involved:
  - **Acute monoarthritis** suggests infection, but gout and trauma are possible.
  - **Asymmetric, oligoarticular** (<5 joints) involvement, particularly of the lower extremities, is typical of OA and ReA.
  - **Symmetric, polyarticular** (≥5 joints) involvement is typical of RA and SLE.
  - Involvement of the **spine, sacroiliac (SI) joints, and sternoclavicular** joints is characteristic of ankylosing spondylitis (AS).
  - In the hands, **distal interphalangeal (DIP) joints** are involved in OA (Heberden's nodes) and in psoriatic arthritis (PsA) but are spared by RA.
  - **Proximal interphalangeal (PIP) joint** involvement is seen in OA (Bouchard's nodes) and RA.
  - **Metacarpophalangeal (MCP) joints** are involved in RA but not in OA.
  - **Acute first metatarsophalangeal (MTP) joint** arthritis is classic for gout (podagra) but is also seen in OA and ReA.
  - Vasculitis and SLE may present with **multiple organ system involvement**, often without major joint complaints.
  - Fibromyalgia presents with **diffuse pain** but without arthritis.
  - Myositis presents with **muscle weakness**, rashes, and, occasionally, peripheral arthritis.

History
- A comprehensive history and physical examination are often enough to make a diagnosis.
- Certain diseases are more frequent in specific **age groups and genders**.
  - SLE, juvenile RA, and GC arthritis are more common in the young.
  - Gout, OA, and RA are more common in middle-aged persons.
  - Polymyalgia rheumatica (PMR) and giant cell arthritis occur in the elderly.
  - Gout and AS are more common in men; gout is rare in premenopausal women.
  - SLE, RA, and OA are more common in women.
- Ask about **pain**, swelling, weakness, tenderness, limitation of motion, stiffness, as well as constitutional symptoms when presented with a musculoskeletal complaint because these clues will help you narrow your diagnosis.
  - For example, joint pain that occurs at rest and worsens with movement suggests an inflammatory process, whereas pain elicited with activity and relieved by rest usually indicates a mechanical disorder such as a degenerative arthritis.
- Inquire about what **medications** they are taking because many have side effects and patients on immunosuppressive drugs are predisposed to developing infections.
  - Some medications may cause a **lupus-like syndrome** (e.g., hydralazine, procainamide), **myopathies** (e.g., statins, colchicine, zidovudine), or **osteoporosis** (e.g., glucocorticoids, phenytoin).
  - **Alcohol** commonly precipitates gout and may rarely cause myopathies and avascular necrosis (AVN).
  - Vasculitis, arthralgias, and rhabdomyolysis may also be seen with **substance abuse** (e.g., cocaine, heroin).
- Certain areas of the United States and Europe have an increased incidence of **Lyme disease**; therefore, it is important to inquire about recent trips to these areas.
- A **family history** may be important in AS, gout, and OA.
- The **review of systems** may identify other organ involvement and support the diagnosis.
  - The **nervous system** may be involved in SLE, vasculitis, and Lyme disease.
  - **Eye involvement** may be severe and occurs in Sjögren's syndrome (SS), RA, seronegative spondyloarthropathies, giant cell arthritis, Behçet's disease, and granulomatosis with polyangiitis (GPA).
  - **Oral mucosal ulcers** are common in SLE, enteropathic arthritis, and Behçet's disease.
  - **Rashes** are seen in SLE, vasculitis, PsA, dermatomyositis (DM), adult-onset Still's disease, and Lyme disease.

○ **Raynaud's phenomenon** is a reversible, paroxysmal constriction of small arteries that occurs most commonly in fingers and toes, and is precipitated by cold and stress. The classic sequence is initial blanching followed by cyanosis and finally erythema due to vasodilation and is accompanied by numbness or tingling. It may be idiopathic or associated with scleroderma, DM, SLE, RA, and mixed connective tissue disease (MCTD).

○ **Pleuritis and pericarditis** may be seen in RA, SLE, MCTD, and adult-onset Still's disease.

○ **Gastrointestinal (GI) involvement** is seen in enteropathic arthritis, **polymyositis** (PM), and scleroderma. The latter may be associated with dysphagia.

Physical Examination

• Tailor the physical examination based on the presenting complaint.

• If the main complaint is arthritis or arthralgia, look for signs of inflammation such as swelling, warmth, erythema over the joint and surrounding structures, tenderness, deformity, limitation of motion, instability of the joint, and crepitus.

• If the pain appears to be nonarticular in origin, examine the surrounding bursae, tendons, ligaments, and bones for tenderness and inflammation.

• If there is suspicion of systemic involvement, make sure to perform a thorough examination so as not to miss any important findings that could help you determine the etiology of their symptoms. In addition to a thorough examination of all the joints, examine the:

○ Hair for alopecia or rashes

○ Skin for discoloration, rash, ulceration, or blistering as well as the nails for pitting

○ Nose and mouth for signs of ulceration

○ Heart and lungs for signs of pericardial or pleural rubs, and so on

○ Abdomen for signs of serositis, pain related to ischemic bowel, and so on

○ Genitalia for ulcerations if there is clinical suspicion for Behçet's disease and/or inflammatory bowel disease

• The back examination should include the spinous processes as well as paraspinal and surrounding muscles. Do not forget to examine the SI joints as well.

Differential Diagnosis

Approach to Monoarthritis

• Common causes of monoarthritis are **infection, crystal-induced arthritis, and trauma** (Table 1-2).

• Acute pain or swelling of a single joint requires immediate evaluation for septic arthritis, which can rapidly destroy the joint if left untreated (see Fig. 1-1).[1]

• It is also important to distinguish pain arising from periarticular structures (tendons, bursa), which usually requires only symptomatic treatment, and cases of referred pain (shoulder pain due to peritonitis or heart disease).

• The history should exclude trauma and can provide clues such as:

○ History of tick bite (Lyme disease)

○ Sexual risk factors (GC arthritis)

○ Colitis, uveitis, and urethritis (seronegative spondyloarthropathies)

• Physical examination usually distinguishes between articular and nonarticular disorders.

• **Perform arthrocentesis in patients with acute monoarthritis** (see Chapter 4). Send synovial fluid:

○ Leukocyte count with differential ($>2,000/mm^3$ suggests an inflammatory process)

○ Gram stain and culture

○ Crystal analysis. A wet mount of the fluid examined under polarizing microscopy may identify crystals, but **the presence of crystals does not exclude infection.**

• Synovial biopsy and arthroscopy are sometimes used to diagnose chronic monoarthritis.

• **Culture other potential sources** of infection (throat, cervix, rectum, wounds, blood).

TABLE 1-2	FEATURES AND CAUSES OF MONOARTHRITIS	
Type	**Features**	**Causes**
Infectious arthritis	Common; acute; may or may not have fever or leukocytosis; synovial fluid culture usually confirmatory in nongonococcal arthritis	Bacteria (gonococci and *Staphylococcus aureus*) most common. Also viruses (HIV, hepatitis B), fungi, mycobacteria, Lyme disease
Crystal-induced arthritis	Common; very acute onset; extremely painful; crystals on microscopic examination of synovial fluid	Monosodium urate crystals (gout), calcium pyrophosphate dihydrate crystals, and others
OA	Common; usually in the lower extremities; synovial fluid is noninflammatory	May be primary or secondary to trauma, hemochromatosis
Trauma	Common; history is diagnostic; occurs rarely in inpatients	Fracture, hemarthrosis, internal derangement
AVN of bone	Uncommon; more common in the hip, knee, shoulder	Risk factors include trauma, glucocorticoid or alcohol use
Tumors	Uncommon	Benign or malignant, primary or metastatic
Systemic diseases with monoarticular onset	Uncommon (follow-up may be needed for diagnosis)	Psoriatic arthritis, SLE, ReA, RA

AVN, avascular necrosis; HIV, human immunodeficiency virus; OA, osteoarthritis; RA, rheumatoid arthritis; ReA, reactive arthritis; SLE, systemic lupus erythematosus.

- Radiographs are useful in cases of trauma and may show OA or chondrocalcinosis in calcium pyrophosphate deposition disease.
- **A patient with synovial fluid that is highly inflammatory requires empiric antibiotic therapy until the evaluation, including cultures, is completed.**

Approach to Polyarthritis
- Polyarthritis is one of the most common problems in rheumatology (see Fig. 1-2).[1]
- The number and pattern of joint involvement suggest the diagnosis (Table 1-3).
- There are many nonarticular causes of generalized joint pain.
  - Disorders of periarticular structures (tendons, bursae) cause joint pain but usually involve a single joint.
  - Myopathies occasionally cause widespread pain, but muscle weakness is the primary symptom of myositis.
  - PMR causes shoulder and pelvic girdle pain with morning stiffness, but there is usually no arthritis on examination; weakness is not a feature of this disease.
  - Neuropathies, primary bone diseases (Paget's disease), and fibromyalgia can also cause widespread pain but are distinguished by history and physical examination.

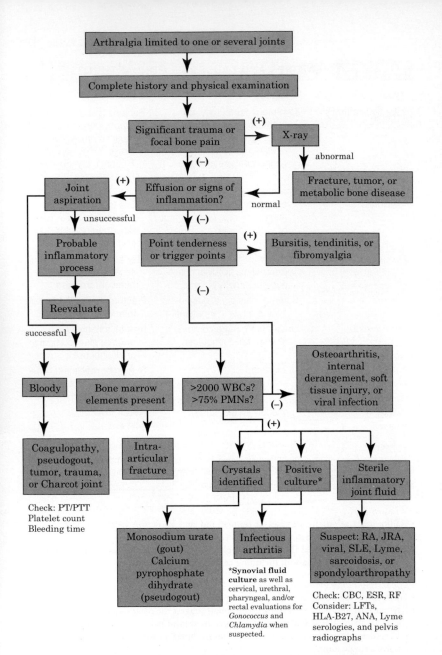

FIGURE 1-1. Approach to monoarthritis. CBC, complete blood count; ESR, erythrocyte sedimentation rate; JRA, juvenile rheumatoid arthritis; LFTs, liver function tests; PMNs, polymorphonuclear cells; PT, prothrombin time; PTT, partial thromboplastin time; RA, rheumatoid arthritis; RF, rheumatoid factor; SLE, systemic lupus erythematosus. (Adapted from American College of Rheumatology ad hoc Committee on Clinical Guidelines. Guidelines for the initial evaluation of the adult patient with acute musculoskeletal symptoms. *Arthritis Rheum.* 1996;39:1.)

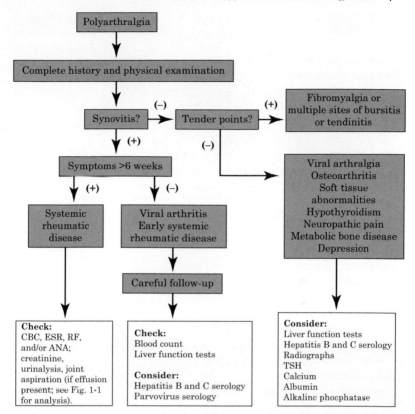

FIGURE 1-2. Approach to polyarthritis. ANA, antinuclear antibody; CBC, complete blood count; ESR, erythrocyte sedimentation rate; RF, rheumatoid factor; TSH, thyroid-stimulating hormone. (Adapted from American College of Rheumatology ad hoc Committee on Clinical Guidelines. Guidelines for the initial evaluation of the adult patient with acute musculoskeletal symptoms. *Arthritis Rheum.* 1996;39:1.)

- **RA** is the prototypical polyarticular arthritis.
  - Given its prevalence (between 0.5% and 1%), it is important to recognize and distinguish RA from other types of arthritis.[2]
  - RA usually begins with **symmetric peripheral arthritis** of multiple small joints of the hands, wrists, and feet that progresses over weeks to months. Morning stiffness is prominent and usually lasts more than 1 hour. Other joints (knees, ankles, shoulders, elbows) are sequentially involved. Involvement of the cervical spine, temporomandibular joint, and sternoclavicular joint may also be seen.
  - Lumbar spine, SI joint, and DIP involvement is not seen.
- **SLE** may present with polyarthritis similar to RA. The arthritis may be intermittent and accompanied by fever, rashes, serositis, and other organ involvement.
- **Viral arthritis** (due to parvovirus B19, hepatitis B, rubella, human immunodeficiency virus [HIV]) may have an acute onset with fever and rashes, and persist for months.

TABLE 1-3	Causes of Polyarthritis

Inflammatory

Polyarticular peripheral (usually symmetric)

RA (usually presents insidiously, additive)

Viral arthritis (usually acute onset)

SLE

PsA (occasionally)

Palindromic rheumatism (recurrent attacks)

Oligoarticular with axial involvement (usually asymmetric, lower extremity joints)

Seronegative spondyloarthropathies (AS, ReA, PsA, and enteropathic arthritis)

Oligoarticular without axial involvement (usually asymmetric)

Lyme disease

Polyarticular gout (more commonly monoarticular)

CPPD

Bacterial endocarditis

Septic arthritis (particularly in patients with RA)

Sarcoidosis

Behçet's disease and relapsing polychondritis (rare)

Rheumatic fever (usually migratory)

Noninflammatory

OA (hands, generalized, posttraumatic; can be secondary to metabolic disease like hemochromatosis, ochronosis, acromegaly)

Sickle cell disease

Hypertrophic osteoarthropathy

Others (rare; leukemia, hemophilia, amyloidosis)

AS, axial spondyloarthropathy; CPPD, calcium pyrophosphate deposition disease; OA, osteoarthritis; PsA, psoriatic arthritis; RA, rheumatoid arthritis; ReA, reactive arthritis; SLE, systemic lupus erythematosus.

- **Palindromic rheumatism** causes recurrent attacks of symmetric arthritis that affect the hands, wrists, and knees and are self-limited over several days.
- The **seronegative spondyloarthropathies** (axial spondyloarthropathy, ReA, PsA, etc.) are characterized by spine and SI joint involvement, enthesopathy (inflammation at sites of tendon insertion to bone), and varying degrees of peripheral joint, eye, skin, and GI involvement.
  - Peripheral joint involvement is usually **asymmetric, oligoarticular**, and of the lower extremities (knee, ankle).
  - **Dactylitis**, diffuse swelling of a digit ("sausage digit"), may be seen in fingers and toes, and is characteristic of ReA and PsA.
  - A symmetric, polyarticular form of PsA exists that is similar to RA.
- Oligoarticular disease may also be seen with Behçet's disease, sarcoidosis, and relapsing polychondritis.
- **Bacterial arthritis** may be polyarticular in patients with preexisting joint damage (RA).

- **GC arthritis** may be migratory and is accompanied by fever, pustular skin lesions, and tenosynovitis.
- Fever and migratory arthralgias or mild arthritis may be seen in early **Lyme disease**, and a persistent oligoarticular arthritis occurs months later.
- **Bacterial endocarditis** often presents with fever and low back pain, along with arthralgias, and may have a positive RF.
- **Gout** is usually monoarticular, but polyarthritis is sometimes seen, particularly later in the disease.
- Pseudogout may present as "pseudo-RA" with bilateral hand and wrist involvement.
- Rheumatic fever occurs after streptococcal infection and is characterized by migratory arthritis of large joints, fever, and extra-articular involvement (carditis, chorea, rash).
- OA is the most common form of noninflammatory polyarthritis.
  - ○ **DIP, PIP, first carpometacarpal (CMC), knees, hips, spine, and first MTP joints** are typically involved.
  - ○ Hemochromatosis predisposes to OA in unusual joints (second and third MCPs).

Approach to Patients with Positive Antinuclear Antibodies

- **Antinuclear antibodies (ANAs)** are autoantibodies that target nucleic acid and nucleoprotein antigens and are usually detected by indirect immunofluorescence (see Chapter 5) (see Fig. 1-3).[3]
- ANAs are **very sensitive** but not specific for SLE. Their absence by current assays practically rules out SLE.
- ANAs are present in other rheumatic diseases (e.g., scleroderma, MCTD, PM, SS), drug-induced lupus (DIL), some infectious diseases (e.g., HIV), and in up to 30% of healthy individuals.[4]
- They are also present in many patients with chronic liver or lung disorders and in those with nonarticular autoimmune diseases such as thyroiditis.
- **An ANA test should be ordered only when you suspect a patient has an underlying autoimmune condition such as SLE.**
- A positive ANA should be followed by a complete history and physical examination to identify those conditions.
  - ○ A history of hydralazine or procainamide use suggests DIL.
  - ○ Myositis, skin changes, and Raynaud's phenomenon suggest MCTD, myositis, or scleroderma.
  - ○ Sicca symptoms (dry eyes and dry mouth) suggest SS.
- **SLE** is a multisystem disease that is diagnosed clinically.
  - ○ Criteria developed for the classification of lupus (see Chapter 12) can be used as a framework for assessing whether a patient has SLE.
  - ○ Certain other diseases (acute HIV infection, endocarditis, autoimmune hepatitis) may fulfill criteria for SLE.
  - ○ High-titer ANAs (>1:640) should be followed by assays for antibodies to certain antigens (double-stranded DNA, Sjögren's syndrome–related antigen A [SSA]/Ro, Sjögren's syndrome–related antigen B [SSB]/La, ribonucleoprotein [RNP], Smith [Sm]) that may be more specific for SLE and other rheumatic diseases.
  - ○ If no definitive diagnosis is made, follow-up may be indicated.
  - ○ Up to 40% of patients referred to a rheumatologist for evaluation of positive ANAs who do not fulfill criteria on presentation do fulfill criteria for SLE after months to years of follow-up.

Approach to Patients with Possible Systemic Vasculitis

- The vasculitides are a heterogeneous group of disorders characterized by inflammation of blood vessels.
- Vasculitis is often suspected in patients with multiple organ involvement. Vessels in the respiratory tract, kidneys, GI tract, peripheral nerves, and skin may be involved to varying degrees depending on the category of vasculitis and the size of the blood vessel involved.

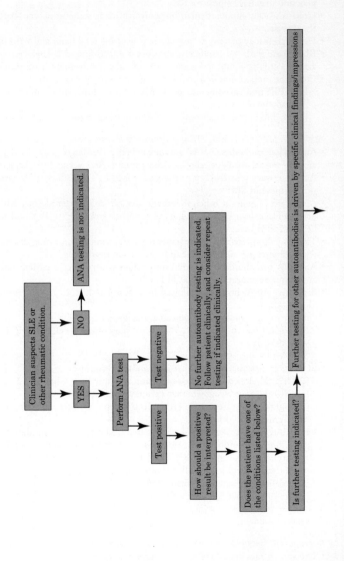

Clinician suspects SLE or
other rheumatic condition.

YES → Perform ANA test

NO → ANA testing is not indicated.

Test positive

Test negative

How should a positive
result be interpreted?

Does the patient have one of
the conditions listed below?

Is further testing indicated?

No further autoantibody testing is indicated.
Follow patient clinically, and consider repeat
testing if indicated clinically.

Further testing for other autoantibodies is driven by specific clinical findings/impressions

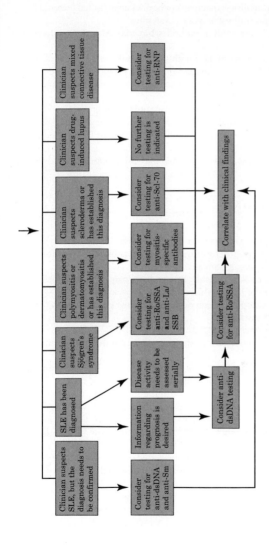

FIGURE 1-3. Approach to a positive ANA. ANA, antinuclear antibody; dsDNA, double-stranded DNA; RNP, ribonucleoprotein; SLE, systemic lupus erythematosus; Sm, Smith; SSA, Sjögren's syndrome–related antigen A; SSB, Sjögren's syndrome–related antigen B. (From Kavanaugh A, Tomar R, Reveille J, et al. Guidelines for clinical use of the antinuclear antibody test and test for specific autoantibodies to nuclear antigens. *Arch Pathol Lab Med.* 2000;124:71–81)

- Perform a complete history and physical examination on these patients.
  - Patients with suspected vasculitis should be questioned about fever, rashes, arthralgias or arthritis, abdominal pain, weight loss, and any underlying rheumatic diseases (SLE, RA).
  - The physical examination should identify other organ system involvement (purpura, peripheral neuropathy, joint abnormalities) that may not be obvious on initial presentation.
- **ANCA** should be ordered if suspecting some types of vasculitis.
  - ANCA is sensitive and specific for some vasculitides but may be seen in infections (such as HIV).
  - Positive ANCA tends to require confirmation with more specific assays for antibodies against myeloperoxidase (MPO) and proteinase-3 (PR3) (see Chapter 5).
- Other lab tests (ANA, complement levels, hepatitis panels, cryoglobulins, urinalysis) may be useful to establish etiology.
- Chest and sinus radiographs may reveal occult respiratory tract involvement.
- Diagnosis may require histologic examination of the skin, nerve, kidney, or lung tissue.
- Infection should be ruled out before treatment with glucocorticoids or immunosuppressive medications.
- Bacterial endocarditis, embolic disease, and cocaine use may mimic vasculitis and therefore should also be considered.

SPECIAL CONSIDERATIONS

Perioperative Considerations

- There are special considerations for patients with rheumatic diseases who undergo elective surgical procedures related to joint deformities that limit mobility, medications the patient is taking, and existing end-organ damage.
- **Joint deformities** in patients with RA, juvenile RA, and AS may include limited jaw opening and cervical spine fusion or laxity, which can contribute to difficult intubation.
  - Patients with RA should have preoperative cervical spine radiographs (lateral in flexion and extension) to detect severe instability.
  - Fiberoptic or awake intubation may be needed.
  - Patients with AS may also have limitations in thoracic expansion that may complicate mechanical ventilation.
- Cystitis, skin infections, and possible sources of bacteremia such as caries should be treated before joint replacement to prevent seeding of the prosthesis.
- Patients with SS are at risk for corneal abrasions in surgical settings and need to receive ocular lubricants before and after surgery.
  - NPO orders may be made more tolerable with artificial saliva.
  - Particular care is needed with intubation, given the usual poor state of dentition in these patients.
- Many patients with rheumatologic diseases are on nonsteroidal anti-inflammatory drugs (NSAIDs). Aspirin and other NSAIDs affect platelet aggregation and should be discontinued 5 to 7 days before surgery. Selective cyclooxygenase-2 (COX-2) inhibitors do not affect platelet aggregation and may be used until the day of surgery.
- Other medications commonly used include glucocorticoids, disease-modifying antirheumatic drugs (DMARDs), and/or biologic agents (see Chapter 9). A consensus statement was published by the American College of Rheumatology and the American Association of Hip and Knee Surgeons in 2017. Briefly,
  - Continue the current dose of nonbiologic DMARDs because the risk of infection and flares decreased with continuation.
  - Hold biologics and schedule surgery at the end of the dosing cycle. Restart these medications once the wound shows evidence of healing and if there are no clinical signs of infection.

- Hold tofacitinib for at least 7 days prior to surgery.
- For severe SLE, continue mycophenolate mofetil, azathioprine, cyclosporine, or tacrolimus. If SLE is not severe, withhold these medications for 1 week prior to surgery.
- Taper steroids if possible to less than 20 mg of prednisone/day. Continue the current daily dose of glucocorticoids through the surgery (this is in contrast to previous statements recommending "stress" dose steroids). This does not apply to juvenile idiopathic arthritis (JIA) patients or patients who receive steroids for adrenal insufficiency or primary hypothalamic disease.
- Prophylaxis against deep vein thrombosis is mandatory in joint replacement patients.
- Aggressive physical therapy is essential for rehabilitation.
- Acute crystalline arthritis is common in the postoperative period, and management may be difficult in patients with renal dysfunction or who cannot have oral intake. In these patients, intra-articular glucocorticoids (after excluding infection) may be an option (see Chapter 21).

FOLLOW-UP

- Many rheumatologic diseases have similar clinical pictures at onset but evolve into distinct patterns over time, and a close follow-up is needed to make a diagnosis.
- A patient with symmetric, peripheral polyarthritis may have a self-limited viral arthritis, but persistence for more than 12 weeks suggests RA.
- Urgent treatment is required in cases with active infection. Other patients may be treated with NSAIDs with referral to a rheumatologist if disease persists.

REFERENCES

1. American College of Rheumatology ad hoc Committee on Clinical Guidelines. Guidelines for the initial evaluation of the adult patient with acute musculoskeletal symptoms. *Arthritis Rheum.* 1996;39:1.
2. Gabriel SE, Michaud K. Epidemiological studies in incidence, prevalence, mortality and comorbidity of the rheumatic diseases. *Arthritis Res Ther.* 2009;11(3):229.
3. Kavanaugh A, Tomar R, Reveille J, et al. Guidelines for clinical use of the antinuclear antibody test and test for specific autoantibodies to nuclear antigens. *Arch Pathol Lab Med.* 2000;124:71–81.
4. Tan EM, Feltkamp TEW, Smolen JS, et al. Range of antinuclear antibodies in "healthy" individuals. *Arthritis Rheum.* 1997;40:1601–1611.

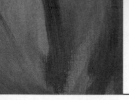

Rheumatologic Joint Examination

2

Colin Diffie and Deborah L. Parks

GENERAL PRINCIPLES

- Musculoskeletal disorders are a common complaint and are the most frequent reason for disability in the population. Knowledge of joint anatomy is fundamental to accurate physical examination.
- The joint examination, if done consistently, can be performed with efficiency and brevity.
- A brief screening examination is presented in Table 2-1.[1]
- More thorough standardized examinations include the 28 and 66 joint count examinations (see Fig. 2-1).

TABLE 2-1	BRIEF JOINT SCREENING EXAMINATION

Upper extremities
   Squeeze across MCP joints collectively and ask patient whether it is painful
   "Make a fist"
   "Touch your fingers to the tip of your thumb"
   "Turn your hands over"
   "Place your hands behind your head"
   "Place your hands behind your back"
Neck and back
   "Touch your chin to your chest"
   "Look up at the ceiling"
   "Turn your head to the left and to the right"
   "Bend over and touch your toes"
Lower extremities
   Squeeze across MTP joints collectively and ask patient whether it is painful
   Perform the FABER maneuver (of hip)
   "Straighten your knee"
   "Step on the gas" (plantar flexion)
   "Pull your foot up" (dorsiflexion)

Note: Examination may be performed in a few minutes. It may be easier to ask the patient to follow the examiner's lead and copy the movements. Any abnormality should be followed by a complete examination.

MCP, metacarpophalangeal; MTP, metatarsophalangeal; FABER, flexion, abduction, and external rotation.

Adapted from: Doherty M, Dacre J, Dieppe P, et al. The "GALS" locomotor screen. *Ann Rheum Dis.* 1992;51:1165–1169.

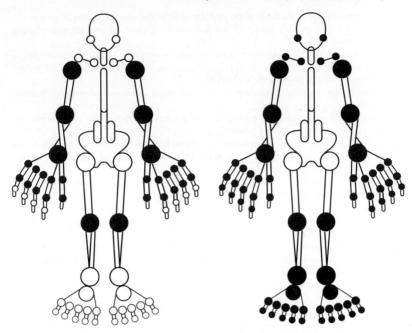

FIGURE 2-1. Standard 28 and 66 joint count examinations. Standardized joint counts. Dark circles represent assessed joints. Note that a 28 joint examination keeps separate tallies for swollen joints and tender joints.

DIAGNOSIS

Clinical Presentation

History
- History should focus on the following points: the onset of the symptoms, insidious versus abrupt, the length of time symptoms have been present, the specific location of the symptoms within or around the joint, aggravating and relieving factors, and if stiffness is present how long it takes for it to resolve with activity. Additional history may include the presence of joint swelling or inflammation, limitation of mobility, and joint instability.
- It is also important to ascertain functional impairment, including how well the patient can perform activities of daily living (e.g., dressing, grooming, cooking) and how the musculoskeletal disorder interferes with occupation or hobbies.

Physical Examination
- In general, the physical examination of the joints should begin with a **visual inspection**, noting alignment, swelling, deformities, and changes in color. It is helpful to compare bilateral structures for symmetry.
- The examination continues with **palpation**.
  ○ Any specific structures of the joint that are tender should be noted, as patients with rheumatologic disease can also have common musculoskeletal complaints.
  ○ Hard swelling around joints may be as a result of bony deformities, whereas tender, "boggy" swelling may be because of synovial inflammation (synovitis). Patients may also have soft-tissue swelling or adipose tissue that they perceive as synovial swelling.

- Simultaneously, notice the **bulk, tone, and strength** of the associated muscle groups.
- Assess **active and passive range of motion**, making note of any pattern of joint involvement.
- Finally, perform **specific provocative tests** for each joint to help identify a source of pain. A good example is Phalen's test for carpal tunnel syndrome. See Chapter 8 for a thorough discussion of various provocative maneuvers.
- Evaluate for periarticular tenderness or swelling, such as from tendinopathy, bursitis, and enthesitis.
  - Pain in a non–joint-centered pattern should prompt evaluation for nonarthritic diseases, such as neuropathy or fibromyalgia.
  - When considering spondyloarthropathy, evaluate for sites of **enthesopathy**. The Leeds Enthesitis Index for psoriatic arthritis evaluates the bilateral Achilles tendon insertion, the medial femoral condyle, and the lateral epicondyle of the humerus. Other common sites include the plantar fascia, the insertions of the patellar tendon on the tibial tuberosity and patella, the medial epicondyle of the humerus, and the supraspinatus insertion.[2]
- **Point-of-care ultrasonography** can be an extension of the physical examination when done by an experienced practitioner.
  - Ultrasound is significantly more sensitive than conventional examination for palpation of synovitis or enthesitis. This can be especially helpful in early disease where radiographs have poor sensitivity.
  - In rheumatoid arthritis (RA), for example, ultrasonographic signs of synovitis correlate with postcontrast synovial enhancement on magnetic resonance imaging (MRI).[3]
  - Synovitis on ultrasound appears as an abnormal hypoechoic intra-articular tissue. It is poorly compressible and nondisplaceable and may have increased signal on Doppler images.
  - Ultrasound may aid with joint injections in selected patients, such as those where landmark palpation is not feasible because of obesity or deformity, or where advanced osteoarthritis (OA) or deformity may impede conventional joint injections.
- **Examining individual joints**
  - **Hands:** Begin with **visual inspection** by instructing the patient to stretch out all fingers with the palms down. Then, palms up, have the patient make a fist and oppose the thumb to the base of the fifth finger. Inspect for visible swelling, erythema, or deformity. For example, subluxations of the metacarpophalangeal (MCP) joints with ulnar deviation of the digits are seen with RA. Lastly, note any atrophy of the lumbrical or thenar muscles, which can suggest nerve compression. **Palpate** each joint for tenderness. If there is finger lag with extension, palpate the flexor tendon for a snapping with extension or the presence of a nodule. Either of these findings may suggest **trigger finger.** Also note **grip strength** and ability to fine pinch. Normal patients should be able to make a completely closed fist.
    - **Heberden's nodes:** Bony nodules that can develop over the distal interphalangeal (DIP) joints and are characteristic of OA
    - **Bouchard's nodes:** Similar to Heberden's nodes, except found on the proximal interphalangeal (PIP) joints (also characteristic of OA)
    - **"Swan neck" deformity:** Hyperextension of the PIP joint with fixed flexion of the DIP joint
    - **"Boutonniere" deformity:** Fixed flexion of the PIP joint with hyperextension of the DIP joint
    - Other findings include **tophi** (hard or soft uric acid deposits seen in chronic gout), **fingernail changes** (seen in psoriatic arthritis), **cuticle abnormalities** (seen in dermatomyositis), and **sclerodactyly** (skin tightness and loss of soft tissue of fingers and toes seen in scleroderma).

- **Wrists:** Passively flex, extend, and deviate the wrists medially (ulnarly) and laterally (radially). Normal range of motion for flexion is 80 degrees and extension is 70 degrees. Note any swelling, warmth, or tenderness along the joint. Synovitis is easiest to palpate dorsally at the distal end of the radius. Chronic inflammatory arthritis may result in subluxation of the wrist, causing prominence of the ulna on the dorsomedial wrist.

- **Elbows:** Important landmarks in the elbow include the lateral epicondyle, the medial epicondyle, the olecranon, and the head of the radius. The elbow joint can be palpated for synovitis in the lateral para-olecranon groove, between the lateral epicondyle and the olecranon, with its distal margin at the head of the radius. Passively flex, extend, pronate, and supinate the forearms. Normal range of motion is extension to 0 degrees (hyperextension occurs with >minus 10 degrees extension) and flexion to 150 degrees (the thumb should be able to touch the shoulder). With the elbow flexed at 90 degrees, the forearms should supinate and pronate to 80 degrees. Palpate along the extensor surface of the ulna and over the olecranon bursa for **rheumatoid nodules.** These fleshy nodules are usually firm, nontender, and mobile with respect to the overlying skin. Gouty **tophi,** which often occur in the same area, are usually more firm. Tenderness over the medial and lateral epicondyles suggests epicondylitis. Finally, observe the **olecranon bursa** for any swelling, warmth, or erythema.

- **Shoulders:** The shoulder is a highly mobile joint with normal flexion and abduction of up to 180 degrees. Dozens of provocative tests have been studied to evaluate for shoulder pathology, with significant interobserver variability, limited sensitivity/specificity, and conflicting definitions.[4] Because of this heterogeneity, ultrasound by an experienced sonographer helps when there is clinical uncertainty. A brief screening test of shoulder range of motion is the **Apley scratch test.** It includes the following maneuvers: to evaluate external rotation and abduction, ask the patient to touch the contralateral scapula by reaching behind the neck. To evaluate internal rotation and adduction, ask the patient to touch the contralateral scapula by reaching behind the back. To evaluate the rotator cuff, perform both impingement and drop arm tests. The **Neer impingement sign** can be elicited by passive forward flexion of the internally rotated arm while the examiner stabilizes the scapula. A positive test produces pain with this maneuver. The **drop arm** test evaluates for a tear of the rotator cuff. The test is performed by placing the patient's shoulder in 90 degrees abduction. Have the patient slowly lower the arm to the side. The test is considered positive if the arm cannot be smoothly lowered to the side.

- **Neck:** Ask the patient to flex and extend the neck. Normal range of motion permits the chin to touch the chest. Ask the patient to turn his or her neck to the right, then to the left. Normal rotation is about 60 degrees. To evaluate lateral flexion, ask the patient to bring his or her ear toward each shoulder. Palpation of the spinous processes should be performed on the basis of the clinical history to assess for tenderness that can suggest infection, fracture, or joint involvement. Examine for tender points in the paraspinal musculature. **Spurling's test** may be performed to help assess if radicular pain from the neck is present. The patient's neck is extended and rotated to the side of the pain and then firm pressure is applied to the top of the head pushing downward. If radicular symptoms are present, it suggests foraminal stenosis as the cause.

- **Back:** Assess the curvature of the spine. The normal spine has three curves: lumbar lordosis, thoracic spine kyphosis, and cervical lordosis. Identify the presence of abnormal lordosis, kyphosis, scoliosis, or lateral tilt of the spine. Palpate for any tenderness along the spine and paraspinal muscles. While the patient is standing, instruct him or her to bend forward, backward, right, and left. If spondyloarthropathy (see Chapter 16) is suspected, perform the modified **Schober test.** With the patient standing, mark two midline points, one 10 cm above the lumbosacral junction (midline between the posterior iliac spines) and the other 5 cm below the junction. The points will be 15 cm apart.

Ask the patient to flex forward and measure the distance between the two points. In a normal individual, the span will increase by ≥5 cm.

○ **Hips:** While the patient is lying supine on the examination table, passively flex one hip and knee while the other leg is held straight. Normal flexion is 120 degrees (the patient should be able to touch the heel to the buttock). While the hip and knee are flexed at a 90-degree angle, rotate the hip to measure hip external and internal rotation. Normal values are 45 degrees for each. Internal rotation is often limited with arthritis of the hip. Note any limitation, crepitus, or pain. Recall that hip pain is referred to the groin. A quick screening maneuver to assess the hip joint is the **FABER test:** Flexion, abduction, and external rotation of the hip are tested by exerting light downward pressure on the knee, while the hip is flexed with the heel touching the opposite knee. Pain suggests hip or sacroiliac joint pathology.

○ **Knees:** Note the alignment of the knees in standing, including valgus or varus deformities. Palpate along the joint margins for tenderness and bony ridges (seen with OA). Palpate the surrounding tendons and bursa. Passively flex and extend the knee while feeling for crepitus. The knee normally extends to 10 degrees of hyperextension and flexes to 135 degrees. Effusions are relatively easy to detect in the knee. Feel for joint effusion by palpating the medial and lateral aspects of the patella while using the other hand (placed proximal to the patella) to gently "milk" fluid toward the patella. One can also assess for fluid with the "bulge" sign: Observe for a "bulge" medial or lateral to the patella as pressure is applied from the opposite side.

○ **Ankles:** Passively flex and extend the ankle (tibiotalar joint) to assess range of motion. Normal dorsiflexion (from the ankle at a 90-degree angle to the leg) is 20 degrees, and normal plantar flexion is 50 degrees. Then medially and laterally deviate the calcaneus to elicit abnormalities of the subtalar joint motion. To test the midtarsal joint, stabilize the heel with one hand, then use the other hand to invert and evert the forefoot. In order to palpate the tibiotalar joint (ankle joint), approach anteriorly with the foot in plantar flexion, as the dome of the talus nestled between the distal tibia and fibula becomes more exposed. Other common sources of pain in the ankle should be palpated and include the anterior talofibular ligament and the posterior tibialis/peroneal tendons.

○ **Metatarsophalangeal joints:** Ask the patient to plantar flex and dorsiflex the toes. Palpate each joint for tenderness, warmth, and effusion. Observe for **hallux valgus,** lateral deviation of the great toe with respect to the first metatarsal. With hallux valgus, the head of the first metatarsal is more prominent and may enlarge on the medial side. Observe for tophi at the first metatarsophalangeal joint.

REFERENCES

1. Doherty M, Dacre J, Dieppe P, et al. The "GALS" locomotor screen. *Ann Rheum Dis.* 1992;51:1165–1169.
2. Sakkas LI, Alexiou I, Simopoulou T. Enthesitis in psoriatic arthritis. *Semin Arthritis Rheum.* 2013;43:325–334.
3. Terslev L, Torp-Pedersen S, Savnik A, et al. Doppler ultrasound and magnetic resonance imaging of synovial inflammation of the hand in rheumatoid arthritis: a comparative study. *Arthritis Rheum.* 2003;48:2434–2441.
4. Hegedus EJ, Goode AP, Cook CE, et al. Which physical examination tests provide clinicians with the most value when examining the shoulder? Update of a systematic review with meta-analysis of individual tests. *Br J Sports Med.* 2012;46:964–978.

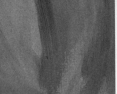

Aspiration and Injection of Joints, Bursae, and Tendon Sheaths

3

Devon M. DiVito, Philip Chu,
Jennifer L. Demertzis, and Deborah L. Parks

GENERAL PRINCIPLES

- Aspiration and injection of joint, bursa, and tendon sheath are fundamental skills for the evaluation and treatment of articular and bursal disease.
- Acute monoarthritis warrants immediate aspiration to evaluate for a septic joint.
- Therapeutic steroid injection should never be performed if there is clinical concern for a septic joint; exclude infection first.
- Procedures on artificial joint replacements are ideally performed in consultation with the treating surgeon.
- Ultrasound (US)-guided aspiration and injection techniques have been shown to be more accurate than landmark (LM)-guided or palpation-guided (PG) procedures,[1] though it is not clear from the literature that image guidance increases efficacy of therapeutic injections.

DIAGNOSIS

Clinical Presentation

- Although most rheumatologic conditions are diagnosed by history and physical examination, confirmation with imaging and/or diagnostic aspiration may be warranted.
- In addition, laboratory evaluation such as a complete blood count (CBC), erythrocyte sedimentation rate (ESR), C-reactive protein (CRP), and prothrombin time (PT)/partial thromboplastin time (PTT)/international normalized ratio (INR) may also be indicated for a complete evaluation prior to performing a diagnostic or therapeutic injection or aspiration.

Indications
- Diagnostic:
  - Evaluation for septic arthritis
  - Undiagnosed acute monoarthritis
  - Monoarticular joint effusion in a patient with polyarticular inflammatory arthritis
  - Evaluation for post-traumatic hemarthrosis
- Intra-articular injection of contrast for arthrography
- Therapeutic intra-articular and/or extra-articular injection (e.g., steroids, hyaluronate)[1-4]

Contraindications
- Cellulitis overlying the target joint, bursa, or tendon sheath is the only absolute contraindication to injection or aspiration.
- Several relative contraindications exist for arthrocentesis and steroid injection, as listed in Table 3-1.[5]
- Anticoagulation status or coagulopathy should be documented; however, evidence indicates that complication rates from arthrocentesis are low in this patient population. Therefore, this should not delay the procedure, especially in the evaluation of septic arthritis.[6,7]

TABLE 3-1	RELATIVE CONTRAINDICATIONS TO ARTHROCENTESIS AND JOINT, BURSA, AND TENDON SHEATH INJECTION
Arthrocentesis	**Intra-articular or Bursal Steroid Injection**
• Platelets < 50,000 • Coagulopathy • Anticoagulant therapy	• Bacteremia • Unstable joint and/or fracture • Neuropathic joint • Prior failure to respond to injection • Joint prosthesis • Tumor

Diagnostic Testing

Introduction to the use of US for joint, bursal, or tendon sheath access:

- The success of joint, bursa, or tendon sheath aspiration or injection depends on the accurate insertion of the needle into the intended location. US guidance has been shown to be more accurate than LM or PG procedures, though it is unclear from the literature whether this increases efficacy for therapeutic injections.[8,9]
- Although operator variability may pose challenges for inexperienced users, the advantages of US include real-time evaluation of anatomy to both target and avoid key structures, real-time manipulation of the needle, navigation through complicated anatomy, and confirmation of needle location.[1-3]
- Appropriate US transducer selection is one of the most important steps for success of the intended procedure:
  - High-frequency (>10 MHz) linear array transducer: shoulder, elbow, wrist, knee, and ankle
  - Very high-frequency (>15 MHz) linear array transducer with small footprint or "hockey-stick" configuration: small superficial structures such as the hand, foot, and acromioclavicular (AC) joint
  - Low-frequency (<10 MHz) linear or curved array transducer: deep structures such as the hip joint or iliopsoas bursa, larger body habitus, and posterior approach for the glenohumeral joint
- Prior to prepping the patient, perform a prescan to confirm appropriate transducer selection, identify the anatomic target and needle trajectory, and anticipate any unexpected findings that may make the procedure more challenging.
- It is important to understand the planes of visualization when using US guidance:
  - Short axis (SAX) or "transverse" provides an anatomical axial view.
  - Long axis (LAX) or "longitudinal" provides anatomical sagittal or coronal views.
- After identifying the target anatomy, prepare the site and use aseptic technique for the remainder of the procedure. The US probe should be sterilely sheathed, and sterile gel or chlorhexidine liquid should be utilized as conductive medium.
- Two guidance techniques are available for needle localization,[1] as listed in Table 3-2.
- Unless specified, we recommend an in-plane approach for all of the following procedures.

General Technique for Joint, Bursa, and Tendon Sheath Access

- Before proceeding, the risks and benefits of the procedure should be discussed and informed consent obtained by the physician performing the aspiration or injection.
- To access the joint space, palpate and define the anatomy of the joint. Mark the desired location of entry by applying pressure to the patient's skin with a retracted ballpoint pen. This will leave a circular impression on the skin.

TABLE 3-2	TECHNIQUES FOR ULTRASOUND NEEDLE GUIDANCE		
	Needle Course	**Needle Visualization**	**Notes**
In-Plane "Longitudinal"	• Needle advanced parallel to the long axis of the transducer • Perpendicular to the US beam	Visualization of the needle along its entire course is possible with this technique if a < 40-degree angle between the transducer and the needle is maintained	This technique poses a challenge when targeting superficial structures
Out-of-Plane "Transverse"	• Needle advanced perpendicular to the long axis of the transducer • Parallel to the US beam	Visualization of the needle is not constant throughout its course; the tip of the needle may only be seen upon entering the target	Inability to correctly gauge the depth of the needle is a risk of this technique

- Sterile gloves are recommended.
- Clean the skin thoroughly and use aseptic technique throughout the procedure.
- Using a 25-gauge needle, infiltrate 1% lidocaine into the skin and subcutaneous tissues for local anesthesia. Alternatively, a short burst (5–10 seconds) of topical ethyl chloride spray may help to alleviate pain prior to use of lidocaine or in place of lidocaine subcutaneous injection.
- Attach the appropriate gauge needle to the desired size syringe for joint aspiration.
  - If aspirated material is especially viscous, a larger syringe will provide greater suction.
  - If there is high resistance to injection, a smaller syringe provides greater injection force.
- Using your previous skin mark and anatomic LMs, carefully introduce the needle into the desired joint or bursal space. During needle advancement into the joint, slightly pull back on the plunger of the syringe to create suction. Aspiration of synovial fluid should result upon entering the joint.
- If injecting a steroid preparation after joint aspiration or if you require more than one syringe for removal of joint fluid, you may change the syringe while leaving the needle in the joint. A hemostat or Kelly clamp can be used to stabilize the hub of the needle while exchanging syringes. Take great care not to withdraw or advance the needle during syringe transfer.
- If joint aspiration is unsuccessful or assistance is needed for anatomically complex joints, US guidance may be useful.
- If injecting superficial bursa, it is wise to enter the skin and bursa in a "Z" line to avoid establishing a drainage track.
- After arthrocentesis, record the amount of aspirated synovial fluid and grossly examine the fluid for viscosity, clarity, and color.
- Send the synovial fluid to the lab for cell count in a liquid ethylenediaminetetraacetic acid (EDTA)-treated tube, routine Gram stain and culture, and crystal analysis. Glucose, protein, autoantibodies, pH, and complement levels from the fluid are rarely helpful and should not be ordered. Acid-fast bacilli, fungal cultures (in a culture bottle/swab), and cytology can be ordered if clinically indicated.

Equipment
- Antimicrobial solution
  ○ Chlorhexidine is proven to be more effective than povidone-iodine in preventing iatrogenic infection and therefore, is the agent of choice.[10,11]
  ○ Povidone-iodine is recommended if the skin is irritated or when entering an intertriginous area.
- Syringe for aspiration or injection, size determined by the target joint and/or amount of injectate
- Hypodermic or spinal needle
  ○ Length based on aspiration or injection target
  ○ Note that if a longer needle is used, a smaller gauge may be required to overcome resistance from the increased needle length.
  ○ For aspiration, an 18-gauge needle is recommended.
  ○ For injection, 20-, 22-, or 25-gauge needles may be used based on the volume of injectate and injection site.
- Ballpoint pen
- Topical ethyl chloride spray and/or 1% lidocaine for subcutaneous anesthesia, injected with a 25-gauge hypodermic needle
- Hemostat or Kelly clamp
- Gloves
- Gauze, bandages
- Alcohol pads
- US if utilizing image guidance

Specimen Collection
- Laboratory testing supplies depend on the procedure being performed and differential diagnosis for diagnostic aspiration.
- Supplies that may be required include glass slides with coverslips, test tube (EDTA is preferred), sterile-untreated container, blood culture bottle, and/or culture transport swab.
- Important considerations:
  ○ Cell count cannot be performed on a coagulated sample and therefore should be submitted in an EDTA-treated test tube.
  ○ Heparin can interfere with cell staining on differential cell count and crystal identification; therefore, heparin-treated specimen containers are not recommended.[12]

TREATMENT

The general technique for the injection of steroids and other agents into joints, bursa, and tendon sheaths is the same as for a diagnostic aspiration. The following sections describe specifics of each procedure based on the anatomic target.

Shoulder

Acromioclavicular Joint
- When utilizing a PG technique, place the patient in the supine or seated position, palpate the clavicle, and follow it distally to its lateral termination. This slight depression is the AC joint articulation. Insert the needle into the AC joint at the superior or anterior aspect of the joint. This space is small, and you may only be able to insert the tip of the needle into the space.
- For US guidance, position the patient supine, arm in neutral position, with the head of the table elevated. Place the transducer in LAX relative to the clavicle. The AC joint can be identified sonographically by translating the probe either laterally along the shaft of the clavicle or medially along the acromion toward the clavicle. Given the superficial position of this joint, out-of-plane needle approach may be preferred.[13]

Glenohumeral Joint
- The glenohumeral joint may be accessed with either an anterior or a posterior approach, with or without US guidance.
- PG
  - **Posterior approach:** With the patient seated, palpate the posterior margin of the acromion. The needle is inserted and directed anteriorly 1 cm below and 1 cm medial to the posterior corner of the acromion. Direct the needle toward the coracoid process until bone is touched at the articular surface.
  - **Anterior approach:** The patient should be seated or supine with the affected shoulder internally rotated. The point medial to the head of the humerus and slightly inferior and lateral to the coracoid process should be located and marked. Introduce and direct the needle posteriorly. Redirect superiorly and laterally until reaching bone at the articular surface.
- US guidance
  - Although the anterior approach is commonly used, multiple studies suggest that injection accuracy is improved with the posterior approach.[8]
  - Technique specifics of both approaches are listed in Table 3-3.[8,9,13]

Subacromial–Subdeltoid Bursa
- PG
  - The posterolateral approach is generally easier and safer. Identify the posterior corner of the acromion. The entry point is 1 cm inferior and medial to this LM.
  - Enter the subacromial–subdeltoid (SA-SD) bursa with the needle directed anteromedially under the acromion.[13]
- US guidance:
  - Position the patient in the lateral decubitus position with the affected side up.

TABLE 3-3	ULTRASOUND-GUIDED GLENOHUMERAL JOINT ACCESS TECHNIQUES	
	Anterior	**Posterior**
Patient position	• Supine, arm in external rotation	• Lateral decubitus, affected side up
Probe placement	• SAX over the proximal humerus	• SAX inferior to the spine of the scapula
Preprocedural visualization of anatomic landmarks	• Rotator cuff interval • Long head of the biceps brachii tendon	• Glenohumeral joint
Needle target	• Plane immediately superior to the biceps tendon and inferior to the coracohumeral ligament	• Adjacent to the glenoid labrum within the glenohumeral joint
Needle trajectory	• Lateral to medial	• Lateral to medial
Notes		• Take care to avoid piercing the glenoid labral cartilage

SAX, short axis.

○ The SA-SD bursa is located by placing the transducer in LAX over the proximal humerus. Look for the tapered appearance of the supraspinatus tendon insertion on the greater tuberosity. The SA-SD bursa is a hyperechoic structure located between the rotator cuff tendons and overlying deltoid muscle; fluid or synovitis within a distended bursa will appear as a hypoechoic material between the hyperechoic deep and superficial margins of the bursa. Use a lateral-to-medial needle trajectory parallel to the rotator cuff to avoid violating the tendon fibers during the procedure.[13]

Biceps Tendon Sheath
• Biceps tenosynovitis results from inflammation of the biceps tendon sheath within the bicipital groove at the level of the proximal humerus.
• With the patient seated, externally rotate the arm. Palpate the biceps tendon in the bicipital groove. To confirm anatomy, flex and extend the elbow to feel the tendon slide within the groove.
• When injecting, aim the needle superiorly to the tendon at a tangential angle. Take care to only inject around the tendon as steroid injection into the tendon itself may result in tendon rupture. There should be no resistance to injection when done appropriately.
• If utilizing US guidance
  ○ Position the patient supine with the shoulder in external rotation.
  ○ Use a high-frequency linear array transducer to identify the biceps tendon in the axial plane by placing the transducer in SAX over the bicipital groove.
  ○ A lateral-to-medial needle approach is recommended, targeting the lateral margin of the bicipital groove, deep to the tendon itself. The needle tip will rest against the bony floor of the bicipital groove.
  ○ Successful injection into the biceps tendon sheath will result in visualization of injected fluid surrounding and lifting the tendon from the underlying bone.[13]

Elbow

Elbow Joint
• Although the elbow joint may be accessed via PG or US guidance, a recent study has shown that US guidance increases injection accuracy rates.[8]
• If utilizing PG, the elbow should be flexed at 90 degrees, and the joint should be entered in the center of the triangle formed by the lateral epicondyle, radial head, and olecranon process. Insert the needle perpendicular to the skin at the joint.
• US guidance
  ○ A posterior or radial approach may be performed, both with similar accuracy.
  ○ Posterior approach:
    ▪ Position the patient prone with forearm hanging over the edge of the table and elbow in 90 degrees of flexion.
    ▪ Place the transducer in SAX over the olecranon to identify the posterior humeral recess located between the olecranon apex and the trochlea.
    ▪ Take note to identify and avoid the ulnar nerve located dorsal to the medial epicondyle.
    ▪ The needle is advanced radial to ulnar, passing under the triceps tendon.
  ○ **Radial approach:** Position the elbow in 40 degrees of flexion with the forearm pronated and palm resting on the table. Place the transducer in LAX to the radius and move the transducer proximally to identify the distinctive contour of the radial head and adjacent radiocapitellar joint. Because of its superficial location, a SAX or an out-of-plane approach may provide a more direct path into the joint.[14]

Olecranon Bursa
• This superficial bursa is located at the extensor surface of the ulna distal to the olecranon process. Position the patient with their arm comfortably flexed or extended and supported.

- Enter the superficial bursa perpendicular to the skin in a "Z" line to avoid establishing a drainage track.
- Try to avoid areas of the elbow with callus because these areas harbor more bacteria.
- If utilizing US guidance, place the transducer in LAX over the olecranon to confirm the presence of bursal fluid superficial to the olecranon fossa. If present, this will be the needle target; in-plane or out-of-plane needle approach may be used.[14]

Tendon Injections
- Common extensor tendon
  - Lateral epicondylitis ("tennis elbow") is caused by degeneration of the common extensor tendon at its origin on the lateral epicondyle of the humerus.
  - For both PG and US-guided approaches, the patient should be seated or supine with the elbow flexed to 90 degrees and the forearm pronated.
  - When injecting around this tendon, enter the skin directly over the prominence of the lateral epicondyle and perpendicular to the skin. Take care not to inject directly into the tendon to avoid iatrogenic rupture from steroid injection.
  - If utilizing US guidance, place the transducer on the lateral elbow in LAX over the radius and identify the common extensor tendon, which will be immediately adjacent to the lateral epicondyle. Advance the needle distal to proximal and target the peritendinous region immediately superficial to the tendon for glucocorticoid injection.[14]
- Common flexor tendon
  - Medial epicondylitis ("golfer elbow") is caused by degeneration of the common flexor tendon at the medial epicondyle of the humerus.
  - For both PG and US-guided approaches, the patient may be seated or supine with the arm abducted 90 degrees and the forearm supinated.
  - When injecting around this tendon, enter half inch distal to the medial epicondyle. Take care not to inject directly into the tendon.
  - If utilizing US guidance, place the transducer on the medial elbow in LAX to identify the common flexor tendon, which will be located immediately adjacent to the medial epicondyle of the humerus. Take note to identify and avoid the ulnar nerve and the ulnar collateral ligament. Advance the needle distal to proximal and target the peritendinous region immediately superficial to the tendon.[14]

Wrist and Hand
- Aspiration and injection of the small joints of the wrist and hand require specific equipment to achieve procedural success and minimize patient discomfort.
- The smallest needle available should be utilized for injection.
  - **Radiocarpal joint:** 25-gauge, 38-mm needle
  - **Metacarpophalangeal (MCP) and interphalangeal (IP) joints:** 25-gauge, 27-mm needle
  - **Extensor tendon compartments:** 22- to 30-gauge needle
- For aspiration, a large-bore needle is still recommended because the fluid may be viscous.
- For US guidance, a high-frequency (>10 Hz) linear array transducer can be used; if available, a small footprint or "hockey-stick" probe is ideal.[15]
- For synovial biopsy of the wrist, a Quick-Core biopsy needle (16–18 gauge, throw length 10 mm) may be utilized to excise tissue for Gram stain, culture, and histopathology.[16]

Radiocarpal Joint
- The radiocarpal joint may be accessed via PG or LM-guided approaches.
- The reported accuracy rates for the respective approaches range from 25% to 74% and 74% to 99%.[8]
- Regardless of the guidance technique, the compartments of the wrist should always be accessed along the dorsal surface.[2]

- The patient may be positioned several ways based on comfort (e.g., prone, supine, or seated with elbow flexed). However, to facilitate entry into the joint, the wrist should always be held in passive flexion. This may be accomplished by placing a rolled towel or other supportive structure underneath the pronated wrist.[2,15]
- PG
  - Palpate the joint between the distal radius and the scaphoid bone. This is on the radial side of the index finger extensor tendon. Mark this joint accurately so as not to injure the extensor tendons of the thumb or index finger.
  - Enter the joint perpendicular to the wrist.
- US guidance
  - Place the transducer on the dorsal wrist in SAX to identify Lister's tubercle; once identified, rotate the transducer 90 degrees to assume a sagittal orientation and identify the radioscaphoid joint in LAX.
  - This orientation will allow for in-plane needle guidance as the needle is advanced distal to proximal to target the space between the second and third extensor compartments. The needle may also be advanced out of plane, given the superficial location of the radiocarpal joint and surrounding extensor tendons.[15]
  - For synovial biopsy, an in-plane SAX approach entering from the ulnar aspect of the joint between the extensor digiti minimi and common extensor tendon sheath is utilized. First distend the radiocarpal joint with 1% lidocaine 3 to 5 mL and then obtain specimen with Quick-Core type needle from the midportion of the joint capsule.[16]

Metacarpophalangeal and Interphalangeal Joints
- The patient should be positioned with hand pronated and fingers in a natural state of flexion.
- The target joint may be injected on the medial or lateral side.
- If using a PG approach, orient the needle perpendicular to the table on either side of the target joint.
- If utilizing US guidance, place the transducer in LAX along the MCP for orientation and then move distally to identify the target joint. Use either in-plane or out-of-plane needle guidance to insert the needle into the joint space. Owing to the superficial location of these joints, a standoff pad of sonographic gel may be helpful for near-field visualization of the intended target.
- Take care not to injure the extensor tendon on the dorsal side of the finger.
- Overdistention of the joint capsule will result in patient discomfort.[15]

Tendon Sheath Injections
- Flexor tendon
  - Trigger finger results from inability of the flexor tendon to glide smoothly within the tendon sheath and may be due to inflammation of the tendon, tendon sheath, or annular pulleys.
  - Flexor tendon sheath injection may be performed via LM or US guidance.
  - **LM guidance:** Place the patient's hand in the supinated position. Inject the flexor tendon sheath at the base of the finger just distal to the metacarpal head. Take care not to inject directly into the tendon.
  - **US guidance:** The forearm should be supinated with the hand in slight extension. Place the transducer in LAX along the target metacarpal, advance the needle distal to proximal using an in-plane approach.[15]
- Extensor carpi ulnaris tendon
  - Extensor carpi ulnaris tendon sheath injection may be performed via a PG technique; however, US guidance is recommended for improved accuracy.
  - The patient may be positioned supine or seated with arm outstretched and the hand resting on the radial side.

- ○ Select a high-frequency probe and place it in SAX to the ulna, just distal to the ulnar styloid, to identify the extensor carpi ulnaris.
- ○ With the bevel directed dorsally, an out-of-plane approach is the most direct route to the target.
- ○ An in-plane approach, superficial to the tendon, may be employed; however, there is increased risk of skin depigmentation and fat atrophy with this approach given its superficial location.[15]
- First extensor compartment (De Quervain's tenosynovitis)
  - ○ The first extensor compartment contains the abductor pollicis longus and extensor pollicis brevis tendons.
  - ○ The patient may be positioned supine or seated with arm outstretched and the hand resting on the ulnar side.
  - ○ With the transducer oriented in SAX to the radius just distal to the radial styloid, perform a prescan to localize the radial nerve and artery and to assess for the presence of an accessory vertical septum, which would subcompartmentalize the first compartment tendons.
  - ○ The needle should be advanced in plane from a palmar approach. The needle should travel just deep to the tendon sheath to avoid the radial artery.[15]

Hip

Femoroacetabular Joint and Iliopsoas Bursa
- Aspiration and injection of the femoroacetabular joint and/or iliopsoas bursa are only done under US or fluoroscopic guidance.
- For both injection sites, special attention must be paid to the identification and avoidance of the femoral neurovascular bundle.
- Please refer to Table 3-4 for specific technique instructions for each site.[2,17]

Trochanteric Bursa
- The trochanteric bursa is located between the femoral trochanteric process and the gluteus medius tendon on the lateral aspect of the hip.
- An inflamed bursa results in point tenderness on top of the femoral trochanter.
- Trochanteric bursa injection may be performed with PG or US-guided approaches.
- Regardless of the guidance method, position the patient in the lateral decubitus position to access the affected side. The patient's hips and knees should be positioned comfortably in a slightly flexed position.
- **PG:** Insert the needle perpendicular to the skin into the site of maximal tenderness. There may be resistance passing through the gluteus medius tendon toward the greater trochanter.
- US guidance
  - ○ Transducer selection is based on patient body habitus.
  - ○ Place the transducer in SAX over the proximal thigh to identify the femoral neck and the greater trochanter laterally. Next, move the transducer posteriorly to identify the posterior facet of the greater trochanter, which is the insertion site of the gluteus medius tendon.
  - ○ If present, distention of the bursa will be seen between the gluteus maximus muscle and the posterior trochanteric facet and superior border of the gluteus medius tendon. This is the target for needle placement.
  - ○ Even in symptomatic patients, the bursa may not be distended, so positive identification of anatomic LMs is important for a successful procedure.
  - ○ The needle should be advanced posterior to anterior.[17]

Knee

Knee Joint
- The knee joint is formed by the articulation of the femur, tibia, and patella. The knee joint capsule extends from the proximal tibia to the supracondylar femur deep to the quadriceps muscle.

TABLE 3-4	HIP JOINT AND ILIOPSOAS BURSAL ACCESS TECHNIQUES	
	Femoroacetabular Joint	**Iliopsoas Bursa**
Patient position	• Supine • Hip neutral or in slight internal rotation	• Supine • Hip neutral
Preprocedural anatomic orientation	• LAX over the proximal thigh to identify the acetabulum and femoral head/neck junction • Take care to locate the femoral neurovascular bundle and avoid it during needle placement	• SAX over the femoral head to identify the iliopsoas muscle and tendon by translating the transducer superiorly and parallel to the inguinal ligament • Identify the iliopsoas tendon, which is a hyperechoic fasciculated structure with anisotropy inferior to the iliopsoas muscle belly; the bursa lies deep to the tendon
Needle target	• Femoral head–neck junction	• Iliopectineal eminence • Plane between the iliopsoas tendon and the acetabulum
Needle trajectory	• Distal to proximal	• Lateral to medial
Notes	• A low-frequency linear or curved transducer may be helpful in patients with large body habitus	• Toggling the transducer to elicit anisotropy may help confirm identification of the iliopsoas tendon

LAX, long axis; SAX, short axis.

- Regardless of the technique used, any resistance during injection indicates incorrect needle position. Stop and reposition the needle before proceeding with injection.
- Please refer to Table 3-5 for review of PG approaches.
- There are several acceptable methods for accessing the knee joint with US guidance; however, the medial/lateral patellofemoral and posteromedial techniques are typically reserved for problem-solving and/or a difficult initial suprapatellar attempt. Please refer to Table 3-6 for a review of these approaches.[2,18]

Knee Bursa Injections
- Prepatellar bursa
  - The prepatellar bursa is located directly over the patella. Cystic swelling at this location represents bursitis.
  - **PG:** Position the patient in the supine position with the knee extended. Enter the bursa on the medial or lateral aspect of the bursa, with the needle parallel to the floor.
  - US guidance
    - The patient should be positioned supine with the knee slightly flexed.
    - Place the transducer in SAX inferior to the patella over the distal patellar tendon to identify the bursa and confirm distention.
    - The needle may be advanced either medial to lateral or lateral to medial.[18]
- Pes anserine bursa

TABLE 3-5	**PALPATION-GUIDED KNEE ASPIRATION AND INJECTION TECHNIQUES**	
	Lateral Suprapatellar Approach	**Medial Approach**
Patient position	Knee extended or flexed up to 90 degrees; quadriceps muscle relaxed	
Bony landmarks to identify target	• Palpate the superolateral aspect of the patella (2 o'clock on the left and 10 o'clock on the right) • Mark the skin one finger width superior and lateral to this location	• Palpate the medial patella • Mark the skin medial to the base of the patella (9 o'clock on the left and 3 o'clock on the right)
Needle trajectory	• Advance the needle into the joint at a 45-degree angle from the skin toward the underside of the superolateral patella	• Advance the needle perpendicular to the skin toward the femoral condyle
Notes	• When using the medial approach, the needle may need to be adjusted inferiorly based on patient anatomy and the presence of severe osteoarthritis • When using the medial approach, the needle must be advanced through the entirety of Hoffa's fat pad to enter the synovial space	

○ Superficial bursa is located 3 cm caudal to the medial joint line of the knee beneath the distal pes anserine tendons (sartorius, gracilis, semitendinosus). Inflammation often results from abnormal gait.

○ **PG:** Position the patient supine on the table. Identify the bursa and its point of maximal tenderness. While staying relatively superficial, enter the bursa perpendicular to the skin.

○ US guidance:

  ▪ With the patient positioned supine and the knee slightly flexed, place the transducer in SAX over the posteromedial thigh to locate the semitendinosus muscle and tendon. Next, translate the transducer distally to identify where the pes anserine tendons insert on the proximal tibia.

  ▪ The bursa will be located deep to the tendons and superficial to the medial collateral ligament and can be accessed with in-plane or out-of-plane needle guidance.

  ▪ Take care to avoid the inferior medial geniculate artery and saphenous nerve.[18]

Ankle and Foot

Tibiotalar Joint
• There are several options for patient positioning using LM- or US-guided approaches. Having the patient bend the ipsilateral knee, plantar flex the ankle, and plant the foot on the table may provide additional stability during the procedure. Alternatively, the leg can be elevated on a towel roll, which allows for manipulation of the ankle joint to optimize positioning for the procedure.

TABLE 3-6	ULTRASOUND-GUIDED KNEE ASPIRATION AND INJECTION TECHNIQUES		
	Suprapatellar	**Medial/Lateral Patellofemoral**	**Posteromedial**
Patient position	Supine with knee flexed		Prone with knee extended
Probe placement	• SAX over the anterosuperior knee	• SAX over the anteromedial or anterolateral knee	• SAX over the posteromedial femoral condyle
Preprocedural visualization of anatomic landmarks	• Suprapatellar recess: located between the quadriceps tendon and the prefemoral fat pad	• Medial/lateral patella • Medial/lateral femoral epicondyle • Patellofemoral recess	• Posteromedial femoral condyle chondral surface • Identify and avoid popliteal neurovascular bundle and saphenous vein
Needle trajectory	• Lateral to medial or medial to lateral	• In-plane: lateral to medial or medial to lateral • Out-of-plane: use walk-down technique	• Medial to lateral between the semimembranosus and gracilis muscles
Notes	• Differentiate synovitis from effusion • Preferred approach for synovial biopsy	• Preferred approach when there is no effusion or the suprapatellar recess is difficult to see	• No effusion • Suprapatellar recess difficult to see • Severe patellofemoral osteoarthritis • Baker's cyst

SAX, short axis.

- PG
  - Palpate the tibialis anterior tendon and the medial malleolus.
  - The needle should enter the skin medial to the tendon and lateral to the mid-superior portion of the malleolus.
  - Direct the needle posteriorly to enter the joint space.
- US guidance
  - Select a high-frequency linear array transducer with a small footprint.
  - Before proceeding, identify the dorsalis pedis artery and the extensor tendons, which should be avoided during the procedure.
  - If in doubt, look for grayscale pulsation of the artery and use color Doppler for confirmation of arterial blood flow.
  - With the transducer in LAX to the talar dome, the tibiotalar joint recess will be seen just medial to the extensor tendon and will have the appearance of the letter "v" in the absence of an effusion.
  - If an effusion is present, there will be dark fluid blunting the tibiotalar joint recess; this is the target for needle placement.

- ○ A SAX orientation and needle trajectory may be beneficial when there are large anterior ankle joint osteophytes that can deflect the needle from the joint during an attempted longitudinal approach.
- ○ This approach is also the preferred method to perform a minimally invasive US-guided synovial biopsy if indicated.[2,19]

Subtalar Joint
- The subtalar joint comprises three facets, and the posterior facet has the largest surface area, allowing for multiple approaches. We recommend an anterolateral approach.
- The patient may be positioned, however is most comfortable, as long as the foot is in mild plantar flexion and inversion to open the subtalar joint.
- Select a high-frequency probe. Place the probe in SAX along the lateral malleolus to identify the talar neck, calcaneus, and the calcaneofibular ligament.
- The opening for the subtalar joint will be located just deep to the calcaneofibular ligament.
- An out-of-plane approach with anterior-to-posterior needle trajectory is recommended.[19]

Sinus Tarsi
- Position the patient in the lateral decubitus position with medial foot resting on the table to expose the lateral foot. A rolled towel or small pillow may be placed under the foot to help invert it slightly. Alternatively, the foot may also be positioned on the edge of the table to facilitate slight inversion.
- The sinus tarsi may be injected via PG just anterior and inferior to the lateral malleolus employing a posteromedial needle trajectory.
- Using US guidance, place the transducer in LAX inferior to the lateral malleolus and translate the probe distally to identify the calcaneocuboid joint. Immediately adjacent to this joint, locate the triangular space between the anterior process of the calcaneus and the neck of the talus—this is the sinus tarsi. An out-of-plane approach is best, given the superficial location of the sinus tarsi.[19]

Metatarsophalangeal Joint
- PG is limited secondary to frequent alteration of anatomy by osteophytes; US guidance is often more tolerable and therefore is the preferred method.
- With the patient posited with knee flexed and foot flat on the table, first perform a prescan to identify the extensor tendon, which should be avoided during the procedure.
- Using a standoff pad of sonographic gel may help optimize the US image for very superficial structures.
- The metatarsophalangeal (MTP) joint may be accessed via an in-plane or out-of-plane approach.[19]

Complications
- The most commonly encountered adverse effects are mild in severity and include pain and bleeding at the injection site.
- Uncommon complications including hemarthrosis, iatrogenic infection,[20] allergic reaction to the equipment or injected medications, and damage to surrounding structures, including tendon rupture and nerve damage, are reported.
- Several complications are unique to the use of steroids (Table 3-7) and should be discussed with patients on a case-by-case basis.[20,21]
- Although serious side effects such as septic arthritis and avascular necrosis have been reported, they are rare.
- Despite limited support in the literature, it is often recommended that therapeutic steroid injections should not be performed more frequently than approximately every 3 months to prevent potential complications such as osteoporosis, avascular necrosis, tissue fragility, and increased risk of infection with subsequent arthroplasty.[22]

| TABLE 3-7 | COMPLICATIONS UNIQUE TO THE USE OF STEROIDS FOR JOINT, BURSA, AND TENDON SHEATH INJECTION |

Unique to the use of steroids

- Postinjection flare[20]
- Hyperglycemia[21]; may occur if significant systemic absorption occurs; caution patients with diabetes mellitus who are at increased risk of this complication

More common with fluorinated steroids[20]:

- Subcutaneous fat atrophy
- Skin discoloration at the injection site

ADDITIONAL RESOURCES

- Recommended therapeutic injectate by anatomic target, refer to Table 3-8
- Recommended steroid preparations for joint injection, refer to Table 3-9

| TABLE 3-8 | RECOMMENDED THERAPEUTIC INJECTATE BY ANATOMIC TARGET |

	Methylprednisolone Acetate (mg)	1% Lidocaine (mL)	Additional Additives (0.25% bupivacaine or 0.5% ropivacaine)	Total Amount of Injectate (mL)
Hip	40–80	2	2	5–6
Knee	40	2–4	2–4	9
Ankle	20–40	1–2	None–2	1.5–2
Shoulder	40	2–5	2	5–9
Acromioclavicular	20	0.5	None	1
Elbow	40	1–2	None–2	2.5
Wrist	20–40	None–1	None–2	0.5–2.5
MCP, PIP	10	None	None	<1
Iliopsoas bursa	40–80	5	2	8–9
Greater trochanter bursa	40	None	2	3
Pes anserine bursa	20	0.5	None	1
Subacromial–subdeltoid bursa	40–80	None or 2–4	None–2	4–6
Biceps tendon sheath	40	1	Varies	2–3
Olecranon bursa	40	3	Varies	3–4
Extensor/flexor tendon	40	2–3	Varies	3–4

MCP, metacarpophalangeal; PIP, proximal interphalangeal.

TABLE 3-9	RECOMMENDED STEROID PREPARATIONS FOR JOINT INJECTIONS	
Steroid	Concentration (mg/mL)	Dose (mg)
Dexamethasone acetate[a]	8	4
Methylprednisolone acetate	20, 40, 80	40
Triamcinolone hexacetonide[a]	20	40
Triamcinolone acetonide[a]	10, 40	40 or 32 mg extended release
Betamethasone acetate[a]	6	6

[a]Fluorinated steroids.

REFERENCES

1. Rand E, Welbel R, Visco CJ. Fundamental considerations for ultrasound-guided musculoskeletal interventions. *Phys Med Rehabil Clin N Am*. 2016;27:539–553.
2. Rastogi AK, Davis KW, Ross A, et al. Fundamentals of joint injection. *AJR Am J Reontgenol*. 2016;207:484–494.
3. Hansford BG, Stacy GS. Musculoskeletal aspiration procedures. *Semin Intervent Radiol*. 2012;29:270–285.
4. Caldwell JR. Intra-articular corticosteroids. *Drugs*. 1996;52:507–514.
5. Yui JC, Preskill C, Greenlund LS. Arthrocentesis and joint injection in patients receiving direct oral anticoagulants. *Mayo Clin Proc*. 2017;92(8):1223–1226.
6. Bashir MA, Ray R, Sarda P, et al. Determination of a safe INR for joint injections in patients taking warfarin. *Ann R Coll Surg Engl*. 2015;97(8):589–591. doi:10.1308/rcsann.2015.0044.
7. Thomsen TW, Shen S, Shaffer RW, et al. Arthrocentesis of the knee. *N Engl J Med*. 2006;354;19. https://www.nejm.org/doi/full/10.1056/NEJMvcm051914. Last accessed 7/28/2018.
8. Daley EL, Bajaj S, Bisson LJ, et al. Improving injection accuracy of the elbow, knee, and shoulder: does injection site and imaging make a difference? A systematic review. *Am J Sports Med*. 2011;39:656–662.
9. Finnoff J, Smith J, Peck E. Ultrasonography of the shoulder. *Phys Med Rehabil Clin N Am*. 2010;21(3):481–507.
10. Lee I, Agarwal RK, Lee BY, et al. Systematic review and cost analysis comparing use of chlorhexidine with care of iodine for preoperative skin antisepsis to prevent surgical site infection. *Infect Control Hosp Epidemiol*. 2010;31:1219–1229.
11. Darouiche RO, Wall MJ, Kamal MF, et al. Chlorhexidine-alcohol versus povidone-iodine for surgical-site antisepsis. *N Engl J Med*. 2010;362(1):18–26.
12. Kjeldsberg C, Knight J. *Body fluids: Laboratory examination of cerebrospinal, seminal, serous and synovial fluids*. 3rd ed. Chicago, IL: American Society for Clinical Pathology. 1993:272–283, 292–293.
13. Pourcho AM, Colio SW, Hall MM. Ultrasound-guided interventional procedures about the shoulder anatomy, indications, and techniques. *Phys Med Rehabil Clin N Am*. 2016;27:555–572.
14. Sussman WI, Williams CJ, Mautner K. Ultrasound-guided elbow procedures. *Phys Med Rehabil Clin N Am*. 2016;27:673–687.
15. Colio SW, Smith J, Pourcho AM. Ultrasound-guided interventional procedures of the wrist and hand Anatomy, indications and technique. *Phys Med Rehabil Clin N Am*. 2016;27:589–605.
16. El-Gabalawy HS. Synovial fluid analyses, synovial biopsy, and synovial pathology. In: Firestein GS, Budd RC, Gabriel SE, et al., eds. *Kelley and Firestein's Textbook of Rheumatology*. 10th ed. Philadelphia, PA: Elsevier Inc.; 2017:784–801.
17. Payne JM. Ultrasound-guided hip procedures. *Phys Med Rehabil Clin N Am*. 2016;27:607–629.
18. Lueders DR, Smith J, Sellon JL. Ultrasound-guided knee procedures. *Phys Med Rehabil Clin N Am*. 2016;27:631–648.

19. Henning PT. Ultrasound-guided foot and ankle procedures. *Phys Med Rehabil Clin N Am.* 2016;27:649–671.

20. Peterson C, Hodler J. Adverse events from diagnostic and therapeutic joint injections: a literature review. *Skeletal Radiol.* 2011;40:5–12.

21. Choudhry MN, Malik RA, Charalambous CP. Blood glucose levels following intra-articular steroid injections in patients with diabetes: a systematic review. *JBJS Rev.* 2016;4(3):e5.

22. McIntosh AL, Hanssen AD, Wenger DE, et al. Recent intraarticular steroid injection may increase infection rates in primary THA. *Clin Orthop Relat Res.* 2006;451:50–54.

Synovial Fluid Analysis

Shuang Song and Deborah L. Parks

4

GENERAL PRINCIPLES

- Synovial fluid analysis is useful in distinguishing between inflammatory, septic, noninflammatory, or hemorrhagic conditions.
- New effusions, suspected septic arthritis, and acutely tender, erythematous, and swollen single joints generally require arthrocentesis and synovial fluid analysis.
- Synovial fluid analysis includes gross inspection, microscopic inspection for crystals and birefringence, cell count and differential, Gram stain, and microbiologic cultures.
- A needle of adequate gauge should be used for arthrocentesis of a larger joint. Large syringes may create high-suction gradients and make aspiration difficult.
- Difficult arthrocentesis may require injection of a small amount of saline to obtain a diluted sample of synovial fluid for culture if infection is highly suspected.
- Less accessible joints, such as the hip, may require fluoroscopy or ultrasound as guidance. For readily accessible joints, in general, whenever available, ultrasound-guided arthrocentesis is still the preferred method because of improved aspiration success, greater synovial fluid yield, and improved clinical outcomes.[1,2]
- **Normal synovial fluid**
  - A small volume of synovial fluid is present in a joint, acting as a lubricant and shock absorber for the joint.
  - Normal synovial fluid is an ultrafiltrate of plasma that contains small amounts of high-molecular weight proteins (fibrinogen, complement, globulin) complexed with hyaluronan, which is the major proteoglycan synthesized by synovial cells.
  - Normal synovial fluid is cleared through the synovial lymphatics that are assisted by joint motion.
- **Gross examination**
  - **Viscosity:** Normal synovial fluid is highly viscous and forms a long string when a drop is expressed from the end of the needle. Inflammation results in degradation of the hyaluronan and loss of viscosity.
  - **Color:** Colorless/straw-colored fluid is normal; abnormal fluid may appear yellow/green, white/cream, brown, blood stained, or hemorrhagic.
  - **Clarity:** Normal fluid is transparent. Increased opacity may be due to increased cells or acellular materials.
- **Cell count and cytology**
  - Normal synovial fluid contains fewer than 180 nucleated cells/mm^3, most of which are desquamated cells.
  - The synovial fluid from arthrocentesis is classified as noninflammatory, inflammatory, and septic (Table 4-1), as well as hemorrhagic that is characterized by large numbers of red blood cells.
  - The predominance of polymorphonuclear leukocytes is typically seen in septic synovial fluid that has >50,000 cells/mm^3, acute crystal-induced arthritis, reactive arthritis, psoriatic arthritis, and active rheumatoid arthritis.
  - The predominance of monocytes and lymphocytes is seen in viral arthritis, lupus, and other connective tissue diseases.

TABLE 4-1	GENERAL ANALYSIS OF SYNOVIAL FLUID			
Examination	Normal	Noninflammatory	Inflammatory	Septic
Viscosity	High	High	Low	Very low
Color	Colorless to straw colored	Straw colored to yellow	Yellow/green, white/cream	Yellow or purulent
Clarity	Transparent	Transparent	Cloudy, rice bodies, black speckles[a]	Cloudy
WBCs/mm^3	<200	<2,000	2,000–50,000	>50,000
Neutrophils	<25%	<25%	Often > 50%	>85%
Differential diagnosis		OA, SLE, amyloidosis, osteonecrosis, Charcot's joint, trauma, tumors, ochronosis, Wilson's disease	RA, PsA, reactive arthritis, crystal-induced arthropathies, SLE, scleroderma, infectious (bacterial, tuberculous, viral, fungal) arthritis	Infectious (most often bacterial but also mycobacterial, viral, fungal) arthritis

[a]Rice bodies, seen in chronically inflamed joints, are composed of cellular debris, fibrin, and collagen precipitate. Black-speckled fluid ("ground-pepper sign") may result from the fragmentation of a prosthetic arthroplasty.

WBCs, white blood cells; OA, osteoarthritis; SLE, systemic lupus erythematosus; RA, rheumatoid arthritis; PsA, psoriatic arthritis.

- ○ Eosinophils in the synovial fluid may be associated with parasitic infection, urticaria, or hypereosinophilic syndrome.
- ○ See Table 4-1 for general analysis of synovial fluid.
- **Polarized microscopy**
  - ○ Birefringence of synovial fluid crystals is evaluated by orientating the polarizer parallel to the long axis of the crystal. Positive birefringence is blue, whereas negative birefringence is yellow. For example, monosodium urate crystals are needle shaped and have strongly negative birefringence, whereas calcium pyrophosphate dihydrate crystals are rhomboid shaped and have weakly positive birefringence.
  - ○ Other synovial crystals that are birefringent (negative or positive) include cholesterol crystals, lipid crystals, and glucocorticoid crystals.
  - ○ Hydroxyapatite crystals are associated with a destructive arthritis "Milwaukee shoulder." These crystals are nonbirefringent and cannot be detected by polarized microscopy.
  - ○ See Table 4-2 for crystal analysis of synovial fluid.
- **Microbiology**
  - ○ **Gram stain:** A Gram stain performed on fresh synovial fluid has a sensitivity of 50% and a specificity of almost 100%. Gram-positive bacteria have the highest yield on a Gram stain.

TABLE 4-2 CRYSTAL ANALYSIS OF SYNOVIAL FLUID

Crystal Type	Disease	Morphology	Birefringence	Color[a]
Monosodium urate	Gout	Needles	Negative	Yellow
CPPD	Pseudogout	Rhomboid, rods	Weakly positive	Blue
Cholesterol	OA, RA	Rectangles	Variable	Yellow, blue
Calcium oxalate	Renal disease	Bipyramidal	Positive	Blue
Hydroxyapatite	OA	Round, irregular	None	None

[a]The color of the crystal when its axis is parallel to the slow axis of the red compensator.
CPPD, calcium pyrophosphate dehydrate; OA, osteoarthritis; RA, rheumatoid arthritis.

- **Microorganism culture**
  - Bacteriologic culture is the gold standard for diagnosing septic arthritis, which has a sensitivity of 75% to 95% and a specificity of 90% in nongonococcal septic arthritis.
  - Bacteriologic cultures determine antimicrobial susceptibility and guide the treatment choices.
- **Polymerase chain reaction (PCR)**
  - PCR is highly sensitive for the detection of microorganisms in synovial fluid, but the specificity varies.
  - PCR is the recommended method for diagnosing gonococcal arthritis and tuberculous arthritis.

REFERENCES

1. Wu T, Dong Y, Song HX, et al. Ultrasound-guided versus landmark in knee arthrocentesis: A systematic review. *Semin Arthritis Rheum.* 2016;45:627–632.
2. Sibbitt WL, Kettwich LG, Band PA, et al. Does ultrasound guidance improve the outcomes of arthrocentesis and corticosteroid injection of the knee? *Scand J Rheumatol.* 2012;41:66–72.

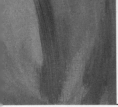

Laboratory Evaluation of Rheumatic Diseases

5

Roseanne F. Zhao and Richard D. Brasington

ERYTHROCYTE SEDIMENTATION RATE

General Principles

- Erythrocyte sedimentation rate (ESR) is the rate of erythrocytes settling in anticoagulated blood; it is a **nonspecific marker of tissue inflammation**. The presence of asymmetric macromolecules produced by the liver during the acute phase response, especially fibrinogen or immunoglobulin, promotes erythrocyte aggregation and increases ESR.
- ESR is affected by many conditions, some of which may be present in patients with rheumatologic diseases.
  - Noninflammatory conditions that tend to raise ESR include anemia (except sickle cell anemia), renal disease (including nephrotic syndrome and glomerulonephritis), hypercholesterolemia, female sex, pregnancy, oral contraceptives, malignancy, thyroid disease, and increasing age.
  - Conditions that can lower ESR include high-dose steroid use, sickle cell anemia, polycythemia, anisocytosis, spherocytosis, microcytosis, hepatic failure, and cachexia.
- ESR is sometimes used to monitor the activity of inflammatory conditions such as systemic lupus erythematosus (SLE) and rheumatoid arthritis (RA), although other markers of disease activity such as clinical signs and symptoms and lab indicators of organ function are more useful.
- ESR is also part of the diagnostic criteria for polymyalgia rheumatic (PMR) and giant cell arteritis (GCA); however, normal values do not exclude disease in the setting of strong clinical suspicion.
- ESR may be normal or decreased in some patients taking biologics, even in the presence of active inflammatory disease; alternative measures of outcome or disease activity should be considered.

Laboratory Assessment

- Anticoagulated whole blood is allowed to stand for 1 hour. The distance between the erythrocyte sediment and top of the tube in millimeters is ESR.
- The presence of acute phase reactants makes the cells fall faster and increases that distance.

C-REACTIVE PROTEIN

General Principles

- C-reactive protein (CRP) is an annular pentameric protein (pentraxin) produced by the liver in response to interleukin-6. Normally present in the serum in trace amounts, CRP **concentrations rapidly increase during inflammation** within 4 to 6 hours, peak at 2 to 3 days, and normalize over a week.
- CRP is induced by pro-inflammatory interleukin (IL)-6 along with IL-1β and tumor necrosis factor α (TNF α), to a lesser extent.
- CRP is a component of the innate immune response whose major function is to recognize foreign pathogens and damaged cells by binding to phosphocholine surfaces, as well as to exposed endogenous ligands including ribonucleoproteins, histones, chromatin,

and lysophosphatidylcholine. Clearance via activation of complement proteins or phago-cytic cells follows.

- Similar to ESR, CRP levels are elevated in either acute or chronic inflammatory states. Unlike ESR, CRP rises and falls rapidly. Obesity, diabetes mellitus, smoking, coronary artery disease, malignancy, and infection may also elevate CRP levels.
- The use of CRP levels in addition to ESR in the rheumatic diseases is limited.
  - In patients with RA, a persistently elevated CRP level may be associated with radio-graphic progression of joint disease and with long-term disability. However, both ESR and CRP are elevated in only 40% of RA patients.
  - CRP levels may also be useful in patients with SLE. In contrast to ESR, CRP levels are usually normal or only mildly elevated in active SLE except in patients with chronic synovitis or acute serositis. In SLE patients with fever in whom synovitis or serositis can be excluded, elevated CRP levels may suggest a bacterial source of inflammation and fever.
- High-sensitivity CRP (hsCRP) allows for the detection of low-grade systemic inflamma-tion, down to levels of 0.3 mg/L compared with the 3 to 5 mg/L range of the regular CRP assay, which can be associated with disease activity.
- Patients taking tocilizumab (IL-6 inhibitor) experience impaired hepatic production of CRP but may still have active disease. Alternative measures of outcome or disease activity should be considered in these patients.

Laboratory Assessment

Nephelometry and enzyme-linked immunosorbent assays (ELISAs) are used to measure CRP.

ANTINUCLEAR ANTIBODIES

General Principles

- Antinuclear antibodies (ANAs) are directed against nuclear antigens. The ANA pattern reflects the different nuclear antigens targeted but is nonspecific. Antibodies against spe-cific nuclear antigens can be tested and have improved specificity for certain diseases.[1]
- ANAs can be useful in the diagnosis of many autoimmune diseases including SLE and other connective tissue diseases (CTDs).
  - The specificities and sensitivities of ANA titers vary by disease and lab assay used. Therefore, one must be cautious in interpreting ANA results.
  - Titers do not correlate with disease activity and remain fairly stable throughout the disease course. **There is no need to repeat ANA test once the diagnosis is clearly established.**
  - Testing should only be performed to support a suspected, specific clinical diagnosis.
  - **While the absence of an ANA virtually excludes a diagnosis of SLE, the presence of ANAs does not establish the diagnosis.**
- Some ANAs, such as anti–double-stranded DNA (anti-dsDNA) antibodies are thought to contribute to disease pathogenesis by cross-reacting with self-antigens or forming im-mune complexes, while most ANAs are not considered pathogenic.

Laboratory Assessment

- ANAs are traditionally detected by indirect immunofluorescence or ELISA. Due to mi-nor variations in assay protocols, the sensitivity and specificity varies on the basis of the assay used and the titer cutoff for a positive result.
  - Higher titers convey increased clinical significance but do not correlate with disease activity.

- ○ ANAs in healthy individuals tend to be of low titers.
- ○ Titers of 1:160 or higher are usually considered positive, with a sensitivity of 90% to 95% in SLE. About a third of normal individuals have a positive ANA test at a titer of 1:40 and 5% have a positive ANA test at 1:160 by indirect immunofluorescence.[2]
- ○ While a negative ANA test by indirect immunofluorescence virtually excludes the diagnosis of SLE, the sensitivity is not as high for ELISA because only a subset of autoantibodies are tested.
- The gold standard for indirect immunofluorescence uses the human epithelial HEp-2 cell line as the substrate.
- ○ This test requires a high level of skill and is subject to observer interpretation. What is classified as a positive ANA test can vary by laboratory.
- ○ Several staining patterns have been described. With the exception of the nucleolar pattern (specific for scleroderma) and the centromere pattern (specific for limited systemic sclerosis [LSSc], also known as calcinosis, Raynaud's, esophageal dysmotility, sclerodactyly, and telangiectasias [CREST]), the ANA staining pattern is generally unhelpful because it is subject to observer interpretation.
- Specific ANAs can be tested by ELISA.
- ○ These ELISA assays contain known antinuclear antigens, coated individually onto 96-well plates, to detect specific ANAs that may be present in human serum.
- ○ Once the ANA is bound to the antigen on the plate, an enzyme-coupled secondary anti-human IgG antibody is used, followed by color detection that can yield a quantitative readout.
- Newer solid-phase assays, such as multiplex bead immunoassays that can simultaneously test for multiple ANAs in the same sample, allow for quantitative, high-throughput analysis. These assays use antigen-coated microspheres in an indirect immunofluorescent assay, with fluorescence signals measured by flow cytometry.
- Reliability and standardization within and between labs and assays remain an ongoing challenge and work in progress.[3-6]

Antibodies against DNA and Histones

Anti-dsDNA and **anti-histone** antibodies were among the first to be discovered and are associated with SLE and drug-induced lupus (DIL), respectively. Virtually all patients with DIL have anti-histone antibodies. Some but not all patients with "native" lupus also have anti-histone antibodies.

Extractable Nuclear Antigens

- Extractable nuclear antigens (ENAs) are **specific antigenic targets for ANAs** that can be extracted from the nucleus using saline.
- These include **anti-Smith (anti-Sm),** which is included in the American College of Rheumatology (ACR) criteria for the diagnosis of SLE, and **anti-ribonucleoprotein (anti-RNP),** which is specific for mixed connective tissue disease (MCTD). **Anti-Ro (anti-SSA)** and **anti-La (anti-SSB)** are associated with Sjögren's syndrome, subacute cutaneous lupus, and neonatal lupus. Other antibodies include **anti–Jo-1,** associated with inflammatory myositis (most commonly polymyositis) as well as anti-synthetase syndrome, and **anti-Scl-70,** specific for scleroderma.
- What is included in the "ENA panel" can vary from lab to lab.
- Patients with negative ANA titers will usually also have negative ENAs, although positive ANA tests do not necessarily result in detectable antibodies to ENAs. **A positive ANA test in a patient with clinically suspected CTD should prompt one to test more specific ENAs.**
- See Table 5-1 for a summary of specific ENAs and disease associations.

TABLE 5-1	AUTOANTIBODIES AND THEIR ASSOCIATED DISEASES	

Antibody	Disease Association	Comments
ANA	SLE, MCTD, SS, PM, DM, scleroderma	Nonspecific (present in 5% of population and prevalence increases with age). Sensitivities: SLE > 95%, MCTD > 95%, SS ~75%, PM/DM > 75%, scleroderma 60%–90%, RA 15%–35%. Also present in other autoimmune disorders, cancer, and infections.
Anti-centromere (pattern of ANA)	LSSc, or CREST	LSSc: specificity 98%, sensitivity 10%–50%. Associated with CREST. May be observed in idiopathic Raynaud's 25%, but some will progress to developing CREST. Staining pattern is easily identifiable on ANA stain as "discretely speckled"
RF	RA	Nonspecific, prevalence increases with age (false-positive in up to 25% of subjects aged >70). Sensitivities: RA 60%–80%, SS 70%, viral hepatitis 25%, bacterial endocarditis 25%, chronic infection, sarcoidosis, malignancy, and cryoglobulinemia. In RA, may have loose correlation with clinical activity and predicts poorer prognosis and extra-articular disease.
ACPA	RA	Highly specific for RA approaching 99%; sensitivity parallels that for RF at ~70%. May be present years before clinically apparent disease. Presence is associated with more severe disease with radiographic damage and extra-articular manifestations.
Anti-dsDNA	SLE	Very specific for SLE, only 50%–80% sensitive. Associated with lupus nephritis and may correlate with disease activity in SLE.
Anti-Sm	SLE	Very specific for SLE, only ~15% sensitive. Associated with lupus nephritis.
Anti-Ro (SSA)	SS	Sensitivities: SS 70%, SLE 25%. Associated with sicca symptoms in other CTDs, extraglandular disease in SS, heart block in neonates with anti-Ro-positive mothers. Correlates with SCLE rash, photosensitivity, or thrombocytopenia in SLE.
Anti-La (SSB)	SS	Sensitivities: SS 40%, SLE 10%. Association with anti-Ro. Correlates with benign course in SLE if no other autoantibody present except ANA.

(continued)

TABLE 5-1	AUTOANTIBODIES AND THEIR ASSOCIATED DISEASES (*continued*)

Antibody	Disease Association	Comments
Anti-U1RNP	MCTD	Detected in 100% of patients with MCTD.
Anti-histone	DIL, SLE	Nonspecific. Sensitivities: DIL > 90%, SLE > 50%.
Anti–Scl-70 (Topoisomerase I)	Scleroderma	Very specific but only 15%–35% sensitive for diffuse systemic sclerosis. Associated with ILD as manifestation of SSc.
Anti–RNA polymerase III	SSc	Very specific but only 20%–25% specific for scleroderma. These antibodies correlate with increased risk for malignant hypertension and renal crisis.
c-ANCA	GPA	Confirm positive values with anti-PR3. Very sensitive (>90%) and specific (99%) for active disease in fulminant GPA but less sensitive in limited GPA (50%). Questionable if levels correlate with disease activity. Less sensitive for MPA 25%, EGPA 33%, and PAN 10%.
p-ANCA	EGPA, MPA	Nonspecific; confirm positive finding with anti-MPO. Sensitivities for anti-MPO: EGPA 50%, idiopathic crescentic glomerulonephritis 64%, MPA 58%, PAN 40%, GPA 24%. Non–anti-MPO p-ANCA present in RA, SLE, PM/DM, relapsing polychondritis, APS, and other autoimmune diseases.
Antibodies to aminoacyl tRNA synthetases		
Anti–Jo-1	PM, DM	Prevalence 15%–25% in DM/PM. Specificity close to 100%. Predicts a constellation of myositis, arthritis, ILD, "mechanic's hands," Raynaud's, and fever (also called antisynthetase syndrome), also seen with other antisynthetase antibodies. More severe muscle disease.
Anti-PL-7	PM, DM	Prevalence <5%. Associated with ILD and gastrointestinal manifestations. Less strongly associated with myositis.
Anti-PL12	ADM, ILD, PM, DM	Prevalence <5%. 90% of patients have early and severe ILD. Less strongly associated with arthritis, mechanic's hands, and myositis.

Antibody	Disease Association	Comments
Anti-EJ	PM, DM	Prevalence <5%.
Anti-OJ	ILD, PM, DM	Prevalence <5%.
Anti-KS	ILD, PM, DM	Prevalence <1%.
Anti-ZO	Myositis	Prevalence <1%.
Anti-YRS	Myositis	Prevalence <1%.
Anti–Mi-2	"Classic" DM	Found in 20%–30% of patients with DM. Associated with V-sign, shawl sign, cuticular overgrowth, good response to therapy and good prognosis. Low frequency of cancer.
Anti-SRP	Necrotizing myositis	<5% sensitive in PM/DM. Prevalence 5%–10%. Associated with acute onset, severe weakness, palpitations, and poor prognosis.
Anti-HMGCR	Necrotizing myositis	Prevalence 5%–10%. Associated with statin-induced disease. Most cases previously referred to as "PM" are more currently considered "autoimmune necrotizing myopathy."
Anti-MDA5	ADM	Hypo/amyopathic, refractory rapidly progressive ILD and severe mucocutaneous ulcerations.
Anti-TIF1γ/α	Malignancy-associated DM	Prevalence 10%–15%.
Anti-NXP2	DM	Usually young-onset severe DM with severe skin disease, calcinosis and dysphagia. Can be associated with GI vasculitis in children which worsens prognosis.
Anti-SAE	DM	"Classic" severe adult-onset DM.
Lupus anticoagulant	Hypercoagulable states, APS	APA; screened for by detecting prolonged PTT or dRVVT that fails to correct with mixing studies and confirmed with phospholipid neutralization studies that confirm a phospholipid-dependent in vitro anticoagulant.
Anti-cardiolipin (aCL)	Hypercoagulable states, APS	APA; association with thrombosis: IgG>>IgM>IgA. Titers tend to correspond with disease activity.
β_2-GPI–dependent aCL	Hypercoagulable states, APS	A type of aCL that binds to complex of β_2-GPI and cardiolipin. Positive values associated with higher risk of hypercoagulable states than non–β_2-GPI–dependent aCL.

(continued)

TABLE 5-1	AUTOANTIBODIES AND THEIR ASSOCIATED DISEASES (*continued*)

Antibody	Disease Association	Comments
Cryoglobulins	HCV, LPD, CTD	Type I: Monoclonal Ig (usually IgM or IgG) that self-aggregate; may have RF activity, associated with LPD. Type II: Monoclonal Ig (usually IgM) with activity against polyclonal IgG (i.e., RF activity), most commonly idiopathic, may be associated with HCV or CTD. Type III: Polyclonal Ig (usually IgM) with activity against polyclonal IgG (i.e., RF activity), most commonly idiopathic, may be associated with HCV or CTD.

ANA, antinuclear antibody; SLE, systemic lupus erythematosus; MCTD, mixed connective tissue disease; SS, Sjögren's syndrome; PM, polymyositis; DM, dermatomyositis; RA, rheumatoid arthritis; LSSc, limited systemic sclerosis; CREST, calcinosis, Raynaud's, esophageal dysmotility, sclerodactyly, and telangiectasias; RF, rheumatoid factor; CCP, cyclic citrullinated peptide; dsDNA, double-stranded DNA; Sm, Smith; SCLE, subacute cutaneous lupus erythematosus; RNP, ribonucleuprotein; DIL, drug-induced lupus; ILD, interstitial lung disease; SSc, systemic sclerosis; RNA, ribonucleic acid; ANCA, antineutrophil cytoplasmic antibody; GPA, granulomatosis with polyangiitis; PR3, proteinase 3; EGPA, Eosinophilic Granulomatous with Polyangiitis; MPA, microscopic polyangiitis; PAN, polyarteritis nodosa; MPO, myeloperoxidase; APS, antiphospholipid syndrome; ADM, amyotrophic dermatomyositis; anti-SRP, anti–signal recognition protein; HMGCR, hydroxy-3-methylglutaryl coenzyme A reductase; MDA5, melanoma differentiation-associated gene 5; TIF1γ/α, transcription intermediary factor 1γ/α; NXP2, nuclear matrix protein 2; SAE, small ubiquitin-like modified 1 activating enzyme; APA, antiphospholipid antibodies; PTT, partial thromboplastin time; dRVVT, dilute Russell's viper venom time; Ig, immunoglobulin; GPI, glycoprotein I; HCV, hepatitis C virus; LPD, lymphoproliferative disease; CTD, connective tissue disease.

RHEUMATOID FACTOR

General Principles

- Rheumatoid factor (RF) is a **polyclonal antibody directed against the Fc portion of immunoglobulin** (Ig), most commonly IgM. IgG and IgA isotypes of RF are very difficult to detect in sera.
- RF is associated with **chronic inflammatory diseases, including RA, other CTDs, and infections** (see Table 5-1).
  - RF has a sensitivity of 60% to 80% for RA and a specificity of about 70%.
  - RF is also elevated in Sjögren's syndrome, hepatitis C infection, multiple myeloma, interstitial lung disease, cryoglobulinemic vasculitis, and sarcoidosis, among other chronic inflammatory and infectious disorders. A small percentage of healthy individuals will also have a positive RF test.
- The role of RF in the pathogenesis of disease is unclear, although one hypothesis suggests that RF initiates immune complexes in the synovium, which activate complement and release chemoattractants that recruit immune cells. RF is often detected prior to the development of arthritis, with an increase in antibody levels prior to onset of disease.[7]

Laboratory Assessment

- RF was classically detected using a latex immunofixation test and reported as a titer.
- Newer methods, including nephelometry and ELISAs, report results in international units.
- The inverse ratio of the nephelometric result correlates roughly with the titer result; for example, 120 IU correlates roughly with a titer of 1:120.
- Only IgM RF testing is routinely available.

ANTI–CITRULLINATED PROTEIN ANTIBODIES

General Principles

- Anti–citrullinated protein antibodies (ACPAs) include antibodies directed against **cyclic citrullinated peptide (CCP)**, filaggrin, vimentin, and fibrinogen, among others yet unidentified. CCP is a synthetic peptide derived from filaggrin that confers high sensitivity and specificity when used to test for antibodies in individuals with RA.
- These peptide/protein targets are unique in that they contain citrulline, an amino acid formed by posttranslational deimination of arginine.
- ACPAs are sensitive (70%) and highly specific (95%) for RA.[8]
- ACPA to **CCPs** are more easily detected and have been detected in the sera of patients with RA up to 10 years prior to the onset of disease. About one-third of patients with RA will be positive for these antibodies but RF negative on presentation.
- There is evidence that these antibodies contribute to disease pathogenesis.
  - In the period leading to onset of disease, antibody levels increase and patients develop additional antibodies to other citrullinated proteins in a phenomenon known as epitope spreading.[7]
  - Higher titers correlate with more erosive disease.[9]
  The stimuli for the induction of these antibodies and mechanisms by which they contribute to disease activity are under investigation and may include mucosal inflammation and the microbiome.

Laboratory Assessment

- The only ACPA that is currently available for clinical testing is anti-CCP antibody.
- Newer generations of an ELISA with CCP have increased the specificity of these tests for RA.

ANTINEUTROPHIL CYTOPLASMIC ANTIBODIES

General Principles

- Antineutrophil cytoplasmic antibodies (ANCAs) are directed against cytoplasmic antigens in human neutrophils.
- ANCAs are not ANAs, although proximity of perinuclear-ANCA (p-ANCA) staining to the nucleus may be mistaken for an ANA. Hence, a positive ANA or p-ANCA test may result in a false-positive result for p-ANCA or ANA, respectively.
- Two distinct staining patterns have been described: cytoplasmic-ANCA (c-ANCA) and p-ANCA.
  - c-ANCA is associated with granulomatosis with polyangiitis (GPA) and p-ANCA is associated with Eosinophilic Granulomatous with Polyangiitis (EGPA), microscopic polyangiitis (MPA), and polyarteritis nodosa (PAN).
  - The specific antigen is proteinase 3 (PR3) for most c-ANCA and myeloperoxidase (MPO) for most p-ANCA.
  - PR3 is a protein present in azurophil granules in neutrophils and is involved in the function and activation of neutrophils. Antibodies to PR3 have high sensitivities and

specificities for active, fulminant GPA. It is believed that neutrophil modification by anti-PR3 antibodies in GPA may account for some of the disease manifestations.

- ○ MPO is a protein involved in the generation of reactive oxygen species and in the modulation of macrophage function. Although p-ANCA and anti-MPO antibodies are present in a large number of diseases, their roles in pathogenesis are poorly understood.
- ○ The presence of PR3 versus MPO antibodies has clinical significance as patients with PR3-ANCA are more likely to relapse.

ANCAs are present in other inflammatory conditions, including autoimmune hepatitis, primary biliary cirrhosis, and ulcerative colitis. Furthermore, they may be induced by certain infections such as *Staphylococcus aureus* and mycobacteria, and by drugs such as propylthiouracil and hydralazine.

Laboratory Assessment

- ANCAs are identified with indirect immunofluorescence staining using ethanol-fixed neutrophils. However, there may be significant variability between different methods.
- Testing for anti-PR3 and anti-MPO antibodies is performed by ELISAs at a reference lab. Current immunoassays have high diagnostic performance.[10]
- According to the 2017 revision of the international consensus on ANCA testing, **PR3 and MPO specific immunoassays may be used for the primary screening of patients suspected of having ANCA-associated vasculitis** without the need for dual testing with indirect immunofluorescence testing.[11] Furthermore, whether or not a patient has PR3 or MPO antibodies is of prognostic significance, with relapsing disease more common in the former case.

MYOSITIS-SPECIFIC ANTIBODIES

General Principles

- The three best-described **myositis-specific antibodies (MSAs)** are **anti–Jo-1** (directed to tRNA histidyl synthetase), **anti–signal recognition protein (anti-SRP)**, and **anti–Mi-2**. Their sensitivities for inflammatory myopathies are low, ranging from 25% to 30%.
- Other important antibodies include those directed against other aminoacyl tRNA synthetases, as well as anti-transcription intermediary factor 1γ (**anti-TIF-1γ**), anti–melanoma differentiation–associated gene 5 (**anti-MDA5**), anti–nuclear matrix protein 2 (**anti-NXP2**), anti–small ubiquitin-like modified 1 activating enzyme (**anti-SAE**), and anti–hydroxy-3-methylglutaryl coenzyme A reductase (**anti-HMGCR**).
- Specific MSA may be associated with certain clinical features and prognosis (see Table 5-1).[12–14]

Laboratory Assessment

These antibodies can be detected by ELISA or multiplex bead immunoassays.

ANTIPHOSPHOLIPID ANTIBODIES

General Principles

- Antiphospholipid antibodies (APAs) are directed against phospholipids and are associated with hypercoagulable and thrombotic states.
- APA is detected by assays for the **lupus anticoagulant (LAC), anticardiolipin antibodies (aCL), anti-β_2-glycoprotein I, and false-positive serologies for syphilis.**
- Of the three APAs, **LAC has the strongest association with hypercoagulation.** The name LAC is derived from the fact that the antibody was first described in patients with SLE

and from its tendency to cause prolonged activated partial thromboplastin time (aPTT) that did not correct with the addition of normal plasma. We now know that LAC can be found in other CTDs or in the absence of a CTD.
- The association between aCL and hypercoagulable states is related to antibody titers and Ig isotype. As a general rule, increased titers of aCL are associated with increased risk of hypercoagulation and thrombosis. IgG aCL carry more risk than IgM aCL, and the risk with IgA aCL is questionable.
- Some aCL bind to complexes composed of phospholipids and β_2-glycoprotein I (β_2-GPI), a natural serum anticoagulant. β_2-GPI–dependent aCL are associated with increased risk of hypercoagulable states.

Laboratory Assessment
- LAC is identified in a stepwise manner using functional phospholipid-dependent clotting assays that reveal a coagulation inhibitor that is neutralized by phospholipids.
  - First, phospholipid-dependent clotting assays such as a dilute prothrombin time, aPTT, kaolin clotting time, or a dilute Russell's viper venom time (dRVVT) are drawn; prolonged times are considered positive results. Each test has different sensitivities in detecting LAC, and **the use of more than one test is recommended.**
  - **The preferred screening test is an aPTT-based test** using silica as an activator in the presence of low levels of phospholipids. A prolonged time suggests the presence of LAC. Positive tests should then be confirmed with a dRVVT. In this assay, Russell's viper venom activates factor X, which leads to the conversion of prothrombin to thrombin, depending on the presence of phospholipids. If an LAC is present, the phospholipids are unavailable and the dRVVT is prolonged.
  - **Mixing studies** are then performed on samples with prolonged times to exclude factor deficiencies. If a prolonged time corrects in mixing studies, the sample is further incubated in different temperatures to exclude a temperature-sensitive inhibitor of coagulation. A sample that does not correct with mixing studies or with **variable-temperature incubation** is identified as having an inhibitor of coagulation. This sample is then incubated with excessive phospholipids to characterize the inhibitor as either a phospholipid-dependent or a phospholipid-independent inhibitor. Excessive phospholipids neutralize the LAC and the prolonged times correct.
  - Although LAC is a phospholipid-dependent inhibitor of coagulation in laboratory assays, the interactions of LAC with phospholipid-rich endothelium and platelets in vivo are thought to activate both platelets and the coagulation cascade, resulting in hypercoagulation and thrombosis.
- **Serologic assays for syphilis such as the venereal disease research laboratory (VDRL) and rapid plasma reagin (RPR) tests detect cardiolipin phospholipids.** When VDRL or RPR test is positive, perform a confirmatory test for antibodies against treponemes such as the fluorescent treponemal antibody absorbed (FTA-ABS) test.
- A false-positive test for syphilis (positive VDRL or RPR test with a nonreactive FTA-ABS) identifies an APA; however, newer ELISAs for aCL have improved sensitivity and specificity and are the preferred method for detection.
- Antibodies to β_2-GPI are detected by IgM and IgG specific ELISAs.
- Testing for all APAs can be influenced by acute thrombotic events and infection. Therefore, positive tests should be repeated in 12 weeks to verify results.
- **False-positive LAC may be seen in patients taking direct oral anticoagulants (DOACs),** which prolong phospholipid-dependent clotting times such as the dRVVT but corrects with excess phospholipids.[15] Testing during trough drug levels or use of an adsorbent to extract DOACs from plasma samples may help reduce the effect of this confounding factor, but more work is needed on this front.

CRYOGLOBULINS

General Principles

- Cryoglobulins are immunoglobulins that are soluble at body temperature but reversibly precipitate at lower temperatures.
- Cryoglobulins are classified into three types. Type I is monoclonal without RF activity. Types II and III are "mixed" with RF activity. In Type II the RF is monoclonal, and in Type III it is polyclonal. Types II and III frequently present as vasculitis. "Essential" cryoglobulinemia is of unknown cause, although many cases have turned out to be associated with hepatitis C.
  - Type I cryoglobulins are monoclonal antibodies, usually of the IgM isotype. They do not typically activate complement. Type I cryoglobulins are observed in **lymphoproliferative disorders** and cause vasoocclusive symptoms.
  - Type II cryoglobulins are a mixture of polyclonal IgG and monoclonal IgM antibodies, while **Type III** cryoglobulins are polyclonal IgG and IgM antibodies. These are associated with **viral hepatitis and CTDs.** As they activate complement, cryoglobulin Types II and III result in **small vessel vasculitis** symptoms.

Laboratory Assessment

- A cryocrit is obtained using a minimum of 10 to 20 mL of fresh venous blood that is drawn into prewarmed test tubes and transported to the lab in sand or water that has been warmed to 37°C. The specimen is allowed to clot at 37°C for 30 to 60 minutes before centrifugation. The supernatant is then stored at 4°C for as long as 7 days. Cryoglobulin Types I and II usually precipitate within 24 hours, whereas Type III may take days.
- Newer methods using electrophoresis can detect and quantify cryoglobulins, but preheated tubes and warm transportation are still required.

COMPLEMENT

General Principles

- The **complement cascade** involves more than 30 proteins and accounts for 15% of the globulin portion of plasma protein.
- Three pathways have been identified: classical, alternative, and leptin.
  - The **classical pathway** involves the opsonization and/or lysis of cells covered with antibodies to cell surface antigens.
  - The **alternative pathway** involves the nonspecific opsonization and/or lysis of foreign cells that lack cell membrane complement regulators.
  - The **mannose-binding lectin pathway** involves the opsonization and/or lysis of foreign cells with mannose groups on the cell membrane.
- The rheumatic diseases that involve immune complex formation and subsequent activation of the classic pathway include SLE, cryoglobulinemic vasculitis, Henoch–Schönlein purpura, and atypical HUS.
- The **total hemolytic complement activity** (CH50) is a functional assay that tests the integrity of the classical pathway. Low total hemolytic complement activity suggests a deficiency of one or more factors.
- C3 and C4 are individual components of the complement cascade and can be measured antigenically.
  - C4 levels in serum typically drop before C3.
  - Low titers of both C3 and C4 are seen in classical pathway activation. However, low C3 with normal C4 suggests alternative pathway elevation.

- In SLE, low C3 and C4 complement levels may correlate with disease activity, especially in lupus nephritis. Conversely, complement proteins may act as acute phase reactants and appear elevated during increased disease activity.
- Not all patients have complement levels that correlate with disease activity, and the pattern of correlation may vary with each patient. Nevertheless, once a pattern is established in a particular patient, levels may be used to monitor disease activity.
- Low C4 levels are present in patients with cryoglobulinemic vasculitis, reflective of complement activation by immune complex deposition.
- Congenital deficiencies in complements C1q and C4 increase the risk for SLE.

The development and emergence of new complement therapeutics, most of which are blocking antibodies, may interfere with the accuracy of current assays that measure complement protein levels or function.[16]

Laboratory Assessment

Complements are measured by ELISA or nephelometry. The **CH50** assay addresses the entire classical complement cascade. The addition of diluted patient serum to antibody-coated sheep red blood cells (RBCs) should result in erythrolysis. CH50 is reported as the amount of serum required to lyse 50% of the RBCs. If the CH50 is undetectable, deficiency of a specific complement component is suspected.

REFERENCES

1. Satoh M, Vázquez-Del Mercado M, Chan EK. Clinical interpretation of antinuclear antibody tests in systemic rheumatic diseases. *Mod Rheumatol.* 2009;19:219–228.
2. Tan EM, Feltkamp TEW, Smolen JS, et al. Range of antinuclear antibodies in "healthy" individuals. *Arthritis Rheum.* 1997;40:1601–1611.
3. Meroni PL, Biggioggero M, Pierangeli SS, et al. Standardization of autoantibody testing: a paradigm for serology in rheumatic diseases. *Nat Rev Rheumatol.* 2014;10:35–43.
4. Pacheco Y, Monsalve DM, Acosta-Ampudia Y, et al. Antinuclear autoantibodies: discordance among four different assays. *Ann Rheum Dis.* 2020;79(1):e6. doi:10.1136/annrheumdis-2018-214693.
5. Pisetsky DS, Spencer DM, Lipsky PE, et al. Assay variation in the detection of antinuclear antibodies in the sera of patients with established SLE. *Ann Rheum Dis.* 2018;77(6):911–913.
6. Mummert E, Fritzler MJ, Sjöwall C, et al. The clinical utility of anti-double-stranded DNA antibodies and the challenges of their determination. *J Immunol Methods.* 2018;459:11–19.
7. Rantapää-Dahlqvist S, de Jong BA, Berglin E, et al. Antibodies against cyclic citrullinated peptide and IgA rheumatoid factor predict the development of rheumatoid arthritis. *Arthritis Rheum.* 2003;48(10):2741–2749.
8. Nishimura K, Sugiyama D, Kogata Y, et al. Meta-analysis: diagnostic accuracy of anti-cyclic citrullinated peptide antibody and rheumatoid factor for rheumatoid arthritis. *Ann Intern Med.* 2007;146:797–808.
9. Berglin E, Johansson T, Sundin U, et al. Radiological outcome in rheumatoid arthritis is predicted by presence of antibodies against cyclic citrullinated peptide before and at disease onset, and by IgA-RF at disease onset. *Ann Rheum Dis.* 2006;65:453–458.
10. Damoiseaux J, Csernok E, Rasmussen N, et al. Detection of antineutrophil cytoplasmic antibodies (ANCAs): a multicentre European Vasculitis Study Group (EUVAS) evaluation of the value of indirect immunofluorescence (IIF) versus antigen-specific immunoassays. *Ann Rheum Dis.* 2017;76(4):647–653.
11. Bossuyt X, Cohen Tervaert JW, Arimura Y, et al. Position paper: Revised 2017 international consensus on testing of ANCAs in granulomatosis with polyangiitis and microscopic polyangiitis. *Nat Rev Rheumatol.* 2017;13:683–692.
12. Mammen AL. Autoimmune myopathies: autoantibodies, phenotypes and pathogenesis. *Nat Rev Neurol.* 2011;7(6):343–354.

13. Ghirardello A, Doria A. New insights in myositis-specific autoantibodies. *Curr Opin Rheumatol.* 2018;30(6):614–622.
14. Satoh M, Tanaka S, Ceribelli A, et al. A comprehensive overview on myositis-specific antibodies: new and old biomarkers in idiopathic inflammatory myopathy. *Clin Rev Allergy Immunol.* 2017;52(1):1–19.
15. Hoxha A, Banzato A, Ruffatti A, et al. Detection of lupus anticoagulant in the era of direct oral anticoagulants. *Autoimmun Rev.* 2017;16(2):173–178.
16. Frazer-Abel A. The effect on the immunology laboratory of the expansion in complement therapeutics. *J Immunol Methods.* 2018;461:30–36.

Imaging of Articular Disease in Rheumatology

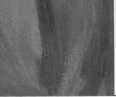

6

Devon M. DiVito, Deborah L. Parks, and
Jennifer L. Demertzis

GENERAL PRINCIPLES

- Although most rheumatologic diseases are diagnosed clinically, imaging can aid in diagnosis and provide objective assessment of disease severity, prognosis, complications, and response to treatment. Modalities useful in the assessment of rheumatologic articular disease include conventional radiography (CR), ultrasound (US), magnetic resonance imaging (MRI), and, to a lesser extent, computed tomography (CT), including dual-energy CT (DE-CT).
- It is important to note that not all features described for each disease are present at any one time and that no individual abnormality is pathognomonic. A summary of characteristic findings is included in Table 6-1.[1]

Conventional Radiography

- CR is the imaging modality of choice for the initial evaluation of most rheumatic conditions because it can evaluate fine bone detail, joint spaces, alignment, and soft-tissue calcifications characteristic of some rheumatic diseases.
- In inflammatory arthritis, CR can detect the late, irreversible sequelae of chronic inflammation such as osseous erosions, joint space narrowing, and malalignment. However, its inability to directly visualize synovitis, articular cartilage loss, bone marrow edema, and tendon disease indicative of active inflammation limits its utility as a prognostic test or indicator of therapeutic response.
- Despite these limitations, CR is universally available and inexpensive, provides a useful baseline for assessing disease progression, and is therefore essential in the evaluation of arthritis.
- A simplified systematic approach using the mnemonic "ABCDS" can be used to interpret bone and joint radiographs:
  - A refers to alignment (e.g., normal, subluxation/dislocation, characteristic malalignment such as boutonniere deformity).
  - B refers to bone (e.g., erosions, osteoporosis, periostitis).
  - C refers to cartilage and joint space (e.g., uniform vs. nonuniform narrowing, ankylosis).
  - D refers to distribution (e.g., proximal vs. distal, symmetric vs. asymmetric).
  - S refers to soft-tissue findings (e.g., effusion, swelling, calcifications).

  A working knowledge of the commonly ordered radiographs for the evaluation of arthritis is recommended to maximize diagnostic yield and minimize unnecessary radiation exposure and cost to the patient (see Table 6-2).[1-3]

Ultrasound

- High-resolution US (>12 MHz) has been increasingly employed to diagnose and evaluate rheumatic disease over the past 10 to 15 years.
- Advantages of US include wide availability, low cost, short examination time for experienced operators, lack of ionizing radiation, and ability to evaluate inflammation in patients who have a contrast allergy or contraindication to MRI.
- Clinically, US has been shown to be more sensitive than physical examination in the detection of joint effusion and synovitis, and can be utilized at point of care by trained rheumatologists.

TABLE 6-1 COMMON IMAGING FINDINGS BY DISEASE

	Osteoarthritis	Erosive Osteoarthritis	Septic Arthritis	Rheumatoid Arthritis	Axial Spondyloarthritis	Peripheral Spondyloarthritis	Gout	CPPD
Distribution	Weight-bearing, repetitive use	Symmetric, distal	Monoarticular	Proximal, symmetric, large and/or small joints	Axial (symmetric SI joints, spine)	Peripheral (asymmetric, distal, and/or SI joints)	Anywhere!	Symmetric, non-weight-bearing
Joint space narrowing	Nonuniform, loose bodies, chronic course	Nonuniform, early aggressive phase	Uniform, rapid	Uniform	Uniform	Uniform, joint space may be preserved even with erosions	Normal, nonuniform	Nonuniform
Bone	Subchondral sclerosis, osteophytes	Osteophytes	Bone loss/destruction adjacent to Soft Tissue (ST) abnormality	Osteoporosis, no bony proliferation	Smooth flowing syndesmophytes, ankylosis	Periostitis, ankylosis, bulky syndesmophytes		Subchondral sclerosis, osteophytes
Cysts, erosions	Subchondral cysts	Central "gull-wing" erosions	Joint-centered erosions	Marginal erosions	Spondylitis, enthesitis	Ill-defined "fluffy" erosions, enthesitis, spondylitis	Well-defined erosions with overhanging edges ("rat-bite")	Large subchondral cysts, out of proportion to degree of joint narrowing
Soft tissue	± Joint effusion	Swelling	Swelling, soft-tissue infection (abscess, ulcer, gas)	Swelling/synovitis, bursitis, rheumatoid (Rh) nodules, tenosynovitis		Dactylitis, nail pitting or onycholysis	Tophus ("lumpy-bumpy"; calcified), bursitis	Chondrocalcinosis

CPPD, calcium pyrophosphate dihydrate deposition.

TABLE 6-2	COMMONLY ORDERED RADIOGRAPHS FOR EVALUATION OF ARTHRITIS	

Joint/Extremity	Typical Views	Specialized Views/Indication
Hand	PA, Oblique, Lateral	Ball-catcher's view: helpful for assessing MCP joint arthritis and erosions
Wrist	PA, Oblique, Lateral	Clenched-fist view: helpful for assessing scapholunate stability in the setting of trauma or CPPD
Foot	AP, Oblique, Lateral	Weight-bearing radiographs should be requested to assess associated alignment abnormalities
Ankle	AP, mortise, Lateral	Weight-bearing radiographs should be requested to assess associated alignment abnormalities
Knee	AP, Lateral	Merchant view: profiles the patellofemoral joint PA-flexed weight-bearing (Rosenberg) view: best for evaluating true degree of cartilage loss along the weight-bearing surfaces of the femorotibial joint
Hip	AP, Frog-leg lateral	Helpful to include a view of the pelvis to compare the joint space to the contralateral side
Sacroiliac joint	PA, Bilateral oblique	Recommend dedicated views of the SI joint. Pelvic radiographs are suboptimal for profiling the SI joint space
Cervical spine	AP, Lateral	Flexion, Extension: Recommended to evaluate for cervical spine instability, particularly in the setting of RA Bilateral Oblique: Recommended to evaluate for neuroforaminal narrowing, particularly in the setting of degenerative disk disease and OA of the facet and uncovertebral joints
Lumbar spine	AP, Lateral, Lateral-coned	Bilateral Oblique: Recommended to evaluate for facet joint OA or suspected pars interarticularis defect(s)

AP, anteroposterior; CPPD, calcium pyrophosphate dihydrate deposition; MCP, metacarpophalangeal; OA, osteoarthritis; PA, posteroanterior; RA, rheumatoid arthritis; SI, sacroiliac.

- US has been shown to be comparable to MRI in the detection of erosions, joint effusions, and synovitis. Unlike MRI, US cannot demonstrate bone marrow edema/osteitis.
- The major disadvantages of US include user dependence and reproducibility; however, these can be offset with dedicated training and a standardized evaluation for each joint.

Although US has been used to evaluate nearly all of the rheumatic diseases discussed below, its applications for osteoarthritis (OA) remain limited.[4]

Magnetic Resonance Imaging

- The superior soft-tissue contrast afforded by MRI allows for a thorough evaluation of all articular and periarticular structures, including synovium, cartilage, tendons and tendon sheaths, muscles and fascia, ligaments, bursae, and bone marrow.
- Like US, MRI has been shown to have higher sensitivity for detecting erosions and synovitis compared to physical examination and CR.
- Disadvantages of MRI include high cost and limited availability. The long examination time and restricted positioning may be difficult for patients with significant joint pain. Pacemakers and other implantable devices are relative contraindications to MRI, limiting use in certain patient populations.[1,5]

Computed Tomography Including Dual Energy

- CT is rarely used to diagnose rheumatic disease because of its limited evaluation of active inflammation, limited soft-tissue contrast, high cost, and high radiation dose.
- However, newer applications such as DE-CT may be useful in diagnosis and quantification of gout.[6,7]

DIAGNOSIS

Osteoarthritis

Primary Osteoarthritis
- Primary OA is the most common joint disease.
- OA commonly affects the hands, feet, knees, hips, and the synovial joints of the lumbar and cervical spine.
- Involvement of the shoulders, elbows, and ankles is uncommon unless there is a history of trauma, repetitive occupational stress, or other preexisting disease.
- Joint involvement can be unilateral or bilateral and is typically asymmetric.
- OA has characteristic CR findings (Table 6-3) that distinguish it from other forms of arthritis.
- Specific CR findings by anatomic target:
  - Hand
    - OA most frequently targets the hand, involving the distal interphalangeal (DIP) and proximal interphalangeal (PIP) joints.
    - Heberden's and Bouchard's nodes refer to osteophyte formation at the DIP and PIP joints, respectively.
    - There is usually sparing of the metacarpophalangeal (MCP) joints.
  - Wrist
    - The first carpometacarpal and scaphotrapeziotrapezoidal ("triscaphe") joints are typical sites of OA in the wrist, often with radial subluxation of the first metacarpal base.
    - Without a history of prior fracture or significant occupational trauma, OA in other joints of the wrist, such as the radiocarpal joint, should suggest a diagnosis other than primary OA.
  - Feet
    - OA most commonly affects the first metatarsophalangeal (MTP) joint.
    - It is often associated with hallux valgus or hallux rigidus (stiffness and painful restriction of dorsiflexion at the first MTP joint).
    - Dorsal osteophytes characteristic of first MTP OA may be best demonstrated on a lateral radiograph.
  - Knee
    - OA of the knees is a growing epidemic secondary to obesity and the aging population.

TABLE 6-3	CHARACTERISTIC CONVENTIONAL RADIOGRAPHY FINDINGS OF PRIMARY OSTEOARTHRITIS

Pertinent Positives	Pertinent Negatives
• Nonuniform joint space narrowing • Osteophyte formation • Subchondral bone formation (sclerosis) • Subchondral bone cysts • Subluxations	• Erosions • Osteopenia

- Joint space narrowing is usually worst in the medial femorotibial compartment with associated varus angulation of the knee, although women often have lateral femorotibial disease due to anatomic valgus alignment of the knee.
- Patellofemoral compartment OA can be seen either in isolation or in conjunction with femorotibial OA.
- Assessment of cartilage loss in the knees is best provided on weight-bearing radiographs. Cartilage loss is present if the joint space is less than 3 mm, narrower than half the space of the other femorotibial articulation in the ipsilateral knee or the same articulation in the contralateral knee, or decreased on weight-bearing compared to non–weight-bearing radiographs. Although joint space width has been shown to correlate with cartilage thickness, narrowing can also occur secondary to meniscal pathology.
- Meniscal tears and cartilage loss can be evaluated directly on MRI. Sequelae of knee OA, such as synovitis and bone marrow edema, are also evaluated on MRI and may be more closely tied to symptomatology than loss of the aneural and avascular articular cartilage that is characteristic of OA.
  - Hip
    - Cartilage loss is usually focal and involves the weight-bearing superolateral aspect of the joint.
    - Diffuse, uniform loss of cartilage with axial migration of the femoral head is more commonly seen in inflammatory arthritis.
  - Spine
    - OA of the spine should not be confused with degenerative disease affecting the intervertebral disks. OA of the spine affects the atlantoaxial, uncovertebral, and facet joints of the cervical spine, and the facet joints of the thoracic and lumbar spine. It demonstrates characteristic features of OA, including nonuniform joint space narrowing, osteophyte formation, and subchondral sclerosis, and can result in neuroforaminal and central canal narrowing.
    - CR is the initial imaging modality for evaluation of OA in the spine. CT, CT myelogram, and/or MR may be indicated for surgical planning or in cases where neurologic symptoms are present to evaluate the effect of bony changes on the spinal cord and nerve roots.
- Ultrasound
  - The hallmark findings of OA may be illustrated with high-resolution US, including:
    - Peripheral marginal osteophytes that appear as a cortical "step off"
    - Joint space loss
    - Joint effusion and/or synovitis
  - Doppler flow may aid in the detection of synovitis.
  - Currently, US is used predominately to assess for joint effusion and synovitis and less commonly to evaluate the articular cartilage.

- Magnetic resonance imaging
  - Allows for a whole-organ approach to the evaluation of OA, including evaluation of synovium, bone marrow, and periarticular soft tissues. MRI can also demonstrate radiographically occult findings such as subchondral insufficiency fractures that may occur in the setting of OA.
  - Whereas most clinical MRI examinations provide a morphologic evaluation of articular cartilage, advanced MRI sequences such as T2 mapping and T1 rho provide a biochemical assessment of articular cartilage that can demonstrate cartilage damage that precedes the morphologic changes seen on traditional MRI. This may eventually allow for detection of at-risk cartilage in OA that may be amenable to early treatment and evaluation for cartilage salvage techniques.[5]
- CT is rarely used in the evaluation of OA, but, when indicated, demonstrates characteristic findings similar to those seen on CR. Most commonly, it is used for presurgical assessment of bony anatomy prior to arthroplasty.

Erosive Osteoarthritis

- Predominantly affects postmenopausal females and has a predilection for the small distal joints of the hands. Unlike typical OA, erosive OA often has a symmetric distribution and rapid course.
- In addition to the hallmark findings of primary OA, erosive OA is characterized by inflammatory changes, specifically central erosions resulting in the classic "gull-wing" deformities. Affected joints may progress to ankylosis, which is rare in primary OA.
- When considering a diagnosis of erosive OA, it is important to exclude the presence of findings that would indicate an alternative inflammatory arthritis, including marginal erosions (rheumatoid arthritis [RA]) or dactylitis (psoriatic arthritis [PsA]).[2,8]

Rapidly Progressive Osteoarthritis

- First described in 1970s, rapidly progressive osteoarthritis (RPOA) is a diagnosis of exclusion characterized by rapid chondrolysis (>2 mm/year) without preexisting arthritis. It most commonly affects the femoroacetabular joint of elderly women.
- Although no consensus exists on the exact etiology of RPOA, it may be the result of a subchondral insufficiency fracture of the femoral head.
- The diagnosis is often made by clinical history in conjunction with serial radiographs, demonstrating rapid joint narrowing, superolateral femoral subluxation, and joint-centered bony remodeling with minimal osteophyte formation.
- On MRI, findings of RPOA include joint effusion and bone marrow edema with remodeling of the femoral articular surface ("hatchet" deformity of the proximal femur).[8,9]
- The rapid joint space loss and bone remodeling of RPOA mimic those of septic arthritis and neuropathic arthropathy. If infection is suspected, arthrocentesis is recommended to confirm the diagnosis.

Rheumatoid Arthritis

- RA is a chronic systemic autoimmune inflammatory disease that presents with musculoskeletal symptoms. Synovitis is the hallmark feature of RA in the musculoskeletal system.
- RA demonstrates a characteristic symmetric distribution affecting the small proximal joints of the hands, wrists, and feet. The cervical spine is the third most commonly affected area, because of the large number of synovial articulations in the cervical spine.
- Although CR remains the mainstay for screening in RA, its inability to detect key findings of active inflammatory disease that precede joint damage has resulted in the increased utilization of US and MRI.
- Both US and MRI are more sensitive for the detection of synovitis and bone erosions compared to clinical examination and CR. MRI is also able to detect bone marrow edema/osteitis, which is a strong predictor of the future presence of erosions.

- Targeted drug therapies in RA have the greatest impact when instituted early in disease. Therefore, it is crucial that patients with active inflammatory arthritis are identified before irreversible joint damage occurs. US and MRI support this approach by allowing for a more sensitive evaluation of all the joints for subtle erosions and synovitis.[4,10]
- Conventional radiography
  - CR findings in RA may be divided into early and late findings, delineated in Table 6-4.
  - The earliest findings are nonspecific and include symmetric periarticular soft-tissue swelling and osteopenia.
  - Erosions are the result of synovial inflammation. They are subtle early in disease and involve the marginal "bare areas" where cartilage is thinnest or absent.
  - Erosions may progress centrally, resulting in severe subchondral articular erosions with associated uniform joint space narrowing later in disease.
  - Periarticular osteopenia observed early in the disease may progress to generalized diffuse osteoporosis.
  - Chronic synovial inflammation results in diffuse uniform cartilage loss and joint space narrowing. Unlike OA, osteophyte formation is not characteristic of RA.
  - Fibrous and osseous ankylosis may occur in end-stage disease, or in patients who present with RA before skeletal maturity. When it occurs, ankylosis is most commonly seen in the carpus, midfoot, and cervical spine.
  - Damage to ligamentous and tendinous structures may result in subluxations and dislocations of affected joints.
- Ultrasound
  - US is increasingly utilized to evaluate patients with RA and has several advantages over CR, including:
    - Increased sensitivity for detecting synovitis. Synovitis is a strong predictor of the development of bone erosions. US can identify synovitis early in RA to initiate drug therapy to prevent bone destruction.
    - Increased sensitivity in detecting erosions. The number of erosions is important to determine as it affects patient classification based on the 2010 American College of Rheumatology/European League Against Rheumatism (ACR/EULAR) recommendations.
    - Identification of extra-articular synovial inflammation such as tenosynovitis and bursitis
    - Differentiation of active disease from remission. US can detect "subclinical" synovitis in the presence of a normal physical examination, which is important in assessing treatment response and managing medical therapy.
  - The major disadvantage of US is the inability to identify bone marrow edema.[4]
- Magnetic resonance imaging
  - With its superior soft-tissue contrast and cross-sectional imaging planes, MRI is the most robust modality for detecting the early changes of RA, including synovitis and

TABLE 6-4	EARLY AND LATE CONVENTIONAL RADIOGRAPHY FINDINGS OF RHEUMATOID ARTHRITIS

Early Findings	Late Findings
• Periarticular soft-tissue swelling • Periarticular osteopenia • Marginal erosions	• Advanced articular erosions • Uniform joint space narrowing • Diffuse osteoporosis • Fibrous and osseous ankylosis (rare)

radiographically occult bone erosions. Detection of synovitis requires administration of intravenous gadolinium contrast agents.
  ○ MRI is the only imaging modality that can detect bone marrow edema/osteitis, which is an important prognostic indicator of future erosions.
  ○ MRI is also the preferred method of imaging musculoskeletal complications of RA and RA therapy, such as tendon ruptures, avascular necrosis, insufficiency fractures, and the sequelae of cervical spine instability.[10]
• CT is not routinely used in the evaluation of RA.

Seronegative Spondyloarthropathies

• Seronegative spondyloarthropathies (SSpAs) are a group of diseases that are rheumatoid factor negative (hence "seronegative") and are correlated with the HLA-B27 haplotype.
• Although synovitis is often present in SSpA, enthesitis (inflammation at the origins and insertions of ligaments, tendons, and joint capsules) is the hallmark finding. Patients may also present with periostitis, dactylitis, erosions ("pencil-in-cup" morphology), ankylosis of affected peripheral joints, and spondylitis and sacroiliitis of the axial skeleton.
• Several classification criteria (e.g., New York criteria, Classification Criteria for Psoriatic Arthritis [CASPAR]) have been developed over the years, the most recent of which was developed by the Assessment of Spondyloarthritis International Society (ASAS) that divides SSpA into two categories based on clinical presentation: axial or peripheral spondyloarthropathy (PSpA).[11]

Axial Spondyloarthropathy
• Subgroup of SSpA that primarily involve the sacroiliac (SI) joints and spine, and are called axial spondyloarthropathies (ASpAs).
• ASAS criteria apply to patients who are less than 45 years of age with inflammatory back pain lasting longer than 3 months.
• In these patients, CR imaging is standard of care. MRI may be obtained in select cases.
• The prototype for the ASpA is ankylosing spondylitis (AS).[11]
• **Ankylosing Spondylitis**
  ○ The most common of the SSpA, AS primarily affects the axial skeleton and less commonly the appendicular skeleton.
  ○ The distribution has classically been described as bilateral and symmetric involving the SI joints first, followed by the spine in an ascending pattern. The hips, knees, shoulders, and small joints may also be affected, particularly in patients with juvenile onset of disease.
  ○ A variety of imaging modalities may be used to evaluate AS.
  ○ Conventional radiography
    ▪ CR imaging should include anteroposterior (AP) and lateral views of the entire spine, and dedicated posteroanterior (PA) and bilateral oblique views of the SI joints to assess for sacroiliitis, which is crucial to the diagnosis. Bilateral symmetric sacroiliitis, ankylosis, syndesmophytes, and ligamentous ossification in the spine ("bamboo spine") are characteristic findings of AS on CR.
    ▪ Erosions and uniform joint space narrowing may be present in large joints, such as the shoulders and hips. Osteopenia, osteophytes, subchondral cysts, and subluxation/dislocation of peripheral joints are rare in AS compared to other inflammatory arthritides.
    ▪ Involvement of the SI joints may be subtle early in disease and is often radiographically occult. Most commonly, sacroiliitis affects the iliac side of the SI joints before the sacral side.
    ▪ CT is more sensitive than CR in demonstrating morphologic findings of chronic sacroiliitis, including erosions and ankylosis. However, it is unable to detect the presence of active SI joint inflammation prior to development of these bony changes.

- The lumbosacral and thoracolumbar junctions are the usual sites of initial spine involvement, with changes progressing in a caudocranial direction.
- Osteitis of the anterior portion of the uncovertebral junction is a common initial finding.
- On lateral radiographs, the vertebrae often look "squared." This is due to erosions at the anterosuperior and anteroinferior vertebral margins, leading to loss of the normal concavity of the anterior facet of the vertebral body.
- Bony sclerosis adjacent to sites of erosion can produce a "shiny corner sign" on CR.
- Ossification of the outer fibers of the annulus fibrosis of the intervertebral disk results in syndesmophytes. In AS, the syndesmophytes are smooth, flowing, and gracile ("bamboo spine"). This can help differentiate AS from other SSpA with spine involvement such as PsA, which have bulky irregular syndesmophytes.
- Enthesitis (bony proliferation and inflammation at sites of tendon and ligament origin and insertion) is notable in AS and other SSpA.
  ○ **Ultrasound:** US is rarely used in the diagnosis of AS because of difficulty evaluating the spine and SI joints. However, it may be used to evaluate for associated peripheral findings, including enthesitis.
  ○ **Magnetic resonance imaging**
    - MRI is ideal for evaluating active sacroiliitis, which is defined as the presence of subchondral or periarticular bone marrow edema at the SI joint in a single location on sequential slices, or multifocal subchondral or periarticular bone marrow edema on a single slice. Synovitis, erosions, enthesitis, and capsulitis may also be present, but are insufficient for diagnosing active sacroiliitis in the absence of bone marrow edema. Intravenous gadolinium contrast is not required for diagnosing bone marrow edema in sacroiliitis but does help detect enthesitis, synovitis, and capsulitis, which may support the diagnosis of axial spondyloarthropathy, particularly early in the course of disease.[12]
    - In general, MRI of the spine is not recommended for diagnosis, but may be used to assess active disease or for problem-solving.
    - MRI may be indicated in the setting of trauma because the rigidity of the spine in ASpA can result in devastating injuries to the spine and spinal cord.
- **Computed tomography:** CT is rarely used for diagnosis of AS, but may be helpful when there is variant SI joint anatomy or in the setting of trauma to evaluate for spinal fractures.[3–5,11]
- **Enteropathic arthritis:** Clinically and radiographically, this arthritis is nearly indistinguishable from that of AS. The key differentiating factor is the presence of inflammatory bowel disease. Enteropathic arthritis is independent of the course of the underlying inflammatory bowel disease.

Peripheral Spondyloarthropathies
- The established ASAS criteria for PSpAs apply to patients who demonstrate predominantly peripheral symptoms with either arthritis, enthesitis, or dactylitis.
- In these patients, additional clinical or imaging findings are required for diagnosis including sacroiliitis on CR, or two of the following: arthritis, enthesitis, or dactylitis.
- Although limited in evaluation of axial inflammatory arthritis, US can assess for inflammation in peripheral joints, including synovitis, joint effusion, erosions, bursitis, tenosynovitis, and enthesitis.
- Like US, MRI is able to assess features of peripheral articular and periarticular inflammation, including synovitis, joint effusion, erosions, bursitis, tenosynovitis, and enthesitis. MRI is the modality of choice for evaluating sacroiliitis and spondylitis and is the only modality that can document the presence of bone marrow edema.
- CT is rarely indicated in PSpA, but may show signs of chronic sacroiliitis, and is important in the evaluation of spine trauma in patients with axial disease.

- The prototype for the PSpA is PsA.[11]
- **Psoriatic Arthritis**
  - PsA predominantly affects the appendicular skeleton in an asymmetric distribution involving the small joints of the hands and feet. Axial involvement of the spine and SI joints occurs less commonly. When present, sacroiliitis is typically asymmetric in PsA, and syndesmophytes in the spine are large and bulky compared to AS. Skin and nail findings of psoriasis usually precede the onset of arthritis.
  - PsA differs from RA radiographically in many important ways, particularly with regard to periosteal bone proliferation (periostitis) and normal bone mineralization.
  - In decreasing order of frequency, PsA involves the hands, feet, SI joints, and spine. DIP joint involvement in the hands also differentiates PsA from RA.
  - Diffuse periarticular soft-tissue swelling (dactylitis) can be striking in the hands and feet, resulting in a "sausage-digit" appearance characteristic of this disease.
  - Erosions are a predominant feature of PsA. In severe cases, erosions can destroy large portions of the underlying bone and give the appearance of a widened joint space because of interposed pannus. The erosions are often ill-defined, distinguishing them from RA and gout. In advanced disease, severe erosions result in "pencil-in-cup" deformities of involved joints.
  - Acro-osteolysis and resorption of the distal phalanges of the hands and feet are characteristic of PsA.
  - Bony proliferation is also relatively unique to PsA. It occurs adjacent to areas of erosions, along the shafts of the bones, across joints, and at tendinous and ligamentous insertion sites ("enthesitis"). Immature bone proliferation appears fluffy and spiculated.
  - The radiographic changes of PsA in the feet are similar to those in the hands. Erosions at the insertion of the Achilles tendon and origin of the plantar fascia due to enthesitis are common.
  - SI joint involvement in PsA is usually bilateral and asymmetric.
  - Bony ankylosis may occur in the SI joints, but it is much less frequent than in AS.
  - Spondylitis usually occurs along with SI joint involvement. Large, bulky, and unilateral or asymmetric paravertebral ossification is a characteristic finding in PsA, which helps distinguish axial involvement in PsA from AS.[3–5,11]
- **Reactive Arthritis (Reiter's Syndrome)**
  - Patients with reactive arthritis (ReA) classically present with a clinical triad of sterile inflammatory arthritis, uveitis or conjunctivitis, and prior urogenital or gastrointestinal infection.
  - ReA has a predilection for the lower extremities. It affects the feet, ankles, knees, and SI joints, with less frequent involvement of the hands, hips, and spine.
  - Many of the radiographic findings in ReA are indistinguishable from those of PsA, with bone erosions, bone proliferation, uniform joint space narrowing, enthesitis, bilateral asymmetric distribution, dactylitis, and lack of osteopenia. Joint ankylosis is less common than in PsA, but enthesitis at the Achilles insertion and plantar fascia origin may be more prominent than in PsA.
  - Clinical correlation is particularly important in differentiating ReA from PsA.[4,5]

Systemic Lupus Erythematosus

- Most commonly affects the hands, hips, knees, and shoulders in a bilateral and symmetric distribution.
- The radiographic appearance is described as deforming nonerosive arthritis with or without osteonecrosis. Classically, systemic lupus erythematosus (SLE) has reducible MCP joint subluxations (Jaccoud's arthropathy).
- In addition to the characteristic CR findings, bone infarcts and/or osteonecrosis can occur secondary to chronic steroid use or, less commonly, in response to vasculitis or a hypercoagulable state associated with SLE. The femoral heads, femoral condyles, tibial plateaus, humeral heads, and tali are the sites most frequently affected by osteonecrosis.

- SLE patients are at increased risk for septic arthritis. Arthrocentesis is recommended for diagnosis if joint infection is suspected.
- Both US and MRI can detect synovitis in SLE. MRI may be used to detect complications of SLE, including osteonecrosis and bone infarcts.
- CT is not commonly used to evaluate SLE.[2]

Crystalline Disease

The deposition of crystals within the articular and periarticular soft tissues defines the rheumatic conditions in this category, including gout, calcium pyrophosphate dihydrate deposition (CPPD) disease, and hydroxyapatite deposition disease (HADD).

Gout

- Gout, the most common crystalline arthropathy, is the result of monosodium urate (MSU) crystal deposition. Although most imaging findings represent gouty articular disease, gout can affect any tissue of the body, including nonarticular bone, tendon, and soft tissue.
- Chronic tophaceous gout is an asymmetric and erosive process with a polyarticular distribution that most commonly involves the feet (especially the first MTP joint), ankles, knees, hands, and elbows.
- In severe cases, gout can lead to secondary OA, disuse osteopenia, and, occasionally, mutilating arthritis.
- Although joint aspiration remains the gold standard for the diagnosis of gout, a variety of imaging modalities are available for the initial evaluation, presumptive diagnosis, quantification of disease, identification of complications, and treatment monitoring.
- Conventional radiography
  - The radiographic findings in acute gouty arthritis are nonspecific and include soft-tissue swelling, joint effusion, and periarticular osteopenia.
  - When the acute arthritic attack subsides, the bone remineralizes and more chronic, slowly progressive bony changes may develop.
  - Although tophi are not radiopaque unless they calcify, they may be detected on CR because of mass effect.
  - Periarticular tophi produce punched-out lesions in adjacent bone with overhanging edges as the bone attempts to remodel around the tophus ("rat-bite" erosions).
  - Because tophaceous gout does not involve the cartilage directly, the joint space is preserved until late in the course of disease. This is a distinguishing feature from other inflammatory arthritides.[2,6,7]
- Ultrasound
  - Several studies have shown the positive role that US plays in the early detection of gout.
  - Characteristic US findings include joint effusion, synovitis, and osseous erosions.
  - MSU crystal deposition along hyaline cartilage may result in the "double-contour sign." This describes the echogenic crystals that deposit on the outer surface of the articular cartilage and parallel the hyperechoic contour of the underlying bone. This finding is specific but not sensitive.
  - Take care not to confuse this finding with CPPD, which has thin hyperechoic bands of crystal deposits within the cartilage (rather than on the cartilage surface).
  - Avoid misinterpreting the normal cartilage interface sign, where the outer surface of the articular cartilage appears hyperechoic because of an adjacent fluid interface.
  - Synovitis associated with gout has been described as heterogeneous but predominately hyperechoic.
  - Floating MSU crystals may be seen in joint fluid; however, this finding is nonspecific for gout.[4,6]
- Magnetic resonance imaging
  - MRI is sensitive for soft-tissue and bone abnormalities that can be seen in gout; however, the findings are nonspecific and may appear similar to those of infection or neuropathic osteoarthropathy.

- ○ Tophi demonstrate intermediate- to low-signal intensity on T1 sequences and heterogeneous signal on T2 sequences with variable enhancement.
- ○ Erosions are identified by bone destruction, but may be difficult to detect because of the variable MR imaging characteristics of adjacent tophi.[6]
- Dual-energy CT
  - ○ DE-CT is a relatively new imaging technique for evaluation of gouty arthritis. It differentiates gout crystals from calcium using specific CT attenuation characteristics of MSU.
  - ○ Advantages
    - Identification and quantification of extra-articular gout
    - Evaluation of joints inaccessible to arthrocentesis or in patients who are unable or unwilling to have joint aspiration performed for definitive diagnosis
    - Earlier initiation or intensification of treatment allowing for improved outcomes and symptom relief[7]
    - Helpful in patients with gout mimics or atypical presentations
  - ○ Limitations
    - Artifacts in postprocessing
    - Less reliable in the diagnosis of acute gout

Calcium Pyrophosphate Deposition Disease
- Also known as pyrophosphate arthropathy and "pseudogout" in the acute setting
- Characteristically involves the radiocarpal joint, second and third MCP joints, and the patellofemoral compartment of the knee
- Chondrocalcinosis is the hallmark of CPPD disease and represents the deposition of crystals within hyaline articular cartilage.
- Conventional radiography
  - ○ CR is the initial imaging modality of choice; however, it is important to note that its sensitivity for the detection of chondrocalcinosis may be as low as 40%.
  - ○ Chondrocalcinosis is most commonly seen in the menisci of the knee and the triangular fibrocartilage of the wrist. Other sites that may be affected include the acetabular labra of the hips, pubic symphysis, and the spine.
  - ○ Chondrocalcinosis is not necessary to make the diagnosis of CPPD arthropathy, and chondrocalcinosis may be caused by other metabolic disorders or senescent change.
  - ○ In acute pseudogout, the usual radiographic findings are soft-tissue swelling and joint effusion. Chondrocalcinosis may or may not be present. The diagnosis is confirmed by the presence of CPPD crystals in aspirated joint fluid.
  - ○ Other CR features of CPPD arthropathy include:
    - Joint space loss and subchondral sclerosis later in the course of disease. Although these features are similar to OA, the distribution differs. CPPD disease is typically bilateral and symmetric, preferentially involving the patellofemoral, radioscaphoid, and MCP joints.
    - Subchondral cysts
      - □ More prominent in CPPD arthropathy than OA
      - □ CPPD cysts appear as clusters of coalescent lucencies of variable size and shape with indistinct margins.
    - As with other non–rheumatoid arthritides, bone mineralization is normal.
  - ○ Important differential considerations based on CR findings include:
    - Neuropathic osteoarthropathy: CPPD arthropathy may be associated with rapid subchondral bone collapse, leading to fragmentation with intra-articular loose bodies, resembling neuropathic osteoarthropathy.
    - Hemochromatosis: Hemochromatosis may be suggested when more diffuse involvement of the MCP joints is observed, including the second through fifth MCP joints.[2]

- Ultrasound
  - High-resolution US has been shown to be both sensitive and specific for the detection of soft-tissue calcifications.
  - CPPD crystals appear as round or amorphous hyperechoic foci within the hypoechoic hyaline cartilage. This is in distinction to the deposits of gout, which traditionally line the hyaline cartilage articular surface.[4]
- MRI is not sensitive for the detection of small calcifications in the articular cartilage and is therefore not recommended for the diagnosis of CPPD disease.
- CT is rarely indicated in the evaluation of CPPD disease, but will demonstrate chondrocalcinosis.[2]

Hydroxyapatite Deposition Disease
- May be idiopathic but may also be secondary to a variety of systemic diseases, which should be excluded in the clinical workup of HADD
- Classically results in periarticular calcium crystal deposition, resulting in calcific tendinitis and bursitis
- Most commonly affects the shoulder including the rotator cuff and biceps tendons and less commonly the hips, wrist, elbow, and spine
- Whereas a single joint distribution is common, multiple joints may be involved at one time or in succession.
- Rarely, HADD may be identified in an intra-articular location. The most classic example of this is Milwaukee shoulder, which is the result of HADD in the glenohumeral joint.[13]
- US
  - Hydroxyapatite crystals may be identified as hyperechoic foci within a tendon or bursae with other signs of inflammation and possible tendinopathy.
  - US-guided needling and aspiration of crystal deposits ("barbotage") may provide symptomatic relief.
- MRI
  - Crystal deposition is identified as globular foci of low-signal intensity on all sequences and should be interpreted in conjunction with CR to confirm the findings.
  - In acute disease, extensive bone marrow and soft-tissue edema may be present and can mimic a tumor or an infection.
- CT is rarely used to diagnose or evaluate HADD. In cases of severe joint destruction such as Milwaukee shoulder, it may assist in surgical planning.[5]

Septic Arthritis
- Septic arthritis is a musculoskeletal emergency with significant morbidity.
- Although clinical presentation may suggest a diagnosis of septic arthritis, any level of suspicion warrants urgent confirmation with joint aspiration so that appropriate treatment may be promptly initiated to minimize complications.
- CR
  - Despite its low sensitivity for demonstrating the early changes of septic arthritis, imaging evaluation of suspected joint infection always begins with CR.
  - The earliest CR findings include:
    - Soft-tissue swelling and joint effusion
    - Marginal erosions from early bone loss adjacent to sites of capsular attachment
    - Synovial hyperemia and early disuse atrophy with periarticular osteopenia
  - Later findings of septic arthritis include uniform joint space narrowing and joint-centered erosions, which are the result of articular cartilage destruction and associated osteomyelitis of the underlying bone.
  - The presence of an already abnormal joint may complicate the interpretation of radiographs.
- Although radiographic features are not specific to the inciting organism, certain findings are common.

- ○ Septic arthritis of any etiology tends to be monoarticular, unless the patient is bacteremic or immunocompromised.
- ○ Bacterial septic arthritis typically results in rapid destruction of articular cartilage and adjacent bone.
- ○ Tuberculous arthritis may present with Phemister's triad: juxta-articular osteoporosis, marginal erosions, and absent or mild joint space narrowing.
- ○ Fungal septic arthritis may have imaging features similar to tuberculous (TB) arthritis, including absent or mild joint space narrowing.
- The MRI appearance of septic arthritis is nonspecific, as similar findings can be seen in inflammatory arthritis and early neuropathic joints. MRI can be used to assess complications of septic arthritis, such as abscess, osteomyelitis, and tissue necrosis. Administration of intravenous gadolinium contrast agents can help distinguish viable (enhancing) from necrotic (nonenhancing) tissue, which has important implications for surgical versus medical management of infection.
- Radionuclide imaging cannot differentiate septic arthritis from inflammatory arthritis but is useful in excluding osteomyelitis.[3,14]

TREATMENT

- Please refer to disease-specific chapters for current evidence-guided treatment regimens.
- Additionally, patients suffering from the above conditions may benefit from US-guided aspiration and/or injection of joints, bursae, and tendon injection. Please refer to Chapter 3 for discussion of available injection procedures.

REFERENCES

1. Brower AC, Flemming DJ. Introduction chapter. In: *Arthritis in Black and White*. 3rd ed. Philadelphia, PA: Saunders; 2012:1–26.
2. Jacobson JA, Gandikota G, Yebin J, et al. Radiographic evaluation of arthritis: degenerative joint disease and variations. *Radiology*. 2008;248:737–747.
3. Jacobson JA, Gandikota G, Yebin J, et al. Radiographic evaluation of arthritis: Inflammatory conditions. *Radiology*. 2008;248:378–389.
4. Taljanovic MS, Melville DM, Gimber LH, et al. High-resolution US of rheumatologic diseases. *Radiographics*. 2015;35:2026–2048.
5. Schweitzer H. The role of radiology in the evolution of the understanding of articular disease. *Radiology*. 2014;273:S1–S22.
6. Gandikota G, Galzebrook KN, Jacobson JA. Advanced imaging in gout. *AJR Am J Roentgenol*. 2013;201:515–525.
7. Gamala M, Linn-Rasker SP, Nix M, et al. Gouty arthritis: decision-making following dual-energy CT scan in clinical practice, a retrospective analysis. *Clin Rheumatol*. 2018;37:1879–1884.
8. Brower AC, Flemming DJ. Arthritis chapter. In: *Arthritis in Black and White*. 3rd ed. Philadelphia, PA: Saunders; 2012:243–260.
9. Boutry N, Paul C, Leroy X, et al. Rapidly destructive osteoarthritis of the hip: MR imaging findings. *Am J Roentgenol*. 2002;179(3):657–663.
10. Sommer OJ, Kladosek A, Weiler V, et al. Rheumatoid arthritis: a practical guide to state-of-the-art imaging, image interpretation, and clinical implications. *Radiographis*. 2005;25:381–398.
11. Chang EY, Chen KC, Huang BK, et al. Adult inflammatory arthritides: What the radiologist should know. *Radiographics*. 2016;36:1849–1870.
12. Özgen A. Comparison of fat-saturated T2-weighted and contrast-enhanced fat-saturated T1-weighted sequences in MR imaging of sacroiliac joints in diagnosing active sacroiliitis. *Eur J Radiol*. 2015;84:2593–2596.
13. Brower AC, Flemming DJ. Hydroxyapatite deposition disease. In: Brower AC, Flemming DJ. *Arthritis in Black and White*. 3rd ed. Philadelphia, PA: Saunders; 2012:325–334.
14. Lin HM, Learch TJ, White EA, et al. Emergency joint aspiration: A guide for radiologists on call. *Radiographics*. 2009;29:1139–1158.

Rheumatologic Emergencies

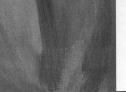

7

Philip Chu and María C. González-Mayda

GENERAL PRINCIPLES

Rheumatologic emergencies, albeit uncommon, present diagnostic challenges and require prompt action.[1] This chapter highlights common rheumatologic emergencies.

INFECTIOUS ARTHRITIS

- The differential diagnosis of **acute monoarthritis** must always include infectious (septic) arthritis. Fever and other constitutional signs are usually present; however, they may be absent in immunosuppressed or geriatric populations. Up to 22% of cases may present as polyarthritis.[2]
- The common mimics of septic arthritis include acute gout or pseudogout, reactive arthritis, hemarthrosis, and primary or metastatic bone tumors.
- Risk factors include abnormal joint architecture, prosthetic joint, increasing age, diabetes mellitus, and immunosuppression.[3]
- The diagnosis of septic arthritis is made unequivocally by synovial fluid analysis.
  - The fluid is sent for cell count and crystals, Gram stain, and culture.
  - **Synovial fluid white blood cell (WBC) counts more than 50,000 are associated with septic joint;** however, partially treated infections or immunosuppression may be associated with lower cell counts.[1]
- **Therapy should not be delayed while awaiting confirmatory diagnosis** because bacterial septic arthritis has a mortality rate of about 10% and serious morbidity.[2]
- **Joints with orthopedic hardware warrant urgent surgical consultation.**
- Empiric antibiotic treatment should include staphylococcal (including methicillin-resistant *Staphylococcus aureus* [MRSA]) and streptococcal coverage. Specific coverage for *Salmonella, Pasteurella,* and gram-negative organisms is to be provided on a case-by-case basis.
- **Removal of purulent material** is essential, either via arthroscopy, open arthrotomy, or closed-needle aspiration.[2]
- See Chapter 35, for a full discussion.

GIANT CELL ARTERITIS

- Giant cell arteritis (GCA) or temporal arteritis is a primary **systemic vasculitis affecting large vessels distal the aortic arch.** It is an often overlooked rheumatologic emergency, and ischemic complications can lead to vision loss in 10% to 15% of patients.[4]
- GCA primarily occurs in patients more than 50 years of age, with peak incidence between the ages of 70 and 80 years.[4]
- The clinical presentation includes **headache, jaw claudication**, fever, **scalp artery tenderness**, and **visual loss.**
- It is often associated with **polymyalgia rheumatica**, which is characterized by aching and stiffness of hip and shoulder girdle muscles.
- Lab studies show a **high erythrocyte sedimentation rate** (ESR > 50 mm/hour) (sensitivity 86%, specificity 27%) and **C-reactive protein** (sensitivity 87%, specificity 31%).

However, up to 4% of patients with biopsy proven GCA may have a normal ESR and CRP.[5]

- Blood cultures are recommended to evaluate infectious causes if the patient is febrile. If clinically indicated, assays for autoantibodies can help evaluate for other rheumatic diseases, and serum protein electrophoresis can evaluate for monoclonal gammopathy.[4]
- Definitive diagnosis requires a **temporal artery biopsy.**
  - Biopsy is positive in 85% to 95% of cases, and a negative biopsy does not rule out GCA.
  - Biopsy can still show histologic abnormalities even after 2 weeks of high-dose steroids; thus, **awaiting biopsy should not delay initiation of treatment** when GCA is suspected.[6]
- Color Doppler ultrasound of the temporal artery can demonstrate a "halo sign," indicating circumferential vascular mural edema (sensitivity 68%, specificity 91%), stenosis, and occlusion. It can provide a noninvasive and rapid approach to initial diagnosis in experienced centers.[7]
- When the diagnosis of GCA is suspected, initiate treatment with high-dose oral prednisone at 1 mg/kg/day.
- If visual symptoms or signs are present, intravenous (IV) pulse therapy with methylprednisolone 1,000 mg for 3 consecutive days is recommended, followed by high-dose oral prednisone.[4]
- Symptoms often rapidly resolve with steroid initiation. Vision loss may be irreversible.
- See Chapter 26, for a full discussion, including subsequent glucocorticoid-sparing therapies.

SCLERODERMA RENAL CRISIS

- Scleroderma renal crisis (SRC) is a severe, sometimes life-threatening complication that occurs in approximately 10% to 15% of patients with diffuse scleroderma.
- SRC is characterized by **rapidly progressive azotemia, malignant hypertension, microangiopathic hemolytic anemia, and thrombocytopenia.**
  - Approximately 10% of patients are normotensive at presentation.[8]
  - Features of hypertensive encephalopathy include headaches, blurry vision, and seizures.[8]
- **Risk factors** include diffuse scleroderma, rapidly progressive skin involvement, early stages (<4 years) of disease onset, presence of **RNA polymerase III antibodies,** presence of new pleural effusion or congestive heart failure, cool ambient temperatures, tendon friction rubs, use of glucocorticoids (>15 mg of prednisone/day), and cyclosporine.[9]
- Differentiating SRC from thrombotic thrombocytopenic purpura (TTP) is critical as the treatments are different. Both diseases can present with microangiopathic hemolytic anemia. TTP is characterized by absent or low serum levels of ADAMTS13 and may have a potential inciting event, such as recent diarrheal illness or chemotherapy.[9]
- The pathogenesis of SRC involves vasculopathy of the arcuate and interlobular arteries, with endothelial cell activation, "onion-skin" hypertrophy, and activation of the renin–angiotensin system.[8,9]
- Treatment involves blood pressure (BP) control with the use of **short-acting angiotensin-converting enzyme (ACE) inhibitor** captopril (initiate at 12.5 mg every 6–8 hours, and uptitrating by 12.5–25 mg increments to a maximum dose of 450 mg/day) with the goal of normalizing the BP (to the patient's previous baseline BP) **within 72 hours.** Once the patient is stabilized, long-acting ACE inhibitors may be used.
- **ACE inhibitors must always be used even in the face of deteriorating renal function.**
- ACE inhibitors started prior to the onset of SRC have not shown any benefit in preventing SRC nor improving mortality.[8]
- Angiotensin receptor blockers (ARBs) and direct renin inhibitors have a theoretical benefit. Dihydropyridine calcium channel blockers can be added if necessary for additional

BP control. Longer-term studies are needed to evaluate the safety and efficacy of endothelin-1 receptor antagonists, such as bosentan.[8]

- **Avoid IV antihypertensives,** such as nitroprusside and labetalol. Avoid β-blockers (may worsen Raynaud's phenomenon).
- Dialysis may be necessary for those patients with severe acute kidney injury.
- See Chapter 15, for a full discussion.

CERVICAL SPINE ABNORMALITIES IN RHEUMATOID ARTHRITIS

- Cervical spine involvement is a common manifestation of rheumatoid arthritis (RA).
- The **atlantoaxial joint is involved** in RA, as chronic inflammation leads to pannus formation, bony erosion, and ligamentous laxity. This can lead to atlantoaxial instability, cranial settling (the odontoid process pushes up into the foramen magnum), and subaxial subluxation.[10]
- Risk factors include seropositivity, erosive disease, rheumatoid nodules, disease-modifying anti-rheumatic drug (DMARD) failure, and steroid use.
- Estimates of cervical instability vary widely and are decreasing due to improved treatment. In one study, the mean disease duration of onset was 12 years. Forty-five percent of RA patients had cervical radiographic changes. Prevalence of anterior atlantoaxial subluxation, cranial settling, and subaxial subluxation was 27%, 11%, and 13%, respectively. Five percent had neurologic deficits.[11]
- Clinical manifestations include **neck pain** at the craniocervical junction, **occipital headache** (compression of the greater and lesser occipital nerves), **sensation of the head falling forward** with flexion, signs of **myelopathy** (muscle atrophy, weakness, paresthesias, spasticity), and signs of vertebrobasilar insufficiency (tinnitus, vertigo, visual disturbance) owing to involvement of the vertebral artery.[10]
- Neurologic deficits can occur even in the absence of pain and, when present, should be addressed urgently.
- Radiographs (anteroposterior, lateral, open-mouth) should be obtained.
- In symptomatic patients, flexion/extension films should be taken only after radiographs have excluded odontoid fracture or severe atlantoaxial subluxation. Anterior atlantodental interval greater than 3 mm is abnormal. **Anterior atlantodental interval greater than 9 mm and posterior atlantodental interval less than 14 mm are associated with increased risk of neurologic injury.**[10]
- As plain radiographs evaluate bony structures, patients with symptoms of cervical instability with negative radiographs or neurologic deficits may warrant **contrast-enhanced magnetic resonance imaging (MRI)** for evaluation of the pannus, cord compression, and nerve roots.
- Most severe instability occurs in flexion, and the **main goal is to prevent flexion** operatively with fusion or nonoperatively with a cervical orthosis.
- Neurologic symptoms should be addressed with a **neurosurgical evaluation** for possible stabilization procedures.
- In addition, patients with cervical spine arthritis are at increased risk of traumatic injury during intubation and should be appropriately managed perioperatively.

TRANSVERSE MYELITIS

- Transverse myelitis is an **inflammatory disorder of the spinal cord.**
- Transverse myelitis can present idiopathically or secondary to other conditions, such as multiple sclerosis (MS), neurosarcoidosis, systemic lupus erythematosus (SLE), antiphospholipid (APL) antibody syndrome, other collagen vascular diseases, paraneoplastic syndromes, and infections.

- Symptoms can present as **pyramidal (motor), sensory, and autonomic disorders,** often developing over hours to days and worsening over days to weeks.
  - Motor weakness follows a pyramidal distribution (flexors of the legs, extensors of the arms).
  - Sensory symptoms present as paresthesias ascending from lower extremities. Pain may or may not be present near the level of the lesion.
  - Autonomic involvement can cause bowel and bladder dysfunction, temperature dysregulation, and labile BPs.
- Initial workup begins with a neurologic examination to help determine the region of spinal cord affected.
- Urgent spinal MRI with gadolinium contrast will help to **first rule out compressive and structural causes** (herniated disk, abscess, hematoma), and brain MRI will help evaluate for MS. The position of the lesion may be higher than the clinical examination localizes; thus, one should also image superior to the suspected level of spinal cord affected.
- Once a compressive etiology is excluded with MRI, **lumbar puncture** and cerebrospinal fluid (CSF) should be obtained for cell count with differential, protein, glucose, oligoclonal bands, and immunoglobulin G (IgG) index. Infectious workup should include bacterial, fungal, and acid-fast bacilli cultures; Venereal Disease Research Laboratory (VDRL); and polymerase chain reaction (PCR) studies for varicella zoster virus (VZV), herpes simplex virus (HSV), cytomegalovirus (CMV), Epstein–Barr virus (EBV), and West Nile virus.
  - If the CSF appears inflammatory (elevated protein, pleocytosis, oligoclonal bands, or elevated IgG index), then demyelinating, infectious, or inflammatory causes should be pursued.
  - Low CSF glucose (<60% of serum glucose) suggests an infection, especially with elevated WBC count. Isolated low CSF glucose can occur in neurosarcoidosis, carcinomatosis, and SLE.
  - Eosinophils can suggest fungal infection, parasitic infection, foreign material, or neuromyelitis optica.
  - Predominantly high neutrophils suggest bacterial or mycobacterial infection.
  - If the CSF is noninflammatory, then vascular, metabolic, neurodegenerative, or neoplastic etiologies are more likely.
- Treatment of transverse myelitis has not been well studied, but high-dose IV methylprednisolone 1,000 mg daily for 3 to 7 days has been recommended.
  - If the response to glucocorticoids is suboptimal, plasma exchange is recommended next.
  - Further immunosuppressive treatment may be indicated based on the most likely underlying disease.
  - Although infectious causes may not be fully excluded, systemic glucocorticoids have been shown to be safe when used concurrently with empiric antibiotics.[12]

CAUDA EQUINA SYNDROME

- Cauda equina syndrome is a rare complication of the seronegative spondyloarthropathies (related to arachnoiditis), in particular ankylosing spondylitis (AS), lumbar disk rupture, spinal or epidural anesthesia, or mass lesions from malignancies or infections.
- In patients with AS, symptoms may be slowly progressive. Cauda equina syndrome from any cause, however, has the potential for rapid onset and progression.
- Symptoms include **severe low back pain, rectal pain, and pain in both legs.**
  - In addition, with progressive disease, patients can develop **saddle anesthesia** with **loss of bladder and bowel control,** poor anal sphincter tone, and impotence.
  - Patients may also develop variable lower extremity, areflexia and asymmetric leg weakness, or loss of sensation.
- Cauda equina syndrome should be **distinguished from sciatica or plexopathy,** which do not involve symptoms of incontinence or impotence.

- **MRI** can help confirm the diagnosis, and **urgent neurosurgical consultation** is required to prevent irreversible neurologic changes.
- **Steroids and localized radiation** treatment may be beneficial with lesions caused by malignancies.

DIFFUSE ALVEOLAR HEMORRHAGE

- Diffuse alveolar hemorrhage is a clinical syndrome characterized by bleeding into the lung alveoli.
- The three histopathologic patterns are pulmonary capillaritis, bland pulmonary hemorrhage, and diffuse alveolar damage. The underlying etiologies include antineutrophil cytoplasmic antibody (ANCA)–associated vasculitis (AAV), microscopic polyangiitis (MPA), pulmonary renal syndromes, SLE, other collagen vascular diseases, idiopathic pulmonary hemosiderosis, bone marrow transplantation, and drugs.
- The clinical presentation includes hemoptysis (may be initially absent in 33% of cases), anemia (or decreasing hemoglobin level), diffuse radiographic infiltrates, and dyspnea progressing to hypoxemic respiratory failure.[13]
- Radiographic findings are nonspecific. Chest x-rays can show patchy or diffuse alveolar opacities. Chest computed tomography (CT) may show ground-glass opacities or areas of consolidation. Hilar and mediastinal adenopathy is not typical but can suggest infection or malignancy.[14]
- Laboratory evaluation should include routine chemistries, liver function tests, complete blood count, coagulation studies, and infectious workup, as well as antinuclear antibodies, anti–glomerular basement membrane (GBM) antibody, ANCA, and complement levels (C3, C4, and CH50).
- Obtain early consult with a pulmonologist to assess the need for **urgent bronchoscopy with sequential bronchoalveolar lavage (BAL)**. BAL fluid can show hemosiderin-laden macrophages, and sequential BAL shows progressively hemorrhagic aliquots.[13]
- Correction of hypoxemia, appropriate control of airway (possibly requiring intubation and mechanical ventilation), and correction of coagulopathies should be addressed immediately.
- In addition to supportive care, treatment is targeted at the underlying disorder. Nevertheless, **high doses of IV glucocorticoids** are the mainstay of initial treatment for many underlying etiologies.
- Other immunosuppressive agents such as cyclophosphamide (AAV, anti-GBM, SLE), rituximab (AAV, anti-GBM), and plasmapheresis (anti-GBM, AAV) have been used for maintenance therapy or refractory cases.[13]

CATASTROPHIC ANTIPHOSPHOLIPID SYNDROME

- Catastrophic antiphospholipid syndrome (CAPS) is the most severe presentation of APS with **acute multiorgan involvement and vascular microthrombi.**
- The diagnosis of "definite CAPS" is made by histopathologic diagnosis, **high-titer APL antibodies**, and failure of **three or more organ systems in 1 week**. Less than three organ system involvement is considered as "probable CAPS."
- This form affects less than 1% of APS patients.
- **Renal complications** (acute renal failure, hypertension, proteinuria) are most common, followed by **pulmonary** (acute respiratory distress syndrome, pulmonary emboli, pulmonary hemorrhage), **neurologic** (cerebral infarcts, encephalopathy, mononeuritis multiplex), **cardiac** (valvular defects, myocardial infarctions), and **skin** (livedo reticularis, purpura) manifestations.
- Possible triggers include **infections**, surgical procedures, subtherapeutic anticoagulation, medications, and SLE flares.[15]

- Differential diagnosis includes TTP/hemolytic–uremic syndrome (HUS); disseminated intravascular coagulation (DIC); hemolysis, elevated liver enzymes, low platelet count (HELLP) syndrome; sepsis; and heparin-induced thrombocytopenia.
- **Mortality rate is high at 30%** but can be reduced with a combination of treatment.
  - Underlying triggers, such as infection, should be treated.
  - Continuous infusion of **unfractionated heparin** is the mainstay of treatment, as heparin inhibits ongoing clotting and may reduce anti-inflammatory activity.
  - IV pulse **glucocorticoids, plasma exchange**, with or without IV **immunoglobulins** are recommended initial treatment in severe cases of CAPS.
  - In refractory cases, rituximab and eculizumab have shown promising results in case reports, that need further validation in larger studies.[15]
- See Chapter 44, for full discussion of the APS.

REFERENCES

1. Slobodin G, Hussein A, Rozenbaum M, et al. The emergency room in systemic rheumatic diseases. *Emerg Med J*. 2006;23:667–671.
2. Mathews CJ, Coakley G. Septic arthritis: current diagnostic and therapeutic algorithm. *Curr Opin Rheumatol*. 2008;20:457–462.
3. Gutierrez-Gonzalez LA. Rheumatologic emergencies. *Clin Rheumatol*. 2015;34:2011–2019.
4. Weyand CM, Goronzy JJ. Clinical practice. Giant-cell arteritis and polymyalgia rheumatica. *N Engl J Med*. 2014;371:50–57.
5. Kermani TA, Schmidt J, Crowson CS, et al. Utility of erythrocyte sedimentation rate and C-reactive protein for the diagnosis of giant cell arteritis. *Semin Arthritis Rheum*. 2012;41:866–871.
6. Achkar AA, Lie JT, Hunder GG, et al. How does previous corticosteroid treatment affect the biopsy findings in giant cell (temporal) arteritis? *Ann Intern Med*. 1994;120:987–992.
7. Arida A, Kyprianou M, Kanakis M, et al. The diagnostic value of ultrasonography-derived edema of the temporal artery wall in giant cell arteritis: a second meta-analysis. *BMC Musculoskelet Disord*. 2010;11:44.
8. Stern EP, Steen VD, Denton CP. Management of renal involvement in scleroderma. *Curr Treat Options Rheumatol*. 2015;1:106–118.
9. Woodworth TG, Suliman YA, Li W, et al. Scleroderma renal crisis and renal involvement in systemic sclerosis. *Nat Rev Nephrol*. 2016;12:678.
10. Gillick JL, Wainwright J, Das K. Rheumatoid arthritis and the cervical spine: A review on the role of surgery. *Int J Rheumatol*. 2015;2015:12.
11. Zhang T, Pope J. Cervical spine involvement in rheumatoid arthritis over time: results from a meta-analysis. *Arthritis Res Ther*. 2015;17:148.
12. West TW. Transverse myelitis—a review of the presentation, diagnosis, and initial management. *Discov Med*. 2013;16:167–177.
13. Lara AR, Schwarz MI. Diffuse alveolar hemorrhage. *Chest*. 2010;137:1164–1171.
14. West S, Arulkumaran N, Ind PW, et al. Diffuse alveolar haemorrhage in ANCA-associated vasculitis. *Intern Med*. 2013;52:5–13.
15. Rodriguez-Pinto I, Espinosa G, Cervera R. Catastrophic antiphospholipid syndrome: The current management approach. *Best Pract Res Clin Rheumatol*. 2016;30:239–249.

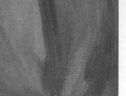

Regional Pain Syndromes

8

Kelvin J. Lee and Lisa A. Zickuhr

GENERAL PRINCIPLES

- Regional pain syndrome refers to pain localized to one area of the body that is not caused by systemic disease. It encompasses many common musculoskeletal sources of pain.
- These syndromes (also called **soft-tissue rheumatic pain syndromes**) occur frequently. They include disorders of bone, cartilage, ligament, muscle, tendon, enthesis (sites where tendons attach to bone), bursa, fascia, and nerve.

Etiology

- Regional pain syndromes may be caused by **trauma, injury from overuse, or degeneration with aging.**
- Consider infections, fractures, or other serious problems (e.g., deep venous thrombosis in a patient with leg pain) in patients who develop regional pain while in the hospital.

DIAGNOSIS

Clinical Presentation

History

- History and physical examination are usually enough to make a diagnosis and **exclude systemic diseases,** such as cancer, infection, and inflammatory arthritis, that may present as regional pain. Signs and symptoms of a systemic process include weight loss, fever, rash, bilateral symptoms, and synovitis (Table 8-1) and should lead to further investigation.
- Question patients about the location, characteristics, and radiation of their pain, duration, presence of numbness or tingling, their ability to function, precipitating events, aggravating and ameliorating factors, underlying diseases, and systemic complaints. It may be helpful to ask the patient to locate the pain with one finger.

Physical Examination

- The physical examination should include **inspection** (looking for atrophy, asymmetry, alignment, swelling, erythema), **palpation** (warmth, crepitus, point tenderness), evaluation of **active and passive ranges of motion,** and a **neurologic examination.**
- Specific maneuvers exist to help identify involvement of specific structures.

TABLE 8-1	FEATURES THAT SUGGEST SYSTEMIC DISEASE
Fever, chills	Pulse abnormalities
Weight loss	Lymphadenopathy
Skin color changes	Neurologic deficits
Bilateral involvement	Muscle wasting or atrophy
Joint warmth, swelling, or tenderness (synovitis)	Laboratory abnormalities

- Always **compare** to the other side and examine at least one joint above and below the suspected involved joint to evaluate for **sources of referred pain.**

Diagnostic Testing

Laboratories
- **Order laboratory tests only if there is suspicion of systemic disease.**
- Tests such as erythrocyte sedimentation rate (ESR), rheumatoid factor (RF), and antinuclear antibodies (ANAs) have a low predictive value in the general population. Abnormal results may be seen in the healthy or in patients with diseases other than inflammatory arthritis.

Imaging
- **Imaging is rarely indicated** at the initial evaluation.
- Plain radiographs do not detect problems of tendons, bursae, or nerves.
- Osteoarthritis (OA) is a very common finding on plain radiographs but may mislead the cause of pain. For example, a patient with OA of the knee on radiographs may have knee pain from anserine bursitis.
- Consider imaging in patients with a history of trauma, atypical symptoms, and lack of improvement with conservative therapy, or if surgery is planned.

Diagnostic Procedures
Electromyogram/nerve conduction velocities (EMG/NCVs) may be helpful in confirming radiculopathy or entrapment neuropathy, especially if surgery is planned.

TREATMENT

- Most regional pain syndromes improve with **conservative treatment.** Table 8-2 presents a general guideline for managing regional pain syndromes.
- Some patients benefit from **assistive devices,** such as splints.
- A referral to **physical or occupational therapy** to increase flexibility, strength, endurance, and alignment may help.
- **Heat or cold application** may also be beneficial.
- When needed, treat pain with medications; however, exercises, physical modalities, and splinting are often more helpful. Medications include nonsteroidal anti-inflammatory drugs (NSAIDs), acetaminophen, muscle relaxants, and opiate analgesics.
- Some conditions improve with intralesional injections of lidocaine or glucocorticoids.
- Reassure patients that most regional pain syndromes are not serious and improve with time.

TABLE 8-2	GUIDELINES FOR MANAGEMENT OF REGIONAL PAIN SYNDROMES

Exclude systemic disease with history and physical examination

Recognize aggravating and ameliorating factors

Provide an explanation of the problem and the likely outcome to the patient

Provide relief from pain

In patients who do not improve, consider other diagnoses and referral

Neck Pain

GENERAL PRINCIPLES

- Neck pain may be due to involvement of the spine or surrounding soft tissues, spinal cord, nerve roots, or referral from other structures or organs (Table 8-3).
- **The majority of neck pain is not serious, and most cases are nonspecific.** The most common causes are cervical strain and/or myofascial pain, whiplash injury, and OA/spondylosis.
- Neck pain is less commonly a result of inflammatory arthritis, such as rheumatoid arthritis (RA) or ankylosing spondylitis (AS).

Etiology

- **Suspect a serious cause of neck pain** (e.g., meningitis, epidural abscess, septic discitis, vertebral osteomyelitis, or metastatic lesions) in patients with a history of fever, intravenous (IV) drug use, weight loss, progressive neurologic findings, or cancer.
- **Cervical strains and/or myofascial pain** can result from overuse, trauma, abnormal posture, sleeping difficulties, and poor workplace ergonomics.
- **Whiplash injury** is a strain caused by abrupt flexion/extension of the neck, usually following an acceleration/deceleration injury. The pain often persists after the acute injury even when no structural abnormality is seen on imaging.

TABLE 8-3	CAUSES OF NECK PAIN

Soft-tissue disorders
Nonspecific neck pain (muscle strain, sprain, spasm)
Whiplash injury
Arthritis[a]
OA and cervical spondylosis
Degenerative disk disease with disk herniation
RA
AS
Juvenile RA
Bone disease[a]
Fracture (due to trauma or osteoporosis) or dislocation
Metastatic lesions
Osteomyelitis
Other
Meningitis
Septic discitis
Thyroiditis
Referred from intrathoracic or intra-abdominal disease.

[a]May be associated with signs and symptoms resulting from radiculopathy or myelopathy.
AS, ankylosing spondylitis; OA, osteoarthritis; RA, rheumatoid arthritis.

- **Spasm** of the cervical musculature is common and often contributes to neck pain.
- **OA/spondylosis** is a common cause of chronic neck pain in adults, especially the elderly.
  - **Spondylosis** refers to **degenerative changes of the spine.**
    - Intervertebral disk desiccation and loss of disk height create abnormal mechanics of the cervical spine.
    - This process causes osteophyte formation the vertebral bodies and facet joints, disk bulging, and vertebral subluxation, the characteristic findings in OA.
  - Osteophytes can cause mechanical pain and **compression of nerve roots.**
  - Neck pain severity may correlate poorly with the degree of radiographic abnormality, especially in younger adults.
- **RA** causes an **erosive synovitis** that can involve the C1 to C2 joints of the neck. This can lead to C1 to C2 subluxation, characterized by pain and signs of spinal cord impingement. It is a medical emergency.
- **AS** also affects the cervical spine, usually following progressive involvement of the lumbar and thoracic spine. The cervical spine becomes less mobile, and fractures may occur after mild trauma.
- **Cervical radiculopathy** is due to encroachment on a nerve root as it exits the intervertebral foramen. Common causes include herniated disks, degenerative disk disease, and OA/spondylosis. Compression of nerve roots can lead to **neck pain and sensory changes that radiate into the arm.** In more severe cases, it can cause motor weakness. Symptoms vary with the root involved (Table 8-4).
- **Cervical spine stenosis** denotes narrowing of the central canal which can lead to **myelopathy.** It can result from congenital abnormalities and spondylosis that narrow the canal and compress the spinal arteries. Initially, patients may have localized neck and arm pain (radiculopathy); however, if the narrowing is more central and compresses the spinal cord, it may lead to myelopathy.
- **Thoracic outlet syndrome** can present as neck and shoulder pain with referred pain to the upper extremities. It is due to compression of the neurovascular bundle as it exits the neck between the anterior and middle scalene muscles, the first rib, and the clavicle or a cervical rib.
- Other nonspinal causes of neck pain include **brachial plexopathy** and **fibromyalgia.**
- **Nonmusculoskeletal causes** of neck pain include angina, aortic dissection, thyroiditis, and peritonsillar/retropharyngeal abscess.

DIAGNOSIS

Clinical Presentation

History
- A good history asks questions that help identify the source of musculoskeletal pain: pain onset, location, duration, symptom quality, radiation, symmetry, sensory changes, motor changes, and aggravating and relieving factors.

TABLE 8-4	NEUROLOGIC FINDINGS IN CERVICAL RADICULOPATHY		
Nerve Root	**Sensory Loss**	**Motor Loss**	**Reflex Loss**
C5	Neck to lateral shoulder, upper arm	Deltoid	Biceps
C6	Lateral arm to thumb, index finger	Biceps	Brachioradialis
C7	Dorsal and palmar forearm, middle finger	Triceps	Triceps
C8	Medial forearm, ring, middle fingers	Finger flexion	—

- The presence of pain in other joints and systemic symptoms are important to diagnose a systemic process.
  - A **history of drug use, infection, or fever** could identify a potential epidural abscess or septic discitis. A history of trauma may suggest fracture; diffuse pain may suggest fibromyalgia; headache and fever may suggest meningitis; and a history of cancer may suggest metastasis.
  - Patients with **RA** or **AS** present with symptoms of the disease in other joints. They will complain of **morning stiffness** that lasts more than an hour.
- A typical history of **spasm/strain** includes pain localized to the neck with symptoms of muscle spasm following trauma, poor posture, or overuse. It is more common in younger adults.
- Neck pain with or without radiculopathy in an older adult is likely due to **spondylosis/OA.**
- Neck pain that radiates into the arm in a dermatomal pattern with associated numbness and paresthesia is highly suggestive of **cervical radiculopathy.** Weakness may or may not be present.
- Clinical manifestations of **cervical myelopathy** include weakness and incoordination of the hands, lower extremity weakness, and gait disturbances. Incontinence is a late finding.
- Patients with **thoracic outlet obstruction** will likely have neurologic symptoms in multiple dermatomes in addition to neck pain. Overhead activities aggravate these symptoms.

Physical Examination
- The physical examination of the patient with neck pain should include cervical **range of motion in all planes** (flexion, extension, rotation, and lateral bending), which normally decreases with age. In RA patients, avoid testing passive range of motion because of the risk of subluxation.
- Palpation for point tenderness is important to detect osteomyelitis and fracture, but it is often also present in mechanical problems. Tender spots and muscle spasms may be noted in cervical paraspinal muscles.
- A **neurologic examination** is crucial to detect the presence of radiculopathy and myelopathy. Radicular compression may lead to sensory changes, weakness, and diminished reflexes depending on the severity in a dermatomal pattern. Neurologic defects may not be detected with mild radiculopathy. As spondylosis can be extensive, more than one cervical root level can be involved. Important findings suggesting myelopathy include upper and lower extremities weakness with hyperreflexia/spasticity and a Babinski's sign in the lower extremities.
- **Spurling's test** is helpful to assess if symptoms in the arm may be related to radiculopathy. The test is performed with cervical extension and rotation to the suspected side while providing axial pressure. This compresses the neural foramina on that side, thereby aggravating nerve compression.
- **Lhermitte's sign** is the sensation of an electric shock down the spine and into the arms and legs with cervical flexion. It may be present in cervical cord compression.
- **Roos hyperabduction/external rotation test** is used to assess for thoracic outlet syndrome. The arm is abducted to 90 degrees and externally rotated to 90 degrees and maintained in this position for 1 minute. The patient opens and closes the hand throughout this time. It is considered positive if it provokes pain and paresthesias.

Diagnostic Testing

Imaging
- Consider imaging in patients with neck pain after trauma, with neurologic findings, and in cases of suspected fractures, metastatic lesions, or infections.
- Plain films may identify osteophytes and intervertebral space narrowing that suggests disk degeneration. **Oblique views** may show narrowing of neural foramina. Occasionally, a cervical rib may be noted, which could support a diagnosis of thoracic outlet syndrome.

- **Open-mouth and lateral flexion/extension radiographs** may be needed to evaluate the atlantoaxial joint for subluxation in RA. If not conclusive, computed tomography (CT) can be ordered.
- **CT and magnetic resonance imaging (MRI)** are more accurate in cases of suspected tumor or infection.
- MRI is the best technique to identify the cause and location of root impingement.
- Radiographic abnormalities are common in the elderly and correlate poorly with symptoms.

Diagnostic Testing
- Nerve conduction studies document the nerve root involved but are seldom necessary unless surgery is contemplated. Surgery has a greater likelihood of improving symptoms if the physical examination, EMG, and radiographic studies all agree on the anatomic location.
- They may also be helpful in determining whether the location of nerve compression is outside the neck.

TREATMENT

- Most mechanical causes of neck pain will resolve with time and **conservative treatment.**
- **Cervical strains:** These cases typically improve with rest. Education on posture, avoidance of repetitive motion, and strengthening will help to treat the underlying cause.
- Treatment of neck **OA** is conservative. Soft cervical collars may provide symptomatic relief. **Use rigid cervical collars only in cases with instability and under close supervision.** NSAIDs are helpful, and local injections and cervical traction are sometimes used. Symptoms may recur periodically with stress of the degenerated structures.
- **Myelopathy:** Progressive myelopathy requires **urgent surgical decompression.**
- **Pharmacologic therapy** includes NSAIDs, acetaminophen, muscle relaxants, opiate analgesics, and gabapentin, depending on the symptoms that are present. Opiates should be used cautiously because of their potential for abuse and side effect profile.
- **Epidural glucocorticoid injections** may be used for cervical radiculopathy, but the data are weak and inconsistent.
- **Physical therapy exercises** improve patient posture to reduce stress/compression on the involved structures, strengthen the surrounding structures, and improve range of motion. Ultrasound and electrical stimulation can also be performed, which may provide some pain relief.
- Specific indications for surgery include bowel/bladder incontinence, worsening neurologic function, progressive myelopathy, and intractable pain and radicular symptoms.[1]

Low Back Pain

GENERAL PRINCIPLES

- Low back pain is very common. It is the **second most common reason to seek medical care.**[2]
- Most patients improve with **conservative treatment**, so education and reassurance are important to prevent unnecessary testing and anxiety.
- The lumbar spinal column is surrounded by vertebral end plates, spinal nerve roots, facet joints, blood vessels, muscles, ligaments, fascia, and sensory nerve fibers in the disks. Any one or a combination of these sites can generate low back pain.
- The major categories of low back pain are mechanical, radicular, inflammatory, infiltrative, and referred.

Etiology

- Many different conditions cause low back pain (Table 8-5).
- **Mechanical disorders** (muscle strains, disk herniation, facet arthritis, etc.) are the most common causes of back pain. **Back strains** may result from overuse, trauma, or poor

TABLE 8-5	DIFFERENTIAL DIAGNOSIS OF LOW BACK PAIN

Mechanical low back pain (97%)

Idiopathic low back pain (lumbago, lumbar strain)

Degenerative disk disease

Osteoarthritis

Spondylosis

Herniated disk

Spinal stenosis

Spondylolysis

Spondylolisthesis

Trauma

Osteoporotic fracture

Neoplasia (<1%)

Metastatic lesions

Multiple myeloma

Lymphoma and leukemia

Primary vertebral tumors

Spinal cord tumors

Infection (<1%)

Osteomyelitis

Paraspinous abscess

Epidural abscess

Septic discitis

Bacterial endocarditis

Rheumatic diseases (<1%)

AS

PsA

ReA

Inflammatory bowel disease–related arthritis

Visceral disease and referred pain (<1%)

Aortic aneurysm

GI disease (pancreatitis, cholecystitis)

Genitourinary (nephrolithiasis, pyelonephritis, pelvic inflammatory disease)

Hip disease

Sacroiliac joint—controversial if not part of an inflammatory arthropathy

AS, ankylosing spondylitis; GI, gastrointestinal; PsA, psoriatic arthritis; ReA, reactive arthritis.

body mechanics. **Herniated disks** can compress nerve roots and cause **radiculopathy** or narrow the spinal canal and cause **myelopathy**. As in the neck, **spondylosis** leads to similar symptoms.

- ○ **Spondylolysis** is a defect of the pars interarticularis that can occur in young patients who are active in sports that require frequent extension, flexion, and rotation of the lumbar spine.
- ○ **Spondylolisthesis** results from a bilateral defect of the pars interarticularis that allows the vertebral body to slip forward relative to the rest of the spine. Etiologies include congenital, developmental, and degenerative causes.
- ○ **Cauda equina syndrome** is the compression of the nerve roots as they exit the distal spinal cord. It is a **surgical emergency.**
- Axial spondyloarthritis (SpA) causes **inflammatory** low back pain. Lumbar spine involvement in RA is rare.
- **Infiltrative causes** of low back pain include cancer and infection. Cancer may present as a metastasis or a local tumor that damages bones and joints or compresses neurologic structures. Infections include osteomyelitis, epidural abscess, and septic discitis. Predisposing conditions include IV drug use, concomitant infection, and endocarditis.
- Visceral disorders can cause **referred back pain.** Examples include abdominal aortic aneurysm and dissection, pancreatitis, cholecystitis, pyelonephritis, nephrolithiasis, and pelvic inflammatory disease.

DIAGNOSIS

Clinical Presentation

History
- **A careful history and physical examination are often enough to identify systemic disease** (Table 8-6).
- Inquire about the nature of the pain, aggravating and relieving factors, and neurologic symptoms.
- Clues to **cancer** in the history are age more than 50 years, history of cancer, unexplained weight loss, lack of relief with bed rest, duration of pain and failure to improve over 1 month, and nocturnal pain.
- Fever, concomitant infections, a history of IV drug use, or onset of low back pain during hospitalization suggest **infection**.
- Morning stiffness of more than 1 hour that improves with exercise, and onset before the age of 40 years, suggests **inflammatory back pain.**
- **Disk herniation** may cause sciatica (pain, numbness, and paresthesias radiating to the lower extremity below the knee).
- Low back pain with bowel and/or bladder dysfunction, saddle anesthesia, and bilateral lower extremity weakness are signs of **cauda equina syndrome** from compression of the sacral nerve roots. Patients with these symptoms should undergo immediate imaging and neurosurgical referral.
- Symptoms of **spinal stenosis** caused by degeneration/spondylosis mimic those of vascular insufficiency and are often referred to as neurogenic claudication. There is typically heaviness or pain in the bilateral buttocks and thighs with walking upright, as this position causes lumbar extension that narrows the spinal canal. The pain is better when patients lean forward to increase lumbar flexion, as happens when walking with a shopping cart. The pain resolves after a very brief period of sitting down, in contrast to the pain of vascular claudication, which may take much longer to resolve.
- **Spondylolisthesis** and **spondylolysis** are often aggravated by lumbar extension. Radicular symptoms are not typically present.
- A history of older age, female sex, thin build, and prednisone use may suggest **osteoporosis with a compression fracture.**

TABLE 8-6	EVALUATION OF SELECTED CAUSES OF LOW BACK PAIN					
	Idiopathic Low Back Pain	Herniated Disk	Spinal Stenosis	AS	Metastases	Spinal Infection
Pain characteristic	Dull, lower back; may radiate to buttocks; improves with rest	Sudden, sharp, intense; radiates below the knee (sciatica); usually unilateral	Pseudoclaudication: Bilateral pain (buttocks, thighs, legs) brought on by standing or walking and relieved by sitting or flexing spine	Insidious, chronic, worse in the morning, improves with exercise	Chronic, severe, not improved with bed rest	Severe, sharp; may radiate to thighs
History	History of lifting or straining	History of lifting or straining	Occurs in patients >60 years with degenerative disease of the spine	Occurs in patients <40 years; may have family history, or history of uveitis or axial arthritis	Age > 50 years, history of cancer, weight loss, failure of conservative management	Immunocompromised patients; history of IV drug abuse, alcohol abuse, infections; fever not always present
Physical examination	May have pain with movement or in certain positions; neurologic examination is normal	Pain radiating down the leg with straight-leg raise; may have altered dermatomal sensation, weakness, or decreased reflexes; 95% S1 root	May have sensory, motor, and reflex abnormalities	Decreased range of motion, arthritis	May show evidence of primary tumor; rule out spinal cord compression in patients with neurologic findings	Neurologic findings present and depend on the level of involvement

(continued)

81

TABLE 8-6	EVALUATION OF SELECTED CAUSES OF LOW BACK PAIN (*continued*)					
	Idiopathic Low Back Pain	Herniated Disk	Spinal Stenosis	AS	Metastases	Spinal Infection
Lab studies	None needed	None needed	None needed	ESR often elevated; HLA-B27 may be present but is not a good screening test	ESR may be elevated	ESR often elevated; positive blood cultures, leukocytosis not always present
Imaging	None needed	MRI recommended in patients with neurologic deficits	MRI may be needed for diagnosis	Radiographs may show sacroiliitis; "bamboo spine" is a late finding	CT or MRI; emergent imaging needed in suspected cord compression	MRI indicated

AS, ankylosing spondylitis; CT, computed tomography; ESR, erythrocyte sedimentation rate; IV, intravenous; MRI, magnetic resonance imaging; SI, sacroiliac.

- Inquire about non–lumbar spine–related symptoms of RA and SpA if an inflammatory cause is suspected.
- A history of vascular disease may suggest abdominal aortic aneurysm or vascular claudication.

Physical Examination
- Lumbar **range of motion** should be assessed in all planes. Often, pain will be worse in flexion with a herniated disc. Pain is likely to be worse in extension with spondylolysis and spinal stenosis. Other sources of back pain can limit range and cause pain in multiple directions.
- Localized tenderness over the midline is seen in **vertebral fractures** caused by osteoporosis, metastatic disease, multiple myeloma, or osteomyelitis. Spinal tenderness can also be present from mechanical causes. Tenderness in the paraspinal muscles may represent spasm or a muscle strain.
- The **general physical examination** may provide clues to underlying systemic disease. Fevers (infection, inflammatory disease, cancer), murmurs (endocarditis), breast masses (metastases), pulsatile abdominal masses, and pulse abnormalities (aortic aneurysm) are important findings.
- The **neurologic examination** should identify spinal nerve root involvement or cord symptoms (Table 8-7). Sphincter tone and saddle anesthesia should be assessed if suspecting cauda equina syndrome.
- A positive **straight-leg raising test** suggests nerve root compression. The test is performed with the patient supine, and the leg is raised with the knee fully extended. A positive test reproduces pain radiating below the knee when the leg is raised. Compare the excursion of the straight-leg raise from one side to other. The involved side will have less range of motion. Low back pain without radiation below the knee does not constitute a positive test.
- **Schober's test** should be performed to help assess for limited flexion with suspected spondyloarthropathy (see Chapter 16).

Diagnostic Testing

Laboratories
Laboratory tests (e.g., ESR, C-reactive protein [CRP], urinalysis [UA], complete blood count [CBC], cultures) may occasionally help exclude systemic disease.

Imaging
- Plain radiographs are often an unnecessary expense for the patient. Do not order them unless red flags are present or if you suspect cancer, fracture, infection, or inflammatory spondyloarthropathy. Degenerative changes in the lumbar spine are often unrelated to the cause of myofascial pain.
- CT scans and MRI are more sensitive than plain radiographs. However, they often reveal abnormalities even in asymptomatic adults. CT and MRI should be reserved for cases

TABLE 8-7	NEUROLOGIC FINDINGS IN LUMBAR SPINAL NERVE ROOT INVOLVEMENT		
Nerve Root	**Sensory Loss**	**Motor Loss**	**Reflex Loss**
L4	Lateral thigh, medial leg to medial malleolus	Knee extension, thigh adduction, foot dorsiflexion	Knee
L5	Posterolateral thigh, lateral leg to dorsal foot	Great toe extension and foot dorsiflexion	—
S1	Posterior leg, lateral, and plantar foot	Plantar flexion of great toe and foot	Ankle

with a strong suspicion of cancer or infection, for patients with persistent neurologic deficits, or when conservative treatment fails. Occasionally, MRI of the sacroiliac (SI) joints is needed to diagnosis sacroiliitis.
- A **bone scan** may reveal a stress injury at the pars interarticularis in a young, active adult.

TREATMENT

- Most patients improve with **conservative treatment** within 12 weeks. Education and reassurance are important to prevent unnecessary testing and anxiety.
- Acetaminophen, NSAIDs, and muscle relaxants are effective for low back pain. Gabapentin may be needed for pain from nerve compression. Opioids should be used sparingly.
- **Physical therapy** benefits patients with persistent pain, strengthening their abdominal and back muscles and reinforcing proper body mechanics.
- Encourage patients to return rapidly to their normal activities, but avoidance of heavy lifting may be prudent until the pain improves.
- **Bed rest does not accelerate recovery** in low back pain or sciatica.
- **Surgical evaluation** should be immediate in patients with cord compression or progressive neurologic deficits. Patients with persistent, disabling pain or neurologic findings may benefit from surgical referral.
- Chronic low back pain is difficult to manage and sometimes requires a multidisciplinary approach to rehabilitation, depression, and substance abuse.

Shoulder Pain

GENERAL PRINCIPLES

- The shoulder is a mobile joint, at the expense of joint stability. The glenoid fossa, labrum ligaments, and rotator cuff provide stability; hence, damage of these structures can reduce stability and lead to further injury and pain.
- The **rotator cuff** is composed of the tendons of the supraspinatus, infraspinatus, teres minor, and subscapularis muscles and attaches to the humeral tuberosities. The supraspinatus lies between the acromion and the humeral head, explaining why pain from rotator cuff disease worsens with elevation of the arm (**impingement**).
- The shoulder girdle is made up of four joints. One of these is the scapulothoracic joint, which is not a true anatomic joint. The remaining three are typically affected in different types of arthritis: glenohumeral joint (affected in RA, calcium pyrophosphate deposition disease [CPPD], septic arthritis, and OA), acromioclavicular (AC) (OA), and sternoclavicular (AS, septic arthritis, and synovitis, acne, pustulosis, hyperostosis, osteitis [SAPHO] syndrome).

Etiology

- There are many causes of shoulder pain (Table 8-8).
- **Impingement** is caused by compression of the rotator cuff tendons and/or subacromial bursa under the coracoacromial arch.
  - The acromion, coracoid process, and coracoacromial ligament form an arch over the humeral head, where the supraspinatus and bursa lie.
  - Abduction elevates the greater tuberosity of the humerus, compressing the rotator cuff tendon insertions against the arch.
  - Normally, the rotator cuff helps to stabilize the humeral head in the glenoid fossa, but with injury, weakness, or tendinopathy of the rotator cuff, the humeral head may translate superiorly during overhead activities, leading to impingement.

TABLE 8-8	**CAUSES OF SHOULDER PAIN**

Periarticular disorders
Rotator cuff tendinitis
Calcific tendinitis
Rotator cuff tear
Subacromial bursitis
Bicipital tendinitis
Adhesive capsulitis
Articular disorders
Inflammatory arthritis (RA)
Glenohumeral arthritis
Acromioclavicular arthritis
Sternoclavicular arthritis
Septic arthritis
Osteonecrosis (of humeral head)
Fractures, dislocations
Neurovascular diseases (usually have neurovascular symptoms)
Brachial plexopathy
Suprascapular nerve entrapment
Thoracic outlet syndrome
Referred pain (should be suspected in cases with normal range of motion)
Cervical spine disease
Intrathoracic or intra-abdominal disease
Other
PMR (usually bilateral)
Fibromyalgia
Reflex sympathetic dystrophy

PMR, polymyalgia rheumatic; RA, rheumatoid arthritis.

- **Rotator cuff tendinopathy is the most common cause of shoulder pain.** It can be acute or chronic and is sometimes associated with calcium deposits in the tendon (calcific tendinitis). Overuse, trauma, age-related degeneration, and osteophytes on the inferior portion of the acromion are other common causes.
- **Subacromial bursitis** may be associated with rotator cuff tendinitis or other abnormal mechanics that cause impingement of the bursa against the acromion or coracoacromial ligament.
- **Rotator cuff tears**, partial or complete, result from trauma or gradual degeneration.
- **Bicipital tendinitis** results from overuse, especially in laborers or weight lifters. A biceps tendon tear may occur in an older adult.
- **Adhesive capsulitis** ("frozen shoulder") is seen in diabetes, inflammatory arthritis, and prolonged shoulder immobilization. The shoulder joint capsule and surrounding structures contract, restricting mobility of the shoulder joint and causing pain.
- **AC OA** may occur with chronic repetitive irritation.

• **Instability** can be primary (i.e., laxity of the patient's connective tissue) or secondary (i.e., damaged ligaments from trauma or dislocation). This instability causes impingement and pain in the surrounding structures.

DIAGNOSIS

Clinical Presentation

History
• **Impingement/subacromial bursitis/rotator cuff tendinopathy:** Pain is usually over the lateral deltoid and worsens with overhead activity. Night pain resulting from difficulty positioning the painful shoulder is common.
• **Rotator cuff tendon tears:** Complete tears cause inability to actively abduct the shoulder.
• **Biceps tendinopathy** usually causes anterior shoulder pain.
• **Adhesive capsulitis** causes a painful shoulder with significant loss of active and passive range of motion.
• **AC arthritis** causes pain over the AC joint that is aggravated by reaching across the body or overhead.

Physical Examination
• **Both passive and active range of motion** should be assessed. In adhesive capsulitis, passive and active range will be decreased, whereas in many other shoulder disorders, active range will be decreased, but passive range will be normal or near normal.
• Palpation of the subacromial space should be performed to assess for bursitis or supraspinatus tenderness. The subscapularis can be palpated anteriorly just inferiolaterally to the coracoid process. The infraspinatus and teres minor can be palpated posteriorly and inferiorly to the acromion. Also palpate the AC joint for tenderness.
• The **impingement sign** is typically positive in supraspinatus tendinopathy, and subacromial bursitis (but may also be seen in other shoulder diseases). The sign is elicited by passively forward flexing the patient's internally rotated arm with the examiner holding down the scapula with the other hand. This produces pain in cases of impingement.
• The **drop arm** test is positive with a large rotator cuff tear. It is performed by placing the arm at 90 degrees abduction and instructing the patient to lower it slowly to the side. The test is positive when the patient is unable to perform the motion smoothly.
• **Biceps tendinitis** is suspected when the bicipital groove along the anterior humeral head is tender on palpation. Pain with supination of the forearm against resistance or forward flexion of the externally rotated arm against resistance is seen.
• Have the patient horizontally adduct the arm across the chest to stress the AC joint. Pain at the AC joint suggests that this joint is irritated.

Diagnostic Testing

Imaging
• Plain films are needed if the history and physical examination suggest a dislocation, fracture, or a primary/metastatic tumor.
• MRI or ultrasound may distinguish between partial and complete rotator cuff tears.

TREATMENT

• Treatment of **rotator cuff/bursitis/impingement injuries** includes rest and specific exercises to strengthen the rotator cuff and improve range of motion. Prolonged immobilization of the shoulder in any shoulder disease should be avoided as it may cause adhesive capsulitis. NSAIDs and local anesthetic with glucocorticoid injections are also used. Surgery may be needed to address the impingement or in cases of acute, full-thickness tears.

- **Biceps tendinitis** and rotator cuff tendinitis are treated with rest and rotator cuff strengthening exercises.
- **Adhesive capsulitis** is treated with NSAIDs, glucocorticoid intra-articular injections, and physical therapy to regain the shoulder's full range of motion. Surgical intervention is rarely necessary.
- The AC joint may be injected if needed, and surgery may be performed if conservative treatment does not help.
- Surgery is necessary to repair complete rotator cuff tears.

Elbow Pain

GENERAL PRINCIPLES

- Elbow pain is usually caused by **periarticular disorders.**
- The elbow joint is frequently involved in RA but rarely in OA.

Etiology

- **Olecranon bursitis** may be septic or idiopathic, resulting from inflammatory conditions (RA, gout, and CPPD), or trauma. It can also be caused by the repetitive, low-pressure trauma of frequently resting on the olecranon.
- **Lateral and medial epicondylitis** are colloquially known as tennis and golfer's elbow, respectively, but may be due to any type of overuse activity. They occur at the origin of the common extensor tendon (lateral epicondylitis) and flexor tendons (medial epicondylitis).
- Overuse of the biceps and triceps tendons can also produce elbow pain.
- **Ulnar nerve entrapment** occurs at the cubital tunnel where the nerve passes through. The nerve can become irritated by direct pressure, repetitive motion, osteophytes, and prolonged elbow flexion.
- Other causes of elbow pain include septic arthritis, RA, gout, pseudogout, and compression of the posterior interosseous nerve just distal to the posterior elbow as it passes through the supinator muscle.

DIAGNOSIS

Clinical Presentation

History

- **Olecranon bursitis** can begin acutely or chronically. If it is infectious, it will be quite painful in a short period of time. Patients will complain of a visible swelling posteriorly that will cause variable pain depending on the cause.
- Patients with medial or lateral **epicondylitis** will complain of pain localized to the respective epicondyle. Pain is aggravated with repetitive use of the hand, often occurring in laborers.
- **Ulnar nerve compression** will produce symptoms of posteromedial elbow soreness that is aggravated by resting on the medial elbow. Tingling and/or numbness will be noted in the fourth and fifth digits. Weakness of the hand muscles is possible.
- Gout pain will be acute with associated swelling. RA will involve other joints. A septic joint will be quite painful with fever present.
- **Posterior interosseous nerve entrapment** may produce symptoms of posterolateral elbow pain with numbness/tingling in the lateral forearm and hand. Weakness of the wrist and finger extensors may occur.

Physical Examination

- Begin the examination by noting flexion, extension, supination, and pronation **range of motion**. Palpate the major tendons at their origins or insertions for tenderness. Visually inspect for joint or bursa swelling, warmth, and erythema.
- **Olecranon bursitis** presents with swelling over the posterior elbow. The surrounding area may be swollen, warm, and erythematous in septic bursitis. Septic bursitis usually does not compromise elbow mobility, but a septic elbow joint does. Septic bursitis should be aspirated (taking care to avoid penetrating into the elbow joint).
- **Lateral epicondylitis** presents with tenderness localized to the lateral epicondyle at the insertion of the common extensor tendon. Pain is exacerbated by resisted wrist extension, forearm supination, and middle finger extension.
- **Medial epicondylitis** is diagnosed by tenderness over the medial epicondyle at the insertion of the flexor tendons and by painful resisted wrist flexion and forearm pronation.
- Percussion of the ulnar nerve in the cubital tunnel and prolonged elbow flexion will produce pain and paresthesia in **ulnar nerve entrapment**. Check the sensation in the fourth and fifth digits.
- **Posterior interosseous nerve entrapment** symptoms can be aggravated with resisted supination with the elbow at 90 degrees and fully flexed. There will be tenderness 5 to 6 cm distal to the lateral epicondyle over the supinator. Weakness is present on testing wrist and finger extension.

TREATMENT

- Nonseptic **olecranon bursitis** due to trauma can be treated with NSAIDs, avoiding aggravating activity and a compression strap. It may need aspiration. It can be injected with glucocorticoids but may recur. Septic bursitis should be treated with antibiotics and may need to be aspirated daily. Surgical incision and drainage may be required.
- Treatment of **lateral and medial epicondylitis** includes NSAIDs, ice, rest, and avoidance of exacerbating activities. A tennis elbow strap may be beneficial. If an inflammatory component is suspected, glucocorticoid injections can produce short-term relief. The injection should not be directly into the tendon to avoid tendon rupture. Surgery to debride degenerative portions of the tendon is an option if conservative treatment fails.
- **Ulnar nerve entrapment** can be treated conservatively with the use of an elbow pad. The pad cushions the posteromedial elbow during the day to reduce pressure on the cubital tunnel. At night, the pad can be rotated so that it is anterior in the cubital fossa. This placement prevents excessive elbow flexion at night. Occasionally, ulnar nerve transposition is required.
- **Posterior interosseous nerve compression** can be treated with rest from offending motions. If symptoms do not improve, then surgery for decompression is possible.

Hand and Wrist Pain

GENERAL PRINCIPLES

- The hand and wrist are common sites of arthritis, both inflammatory (i.e., RA, lupus, psoriatic arthritis [PsA], etc.) and noninflammatory (OA). The presence or absence of synovitis, joint deformities, and the specific joints involved offer clues to the diagnosis.
- OA typically affects the proximal and distal interphalangeal joints and the first carpometacarpal (CMC) joints.
- RA affects the wrist, metacarpophalangeal (MCP), and the proximal interphalangeal joints, sparing the distal interphalangeal joints and the first CMC.

- Hand and wrist pain may also be due to periarticular disorders and infections.
- Unilateral pain is often a result of trauma, overuse, or infection; consider arthritis or systemic diseases in patients with bilateral pain.

Etiology

- **Carpal tunnel syndrome** (CTS) commonly causes hand pain. The median nerve and the flexor tendons pass through a tunnel at the wrist limited by the carpal bones and the transverse carpal ligament. CTS may be idiopathic but is also seen in pregnancy, RA, diabetes, obesity, myxedema, and disorders that encroach on the nerve (osteophytes, tophi, amyloid deposits).
- The **ulnar nerve,** as discussed earlier, may become entrapped at the elbow, causing hand pain and numbness or paresthesias of the ulnar side of the ring and little fingers. Compression of the ulnar nerve at the wrist causes similar symptoms and may be due to trauma or fracture of the carpal or fifth metacarpal bones.
- **De Quervain's tenosynovitis** is the inflammation of the extensor pollicis brevis and abductor pollicis longus tendons at the level of the radial styloid. It may be due to repetitive thumb pinching while moving the wrist, such as in guitar playing.
- **Tenosynovitis and tendinopathy** may also occur in other flexor and extensor tendons. Localized pain and tenderness on palpation and with resisted movement are seen. Tenosynovitis/tendinopathy may be due to overuse, trauma, RA, or idiopathic.
- **Infectious tenosynovitis** may be seen in gonococcal arthritis and as a result of puncture wounds.
- **Ganglions** are the most common soft-tissue tumors of the hand and wrist. They are mucin-filled cysts that arise from adjacent tendon sheaths or joint capsules. They usually appear on the dorsal aspect and are painless but may limit movement if large.
- **Trigger finger** is a common cause of hand pain and discomfort. Trigger finger is due to thickening of the retinacular pulley in the palm or a fibrous nodule on the tendon that interferes with flexion. The thumb, ring, and long fingers are most commonly affected. Glucocorticoid injections or surgery is helpful.
- **Dupuytren's contracture** is a thickening and shortening of the palmar fascia, resulting in visible thickening and cording of the palm that is usually painless. The ring finger is affected most frequently. It may be idiopathic and is also seen in diabetics or in patients with chronic alcohol abuse.

DIAGNOSIS

Clinical Presentation

History

- **CTS:** Pain and tingling of the hand is characteristic but may extend to the wrist, forearm, arm, and, sometimes, shoulder. Numbness and paresthesias are felt in the distribution of the median nerve (thumb, index, and middle fingers; radial aspect of ring finger). The hand may be weak and clumsy and feel swollen. Bilateral disease is common. Women are affected more frequently.
- Patients with **de Quervain's tenosynovitis** will complain of radial-sided wrist pain that is worse with gripping tightly and may note swelling over the radial styloid.
- **Tendinopathy** presents with pain localized to a tendon that is aggravated by activity and relieved with rest.
- Patients with **infectious tenosynovitis** will complain of significant pain and swelling along the tendon. Fever may also be present, depending on the acuity of the infection.
- Patients with **trigger finger** note painful clicking in the palm and locking of the finger in flexion. These symptoms may be intermittent.

Physical Examination
- To diagnose **CTS**, the examination should identify median nerve involvement and exclude cervical or brachial plexus abnormalities. Weakness and atrophy of the thenar muscles are usually late findings. Tinel's and Phalen's signs may be present but are neither sensitive nor specific. **Tinel's sign** is distal paresthesias produced by sharp tapping over the median nerve at the wrist. **Phalen's sign** is reproduction of symptoms when the wrists are held flexed against each other. The **flick sign** may be more accurate: When asked "What do you actually do with your hand(s) when the symptoms are at their worst?" patients with CTS do a flicking movement with their hand(s) similar to how someone would shake water off their hands.[3]
- **Finkelstein's test** is positive in **de Quervain's tenosynovitis** when passive ulnar deviation of the wrist while the fingers are flexed over the thumb reproduces pain.
- Tenosynovitis/tendinopathy can be diagnosed by localized pain and tenderness on palpation and with resisted movements. Infectious tenosynovitis will display edema, warmth, and erythema with likely surrounding cellulitis and drainage.
- On examination of **trigger finger,** difficulty extending the finger from flexion is noted. A palpable nodule may be felt.
- **Dupuytren's** presents with a lump in the hand and difficulty extending the fingers. The contraction worsens with time.

Diagnostic Testing

Imaging
Order radiographs in patients with hand trauma and visible abnormalities of the joints.

Diagnostic Testing
Nerve conduction studies are usually diagnostic in unclear cases of CTS.

TREATMENT

- Treatment of **CTS** begins with conservative measures, including nighttime splinting in a wrist cock-up splint, rest, and NSAIDs. Careful injection with glucocorticoids is helpful. Surgical release of the transverse carpal ligament is beneficial if conservative measures fail.
- **De Quervain's tenosynovitis** responds to rest, ice, NSAIDs, and a forearm-based thumb spica splint. Surgical release or local glucocorticoid injection may be indicated in refractory cases.
- **Tenosynovitis and tendinopathy** are treated with rest, ice, and NSAIDs.
- **Infectious tenosynovitis** requires drainage and antibiotics.
- **Dupuytren's contracture** benefits from stretching and glucocorticoid injections in the initial stages, but surgery may be needed to release chronic contractures.
- **Ganglions** are treated with aspiration and surgical excision if they limit motion or are cosmetically unacceptable.
- Glucocorticoid injections or surgery is helpful for **trigger finger.**

Hip Pain

GENERAL PRINCIPLES

- Hip pain is a very common complaint and may be due to articular and periarticular disorders or may be referred from other structures (Table 8-9).
- Different disorders cause pain in different areas around the hip joint, which may be useful for diagnosis. Ask the patient to point to the location of maximal pain.

TABLE 8-9	CAUSES OF HIP PAIN

Articular disorders
Noninflammatory
OA
Osteonecrosis (AVN) of the femoral head
Fracture
Labral tear
Hip impingement
Inflammatory
Seronegative spondyloarthropathies
Septic arthritis
Juvenile RA
RA (usually late in the disease)
Periarticular disorders
Trochanteric bursitis
Ischiogluteal bursitis
Iliopsoas bursitis
Septic bursitis
Referred pain
Lumbar spine OA and sciatica
Spinal stenosis
Sacroiliitis
Knee disorders
Vascular insufficiency
Meralgia paresthetica

AVN, avascular necrosis; OA, osteoarthritis; RA, rheumatoid arthritis.

Etiology

- **Hip OA** is a very common cause of hip pain and increases with age. True hip joint arthritis usually causes **pain in the anterior groin** that worsens with weight bearing (see Chapter 2).
- Lumbosacral spine and SI joint disease cause **buttock pain,** as do spinal stenosis and vascular insufficiency.
- The hip joint is affected in RA (usually late in the disease) and in juvenile RA and the seronegative spondyloarthropathies.
- **Fractures** of the femoral neck are common in elderly women with osteoporosis and may occur after a fall.
- **Avascular necrosis (AVN)** commonly affects the hip joint. It is seen in patients with sickle cell anemia, lupus, alcoholics, and long-term steroid use. Refer patients with fractures and osteonecrosis for orthopedic consultation.
- **Trochanteric bursitis** is a very common cause of pain over the **lateral aspect** of the pelvis. It is more common in the elderly and is often associated with OA of the lumbar spine or hip.

- **Ischiogluteal bursitis** is caused by trauma or prolonged sitting on hard surfaces.
- **Iliopsoas bursitis** is caused by inflammation of the bursa located between the hip joint and the overlying psoas muscle. **Anterior thigh and groin pain** is present.
- **Meralgia paresthetica** is caused by compression of the lateral femoral cutaneous nerve at the groin. This condition is seen in pregnant or obese patients and in people who wear tight garments or heavy belts. Eliminating the source of compression and, occasionally, glucocorticoid injections are useful.
- **Labral tears** of the hip are more common in young active patients. They may occur with trauma or insidiously. Patients complain of **groin pain** that worsens with activity.
- **Piriformis syndrome** is a compression of the sciatic nerve as it passes deep to or through the piriformis and can cause **pain in the buttock,** with numbness and tingling in the leg in a nondermatomal pattern.

DIAGNOSIS

Clinical Presentation

History
- **Hip arthritis** will cause pain in the groin that is aggravated with weight-bearing activities. Patients will also note decreased range of motion when attempting to sit with legs crossed.
- OA of the lumbar spine can refer pain to the buttock, and patients will often complain that this is hip pain.
- **AVN** of the hip will present with groin pain that is aggravated with weight bearing.
- Patients with **trochanteric bursitis** will complain of pain that is worse with lying on the affected side, walking, climbing stairs, and rising from a seated position.
- In **ischiogluteal bursitis,** the pain is over the buttocks, may radiate down the thigh, and is worse with sitting. As this is the origin of the hamstring muscles, the differential diagnosis includes hamstring tendinopathy.
- **Meralgia paresthetica** causes anterior or lateral thigh pain that can be accompanied by numbness or paresthesias.
- **Labral tears** typically cause chronic hip pain in a younger patient that is often difficult to diagnose. Activity aggravates symptoms.
- **Piriformis syndrome** presents with complaints of buttock pain with paresthesia and pain in the posterior leg.

Physical Examination
- Hip arthritis is identified by decreased range of motion and pain in the groin with combined flexion/adduction and internal rotation. Combined flexion/abduction/external rotation (**FABER test**) can also illicit pain in the groin.
- Pain originating in the hip joint generally will be aggravated by combined flexion/internal rotation and adduction. The FABER test will also provoke symptoms.
- On examination of **trochanteric bursitis,** localized tenderness with palpation of the trochanteric area (the uppermost area with the patient lying on his or her side) and pain with resisted abduction are seen.
- **Iliopsoas bursitis** is identified by a combination of pain with palpation or with hyperextension or with resisted flexion. Ischiogluteal bursitis is noted with palpation over the ischium.
- **Labral tear** symptoms can be elicited with the FABER test.
- In **piriformis syndrome,** the posterior buttock will be tender, and stretching of the piriformis muscle may aggravate the symptoms.

Diagnostic Testing

Imaging
- Imaging is reserved for cases of trauma and suspected fracture, for patients with risk factors for AVN, and for patients with chronic hip pain.
- MRI is useful to establish the presence of a labral tear.

TREATMENT

- **Trochanteric bursitis** treatment consists of stretching exercises, weight loss, and NSAIDs. Injection of the trochanteric bursa area with lidocaine and glucocorticoids is a relatively simple procedure and may bring relief.
- Both **ischiogluteal and iliopsoas bursitis** respond to conservative measures of rest, NSAIDs, and, potentially, glucocorticoid injections.
- **Meralgia paresthetica** can be addressed by eliminating the source of compression. Occasionally, glucocorticoid injections are useful.
- **Labral tears** can be treated with arthroscopic surgery.
- **Piriformis syndrome** is treated with stretching, massage, and, if recalcitrant, surgery.

Knee Pain

GENERAL PRINCIPLES

- Knee pain is a very common complaint and can be due to articular or periarticular disorders (Table 8-10).
- Common arthritides such as OA, RA, and gout frequently affect the knee.

Etiology

- **Knee OA** is a very common cause of knee pain. It is insidious in onset but often originates from a previous trauma that damaged the normal cartilage or created abnormal mechanics in the knee.

TABLE 8-10	CAUSES OF KNEE PAIN

Articular disorders

Noninflammatory

OA

Internal derangement (due to meniscal cartilage or cruciate ligament injuries)

Osteonecrosis (AVN)

Fracture

Inflammatory

RA

Gout and calcium pyrophosphate deposition disease

Seronegative spondyloarthropathies

Viral arthritis

Septic arthritis

Periarticular disorders

Bursitis (anserine, prepatellar, infrapatellar)

Tendinitis (patellar, quadriceps)

Patellofemoral pain syndrome

Popliteal cysts

AVN, avascular necrosis; OA, osteoarthritis; RA, rheumatoid arthritis.

- There are multiple intra-articular structures (articular cartilage, meniscal cartilage, cruciate ligaments) that may degenerate with age, overuse, or trauma and lead to internal derangement.
- Knee pain may be **referred from hip disorders.**
- **Anserine bursitis** is inflammation of the pes anserinus bursa that often becomes inflamed with athletic activity.
- **Prepatellar and infrapatellar bursitis** are common in people who spend a lot of time on their knees. This bursitis is occasionally septic (especially after breaks in the skin).
- **Tendinopathy:** Degeneration of the tendons around the knee may occur with overuse. Tendinitis may occur with inflammatory arthritis.
- **Patellar tendinopathy** is seen in young athletes who engage in repetitive jumping or kicking (jumper's knee). Pain is over the patellar tendon.
- **Popliteal tendinopathy** causes posterolateral knee pain.
- The quadriceps and patellar **tendons may rupture** due to trauma and repetitive injuries and in patients with RA and lupus, and those who are receiving glucocorticoids. Sudden pain and inability to extend the knee are the symptoms.
- **Iliotibial band syndrome** is due to friction as the band passes over the lateral femoral condyle with flexion and extension. Repeated motions such as running promote repetitive friction. Excessive pronation may increase the amount of stress on the band as it passes over the condyle.
- **Patellofemoral pain** is thought to be due to malalignment (poor positioning of the patella) as it moves up and down the trochlear groove of the femur during flexion and extension. Softening of the cartilage with some non–full-thickness breakdown may occur resulting in **chondromalacia patellae.**
- **Popliteal cysts** (Baker's cysts) may be seen in patients with OA or RA and often communicate with the knee joint cavity.
- **Osgood–Schlatter disease** is seen in adolescents and presents with pain at the site of the insertion of the patellar tendon to the tibial tuberosity.
- **Osteochondritis dissecans** occurs most often in the teenage years and is due to focal necrosis of the subchondral bone. The overlying cartilage is thereby fragile, and fragments of cartilage and bone can break off and form a loose body in the joint. It usually occurs in patients involved in athletics.
- Other less common causes of knee pain can include a **synovial plica,** which can be irritated and cause anteromedial knee pain. **Pigmented villonodular synovitis** is an overgrowth of the synovial lining of a joint and can occur in the knee. It leads to vague knee pain and swelling.

DIAGNOSIS

Clinical Presentation

History
- **OA** symptoms include morning stiffness that lasts less than 30 minutes and pain that worsens with use and improves with rest.
- Suspect **internal derangement** in patients, often young adults, who complain of "locking" or "catching" sensations after trauma (particularly sports injuries). Commonly, they will report acute, painful swelling (due to hemarthrosis) at the time of injury. They may also note the knee giving way with pivoting after an anterior cruciate ligament tear.
- Medial knee pain occurs with **anserine bursitis.** Pain is noted with using stairs and may improve after a few minutes of activity.
- **Prepatellar bursitis** presents as pain (and occasionally erythema, warmth, swelling) anterior to the patella.
- **Popliteal cysts** (Baker's cysts) may be asymptomatic or cause swelling in the posterior knee. A ruptured cyst can dissect down the calf and mimic deep venous thrombosis.

- Lateral knee pain occurs with **iliotibial band syndrome.** It is typical in runners and bikers.
- Anterior knee pain aggravated by activity can reflect **patellofemoral pain.** It is characterized by pain in the patellar region that is worse with using stairs and running. **Osgood–Schlatter disease**, or osteochondritis of the tibial tubercle, typically occurs in pubertal males involved in sports. Repetitive traction of the patellar tendon causes reactive bony proliferation where the patellar tendon inserts onto the tibia. **Patellar tendinopathy** can cause anterior knee pain with activity as well.
- Posterior knee pain can result from hamstring tendinitis, popliteal tendinitis, or Baker's cyst.
- Knee pain occurs in **osteochondritis dissecans** when cracks form the articular cartilage and underlying bone. There may be symptoms of catching or limited range of motion if a loose body is present.

Physical Examination
- On physical examination of the **osteoarthritic knee,** tenderness along the joint line, small effusions, and crepitus may be found. There may be decreased range of motion (scc Chapter 11).
- Specific maneuvers on physical examination may detect damage to the internal structures with internal derangement.
- Palpation is helpful in locating the specific structure involved.
- **Arthrocentesis** is relatively simple to perform on the knee and should be done in cases of monoarthritis to exclude infection, crystal-induced arthritis, or hemarthrosis.
- In **anserine bursitis,** the anserine bursa is point tender to palpation just inferior to the medial joint line. Swelling is not usually appreciated.
- **Prepatellar bursitis** will present as a large swelling anterior to the patella. It may be red and warm, suggesting possible infection.
- The popliteal tendon will be tender to palpation in the posterolateral knee with tendinopathy. Resisted knee flexion with the tibia externally rotated may reproduce pain.
- In **iliotibial band syndrome,** there is point tenderness over the band at the lateral condyle of the femur. Swelling is not typically present.
- **Patellofemoral pain** can be identified by palpating for tenderness on the posterior surface of the patella, while the knee is extended and the quadriceps are relaxed. The pain can also be reproduced when the patella is held immobile, while the patient contracts the quadriceps muscle.
- Tenderness and a prominent size of the tibial tuberosities will be noticed with **Osgood–Schlatter disease.**
- With the patient lying prone with both knees extended, a swelling in the popliteal fossa will be notable if **Baker's cyst** is evident.

Diagnostic Testing
Imaging
- In general, reserve imaging for post-traumatic pain and for patients with chronic pain. Ligament and meniscal tears are noted with MRI.
- **Ultrasound** can be used to diagnose **Baker's cyst** and to rule out more serious pathology, such as a popliteal artery aneurysm or a soft-tissue tumor.
- Plain films can identify **osteochondritis dissecans**. Then, MRI can be used to determine the extent and stability of the lesion.

TREATMENT

- **Anserine bursitis** treatment includes rest, ice, and stretching. If symptoms do not improve, then glucocorticoid injections can be helpful.
- In **prepatellar bursitis,** recommend avoiding kneeling to help resolve the bursitis. However, aspiration may be needed in cases with abundant fluid. Surgical excision may be necessary for frequent recurrences.

- **Patellar tendinitis** treatment is rest, ice application, and stretching exercises. Glucocorticoid injections are contraindicated due to the risk of tendon rupture.
- **Popliteal tendinopathy** responds to hamstring strengthening. Be sure to rule out an acute ligamentous injury to the knee if the injury is traumatic.
- **Rupture** of the patellar tendon and quadriceps tendon require surgical repair.
- **Iliotibial band syndrome** is treated with rest, physical therapy, and orthotics. Glucocorticoid injections may be needed if no improvement occurs with therapy. Surgery is a last resort.
- **Patellofemoral pain** is treated initially with rest from aggravating activities. Gradual pain-free strengthening of the quadriceps muscle and hip abductors is recommended. Orthotics may help improve knee alignment in those with increased pronation. Patellofemoral supports may provide some patients relief.
- Treatment of **Osgood–Schlatter** syndrome is rest from offending athletic activities. It usually resolves as the patient grows older.
- A symptomatic **Baker's cyst** can be treated with aspiration and injection of the knee joint with glucocorticoids.
- Treatment of **osteochondritis dissecans** is conservative or surgical depending on the extent of the lesion.

Ankle and Foot Pain

GENERAL PRINCIPLES

- Ankle and foot pain are common problems from periarticular disorders, arthritis, or trauma and are often worsened by **inappropriate footwear.**
- The history and physical examination usually lead to a diagnosis. A history of diabetes, peripheral neuropathy, or peripheral vascular disease is particularly important.

Etiology

- Arthritis frequently affects the ankle and foot. **OA spares** the ankle but often involves the first metatarsophalangeal (MTP) joint, causing lateral deviation (**hallux valgus** or **bunion**). Bunions are more common in women.
- **RA** affects the ankle and forefoot in most patients. Bilateral ankle pain and synovitis and forefoot pain usually accompanies other joint involvement.
- The first MTP is the most commonly affected joint in acute **gout** (podagra).
- Motor, sensory, and autonomic neuropathies (seen in diabetic and other peripheral neuropathies) may lead to severe joint deformities in **neuropathic arthropathy (Charcot joint).**
- **Ankle sprains** are very common in outpatients and usually follow ankle inversion.
- **Stress fractures** are common causes of foot pain and occur as a result of overuse. They affect the second or third metatarsals most frequently.
- **Plantar fasciitis** is the most common cause of plantar foot pain and is due to inflammation of the plantar fascia at its insertion into the calcaneus. It may be idiopathic, owing to overuse/running, or a form of enthesitis in SpA (see Chapter 16).
- **Achilles tendinitis** occurs when the Achilles tendon becomes inflamed because of trauma or overuse (dancers, runners). The **tendon may rupture** from trauma or as a side effect of medications (glucocorticoids or quinolone antibiotics). Rupture is a known complication of injection of the Achilles tendon with glucocorticoids.
- **Achilles enthesitis** occurs when the tendon's insertion site into the calcaneus is inflamed. It is characteristic of SpA.
- **Achilles bursitis** occurs with inflammation of the retrocalcaneal bursa, which sits proximal and anterior to the tendon insertion.

- **Posterior tibial tendinitis** causes pain along the tendon near the medial malleolus.
- **Peroneal tendinitis** causes pain anterior to the lateral malleolus.
- **Tarsal tunnel syndrome** is characterized by pain, numbness, and paresthesias of the sole. The posterior tibial nerve is compressed at the flexor retinaculum, posterior to the medial malleolus.
- **Morton's neuroma** is due to compression of an interdigital nerve, most commonly between the third and fourth toes. It causes forefoot pain and numbness and tingling of these toes. It occurs more frequently in middle-aged women and is exacerbated by walking and by wearing narrow shoes or high heels.
- **Metatarsalgia** (pain arising from the metatarsal heads) may be due to high heels, everted foot, arthritis, trauma, or deformities and is quite common.

DIAGNOSIS

Clinical Presentation

History
- **Stress fractures** become more painful as an activity continues.
- **Plantar fasciitis** causes pain that is worse in the morning, especially when the patient first stands up. Pain occurs after prolonged standing or walking.
- **Tendinitis** is often most painful when beginning an activity and then becomes less painful as the area "warms up."
- Patients often feel a pop as if they have been "shot" when the Achilles ruptures.

Physical Examination
- The physical examination should include inspection (looking for deformities, abnormal calluses), palpation (of tender areas), sensory testing, and evaluation of distal pulses.
- **Examine the patient's footwear.** Signs of abnormal (or unilateral) wear or frequent use of high heels or narrow pointed shoes are important clues.
- Tophi and deformities at the first MTP joint suggest chronic **gout.**
- **Ankle sprains** present with edema and tenderness to palpation over the ligament(s) involved. Valgus and varus testing provokes ligament injury.
- Palpation of the involved bone will produce tenderness with a **stress fracture.**
- Tenderness over the distal edge of the plantar surface of the calcaneus will be present in **plantar fasciitis.**
- Tenderness over the tendon will be present with Achilles tendinitis. Patients will have difficulty walking and dorsiflexing the foot.
- **Rupture of the Achilles tendon** can be noted as an anatomical defect but also by the **Thompson's test.** The patient lies prone with the knee extended. Squeezing the calf muscle will cause plantar flexion if the tendon is intact. If the tendon is ruptured, plantar flexion will not occur.
- Tenderness just proximal to the insertion of the Achilles and between the tendon and the calcaneus will be present with **retrocalcaneal bursitis.** In **tarsal tunnel syndrome,** tapping over the nerve as it passes around the medial malleolus may reproduce symptoms. The area may be tender to palpation.
- Squeezing the metatarsal heads together can aggravate the pain of **Morton's neuroma.**
- Palpation over the metatarsal heads reveals tenderness in **metatarsalgia.**

Diagnostic Testing

Imaging
- Radiographs are rarely useful, except in cases of trauma.
- According to the Ottawa guidelines for ankle sprains, **obtain radiographs** to rule out fracture in patients with medial or lateral malleolar tenderness or with inability to bear weight after the event or in the emergency department (ED).

- The Ottawa guidelines for foot injuries recommend plain films to rule out fracture if there is pain in the midfoot after the injury and if any of the following are present: There is tenderness at the base of the fifth metatarsal or the navicular, or if the patient cannot bear weight after the event or in the ED.
- Radiographs sometimes do not detect stress fractures. Bone scan or MRI may be used for diagnosis.

Diagnostic Testing
When considering surgery for tarsal tunnel syndrome, electrodiagnostic testing will help confirm the diagnosis.

TREATMENT

- Treatment of foot and ankle pain is conservative. Rest, stretching exercises, and NSAIDs are frequently used.
- **Orthoses and appropriate footwear** are an essential part of care in many cases. Assistance from podiatrists and orthotists is invaluable.
- A shoe with a wide toe box provides symptomatic relief for **bunions,** but surgery is often performed for cosmetic reasons.
- **Stress fractures** are treated conservatively with immobilization in a boot or splint. Stress fractures in the navicular require strict non–weight bearing.
- **Ankle sprains** are initially treated with rest, ice, compression, and elevation, followed by range of motion and strengthening exercises.
- **Plantar fasciitis** is treated with stretching of the calf muscles, heel inserts/orthotics, and NSAIDs. Occasionally, glucocorticoid injections are used.
- Treatment of **Achilles tendinitis** is conservative, but **rupture** requires surgical evaluation. Retrocalcaneal bursitis treatment includes rest and NSAIDs.
- **Posterior tibial and peroneal tendinopathy** respond well to rest. Arch supports/orthotics help to decrease pronation and the stress that it causes on these tendons.
- In **tarsal tunnel syndrome,** glucocorticoid injections are helpful but should be done carefully. If excessive pronation is present, orthotics should be provided. Surgical decompression may be needed.
- Properly fitting footwear with sufficient width or a metatarsal pad is helpful in treating **Morton's neuroma.** Glucocorticoid injections are sometimes used for relief. Some patients require surgery.
- Proper footwear and a metatarsal pad are helpful in treating **metatarsalgia.**

REFERENCES

1. Carette S, Fehlings MG. Clinical practice. Cervical radiculopathy. *N Engl J Med.* 2005;353:392–399.
2. Deyo RA, Weinstein JN. Low back pain. *N Engl J Med.* 2001;344:363–370.
3. Shoen RP, Moskowitz RW, Goldberg VM. *Soft Tissue Rheumatic Pain: Recognition, Management, Prevention.* 3rd ed. Philadelphia, PA: Lea & Febiger; 1996.
4. Reveille JD. Soft-tissue rheumatism: diagnosis and treatment. *Am J Med.* 1997;102:23–29.

Drugs Used for the Treatment of Rheumatic Diseases

9

Divya Jayakumar and
María C. González-Mayda

GENERAL PRINCIPLES

- Although rheumatologic diseases encompass a wide range of organ systems, there are a relatively limited number of drug classes for treatment.
- The main classes of medications used in rheumatology include:
  - Analgesics
  - Salicylates/nonsteroidal anti-inflammatory drugs (NSAIDs)/cyclooxygenase-2 (COX-2) inhibitors
  - Glucocorticoids (GCs)
  - Disease-modifying antirheumatic drugs (DMARDs)
  - Biologics
  - Gout medications
    - Urate-lowering agents
    - Anti-inflammatory
  - Osteoporosis medications

ANALGESICS

- Analgesics largely **reduce pain**, not inflammation. Consequently, their use is limited in rheumatology as many diseases are strongly inflammatory.
- Analgesics are very useful for **osteoarthritis (OA)**, given their minimal side-effect profiles.
- Medications:
  - **Acetaminophen**
    - **Dosage:** 325 to 650 mg orally (PO) q4 to 6h or 1,000 mg PO q6 to 8h. Limit to 4 g/24 hours in liver-competent patients and ≤ 2 g/24 hours with hepatic insufficiency.
    - **Mechanism:** Largely unclear, although it inhibits prostaglandin synthesis in central nervous system (CNS). There may also be inhibition of COX isoenzymes.
    - **Side effects:** It is generally well tolerated. Combination with hepatotoxic agents, such as ethanol, potentiates hepatotoxicity. It can increase international normalized ratio (INR) when large doses are given with warfarin.
    - **Contraindications/precautions:** Chronic alcohol use, liver disease, and glucose-6-phosphate dehydrogenase (G6PD) deficiency. Food and Drug Administration (**FDA**) **pregnancy category: C.** Though it crosses the placenta, there is no increased teratogenicity in pregnancy. Acetaminophen is also excreted in breast milk and is acceptable in usual recommended doses.
  - Tramadol
    - **Dosage:** 50 to 100 mg PO q4 to 6h
    - **Mechanism:** Inhibits ascending pain pathways by binding to μ-opiate receptors in CNS. Also inhibits norepinephrine and serotonin reuptake.
    - **Side effects:** Somnolence, dizziness, headache, nausea, and vomiting
    - **Contraindications/precautions:** History of alcohol or drug use, chronic respiratory disease, liver disease, concomitant use of tricyclic antidepressants (TCAs), monoamine oxidase inhibitors (MAOIs), selective serotonin reuptake inhibitors (SSRIs),

and seizure disorder. **FDA pregnancy category: C.** Use only if benefits outweigh risks, because neonatal seizures and withdrawal syndrome and fetal death have occurred.

▪ **Tramadol has a synergistic effect on pain when combined with acetaminophen.** They are often prescribed together.

SALICYLATES/NSAIDS/COX-2 INHIBITORS

- Used for anti-inflammatory, antipyretic, and analgesic purposes
- These drugs work by **inhibiting COX**, with other unidentified mechanisms likely contributing to effect.
- Salicylates and NSAIDs block COX-1 and COX-2 nonspecifically, whereas COX-2 inhibitors predictably inhibit only COX-2.
- COX converts arachidonic acid to prostaglandins, leukotrienes, or thromboxanes, leading to a complex response involving both pro-inflammatory and anti-inflammatory actions.
- COX-2 is an inducible enzyme that leads to a pro-inflammatory phenotype.
- Adverse effects seen with salicylates and NSAIDs are diverse, including
  - **Gastrointestinal (GI):** Gastritis and ulcer formation that can lead to perforation (particularly with age >65, smoking, higher duration and dose of NSAIDs; risk = 1% per patient year)
  - **Renal:** Hypertension, hyperkalemia, reduction in efficacy of diuretics and antihypertensives, edema (due to vasoconstriction along with water and sodium retention), and, rarely, interstitial nephritis (with long-term, chronic use)
  - **CNS:** Headaches, aseptic meningitis, tinnitus (with acetylsalicylic acid [ASA]), altered mental status, and aseptic meningitis
  - **Hepatic:** Transaminitis and Reye's syndrome in children with viral illness
  - **Hematologic:** Impaired platelet aggregation (reversible, except with salicylates) and anemia (usually from GI blood loss)
  - **Hypersensitivity reactions: Samter's triad of nasal polyps, asthma, and hypersensitivity to all NSAIDs** is due to excessive leukotriene production after NSAID administration. Other hypersensitivity reactions, such as rash, can also occur separately from Samter's triad.
  - **COX-2 inhibitors reduce GI events by 20% to 40% and do not inhibit platelet aggregation.** Renal and hypersensitivity reactions are equal to NSAIDs.
  - **Pregnancy:** Avoid in early and late pregnancy because it may cause premature closure of ductus arteriosus.
  - See Table 9-1 for a list of medications.

TABLE 9-1	NSAIDs AND SELECTIVE COX-2 INHIBITORS	
Classification	**Drug**	**Dosage (PO, Adult Dose Unless Indicated)**
Carboxylic acid: acetylated[a]	Aspirin	2,400–5,400 mg/day in 4 divided doses
Carboxylic acid: nonacetylated salicylates[a]	Salsalate	3 g/day in 2–3 divided doses
	Diflunisal	500–1,500 mg/day in 2 divided doses
	Choline salicylate	870–1,740 mg/dose given qid
	Choline magnesium trisalicylate	1–3 g/day in 2–3 divided doses

Classification	Drug	Dosage (PO, Adult Dose Unless Indicated)
Carboxylic acid: acetic acids	Etodolac	Immediate release: 800–1,200 mg/day in 2–4 divided doses
		Sustained release: 400–1,000 mg once daily
	Diclofenac	Immediate release: 100–200 mg/day in 2–3 divided doses
		Sustained release: 100–200 mg once daily
	Diclofenac and misoprostol[b]	150–200 mg/day (diclofenac) in 3 divided doses
	Indomethacin	Immediate release: 50–200 mg/day in 2–3 divided doses
		Sustained release: 75 mg once or twice daily
	Ketorolac[c]	PO: 10 mg q4–6h; IM/IV: 30–60 mg × 1, followed by 15–30 mg q6h
	Nabumetone	1,000–2,000 mg in 1–2 divided doses
Propionic acids	Fenoprofen	900–3,200 mg/day in 3–4 divided doses
	Flurbiprofen	200–300 mg/day in 2–4 divided doses
	Ibuprofen	OTC dose: 200–400 mg q4–6h; prescription dose: 1,200–3,200 mg/day in 3–4 divided doses
	Ketoprofen	OTC dose: 12.5 mg q4–6h; prescription dose: 150–300 mg/day in 3–4 divided doses
		Extended release: 200 mg once daily
	Naproxen	Immediate release: 500–1,500 mg/day in 2–3 divided doses
		Extended release: 750–1,500 mg once daily
	Naproxen sodium	OTC: 220 mg bid–tid; prescription: 550–1,375 mg/day in 2–3 divided doses; may increase to 1,650 mg/day for limited periods of time only
	Oxaprozin	600–1,800 mg/day; doses <1,200 mg/day in 1–2 divided doses; doses >1,200 mg/day in 2–3 divided doses
Fenamates	Meclofenamate	200–400 mg/day in 3–4 divided doses
	Mefenamic acid[d]	250 mg q6h
Oxicams	Meloxicam	7.5–15 mg once daily
	Piroxicam	10–20 mg/day
Selective COX-2 inhibitors[e]	Celecoxib[e]	OA: 100–200 mg/day in 1–2 doses; RA: 200–400 mg/day in 2 divided doses

[a]Salicylate level may be used to monitor therapy (target level is 15–30 mg/dL).
[b]Risk of gastric ulcer is decreased relative to other traditional NSAIDs.
[c]Not indicated for use exceeding 5 days because of increased risk of side effects, including GI bleed; adjust dose based on weight and age.
[d]Not indicated for use exceeding 1 week.
[e]Caution in patients with a history of hypersensitivity to sulfonamides.
bid, twice daily; COX-2, cyclooxygenase-2; NSAIDs, nonsteroidal anti-inflammatory drugs; OA, osteoarthritis; PO, orally; qid, four times a day; RA, rheumatoid arthritis; tid, three times a day.

GLUCOCORTICOIDS

- GCs, also referred to as corticosteroids or steroids, remain one of the most effective anti-inflammatory and immunosuppressive medications. They also possess significant toxicity with prolonged use.
- Patients taking alternate-day GC therapy, low-dose prednisone (<5 mg/day), or GCs less than 3 weeks usually do not have suppression of the hypothalamic–pituitary axis (HPA). Anyone who is on ≥20 mg/day or has clinical Cushing's syndrome is assumed to have HPA suppression. Otherwise, there is variable suppression of the HPA.
- **Medications: Prednisone (PO), prednisolone (PO), hydrocortisone (PO/intramuscular [IM]/IV), methylprednisolone (IV/intra-articular), dexamethasone (PO/IV/IM), and triamcinolone (intra-articular)** (see Table 9-2 for equivalent doses of GCs)[1]
  - **Dosage:** Highly dependent on disease and clinical situation (Table 9-3)[2]
  - **Mechanism:** Effects are pleiotropic and include inhibition of leukocyte trafficking, restriction of leukocyte access to inflamed tissue, attenuated production of inflammatory humoral mediators, and inhibition of various functions of leukocytes, fibroblasts, and endothelial cells

TABLE 9-2	COMPARISON OF REPRESENTATIVE GLUCOCORTICOID PREPARATIONS			
	Approximate Equivalent Dose[a], mg	Relative Anti-inflammatory Activity	Relative Mineralocorticoid Activity	Duration of Action, Hours
Cortisol[b]	20	1	1	8–12
Cortisone acetate	25	0.8	0.8	8–12
Hydrocortisone	20	1	1	8–12
Prednisone	5	4	0.8	12–36
Prednisolone	5	4	0.8	12–36
Methylprednisolone	4	5	0.5	12–36
Triamcinolone	4	5	0	12–36
Fludrocortisone[c]	—	10	125	12–36
Dexamethasone	0.75	30	0	36–72

[a]Equivalent dose shown is for oral or IV administration. Relative potency for intra-articular or intramuscular administration may vary considerably.

[b]Data for cortisol, endogenous glucocorticoid hormone, are included for comparison with synthetic preparations listed.

[c]Fludrocortisone is not used for anti-inflammatory effect.

Adapted from: Schimmer BP, Parker KL. Adrenocorticotropic hormone; adrenocortical steroids and their synthetic analogs; inhibitors of the synthesis and actions of adrenocortical hormones. In: Brunton LL, Lazo J, Parker K, eds. *The Pharmacological Basis of Therapeutics.* Vol. 11. New York, NY: McGraw-Hill; 2005:27–28.

TABLE 9-3	APPROXIMATE DOSAGES OF GLUCOCORTICOIDS FOR VARIOUS CLINICAL SITUATIONS AND POTENTIAL ADVERSE EFFECTS		
Terminology	**Dosage**[a]	**Clinical Application**	**Adverse Effects**
Low	≤7.5	Maintenance therapy	Few
Medium	>7.5 to ≤30	Initial therapy for mild-to-moderate disease such as rash or arthritis	Dose dependent and considerable if treatment given for longer periods of time
High	>30 to ≤100	Initial therapy for moderate-to-severe (non–life-threatening) disease such as nephritis or vasculitis	Cannot be administered for long-term therapy owing to severe side effects
Very high	>100	Initially given in severe, acute, and/or life-threatening exacerbations of rheumatic diseases	Cannot be administered for long-term therapy owing to dramatic side effects
Pulse therapy	>250 for 1 or several days	Particularly severe and/or potentially life-threatening forms of rheumatic diseases	High proportion of cases have a relatively low incidence of side effects

[a]Dosage is given in milligrams of prednisone equivalent per day.

Adapted from: Buttgereit F, Burmester GR. Glucocorticoids. In: Klippel JH, Stone JH, Crofford LJ, et al., eds. *Primer on the Rheumatic Diseases.* 13th ed. New York, NY: Springer Science+Business Media; 2008:644–650.

- ○ **Side effects:** Adverse effects are **usually seen with doses ≥10 mg/day** and may impact the following systems:
  - ▪ Musculoskeletal (myopathy)
  - ▪ Endocrine (hyperglycemia, weight gain, iatrogenic Cushing's syndrome, secondary osteoporosis)
  - ▪ Cardiovascular (dyslipidemia, hypertension)
  - ▪ Dermatologic (acne, purpura, and cutaneous atrophy due to catabolic effects)
  - ▪ Ophthalmologic (cataracts, glaucoma)
  - ▪ Infectious (overall relative risk of infection is 2.0, but is dose dependent)
  - ▪ Psychological (psychosis, minor mood disturbances)
- ○ **Contraindications/precautions:** Systemic infection (especially fungal), heart failure (due to fluid retention), diabetes mellitus (hyperglycemia), hepatic impairment, acute myocardial infarction (risk of myocardial rupture), and myasthenia gravis (exacerbation of symptoms may occur). **FDA pregnancy category: D.** Teratogenicity (oral clefts, low birth weight) occurs with first-trimester use. When essential in pregnancy, use lowest effective dose for shortest duration of time.
- ○ **Special considerations:** For patients with suspected HPA suppression, GCs must be tapered off gradually, not discontinued abruptly, to allow for recovery of the HPA. In addition, those undergoing major surgery may need stress-dose GCs until 48 hours postoperatively and should be monitored for signs of adrenal insufficiency.

DISEASE-MODIFYING ANTIRHEUMATIC DRUGS

- This group of medications has both anti-inflammatory and immunomodulatory effects, with highly variable clinical responses.
- They are usually used as steroid-sparing therapy and have a slow onset of action.
- There is a high rate of discontinuation due to lack of efficacy or drug toxicity.
- Medications
  - **Hydroxychloroquine (HCQ)**
    - **Dosage:** 5 mg/kg/day or less, of real body weight, which is usually 200 to 400 mg PO qday. The 400-mg dose can be split into 200 mg twice daily (bid).
    - **Mechanism:** It inhibits neutrophil trafficking and complement-dependent antigen–antibody responses. It also interferes with lysosomal enzymes.
    - **Onset of action:** 4 to 6 weeks
    - **Side effects:** This drug is generally well tolerated, but some patients may have indigestion or hypersensitivity rash. Retinopathy and bone marrow suppression are rare complications.
    - **Contraindications/precautions:** It carries a **boxed warning** for use by experienced physicians only. History of hypersensitivity or visual changes on related therapy, G6PD deficiency, psoriasis (may worsen on therapy), and macular degeneration are contraindications to its use. HCQ is cleared by the kidneys; hence, renal dysfunction raises risk of toxicity. Concomitant use with tamoxifen increases the risk of toxicity. **FDA pregnancy category:** C. HCQ crosses the placenta; however, there has been no increase in miscarriages, congenital malformations, or teratogenicity in patients who continue the drug during pregnancy. Low concentrations of the drug are found in breast milk and are compatible with breastfeeding.
    - **Monitoring:** As per the 2016 American Academy of Ophthalmology recommendations, baseline ophthalmologic examination followed by annual examinations is required for high-risk patients. All other patients can have a baseline ophthalmologic examination and annual screening starting 5 years after therapy initiation.[3]
  - **Methotrexate**
    - **Dosage:** Start with 10 to 15 mg/week (PO/subcutaneous [SC]), and increase 5 mg q2 to 4 weeks as needed to a maximum of 20 to 25 mg/week. At doses above 15 mg/week, better absorption is seen with SC methotrexate without an increase in adverse events.
    - **Mechanism:** It inhibits dihydrofolate reductase, acting as folate antimetabolite that inhibits DNA synthesis and repair.
    - **Onset of action:** 3 to 6 weeks, but additional improvement can be seen up to 12 weeks.
    - **Side effects:** Anorexia, nausea, diarrhea, stomatitis, alopecia, and transaminitis are not rare, and all can be reduced with administration of folic acid 1 mg daily; pneumonitis and infection are much less common.
    - **Contraindications/precautions:** There is a **boxed warning** for acute renal failure, bone marrow suppression, dermatologic reactions (including toxic epidermal necrolysis), diarrhea/stomatitis, hepatotoxicity, lymphomas, infections, pneumonitis, and ascites/pleural effusions (reduced elimination of methotrexate). Chronic alcohol use is a contraindication. **This medication is also FDA pregnancy category: X.** Positive evidence of human fetal risk based on adverse reaction data from investigational or marketing experience and studies in humans contraindicates its use in pregnant women with psoriasis or rheumatoid arthritis (RA). Breastfeeding is contraindicated.
    - **Monitoring:** A baseline complete metabolic profile (CMP), complete blood count (CBC), hepatitis panel, and chest radiographs are required. CMP and CBC should

be done q4 weeks for the first 3 months, then q8 to 12 weeks over the next 3 to 6 months, then q12 weeks thereafter. Liver biopsy should be performed if persistent hepatic function profile (HFP) abnormalities, alcoholism, or chronic hepatitis B or C, and pulmonary function tests if lung toxicity is suspected.

○ **Leflunomide**
  ▪ **Dosage:** 10 to 20 mg PO daily
  ▪ **Mechanism:** It inhibits dihydroorotate dehydrogenase, inhibiting de novo pyrimidine synthesis. This affects proliferation and also reduces inflammation.
  ▪ **Onset of action:** 4 to 8 weeks
  ▪ **Side effects:** These include diarrhea, alopecia, hepatitis, rash, infection, hypertension, and headache.
  ▪ **Contraindications/precautions:** There is a **boxed warning** for severe liver injury. Renal or hepatic impairment, chronic alcohol use, and preexisting bone marrow suppression are contraindications to its use. **FDA pregnancy category: X. It is teratogenic.** Studies in animals or humans have demonstrated fetal abnormalities and/or there is positive evidence of human fetal risk based on adverse reaction data from investigational or marketing experience, and **the risks involved in use of the drug in pregnant women clearly outweigh potential benefits.** If a woman on leflunomide wishes to conceive, active metabolite levels should be below 0.02 mg/L $\times$ 2 (2 weeks apart), after which three menstrual cycles must be completed before conception. As the metabolites may remain in the body for years, a cholestyramine washout is essential (8 g three times a day [tid] for 11 days).
  ▪ **Monitoring:** Screen for pregnancy prior to therapy. Baseline CMP and CBC are required. Blood pressure, CMP, phosphate (leflunomide can occasionally increase renal excretion of phosphate), and CBC should be monitored q4 weeks for first 6 months, then q12 weeks. Discontinue leflunomide and initiate cholestyramine therapy if transaminitis likely leflunomide-induced (alanine aminotransferase [ALT] ≥3 times upper limit of normal [ULN]) or other serious adverse effects occur.

○ **Sulfasalazine**
  ▪ **Dosage:** Start with 500 to 1,000 mg PO daily, increasing weekly as needed to 2 to 3 g/day divided in two equal doses.
  ▪ **Mechanism:** Exact mechanism of action is unknown; however, it is felt to have both anti-inflammatory and immunomodulatory effects.
  ▪ **Onset of action:** 8 to 12 weeks
  ▪ **Side effects:** Headache, rash, anorexia, dyspepsia, nausea, vomiting, reversible oligospermia, dizziness, bone marrow suppression, and transaminitis may all occur. GI symptoms are less common with the enteric-coated form of the drug.
  ▪ **Contraindications/precautions:** Sulfa allergy, G6PD deficiency, renal or hepatic impairment, and GI or genitourinary (GU) obstruction. **FDA pregnancy category: B.** Sulfasalazine can be given to women of childbearing age because it does not seem to cause spontaneous abortions or fetal abnormalities, though it is found in similar concentrations in the fetus.
  ▪ **Monitoring:** Baseline CMP and CBC are required and should be repeated q2 weeks for first 3 months, q4 weeks for the next 3 months, then q12 weeks thereafter.

○ **Azathioprine**
  ▪ **Dosage:** Start with 1 mg/kg/day PO daily or divided bid for 6 to 8 weeks, then increase by 0.5 mg/kg q4 weeks as needed until response or up to a maximum of 2.5 mg/kg/day.
  ▪ **Mechanism:** This drug antagonizes purine metabolism, with 6-thioguanine nucleotides mediating most of the effects.

- **Onset of action:** 6 to 8 weeks
- **Side effects:** Leukopenia, nausea, vomiting, diarrhea, myalgia, malaise, dizziness, hepatotoxicity, and HFP abnormalities may all occur and are usually dose dependent.
- **Contraindications/precautions: Boxed warning** for use by experienced physicians only and increased risk of neoplasia (lymphoma, skin cancer) with history of treatment with alkylating agents (cyclophosphamide, chlorambucil, melphalan). **FDA pregnancy category: D.** Azathioprine crosses the placenta; however, pregnant women treated with azathioprine had a similar rate of fetal malformation as the general population. Because data are limited, azathioprine may be considered when benefits of disease control outweigh risks of prematurity.
- **Monitoring:** Thiopurine methyltransferase (TPMT) genotyping or phenotyping prior to therapy can help guide initial dosing. CBC and CMP should be done at baseline. CBC should be repeated weekly during the first month, q2 weeks during months 2 and 3, then monthly, with CMP q3 months.

○ **Mycophenolate mofetil**
- **Dosage:** Start with 500 mg PO bid and increase by 1,000 mg q3 to 4 weeks as needed to a maximum dose of 1,500 mg PO bid. Mycophenolate sodium (Myfortic) 180 mg is equivalent to mycophenolate mofetil (Cellcept) 250 mg.
- **Mechanism:** Inhibits de novo guanosine nucleotide synthesis by blocking inosine monophosphate dehydrogenase (IMPDH), thereby reducing lymphocyte proliferation.
- **Onset of action:** Peak levels of active metabolites occur 1 to 2 hours, with a half-life of 16 hours.
- **Side effects:** The most common adverse effect is nausea. The following may also occur: hypertension or hypotension, edema, chest pain, tachycardia, pain, headache, insomnia, infection, dizziness, anxiety, hyperglycemia, hypercholesterolemia, hypomagnesemia, hypokalemia, abdominal pain with nausea and vomiting, diarrhea and/or constipation, dyspepsia, bone marrow suppression, acute renal failure, dyspnea, and pleural effusion.
- **Contraindications/precautions:** There is a **boxed warning** for use by experienced physicians only. The drug is associated with increased risk of infections, lymphoma, and skin malignancy. **FDA pregnancy category: D.** Women of childbearing potential must use contraception because drug exposure has been associated with pregnancy loss and congenital malformations. It should be used with caution in peptic ulcer disease and renal impairment.
- **Monitoring:** CBC is required at baseline and weekly during the first month, q2 weeks during months 2 and 3, then monthly. CMP is done at baseline and then q3 months.

○ **Cyclophosphamide**
- **Dosage:** Dose and route of administration are highly dependent on the severity of a disease and must be administered with the input of a rheumatologist. If PO, 1 to 2 mg/kg/day every AM is the usual starting dose; if IV, 0.25 to 1.0 g/m^2 monthly.
- **Mechanism:** This is an alkylating agent, interfering with DNA synthesis.
- **Onset of action:** 4 to 7 days
- **Side effects:** Alopecia, sterility, nausea, vomiting, diarrhea, mucositis/stomatitis, **acute hemorrhagic cystitis** (reduced with concurrent administration of Mesna IV), bone marrow suppression, infection, headache, rash, and **bladder transitional cell carcinoma** may all occur.
- **Contraindications/precautions:** Use is contraindicated with depressed bone marrow function and infection. Exercise caution with severe renal or hepatic impairment. **FDA pregnancy category: D.** It is teratogenic and can cause birth defects, miscarriage,

and fetotoxicity in newborns. Advise women of reproductive age to avoid pregnancy and to use effective contraception for up to 1 year.

- **Monitoring:** CBC, CMP, and urinalysis (UA) are required at baseline and at least weekly until the dose is stable, then monthly. Lymphopenia is common and is not an indication to reduce dose. Neutropenia should be avoided by dose reduction.

○ Cyclosporine

- **Dosage:** For RA, start with 2.5 mg/kg/day PO divided bid. Can increase by 0.5 to 0.75 mg/kg/day after 8 weeks depending on clinical response. Additional dosage increases can be done again at 12 weeks as needed to a maximum of 4 mg/kg/day. For lupus nephritis, start at 4 mg/kg/day for 1 month, then reduce the dose by 0.5 mg/kg q2 weeks until reaching a maintenance dose of 2.5 to 3 mg/kg/day.
- **Mechanism:** This drug blocks interleukin (IL)-2 production and release from T lymphocytes.
- **Onset of action:** 4 to 12 weeks
- **Side effects:** Common adverse effects include hypertension and edema. Headache, hirsutism, hypertriglyceridemia, nausea, diarrhea, dyspepsia, tremor, renal failure, and infection may also occur.
- **Contraindications/precautions:** There is a **boxed warning** for use by experienced physicians only. Patients should be monitored for development of hypertension, infection, malignancy (lymphoma and skin), nephrotoxicity, and skin cancer. **FDA pregnancy category: C.** No adequate controlled studies available on pregnant women. It should not be used in pregnancy unless potential benefits outweigh risks because it causes premature births and low birth weight.
- **Monitoring:** Baseline studies should include blood pressure and creatinine. Thereafter, monitor creatinine q2 weeks for the first 3 months, then monthly. If hypertension develops, decrease dose by 25% to 50%; if hypertension persists, discontinue the drug. No additional benefit has been seen in monitoring cyclosporine levels.

BIOLOGICS

- Biologics represent a novel class of therapeutics that take advantage of modern recombinant protein engineering techniques that selectively block a pathway important in immunity.
- Biologics have revolutionized the treatment of many rheumatic conditions, leading to response rates that have been unmatched with prior therapies. These medications have the potential to reactivate prior infections, which can cause significant morbidity and mortality.
- Prior to initiating any biologic, ensure patient is **up to date with vaccinations, especially live vaccines. Also ensure they have been screened for tuberculosis (TB), hepatitis B, and hepatitis C.** Biologic use is discouraged with any of these infections. Also inquire about history of malignancy (lymphoma, melanoma), demyelinating disease, and pregnancy.
- **Live virus vaccines are contraindicated once a biologic has been initiated. Annual inactivated influenza vaccine and age-appropriate pneumococcal, meningococcal, and Haemophilus influenzae B vaccine is encouraged. Inactivated zoster vaccine is available; however, no studies are available on immunocompromised patients.**
- Nomenclature in biologics[4]:
  ○ **-cept:** Receptor drug preventing ligand from binding to its receptor
  ○ **-ximab:** Chimeric monoclonal antibody (mAb)
  ○ **-zumab:** Humanized mAb
  ○ **-mumab:** Completely humanized mAb

○ **-ra:** Receptor antagonist
○ **-tinib:** Inhibitor
- Anti–tumor necrosis factor (TNF) therapies
  ○ **Etanercept**
    ▪ **Dosage:** The usual dose is 50 mg SC qweek, but it can be split into 25 mg SC 2×/week. It can be given either alone or in combination with methotrexate, leflunomide, or sulfasalazine to improve efficacy.
    ▪ **Mechanism:** It is a soluble TNF receptor linked to the Fc portion of humanized immunoglobulin G1 (IgG1), limiting the amount of TNF-α that can bind to endogenous TNF receptors.
      □ **Onset of action:** 1 to 2 weeks
  ○ **Adalimumab**
    ▪ **Dosage:** The usual dose is 40 mg SC q2 weeks, but it can be used 40 mg SC weekly. It can be given either alone or in combination with methotrexate, leflunomide, or sulfasalazine to improve efficacy.
    ▪ **Mechanism:** It is a recombinant mAb that binds to soluble TNF-α, preventing it from binding to its receptor.
    ▪ **Onset of action:** 4 to 6 weeks
  ○ **Infliximab**
    ▪ **Dosage:** Start with 3 mg/kg intravenous (IV) at 0, 2, and 6 weeks, then q8 weeks thereafter. Dosing can range from 3 to 10 mg/kg, repeated q4 to 8 weeks. It is usually given with methotrexate, leflunomide, or sulfasalazine to improve efficacy and to help prevent the formation of anti-infliximab antibodies.
    ▪ **Mechanism:** It is a chimeric mAb against TNF-α, thus neutralizing activity.
      □ **Onset of action:** 2 to 3 weeks
  ○ **Certolizumab pegol**
    ▪ **Dosage:** Start with 400 mg SC at weeks 0, 2, and 4, then 200 mg SC q2 weeks. Maintenance dose is 200 mg q2 weeks or 400 mg q4 weeks.
    ▪ **Mechanism:** A mAb consisting of a pegylated humanized antibody Fab (antigen-binding fragment) of TNF-α. The pegylation prolongs its half-life. It can be given either alone or in combination with methotrexate, leflunomide, or sulfasalazine to improve efficacy.
    ▪ **Onset of action:** 4 to 8 weeks
  ○ **Golimumab**
    ▪ **Dosage:** It can be given as 50 mg SC monthly or as an infusion of 2 mg/kg at 0, 4, and q8 weeks thereafter. Methotrexate is used as an adjunct for RA, and DMARDs are optional for psoriatic arthritis (PsA) and ankylosing spondylitis (AS).
    ▪ **Mechanism:** It is a humanized anti-TNF mAb that binds to both transmembrane and soluble forms of TNF-α, preventing it from binding to its receptor. It can be given either alone or in combination with methotrexate, leflunomide, or sulfasalazine to improve efficacy.
    ▪ **Onset of action:** 4 to 8 weeks
  ○ FDA-approved indications for anti-TNF therapies
    ▪ All anti-TNF therapies are approved for RA, PsA, and AS.
    ▪ Etanercept and adalimumab are approved for polyarticular juvenile idiopathic arthritis (JIA).
    ▪ Adalimumab is also approved for noninfectious uveitis.
    ▪ Anti-TNF therapy, with the exception of etanercept, is approved for Crohn's or ulcerative colitis or both.
    ▪ Off-label uses include reactive arthritis, Behçet's disease, TNF receptor–associated periodic fever syndrome (TRAPS), sarcoidosis, relapsing polychondritis, adult-onset

Still's disease, pyoderma gangrenosum, SAPHO (synovitis, acne, pustulosis, hyperostosis, and osteitis) syndrome, and hidradenitis suppurativa.

- Not useful in systemic lupus erythematosus (SLE), Sjögren's syndrome, antineutrophil cytoplasmic antibody (ANCA)–associated vasculitis, and giant cell arteritis.
  - Side effects of anti-TNF therapies: Injection site/infusion reactions (the latter seen mainly with infliximab), headache, nausea, rash, infections (including TB and fungal), malignancy (lymphoma in children,[5] skin cancer), demyelinating conditions, hepatotoxicity, palmoplantar psoriasis (most seen with infliximab), ANA positivity, and drug-induced lupus may occur.
  - Contraindications/precautions for anti-TNF therapies
    - There is a boxed warning for infection, malignancy, and TB. Use only with extreme caution with infection (hepatitis B can reactivate), seizure disorder, and alcoholic hepatitis (etanercept). Avoid usage in heart failure, demyelinating disease (multiple sclerosis, Guillain–Barré syndrome), optic neuritis, bone marrow abnormalities, or concurrent use of biologic agents.
    - Avoid etanercept in uveitis and inflammatory bowel disease–associated arthritis.
    - FDA pregnancy category: B. No adequate controlled studies available on pregnant women; hence, it should be used during pregnancy only if clearly needed.
- B-cell modulating agents
  - Rituximab
    - Dosage: For RA, infuse 1 g IV at 0 and 2 weeks, then again q6 to 12 months. Redosing usually occurs when the patient relapses, though some studies suggest a preset q6-month regimen may work better. For ANCA-associated vasculitis induction therapy, infuse 375 mg/m^2 once weekly for four doses. Once vasculitis remission has been achieved, the dose can be changed to a 500-mg infusion at 0 and 2 weeks q6 months with further taper depending on clinical response. Monitoring B-cell levels in blood is not useful.
    - Mechanism: It is a chimeric mAb against CD20 antigen on B cells, leading to peripheral B-cell depletion. Though plasma cells are preserved, some patients can develop hypogammaglobulinemia with repeat rituximab exposure.
    - Onset of action: Can vary. Half-life of 18 to 23 days
    - FDA-approved indications in rheumatology: RA (after methotrexate and anti-TNF failure) along with ANCA-associated vasculitis: granulomatosis with polyangiitis and microscopic polyangiitis. It is also FDA approved for various non-Hodgkin's lymphomas, chronic lymphoid leukemia, and pemphigus vulgaris.
    - Side effects: Headache, fever, infusion reactions, rash, nausea, abdominal pain, bone marrow suppression (especially in RA patients), weakness, hypogammaglobulinemia, infection, and cough may all occur. There are rare but well-documented reports of JC virus reactivation, leading to progressive multifocal leukoencephalopathy (PML).
    - Contraindications/precautions: There is a boxed warning for infusion reactions, mucocutaneous reactions, and PML. Use only with extreme caution with infection (hepatitis B can reactivate) and history of cardiovascular disease. Late-onset neutropenia, hypogammaglobulinemia, bowel obstruction, and perforation have also been reported. Do not give concurrently with other biologics. No live vaccines should be administered while receiving rituximab. Inactivated vaccines when indicated should be given 4 weeks prior to rituximab infusion. FDA pregnancy category: C. No adequate controlled studies available on pregnant women. B-cell lymphocytopenia can occur in infants exposed in utero. Avoid use unless benefits outweigh risks.
    - Monitoring: Baseline hepatitis panel and CBC. Repeat CBC q3 months. Can consider obtaining baseline quantitative immunoglobulin levels and repeating them if patient develops recurrent infections.

- ○ **Belimumab**
  - ▪ **Dosage:** Start with 10 mg/kg IV q2 weeks for the first three doses, then q4 weeks thereafter. SC dose is 200 mg once weekly.
  - ▪ **Mechanism:** This is a humanized IgG1λ mAb to human B-lymphocyte stimulator (BLyS), which prevents it from binding its receptors on B cells. BLyS is a major survival signal for B cells, and BLyS blockade attenuates B-cell survival.
  - ▪ **Onset of action:** 8 to 16 weeks
  - ▪ **FDA-approved indication in rheumatology:** SLE. Most effective in patients with active serologies (low C3/C4, elevated anti–double-stranded DNA antibody).
  - ▪ **Side effects:** Nausea/vomiting, diarrhea, chest pain/shortness of breath, depression, anxiety, suicide, migraine headache, nasopharyngitis, bronchitis, and leukopenia may occur. Infection, infusion reactions, and malignancy were not increased over placebo rate.
  - ▪ **Contraindications/precautions:** Do not redose if the patient has had a prior anaphylactic reaction. **FDA pregnancy category: C. Live vaccines should not be administered 30 days prior or concurrently** with belimumab. **FDA pregnancy category: C.** No adequate controlled studies available on pregnant women. Avoid use unless benefits outweigh risks.
- • **T-cell modulating agents**
  - ○ **Abatacept**
    - ▪ **Dosage:** The dose of this IV medication is weight dependent: less than 60 kg: 500 mg; 60 to 100 kg: 750 mg; more than 100 kg: 1,000 mg. Administer it at 0, 2, and 4 weeks, then q4 weeks. SC dosing consists of 125 mg once weekly.
    - ▪ **Mechanism:** It is a fusion protein made up of Fc fragment of IgG1 and extracellular domain of CTLA-4 (cytotoxic T-lymphocyte antigen-4). It binds to CD80/CD86 on antigen-presenting cells, thus preventing T-cell costimulation and activation.
    - ▪ **Onset of action:** 2 months
    - ▪ **FDA-approved indications in rheumatology:** RA, PsA, and polyarticular JIA (inadequate responders to DMARDs)
    - ▪ **Side effects:** Headache, nausea, infection, hypertension, and exacerbations of chronic obstructive pulmonary disease (COPD) may occur.
    - ▪ **Contraindications/precautions:** Avoid with concurrent use of other biologics. Caution with malignancy, infections, and COPD. **FDA pregnancy category: C.** No adequate controlled studies available on pregnant women. Avoid use unless benefits outweigh risks.
- • **Janus kinase (JAK) inhibitors**
  - ○ **Tofacitinib**
    - ▪ **Dosage:** Immediate release: 5 mg PO bid. Extended release: 11 mg once daily. In moderate renal or liver disease, reduce to 5 mg once daily.
    - ▪ **Mechanism:** Small molecule that predominantly inhibits JAK 1 and JAK 3, reducing phosphorylation and activating signal transducers along with transcription of growth factors and cytokines.
    - ▪ **Onset of action:** 4 to 6 weeks
    - ▪ **FDA-approved indications in rheumatology:** RA and PsA. It is also FDA approved for ulcerative colitis.
    - ▪ **Side effects:** Headache, nasopharyngitis, diarrhea, infection, malignancy, lipid abnormalities, and transaminitis may occur.
    - ▪ **Contraindications/precautions:** Avoid with concurrent use of other biologics. Herpes zoster infection may be increased. Stop drug for lymphopenia less than 500/mm^3, absolute neutrophil count (ANC) less than 1,000/mm^3, and hemoglobin drop more than 2 g/dL. Caution with lipid abnormalities drug interactions with rifampin and

ketoconazole/fluconazole. **FDA pregnancy category: C.** No adequate controlled studies available on pregnant women. Avoid use unless benefits outweigh risks.
- **Other JAK inhibitors under investigation:** Peficitinib (JAK 1/JAK 3) and filgotinib (JAK 1)
- **Monitoring:** Baseline purified protein derivative (PPD), hepatitis panel, CBC, CMP, and fasting lipid panel (FLP). Repeat CBC, CMP, and FLP around 6 weeks, then CBC and CMP q3 months thereafter.
○ Baricitinib
  - **Dosage:** 2 mg daily
  - **Mechanism:** Small molecule that predominantly inhibits JAK 1 and JAK 2, reducing phosphorylation and activating signal transducers along with transcription of growth factors and cytokines.
  - **Onset of action:** 4 to 6 weeks
  - **FDA-approved indications in rheumatology:** RA
  - **Side effects:** Upper respiratory tract infection, transaminitis, infection, malignancy, lipid abnormalities, and thrombosis
  - **Contraindications/precautions:** Avoid with concurrent use of other biologics. Risk of herpes zoster infection may be increased. Stop drug for lymphopenia less than 500/mm^3, ANC less than 1,000/mm^3, and hemoglobin drop more than 2 g/dL. Caution with lipid abnormalities and thrombosis. **Pregnancy:** Limited data available, animal reproduction studies showed adverse events.
  - **Monitoring:** Similar to tofacitinib
○ Upadacitinib
  - **Dosage:** 15 mg once daily
  - **Mechanism:** Small molecule that preferentially inhibits JAK-1 over JAK-2, -3, and non-receptor tyrosine-protein kinases, although it is not entirely specific for JAK-1. This inhibition thereby reduces phosphorylation and activates signal transducers along with transcription of growth factors and cytokines.
  - **Onset of Action:** 4-6 weeks
  - **FDA-approved indications in Rheumatology:** RA
  - **Side effects:** Upper respiratory tract infection, nausea, transaminitis, infection, malignancy, lipid abnormalities, thrombosis
  - **Contraindications/precautions:** Avoid with concurrent use of other biologics. Can cause an increased risk of infections, including bacterial, tuberculosis, Herpes zoster and invasive fungal infections. Stop drug for lymphopenia <500/mm3, ANC< 1000/mm3, hemoglobin drop >2g/dL. Caution with lipid abnormalities. Increased thrombosis risk. **Pregnancy:** Limited data available, animal reproduction studies showed in utero exposure may cause fetal harm
  - **Monitoring:** Similar to Tofacitinib[6]
• IL-1 blockade
  ○ Anakinra
    - **Dosage:** 100 mg SC once daily
    - **Mechanism:** It is a recombinant IL-1 receptor antagonist, leading to IL-1 inhibition.
    - **Onset of action:** 1-2 weeks
    - **FDA-approved indications in rheumatology:** RA and neonatal onset multisystem inflammatory disease (NOMID) and acute gout (off-label)
    - **Side effects:** Headache, injection site reactions, infection, nausea, vomiting, diarrhea, abdominal pain, neutropenia, and flulike syndrome may occur.
    - **Contraindications/precautions:** Avoid with concurrent use of other biologics. Caution with renal impairment, malignancy, infections, asthma, and bone marrow suppression. **FDA pregnancy category: B.** No adequate controlled studies available on pregnant women; hence, avoid use unless clearly indicated.

- **Monitoring:** Baseline PPD, CMP, and CBC. CBC monthly for 3 months, then q3 months.
  - ○ Rilonacept
    - ▪ **Dosage:** 320 mg SC loading dose, followed by 160 mg SC weekly
    - ▪ **Mechanism:** Acts as a decoy receptor binding to IL-1β and blocking its signaling. It also binds to IL-1α and IL-1 receptor antagonist with less affinity.
    - ▪ **Onset of action:** 6 weeks
    - ▪ **FDA-approved indication in rheumatology:** Cryopyrin-associated periodic syndromes (CAPSs)
    - ▪ **Side effects:** Injection site reaction, infections, and cough
    - ▪ **Contraindications/precautions:** Avoid with concurrent use of other biologics. Caution with infections, malignancy, hyperlipidemia, asthma, and bone marrow suppression. **FDA pregnancy category: C.** No adequate controlled studies available on pregnant women. Animal studies showed fetal harm.
  - ○ Canakinumab
    - ▪ **Dosage:** more than 40 kg: 150 mg SC q8 weeks
    - ▪ **Mechanism:** Recombinant, humanized IL-1β mAb of the IgG1/κ isotype
    - ▪ **Onset of action:** 8 days
    - ▪ **FDA-approved indications in rheumatology:** CAPS, TRAPS, Muckle–Wells syndrome, hyper-IgD periodic fever syndrome, mevalonate kinase deficiency, familial cold urticaria, systemic JIA, and familial Mediterranean fever
    - ▪ **Side effects:** Nasopharyngitis, diarrhea, vertigo, and injection site reactions
    - ▪ **Contraindications/precautions:** Avoid with concurrent use of other biologics. Caution with infections, malignancy, and bone marrow suppression. **FDA pregnancy category: C.** No adequate controlled studies available on pregnant women. Avoid use unless clearly needed.
- **IL-6 blockade**
  - ○ Tocilizumab
    - ▪ **Dosage:** For IV use, start with 4 mg/kg q4 weeks. The dose can increase to 8 mg/kg, up to 800-mg infusion. For SC usage, give 162 mg SC weekly for more than 100 kg and 162 mg SC every other week for less than 100 kg.
    - ▪ **Mechanism:** It is a humanized IL-6 receptor inhibitor that binds to both the soluble and membrane-bound IL-6 receptors, hindering IL-6–mediated signaling.
    - ▪ **Onset of action:** 2 weeks
    - ▪ **FDA-approved indications in rheumatology:** RA, systemic and polyarticular JIA, and giant cell arteritis
    - ▪ **Side effects:** Headache, infusion or injection site reactions, infection, nausea, vomiting, diarrhea, abdominal pain, hepatotoxicity, rash, hypertriglyceridemia, and **GI perforation** (especially with concurrent NSAID use) may occur.
    - ▪ **Contraindications/precautions:** Avoid concurrent use with other biologics. There is a **boxed warning** for infections, including TB. Avoid use in patients taking NSAIDs, or with a history of diverticulosis or peptic ulcer disease, active hepatic disease, or hepatic impairment. Patients should be monitored for bone marrow suppression and demyelinating disease. **FDA pregnancy category: C.** No adequate controlled studies available on pregnant women.
    - ▪ **Monitoring:** CBC, CMP, and lipid panel should be checked at baseline and q4 to 8 weeks (lipid panel can be checked q6 months following initiation).
      - □ If transaminases more than 1 to 3× ULN, reduce dose to 4 mg/kg or hold therapy until they normalize. If transaminases more than 3 to 5× ULN, discontinue until they are less than 3× ULN, then resume at 4 mg/kg. If increase is persistent, permanently discontinue therapy.

- □ If transaminases more than 5× ULN, discontinue therapy. If ANC 500 to 1,000 cells/mm³, hold therapy until ANC more than 1,000 cell/mm³ and restart at 4 mg/kg. If ANC less than 500 cells/mm³, discontinue therapy.
  - □ If platelets 50,000 to 100,000 cells/mm³, hold therapy until platelets more than 100,000 cell/mm³ and restart at 4 mg/kg. If platelets less than 50,000 cells/mm³, discontinue therapy.
  - □ **Other IL-6 blockers:** Sarilumab
- ○ **Sarilumab**
  - ▪ **Dosage:** 200 mg SC every 2 weeks. Can reduce dose to 150 mg SC every two weeks if neutropenia, transaminitis or thrombocytopenia occur.
  - ▪ **Mechanism:** Humanized IL-6 receptor inhibitor that binds to both the soluble and membrane-bound IL-6 receptors, hindering IL-6–mediated signaling.
  - ▪ **Onset of Action:** 2 weeks
  - ▪ **FDA-approved indications in Rheumatology:** RA
  - ▪ **Side effects:** Hepatotoxicity, injection site reactions, hypertriglyceridemia, infection, neutropenia/leukopenia, thrombocytopenia and rarely GI perforation (especially with concurrent NSAID or steroid use) may occur.
  - ▪ **Contraindications/precautions:** Avoid concurrent use with other biologics. There is a boxed warning for infections, including TB. Avoid use in patients taking NSAIDs, or with a history of diverticulosis or peptic ulcer disease, active hepatic disease, or hepatic impairment. Patients should be monitored for bone marrow suppression and elevation in lipid levels.
  - ▪ **FDA pregnancy category: C.** There are no adequate controlled studies available on pregnant women.
  - ▪ **Monitoring:** Similar to Tocilizumab[7]
- • **IL-12 and IL-23 blockade**
  - ○ **Ustekinumab**
    - ▪ **Dosage:** ≤100 kg: 45 mg SC at 0 and 4 weeks, q12 weeks thereafter; more than 100 kg: 90 mg at 0 and 4 weeks, q12 weeks thereafter
    - ▪ **Mechanism:** Humanized IgG1/κ mAb that binds to the P40 subunit of IL-12 and IL-23, preventing their binding to shared receptor.
    - ▪ **Onset of action:** 2 weeks
    - ▪ **FDA-approved indications in rheumatology:** Psoriasis and PsA. It is also FDA approved for Crohn's disease.
    - ▪ **Side effects:** Nasopharyngitis, nonmelanoma skin cancers, and mycobacterial, fungal, and salmonella infections
    - ▪ **Contraindication/precautions:** Avoid concurrent use with other biologics. Caution with infections, malignancy, and, rarely, reversible posterior leukoencephalopathy syndrome (RPLS). **FDA pregnancy category: B.** No adequate controlled studies available on pregnant women. Use only if benefits outweigh risks.
- • **IL-17 blockade**
  - ○ **Secukinumab**
    - ▪ **Dosage:** 150 mg SC at 0, 1, 2, 3, and 4 weeks, followed by 150 mg SC q4 weeks. Can also increase to 300 mg SC q4 weeks depending on clinical response.
    - ▪ **Mechanism:** Humanized IgG1 mAb that binds to IL-17A
    - ▪ **Onset of action:** 1 week. Half-life of 22 to 31 days
    - ▪ **FDA-approved indication in rheumatology:** Psoriasis, PsA, and AS
    - ▪ **Side effects:** Nasopharyngitis, diarrhea, and infections
    - ▪ **Contraindications/precautions:** Avoid use in inflammatory bowel disease, infections, and concurrent use of biologics. **FDA pregnancy category: B.** No adequate controlled studies available on pregnant women. Use only if benefits outweigh risks.

○ Ixekizumab
- **Dosage:** 160 mg once, followed by 80 mg at weeks 2, 4, 6, 8, 10, and 12, and 80 mg monthly afterward
- **Mechanism:** Humanized IgG4 mAb that binds to IL-17A
- **Onset of action:** 4 days
- **FDA-approved indication in rheumatology:** Psoriasis and PsA
- **Side effects:** Infection and neutropenia
- **Contraindications/precautions:** Avoid use in inflammatory bowel disease, infections, and concurrent use of biologics. **FDA pregnancy category: C.** No adequate controlled studies available on pregnant women.

• **Complement-targeted therapy**
  ○ Eculizumab
  - **Dosage:** For atypical hemolytic–uremic syndrome (AHUS), start with 900 mg weekly with four doses followed by 1,200 mg at week 5 and q2 weeks thereafter.
  - **Mechanism:** Humanized mAb that attaches with high affinity to complement protein C5, inhibiting its cleavage to C5a and C5b, thus preventing the development of the terminal complement complex C5b-9 (MAC complex).
  - **Onset of action:** ≤1 week
  - **FDA-approved indications in rheumatology:** AHUS. It is also FDA approved for paroxysmal nocturnal hemoglobinuria and generalized myasthenia gravis.
  - **Side effects:** Headache, infusion reactions, infections, diarrhea, and leukopenia
  - **Contraindications/precautions:** Meningococcemia is a feared side effect, avoid in unvaccinated patients (unless risk of treatment delay outweighs benefits). **FDA pregnancy category: C.** No adequate controlled studies available on pregnant women. Use only if benefits outweigh risks.

• **Phosphodiesterase inhibitor**
  ○ Apremilast
  - **Dosage:** Start at 10 mg/day with uptitration to 30 mg PO bid.
  - **Mechanism:** Phosphodiesterase 4 (PDE4) inhibitor, resulting in increased intracellular cyclic adenosine monophosphate (cAMP) levels
  - **Onset of action:** 4 weeks
  - **FDA-approved indications in rheumatology:** Psoriasis and PsA
  - **Side effects:** Diarrhea, nausea, and headache
  - **Contraindications/precautions:** Caution of weight loss and suicidal risk in patients with depression. **FDA pregnancy category: C.** No adequate controlled studies available on pregnant women. Use only if benefits outweigh risks.
  - **Can combine with another biologic if needed**

BIOSIMILARS

Biosimilars are biologics produced by a different manufacturer from the original innovator, which are similar in quality, safety, and efficacy to the original biologic. They are not identical to the original products, having no access to the originator's purification process; hence, concerns of safety and efficacy have been raised. A 2016 systematic review of various clinical trials and observational studies supports similar clinical responses and adverse events for these drugs when compared to their reference products.[8]

GOUT MEDICATIONS

• Understanding which medications should be used during **flares** versus **maintenance periods** is the key to treating gout (see Chapter 21).

- In general, drugs used for acute flares possess anti-inflammatory activity, while maintenance drugs work on reducing uric acid levels either by reducing uric acid synthesis (xanthine oxidase inhibitors) or increasing uric acid excretion (uricosuric agents).
- **Treatment of acute flares:**
  - GCs (see the section "Glucocorticoids" above)
  - NSAIDs/COX-2 inhibitors (see the section "NSAIDs/COX-2 inhibitors" above). **Avoid use of aspirin** because of the paradoxical effect of salicylates on serum urate (uric acid retention at low doses and uricosuria at high doses).
  - Colchicine
    - **Dosage:** Flare treatment—start with 1.2 mg PO, followed by 0.6 mg PO 1 hour later (most effective in the first few hours of gout flare). Then, 0.6 mg PO bid for the next 1 or 2 days, followed by several days of 0.6 mg PO qday. Prophylaxis—0.6 mg PO qday or bid. For creatinine clearance less than 30 mL/min, reduce dosage to 0.3 mg once daily or 0.6 mg q48h.
    - **Mechanism:** Colchicine impedes β-tubulin polymerization into microtubules. This leads to decreased migration of neutrophils to an inflamed area.
    - **Side effects:** Abdominal pain, nausea, vomiting, diarrhea, pharyngolaryngeal pain, hepatotoxicity, bone marrow suppression, and myotoxicity (including rhabdomyolysis) may occur and are generally dose related.
    - **Contraindications/precautions:** Avoid use when concurrently administered with strong CYO3A4 inhibitors or P-glycoprotein in the presence of hepatic or renal impairment. Use caution with renal and liver impairment, bone marrow dysfunction, use of protease inhibitors, cyclosporine, diltiazem, verapamil, fibrates, and statins. **FDA pregnancy category: C.** No adequate controlled studies available on pregnant women. Use only if benefits outweigh risks.
  - Anakinra (**off-label use;** see also under Biologics: IL-1 blockade above).
    - **Dosage:** 100 mg SC daily for 3 days
- **Long-term treatment**
  - Allopurinol
    - **Dosage:** The range is 50 to 800 mg PO daily, and dose is adjusted to maintain serum uric acid less than 6 mg/dL. Doses more than 300 mg should be divided into 2 doses. **Do not begin therapy during acute gouty flares. If a flare occurs in a patient already taking allopurinol, continue allopurinol.**
    - **Mechanism:** It inhibits xanthine oxidase, thereby reducing uric acid production.
    - **Side effects:** Rash may occur and may be associated with life-threatening complications of **toxic epidermal necrolysis and allopurinol hypersensitivity syndrome** (AHS), which presents as rash, fever, hepatitis, eosinophilia, and acute renal failure. This syndrome is associated with HLA-B*58:01 and is more commonly seen in Korean, Han Chinese, and Thai patients.[9] Gout flares, diarrhea, nausea, hepatotoxicity, and, rarely, bone marrow suppression may also occur.
    - **Contraindications/precautions:** Use with caution with renal and liver impairment, bone marrow dysfunction, use of angiotensin-converting enzyme (ACE) inhibitors or diuretics (because of increased risk of hypersensitivity), amoxicillin or ampicillin (because of rash risk), or azathioprine or mercaptopurine (bone marrow suppression). **FDA pregnancy category: C.** No adequate controlled studies available on pregnant women. Use only if benefits outweigh risks.
    - **Monitoring:** Check serum uric acid levels q4 to 6 weeks while dose adjustments are being made. Once uric acid goal is reached, then can check a uric acid level q6 months to 1 year afterward. CBC and CMP can be done intermittently.
  - Febuxostat
    - **Dosage:** The range is 40 to 80 mg PO once daily. **Do not begin therapy during acute gouty flares. If a flare occurs in a patient already taking febuxostat, continue**

febuxostat. Use in patients who fail to respond to allopurinol or have severe allopurinol toxicity.

- **Mechanism:** It inhibits xanthine oxidase, thereby reducing uric acid production. Unlike allopurinol, it is not a purine base analog.
- **Side effects:** Hepatotoxicity, nausea, arthralgia, gout flares, and rash may occur.
- **Contraindications/precautions:** Avoid use in severe renal and liver impairment, **cardiovascular disease,** azathioprine, or mercaptopurine.
- **Monitoring:** Obtain CMP at baseline, 2 months after initiation and then intermittently. **FDA pregnancy category: C.** No adequate controlled studies available on pregnant women. Use only if benefits outweigh risks.

○ Probenecid
- **Dosage:** Start at 250 mg PO bid for 1 week, then either 250 to 500 mg/day or 500 mg/month up to a maximum dose of 2 to 3 g/day. **Do not begin therapy during acute gouty flares. If a flare occurs in a patient already taking probenecid, continue probenecid.**
- **Mechanism:** This is a uricosuric drug, which competitively inhibits reabsorption of uric acid at the proximal convoluted tubule.
- **Side effects:** Rash, gout flares, GI intolerance, and uric acid stone formation may occur.
- **Contraindications/precautions:** Use with caution with renal impairment, peptic ulcer disease, and concurrent use of penicillins and salicylates. **Pregnancy category: B.** Probenecid crosses the placenta; however, animal reproduction studies have not shown it to cause harm to the fetus. No adequate controlled studies in pregnant women.
- **Monitoring:** Prior to initiation, 24-hour urinary uric acid can be checked to identify under-excreters (<700 mg) who are good candidates for therapy. Serum uric acid levels can be monitored until the goal is achieved. CBC and CMP can be checked intermittently.

○ Lesinurad
- **Dosage:** 200 mg PO once daily (can combine use with xanthine oxidase inhibitor)
- **Mechanism:** Inhibits function of renal urate reabsorption transporters (URAT1 and OAT4)
- **Side effects:** Headache, acid reflux, gout flare, and renal failure
- **Contraindications/precautions:** There is a **boxed** warning of acute renal failure, which was more common when lesinurad was given alone. **FDA pregnancy category:** No adequate controlled studies in pregnant women.
- **Monitoring:** Uric acid can be monitored q2 to 5 weeks until the goal is achieved, and CMP can be checked periodically.

○ Pegloticase
- **Dosage:** 8 mg IV q2 weeks. Use as induction therapy in severe tophaceous gout and excessive hyperuricemia
- **Mechanism:** Recombinant mammalian uricase biologic that converts uric acid to allantoin, which is significantly more soluble
- **Side effects:** Anaphylaxis (7%), infusion reactions (urticaria, dyspnea, chest discomfort), and gout flares
- **Contraindications/precautions:** There is a **boxed** warning of **anaphylaxis** and infusion reactions. Premedicate with antihistamines and glucocorticoids, and closely monitor serum uric acid levels prior to each infusion. Discontinue therapy if uric acid levels more than 6 mg/dL, on two consecutive draws, as this indicates the formation of **anti-pegloticase antibodies** and increases the risk of an infusion reaction. Avoid use of concomitant urate-lowering therapy, which may mask antibody-mediated

increases in uric acid. Pegloticase is contraindicated in **G6PD deficiency** (hemolysis, methemoglobinemia). Rare occurrence of exacerbation of heart failure. **FDA pregnancy category: C.** No adequate controlled studies available on pregnant women. Use only if benefits outweigh risks.

- **Monitoring:** Serum uric acid and G6PD levels as indicated above

OSTEOPOROSIS MEDICATIONS

- Virtually, all patients with rheumatic diseases are at risk for osteoporosis, especially those on long-term GC therapy.
- Treatment options include calcium and vitamin D supplementation, bisphosphonates, calcitonin, hormone replacement therapy, parathyroid hormone (PTH) supplementation, and receptor activator of nuclear factor κ-B ligand (RANKL) inhibition.

Vitamin and Mineral Supplementation

- **Calcium carbonate**
  - **Dosage:** 1,000 to 1,200 mg PO qday (elemental calcium). This should be taken with food to improve absorption.
  - **Mechanism:** Supplementation of nutritional element
  - **Side effects:** Abdominal pain, nausea, vomiting, diarrhea or constipation, flatulence, hypophosphatemia, hypercalcemia, milk–alkali syndrome, and renal failure may occur.
  - **Contraindications/precautions:** Avoid use in hypoparathyroid patients and those with a history of calcium-containing renal stones. Additional supplementation over the recommended daily allowance has resulted in increased cardiovascular disease.[10]
  - **Special considerations:** For those on a proton pump inhibitor (PPI) or an H_2 blocker for gastroesophageal reflux disease (GERD), use of **calcium citrate** is recommended.
- **Vitamin D** (D3 = cholecalciferol, D2 = ergocalciferol)
  - **Dosage:** Cholecalciferol: 800 to 1,000 IU/day, unless 25-hydroxyvitamin D [25(OH)D] levels are low (<30). Then, given ergocalciferol 50,000 IU once weekly to once monthly.
  - **Mechanism:** Supplementation
  - **Side effects:** Hypercalcemia, hypercalciuria, and nephrolithiasis may occur.
  - **Contraindications/precautions:** Use with caution in those with hypercalcemia, sarcoidosis, or malabsorption syndrome.
  - **Special considerations:** Some data suggest that cholecalciferol increases 25(OH)D levels more effectively than ergocalciferol. Calcitriol (1,25-dihydroxycholecalciferol) also increases 25(OH)D levels but frequently causes hypercalcemia and/or hypercalciuria, and its use is not recommended (except in chronic dialysis).

Bisphosphonates

- General principles
  - **Mechanism:** These drugs inhibit bone resorption by their actions on osteoclasts and osteoclast precursors.
  - All bisphosphonates should be given on an empty stomach because absorption of drug is less than 1% of dose. Patients are advised to remain upright for 30 minutes to minimize the risk of reflux.
  - Caution is advised with patients experiencing upper GI disease or esophagitis, and chronic kidney disease. If creatinine clearance is less than 30 to 35 mL/minute, avoid use.
  - Limit treatment to 3 to 5 years maximum to reduce risk of **atypical fractures of the femur.** However, recent studies support continuation of bisphosphonate use in patients with persistently increased risk of fracture.[11]
  - Regarding pregnancy, there are no adequate controlled studies available on pregnant women.

- Oral formulations
  - **Class side effects:** Hypocalcemia, hypophosphatemia, headache, GERD, abdominal pain, nausea, diarrhea/constipation, myalgias, and arthralgias
  - **Contraindications/precautions:** Avoid use in those with stage 3 or greater chronic kidney disease, hypocalcemia, and esophageal abnormalities, which would delay esophageal emptying, and those who cannot remain upright for at least 30 minutes after administration. Use caution in those who experience musculoskeletal pain and GI irritation, or have had recent oral surgery (need dental examination prior to therapy because of risk of osteonecrosis of the jaw).
  - **Alendronate:** Dosage: 10 mg PO qday or 70 mg PO qweek. For prophylaxis, 5 mg PO qday or 35 mg PO qweek.
  - **Risedronate:** Dosage: 5 mg PO qday, 35 mg PO qweek, or 150 mg PO qmonth
  - **Ibandronate:** Dosage: 2.5 mg PO qday or 150 mg PO qmonth. Also, IV formulation (see below)
- IV formulations
  - **Class side effects:** A self-limited flulike reaction lasting 3 to 4 days is common after infusion. Bone pain, edema, hypertension, fatigue, fever, headache, hypocalcemia, renal failure, dyspnea, GERD, abdominal pain, diarrhea/constipation, nausea, myalgias, and arthralgias may occur.
  - **Contraindications/precautions:** Avoid use in those with stage 3 or greater chronic kidney disease or hypocalcemia. Use caution in those who experience musculoskeletal pain, GI irritation, and recent oral surgery (dental examination prior to therapy because of risk of osteonecrosis of the jaw). Patients with aspirin-sensitive asthma may develop bronchospasm from taking zoledronic acid.
  - **Ibandronate:** Dosage: 3 mg IV q3 months
  - **Zoledronic acid:** Dosage: 5 mg IV annually
  - **Pamidronate:** Dosage: 60 mg IV q3 months

Selective Estrogen Receptor Modulators

- **Raloxifene**
  - **Dosage:** 60 mg PO qday
  - **Mechanism:** It binds to estrogen receptors, exhibiting both agonist and antagonist properties, inhibiting bone resorption. It also reduces total and low-density lipoprotein (LDL) cholesterol (but not the risk of coronary artery disease [CAD]) and reduces risk of breast cancer.
  - **Side effects:** Hot flashes, flulike syndrome, infections, leg cramps, arthralgias, edema, **venous thromboembolic disease**, and fatal stroke may occur.
  - **Contraindications/precautions:** There is a **boxed warning** for stroke risk and thromboembolic disease. Use with caution in those who have renal or liver impairment, hypertriglyceridemia, concurrent estrogen therapy, and unexplained uterine bleeding. Contraindicated in pregnancy.

Parathyroid Hormone Therapy

- **Teriparatide**
  - **Dosage:** 20 μg SC qday
  - **Mechanism:** This is an "anabolic" agent, which stimulates bone growth and activates bone remodeling. It stimulates pre-osteoblasts to mature into osteoblasts.
  - **Side effects:** Hypercalcemia, hypercalciuria, hypotension, tachycardia, muscle cramps, and hyperuricemia may occur, and there is a theoretical risk of osteosarcoma.
  - **Contraindications/precautions:** There is a **boxed warning** for **osteosarcoma risk.** Use with caution in those who have renal or liver impairment, coronary artery disease, and urolithiasis. Limit use to 2 years. **FDA pregnancy category: C.** There are no adequate controlled studies available on pregnant women.

RANK Ligand Therapy

- **Denosumab**
  - **Dosage:** 60 mg SC q6 months
  - **Mechanism:** This is a humanized mAb to RANKL that reduces osteoclastogenesis, leading to decreased bone resorption.
  - **Side effects:** Musculoskeletal pain, dermatitis, eczema, hypercholesterolemia, cystitis, infections, and hypocalcemia may occur.
  - **Contraindications/precautions:** Do not use in hypocalcemic patients. Use with caution in those with renal impairment. Contraindicated in pregnancy.

Other Therapies

- **Calcitonin**
  - **Dosage:** 200 IU intranasally (one nostril) qday, or 100 IU SC/IM qday.
  - **Mechanism:** It binds to osteoclasts and prevents bone resorption.
  - **Side effects:** Rhinitis, flushing, nausea, and musculoskeletal pain are fairly common. Nasal mucosal erosion may develop with intranasal administration, particularly in those older than 65 years.
  - **Contraindications/precautions:** Temporarily discontinue if nasal ulcers develop. Calcitonin nasal spray was recently removed from the European market because of prostate cancer risk; however, a review by the FDA found no conclusive evidence to discontinue this drug. **FDA pregnancy category: C.** There are no adequate controlled studies available on pregnant women.
- Upcoming osteoporotic therapies
  - **Romosozumab:** Humanized mAb that blocks sclerostin, which is an osteoblast inhibitor.

REFERENCES

1. Schimmer BP, Parker KL. Adrenocorticotropic hormone; adrenocortical steroids and their synthetic analogs; inhibitors of the synthesis and actions of adrenocortical hormones. In: Brunton LL, Lazo J, Parker K, eds. *The Pharmacological Basis of Therapeutics*. Vol. 11. New York, NY: McGraw-Hill; 2005:27–28.
2. Buttgereit F, Burmester GR. Glucocorticoids. In: Klippel JH, Stone JH, Crofford LJ, et al., eds. *Primer on the Rheumatic Diseases*. 13th ed. New York, NY: Springer Science+Business Media; 2008:644–650.
3. Marmor MF, Kellner U, Lai TY, et al. Recommendations on screening for chloroquine and hydroxychloroquine retinopathy (2016) revision. *Ophthalmology*. 2016;123(6):1386–1394.
4. West SG. *Rheumatology Secrets*. 3rd ed. Philadelphia, PA: Elsevier; 2015:633.
5. Diak P, Siegel J, Grenade LL, et al. Tumor necrosis factor alpha blockers and malignancy in children: forty-eight cases reported to the Food and Drug Administration. *Arthritis Rheum.* 2010;62(8):2517–2524.
6. FDA. Drugs@FDA: FDA-Approved Drugs. https://www.accessdata.fda.gov/scripts/cder/daf/index.cfm?event=overview.process&varApplNo=211675
7. FDA. Reference ID: 4101405. https://www.accessdata.fda.gov/drugsatfda_docs/label/2017/761037s000lbl.pdf
8. Chingcuanco F, Segal JB, Kim SC, et al. Bioequivalence of biosimilar tumor necrosis factor-α inhibitors compared with their reference biologics: A systematic review. *Ann Intern Med.* 2016;165(8):565–574.
9. Dean L. Allopurinol therapy and HLA-B*58:01 genotype. Medical genetics summaries [Internet]. Created: March 26, 2013; Last Update: March 16, 2016. https://www.ncbi.nlm.nih.gov/books/NBK127547/. Last accessed 11/5/19.
10. Anderson JB, Kruszka B, Delaney JA, et al. Calcium intake from diet and supplements and the risk of coronary artery calcification and it's progression among older adults: 10-year follow up of the Multi-Ethnic Study of Atherosclerosis (MESA). *J Am Heart Assoc.* 2016;5(10):1–13.
11. Black DM, Schwartz AV, Ensrud KE. Effects of continuing or stopping alendronate after 5 years of treatment: the Fracture Intervention Trial Long-term Extension (FLEX): a randomized trial. *JAMA.* 2006;296(24):2927–2938.

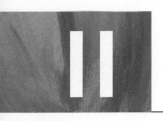

Core Rheumatologic Diseases

Rheumatoid Arthritis

Jaime Flores-Ruiz and Prabha Ranganathan

10

GENERAL PRINCIPLES

Definitions

- Rheumatoid arthritis (RA) is an **inflammatory symmetric polyarthritis**, which untreated can lead to erosions, joint space loss, and destruction of the affected joints.
- RA causes progressive disability, systemic complications, and early death.
- On rare occasions, RA is self-limited but more often is chronic, disabling, and sometimes associated with **systemic manifestations**.

Epidemiology

- RA affects approximately 0.5% to 1% of the adult population.[1]
- The incidence of RA increases with **age** and is four to five times higher in **females** than that in males younger than 50 years but older than 60 to 70 years, the female-to-male ratio is only about 2:1.[2,3]
- Certain shared epitopes in the DR1 allele of the class II major histocompatibility (MHC) region are associated with RA susceptibility, severity, and treatment response.[4]

Etiology

Etiology is unknown. It has been hypothesized that a combination of genetics and environmental triggers (including smoking and infection) leads to inflammation and autoimmunity.[5]

Pathophysiology

- Although the etiology of RA is still unknown, there have been major strides in understanding how the inflammatory process leads to joint destruction.
- Evidence supports initial T-cell activation triggered by an unknown antigen, leading to joint inflammation and destruction.
- RA is characterized by **synovial inflammation** with hyperplasia and increased vascularity (**pannus formation**). The synovium shows leukocytic infiltration, increased expression of adhesion molecules, proteolytic enzymes, cytokines (including tumor necrosis factor [TNF]-α and interleukins [IL]-1, 6, and 17), and activated T and B cells. These provide potential targets for blockade and therapy.[5]
- B lymphocytes act as antigen-presenting cells in the synovium. They also produce antibodies and secrete pro-inflammatory cytokines. B-cell depletion therapy has been shown to be beneficial in patients with RA.
- The synovial membrane enlarges to become the pannus and begins to invade the cartilage and bone. Finally, proliferation of the pannus leads to profound cartilage destruction, subchondral bone erosions, and periarticular ligament laxity. Cytokine-stimulated osteoclast activity also contributes to the **erosions and periarticular osteopenia** found in RA.
- Various citrullinated proteins are present in the rheumatoid joint, including fibrinogen, collagen, and fibronectin, and have recently been implicated in the pathophysiology of RA. The process of citrullination involves conversion of arginine to citrulline by the

enzyme peptidylarginine deiminase (PADI). Of the four isoforms, PADI 2 and PADI 4 are most abundant in the inflamed synovium. In RA, increased citrullination occurs in the inflamed synovium, and antibodies directed against these citrullinated proteins (**anti–cyclic citrullinated peptide [anti-CCP] antibodies**) are produced by resident B cells.

DIAGNOSIS

Clinical Presentation

History

- The presentation and course of RA is variable. Typically, patients present with an insidious onset of **symmetric joint pain, swelling, and morning stiffness** worsening over several weeks. Less common presentations include acute, rapidly progressive polyarthritis and, more rarely, monoarthritis.
- RA commonly involves the **small joints of the hands** (wrists, metacarpophalangeal [MCP] joints, and proximal interphalangeal [PIP] joints) **and feet** (metatarsophalangeal [MTP] joints). Large joints can also be involved and include the shoulder, knee, ankle, elbow, and hip.
- The severity and duration of morning stiffness often correlates with the overall disease activity.
- Generalized malaise and fatigue can often accompany active inflammation.
- Through the course of RA, patients often experience a waxing and waning pattern of synovitis coupled with progressive structural damage, leading to significant deformities and disabilities with advanced disease. Extensive joint damage can lead to functional limitations in joints as well as neurologic compromise, leading to symptoms of muscle weakness and atrophy.
- Most of the articular destruction occurs in the early years of disease. Hence, it is **important to diagnose and treat RA early**.

Physical Examination

- Physical findings in RA involve the identification of symmetric joint inflammation early in the course of the disease and manifestations of joint destruction with chronic disease.
- Active **synovitis** is characterized by warmth, swelling, pain, and palpable effusions. **Synovial proliferation** is appreciated on physical examination by the presence of soft or rubbery tissue around the joint margins. **Joint warmth** is frequently appreciated, although redness is uncommon.
- **Range of motion** can be restricted in the joints with significant effusions, including deeper joints that may not demonstrate other signs of inflammation. Chronic joint destruction with significant degree of cartilage loss produces **crepitus** on palpation.
- Specific articular manifestations follow:
  - The **wrists** are involved in most patients and, over time, can lead to radial–ulnar subluxation and subluxation of carpal bones with radial deviation. Synovitis at the wrist can lead to **median nerve entrapment,** resulting in carpal tunnel syndrome (CTS) or, more rarely, **ulnar nerve entrapment,** resulting in Guyon's canal syndrome.
  - In the **hands,** the **MCPs** are commonly involved and, with extensive damage, may lead to **ulnar deviation** of the hand. The **PIP** joints are often involved with **sparing of distal interphalangeal (DIP) joints.** Chronic inflammation with destruction of surrounding tendons can lead to **Z-shaped thumb** (hyperextension of first interphalangeal joints with palmar subluxation of first MCP), **swan-neck** (hyperextension at PIP, flexion at DIP), and **boutonniere** (flexion at PIP, hyperextension of DIP) deformities. Tenosynovitis of finger tendon sheaths can lead to nodule formation with subsequent catching or tendon rupture.

- **Elbow** involvement is evident by fullness at the radial–humeral joint with the tendency of patients to maintain the joint in flexion. Over time, this can lead to flexion contractures. In addition, inflammation can lead to **compressive neuropathy of the ulnar nerve** with paresthesias and weakness in the ulnar distribution.
  - Involvement of the **shoulder** usually manifests as loss of range of motion, with decreased abduction and limited rotation. Effusions are difficult to appreciate because the shoulder joint lies underneath the rotator cuff. Pain in the shoulder can lead to limited range of motion, and adhesive capsulitis, or frozen shoulder, can develop rapidly.
  - **Cervical spine** involvement with RA is common. Inflammation with involvement of the odontoid process, lateral masses, or tenosynovitis of the transverse ligament can lead to **C1–C2 cervical instability.** This may manifest with neck stiffness, with decreased range of motion. Compression of the cord, nerve roots, or vertebral arteries can occur, leading to neurologic compromise, and may require emergent stabilization. RA involvement of the thoracic and the lumbar spine is rare.
  - **Hip** involvement with RA is also common, but symptoms are often delayed. When present, examination findings include decreased range of motion and pain radiating to the groin, thigh, buttock, low back, or knee.
  - Involvement of the **knee** includes detectable effusions and synovial thickening. Prolonged inflammation can lead to significant instability. Posterior herniation of the joint capsule can result in a **popliteal (Baker's) cyst,** and rupture can mimic thrombophlebitis.
  - Because these are weight-bearing joints, RA involvement of the **foot and ankle** is often symptomatic. The joints most commonly affected include the MTP, talonavicular, and ankle joints. MTP joints can develop cock-up deformities with subluxation of the MTP fat pads, causing pain with ambulation. Inflammation of the talonavicular joint and ankle joints results in eversion of the foot and can cause nerve entrapment, resulting in paresthesias of the sole.
- With the discovery of more effective treatments, extra-articular manifestations of RA occur much less commonly than in previous decades. However, severe RA can manifest with sequelae of systemic inflammation, especially in rheumatoid factor (RF)–positive patients. Common extra-articular manifestations follow:
  - **Skin** manifestations include formation of subcutaneous **rheumatoid nodules and vasculitic skin ulcerations.** Rheumatoid nodules typically form during active inflammation over pressure points in the bursae and tendon sheaths. Common sites include the olecranon bursa, the extensor surface of the forearm, the Achilles tendon, and the tendons of the fingers.
  - **Ocular** involvement usually involves **sicca symptoms** of dry eyes (and dry mouth in Sjögren's syndrome) but can include **episcleritis** or a more concerning **scleritis** and scleromalacia perforans.
  - **Pulmonary** involvement of RA may include interstitial fibrosis, pulmonary nodules, pleuritis, or bronchiolitis obliterans organizing pneumonia. Interstitial fibrosis generally involves the lower lung fields and is often not clinically symptomatic, but it may be severely debilitating in some cases.
  - **Neurologic** manifestations of RA are usually related to nerve entrapment or cervical spine instability. Vasculitis of vasa vasorum can lead to symptoms of **mononeuritis multiplex.**
  - **Cardiac** involvement may include pericardial effusions, pericarditis, valvular lesions, conduction defects, or cardiomyopathy.
  - **Gastrointestinal (GI)** and **renal** manifestations of RA are rare. Amyloidosis can sometimes occur, affecting these organs.
  - Hepatic involvement may include nodular regenerative hyperplasia or portal fibrosis.
  - Hematologic effects of RA include hypochromic–microcytic anemia, **Felty's syndrome** (the triad of leukopenia, lymphadenopathy, and splenomegaly), cryoglobulinemia, and the large granular lymphocyte syndrome.

Diagnostic Criteria

- The diagnosis of RA involves the accumulation of clinical, laboratory, and radiologic features that develop over the course of the disease. Early RA is often difficult to diagnose definitively, yet it can usually be confirmed as the disease progresses.
- The American College of Rheumatology/European League Against Rheumatism classification criteria for RA are presented in Table 10-1.[6]

TABLE 10-1	THE 2010 AMERICAN COLLEGE OF RHEUMATOLOGY/EUROPEAN LEAGUE AGAINST RHEUMATISM CLASSIFICATION CRITERIA FOR RHEUMATOID ARTHRITIS	
Target population (Who should be tested?):		**Score**
1. Patients with at least 1 joint with definite clinical synovitis (swelling)[a]		
2. Patients with the synovitis not better explained by another disease[b]		
Classification criteria for RA (score-based algorithm: Add score of categories A–D; a score of ≥6/10 is needed for classification of a patient as having definite RA)[c]		
A. Joint involvement[d]		
1 large joint[e]		0
2–10 large joints		1
1–3 small joints (with or without involvement of large joints)[f]		2
4–10 small joints (with or without involvement of large joints)		3
>10 joints (at least 1 small joint)[g]		5
B. Serology (at least 1 test result is needed for classification)[h]		
Negative RF and negative anti-CCP antibody		0
Low-positive RF or low-positive anti-CCP antibody		2
High-positive RF or high-positive anti-CCP antibody		3
C. Acute-phase reactants (at least 1 test result is needed for classification)[i]		
Normal CRP and normal ESR		0
Abnormal CRP or abnormal ESR		1
D. Duration of symptoms[j]		
<6 weeks		0
≥6 weeks		1

[a]The criteria are aimed at classification of newly presenting patients. In addition, patients with erosive disease typical of rheumatoid arthritis (RA) with a history compatible with prior fulfillment of the 2010 criteria should be classified as having RA. Patients with long-standing disease, including those whose disease is inactive (with or without treatment) who, based on retrospectively available data, have previously fulfilled the 2010 criteria, should be classified as having RA.

[b]Differential diagnoses vary among patients with different presentations but may include conditions such as systemic lupus erythematosus, psoriatic arthritis, and gout. If it is unclear about the relevant differential diagnoses to consider, an expert rheumatologist should be consulted.

cAlthough patients with a score of <6 of 10 are not classifiable as having RA, their status can be reassessed, and the criteria might be fulfilled cumulatively over time.

dJoint involvement refers to any swollen or tender joint on examination, which may be confirmed by imaging evidence of synovitis. DIP joints, first carpometacarpal joints, and first MTP joints are excluded from assessment. Categories of joint distribution are classified according to the location and number of involved joints, with placement into the highest category possible based on the pattern of joint involvement.

e"Large joints" refer to the shoulders, elbow, hips, knees, and ankles.

f"Small joints" refer to the MCP joints, proximal interphalangeal joints, second through fifth MTP joints, thumb interphalangeal joints, and wrist.

gIn this category, at least one of the involved joints must be a small joint; the other joints can include any combination of large and additional small joints, as well as other joints not specifically listed elsewhere (e.g., temporomandibular, acromioclavicular, sternoclavicular).

hNegative refers to IU levels that are less than or equal to the ULN for the laboratory and assay; low positive refers to IU values that are more than three times the ULN for the laboratory and assay. Where RF information is only available as positive or negative, a positive result should be scored as low positive for RF.

iNormal and abnormal values are determined by local laboratory standards.

jDuration of symptoms refers to patient self-report of the duration of signs or symptoms of synovitis (e.g., pain, swelling, tenderness) of joints that are clinically involved at the time of assessment, regardless of treatment status.

RA, rheumatoid arthritis; RF, rheumatoid factor; CCP, cyclic citrullinated protein; CRP, C-reactive protein; ESR, erythrocyte sedimentation rate; ULN, upper limit of normal; MTP, metatarsophalangeal; DIP, distal interphalangeal; MCP, metacarpophalangeal.

From: Aletaha D, Neogi T, Silman A, et al. 2010 rheumatoid arthritis classification criteria: An American College of Rheumatology/European League Against Rheumatism collaborative initiative. *Arthritis Rheum.* 2010;62:2569–2581.

- These criteria were designed for inclusion of patients in research studies and not for routine clinical diagnosis. However, they can serve as diagnostic guidelines for evaluation of patients with suspected RA.
- This classification system focuses on features at earlier stages of disease that are associated with persistent and/or erosive disease. This will focus attention on **the important need for early diagnosis and treatment to prevent or minimize the occurrence of undesirable sequelae.**

Differential Diagnosis

- The other common causes of **symmetric inflammatory polyarthritis** are systemic lupus erythematosus (SLE), psoriatic arthritis, and viral (parvovirus B19 and hepatitis B and C associated) arthritis.
- Other causes of **inflammatory arthritis that are less symmetric** and typically oligoarticular or monoarticular include gout, pseudogout, septic arthritis, HLA-B27–associated spondyloarthropathies, and adult-onset Still's disease.
- Conditions with **noninflammatory polyarthralgias** should not be confused with RA, such as fibromyalgia, osteoarthritis, malignancy, hypothyroidism or hyperthyroidism, or hyperparathyroidism.
- **Palindromic rheumatism** is a condition similar to RA in which patients develop recurrent attacks of acute, self-limited arthritis.
  - Attacks usually last hours to a few days and may involve any set of joints.
  - Laboratory tests are nonspecific, and synovial fluid analysis reveals an inflammatory reaction.

  ○ Joint damage and systemic manifestations are rare.
  ○ Diagnosis is based on the presence of a relapsing and remitting course of arthritis.
  ○ **Many patients with palindromic rheumatism later progress to develop RA.**
  ○ Treatment is similar to that for RA. Nonsteroidal anti-inflammatory drugs (NSAIDs) may provide pain relief. Glucocorticoids and some disease-modifying antirheumatic drugs (DMARDs) may also be beneficial.
- **Relapsing seronegative symmetrical synovitis with pitting edema (RS3PE)** is a condition usually characterized by the sudden onset of polyarthritis associated with pitting edema of the hands and/or feet.
  ○ Laboratory markers of inflammation are variable, and RF is absent.
  ○ Synovitis is commonly present but rarely leads to joint destruction.
  ○ Treatment involves the use of low-dose glucocorticoids (prednisone, 5–10 mg a day), typically with dramatic improvement of symptoms. NSAIDs and hydroxychloroquine may also provide symptomatic relief and may be useful as steroid-sparing agents.
  ○ **RS3PE may be related to polymyalgia rheumatica and sometimes occur in association with malignancies.**

Diagnostic Testing

Laboratories
- Laboratory evaluation should include a baseline complete blood count (CBC), electrolyte panel, creatinine, hepatic function panel (HFP), urinalysis (UA), and stool occult blood to assess general organ function and comorbidities before initiating medications.
- Serologic markers for RA, including RF and **anti-CCP** antibodies, should be tested. Anti-CCP antibodies have been found in the serum of affected patients years before the onset of clinically apparent disease and are more specific for RA than RF.[7]
- RF should be drawn at baseline and repeated 6 to 12 months later if initially negative, as **approximately 50% of RA patients are positive in the first 6 months of illness and 85% become positive over the first 2 years.** Once RF is positive and the diagnosis of RA is made, there is no need to repeat this test.
- **A low-titer RF can be associated with other chronic inflammatory conditions** such as bacterial endocarditis, hepatitis C with cryoglobulinemia, and primary biliary cirrhosis. A high-titer RF usually indicates RA.
- The sensitivity and specificity of RF for the diagnosis of RA are roughly 66% and 82%, respectively.
- The sensitivity of anti-CCP antibodies for the diagnosis of RA is 70%, but specificity is 95%, superior to RF.
- **Up to 35% of patients with a negative RF at presentation will test positive for anti-CCP antibody.**
- A small number of RA patients (10%–15%) will remain seronegative (RF and CCP antibody negative) throughout the course of the disease.
- Twenty percent to 30% of RA patients have a **positive antinuclear antibody (ANA)**, but this is at a low titer. **Erythrocyte sedimentation rate (ESR)** and **C-reactive protein (CRP)** are markers of inflammation and may be useful to monitor disease activity, although they are not specific for RA.
- The synovial fluid in RA patients is inflammatory. Arthrocentesis is useful to rule out infectious and crystalline arthritis, if these are suspected, particularly if one joint is inflamed out of proportion compared to the others.

Imaging
- **Radiographs** of involved joints may be uninformative early in disease but can be used to monitor disease progression and treatment responses. Early findings include periarticular **osteopenia**. Late findings include **erosions** and symmetric joint space narrowing.

- **Magnetic resonance imaging (MRI) and ultrasound** have been proven to be **more sensitive** methods for detecting **early joint erosions**, synovitis, and tenosynovitis (refer to Chapter 6).
- Of note, plain radiographs of the feet are more likely to show erosions with early RA than hands.

TREATMENT

- The goals of treatment of RA are to alleviate pain, control inflammation, preserve and improve activities of daily living, and prevent progressive joint destruction.
- **Early recognition of disease and pharmacologic treatment provides the cornerstones for the management of RA**; hence, early referral to a rheumatologist is imperative.
- Medical treatment includes the use of NSAIDs, DMARDs, and glucocorticoids.
- Equally important in the management of RA is nonpharmacologic treatment, including patient education, physical therapy, occupational therapy, orthotics, and surgery.

Medications

Nonsteroidal Anti-inflammatory Drugs

- The use of **NSAIDs** in high doses can help alleviate symptoms from pain and inflammation in most patients with RA.
- Patients should be closely monitored for toxicities, especially GI ulcerations and renal dysfunction.
- Some patients may benefit from selective cyclooxygenase (COX)-2 inhibitors that have documented reduced GI toxicities or addition of GI prophylaxis in the form of misoprostol or proton pump inhibitors.
- **NSAIDs do not prevent progression of bone and cartilage damage**; therefore, current treatment strategies recommend NSAID use in combination with DMARDs for initial therapy.
- For details on dosing, toxicities, and monitoring of specific agents, see Chapter 9.

Glucocorticoids

- Glucocorticoids in low doses (e.g., prednisone, 5–10 mg a day) are extremely effective for promptly reducing the symptoms of RA and are useful in helping patients recover their previous functional status.
- Unfortunately, short courses of oral glucocorticoids produce only interim benefit, and chronic therapy is often necessary to maintain symptom management.
- Glucocorticoids are appropriate in patients with significant limitations in their activities of daily living, particularly early in the course of disease while awaiting the efficacy of slow-acting DMARDs.
- **Every effort should be made to taper to the lowest possible dose and to eliminate steroid therapy when feasible.**
- Toxicities of glucocorticoids are well known and include weight gain, cushingoid features, osteoporosis (for details on treatment and prevention of osteoporosis related to glucocorticoids, see Chapter 48), avascular necrosis (AVN), infection, diabetes mellitus, hypertension, and increases in serum cholesterol levels. Keeping the daily dose of prednisone at ≤5 mg a day can often reduce toxicities.
- Glucocorticoid doses should be slowly tapered over several months to avoid adrenal insufficiency.

Disease-Modifying Antirheumatic Drugs

- **DMARDs can slow or arrest the progression of RA.** DMARDs should be **instituted early** (within the first few weeks to 3 months of diagnosis).

- Treatment with DMARDs should be aimed at remission or low disease activity.
- **Many of the DMARDs have significant potential toxicities and may take several months to attain optimal clinical benefit**; therefore, careful monitoring for side effects and symptom relief is required.
- For severe disease flares, the use of oral glucocorticoids may also be necessary while waiting for optimal benefit from DMARDs.
- The choice of an initial DMARD is based on disease severity and the presence of erosive disease and anti-CCP antibodies; the latter are typically associated with a more aggressive disease course. Following is a list of commonly used DMARDs with associated toxicities and monitoring recommendations.
- For details on dosing, toxicities, and monitoring of specific agents, see Chapter 9.

Conventional Synthetic DMARDs
- **Oral methotrexate (MTX) is considered to be the DMARD of choice for most patients** and is imperative in patients with rapid disease progression or functional limitations.
  - From a starting dose of 7.5 to 10 mg once a week, the dose may be increased to 20 mg weekly rapidly.
  - If MTX is at least partially effective, it is continued as background therapy while other agents are added.
  - Common side effects include stomatitis, nausea, diarrhea, and hair loss.
  - Supplementation with folic acid, 1 to 2 mg daily, can reduce such side effects without significantly reducing efficacy.
  - Bone marrow suppression is uncommon, but it may occur at low doses in elderly patients.
  - The risk of liver toxicity is increased by alcohol consumption, preexisting liver disease, and, possibly, by diabetes and obesity.
  - Important contraindications to MTX therapy include liver disease, abnormal liver function tests, and regular alcohol consumption.
  - Liver tests (serum aspartate aminotransferase [AST], alanine aminotransferase [ALT], and albumin) and blood counts are checked every month until the dose is stable and every 2 to 3 months thereafter.
  - A liver biopsy is performed in patients with persistent elevation of liver transaminases or decrease in serum albumin to rule out MTX-induced hepatotoxicity.
  - MTX is to be avoided in patients with serum creatinine of greater than 2.0 mg/dL, as such patients are at higher risk of toxicity because of impaired renal clearance of the drug. Women of childbearing age must use appropriate contraceptive measures because of the teratogenic effects of this drug.
  - MTX is contraindicated in women who are pregnant, contemplating being pregnant or not using adequate contraceptives.
- **Hydroxychloroquine** is effective in mild-to-moderate, nonerosive RA, at doses of 200 to 400 mg/day, but not to be used in patients with moderate-to-severe renal or hepatic insufficiency.
  - Macular toxicity is extremely unusual if the dose does not exceed 5 mg/kg/day, and it rarely occurs before 5 years of treatment.
  - Nonetheless, an ophthalmologist should perform a baseline examination and monitor the patient every 6 to 12 months.
  - Nausea and skin discoloration occur occasionally.
- **Sulfasalazine** should be started at 500 mg twice daily and gradually increased to 2 to 3 g daily in divided doses.
  - An enteric-coated preparation improves GI tolerability.
  - Monitoring for neutropenia and hepatotoxicity should be performed every 1 to 3 months.
  - GI intolerance because of nausea or abdominal pain may occur.

- Sulfasalazine should be avoided in patients with sulfa allergies or glucose-6-phosphate dehydrogenase deficiency.
- **Leflunomide** is a pyrimidine synthesis inhibitor with efficacy comparable to MTX in treatment of RA.
- Diarrhea, nausea, and hair loss are common side effects. Liver tests need to be monitored every 1 to 3 months.
- The effective starting dose is 20 mg/day, which can be reduced to 10 mg/day if the medication is not tolerated or if transaminase levels become elevated.
- **Triple therapy**, that consists of MTX, sulfasalazine, and hydroxychloroquine, is a possible option if there is inadequate response to at least one DMARD.[8] "Triple therapy" is noninferior to TNF-α antagonists plus MTX, with the advantages of being oral and cheaper.[9,10]
- Others nonbiologic DMARDs less commonly used to treat RA include cyclosporine, gold salts, azathioprine, penicillamine, and cyclophosphamide (the latter for rheumatoid vasculitis).

Biologics and Targeted Synthetic DMARDs

- Biologic or targeted synthetic therapy should be initiated when adequate disease control is not achieved with conventional synthetic DMARDs.
- These include **TNF-α antagonists, non–TNF-α–mediated biologic agents**, and **Janus kinase (JAK) inhibitors**.
- The five currently available TNF-α antagonists are etanercept, infliximab, adalimumab, golimumab, and certolizumab. Non–TNF antagonizing biologics include anakinra, rituximab, abatacept, tocilizumab, and sarilumab. The JAK inhibitors are tofacitinib and baricitinib.
- **Many patients who do not respond to one TNF-α antagonist may respond to a different agent in the same class.**
- Combination regimens of conventional synthetic DMARDs plus biologic or targeted synthetic agents are increasingly popular treatment regimens. If tolerated, MTX should be part of every combination.
- **TNF-α antagonists are the initial biologic therapies used in RA patients who fail oral DMARDs. They are often administered in conjunction with MTX therapy**, as there is more effective disease control with combination therapy.[9–13]
  - **Etanercept** is a recombinant DNA-derived protein composed of TNF receptor linked to the Fc portion of human IgG1. Etanercept binds TNF and blocks its interaction with cell-surface receptors.[9,10,14]
  - **Infliximab** is a chimeric human–murine monoclonal antibody to TNF.[12,13]
  - **Adalimumab and golimumab** are fully human monoclonal antibodies to TNF.[15–17]
  - **Certolizumab** pegol is made of Fab antigen-binding domain of a humanized anti-TNF antibody, which is pegylated allowing for delayed elimination and an extended half-life.[18]
- **Non–TNF-α inhibitor biologic agents** are indicated for patients with an inadequate response to TNF-α antagonists.
  - **Anakinra** is an IL-1 receptor antagonist.[19]
  - **Rituximab** is a monoclonal antibody directed against the CD20 antigen on B lymphocytes.[20,21]
  - **Abatacept** is a selective costimulation modulator that inhibits T-lymphocyte activation by blocking the interaction between antigen-presenting cells and T cells.[22,23]
  - **Tocilizumab** and **sarilumab** are humanized monoclonal antibodies against the IL-6 receptor.[24–27]
- **JAK inhibitors, tofacitinib and baricitinib,** are oral DMARDs indicated for patients with an inadequate response to biologic DMARDs.[28–31]
- For details on dosing, toxicities, and monitoring of specific agents, see Chapter 9. A few important side effects of the TNF-α antagonists are discussed here.

- **Serious infections** have occurred rarely with the TNF-α antagonists.
  - TNF-α antagonists are **contraindicated in patients with indolent chronic infections** such as osteomyelitis or tuberculosis (TB), and in anyone with an active infection.
  - **Screening for latent TB** should be performed with a γ interferon release assay before beginning therapy with a TNF antagonist, and patients who test positive for latent TB should be treated with isoniazid before beginning therapy. Also, annual testing for latent TB is now recommended during treatment with a TNF-α antagonist.
  - Treatment with TNF-α antagonist should be temporarily suspended in patients undergoing surgery.
- **TNF-α antagonists should be used with extreme caution in patients with congestive heart failure or significant coronary artery disease.**
- Rare side effects include demyelinating disorders and lupus-like syndromes, with positive antibodies such as ANA, with or without other features of SLE.
- There is no consensus at the present time regarding the risk of lymphoma and malignancy with the use of these drugs, but if their use is warranted in patients with these conditions, these patients need to be monitored closely.

Other Nonpharmacologic Therapies

- **Ancillary medical services** can augment treatment strategies for patients with RA at any stage of disease.
- **Occupational therapy** usually focuses on the hand and wrist, and can help patients with splinting, work simplification, activities of daily living, and assistive devices.
- **Physical therapy** assists in stretching and strengthening exercises for large joints such as the shoulder and knee, gait evaluation, and fitting with crutches and canes. Moderate exercise is appropriate for all patients and can help reduce stiffness and maintain joint range of motion.

Surgical Management

- **Orthopedic surgery** to correct hand deformities and replace large joints such as the hip, knee, and shoulder may benefit patients with advanced disease.
- The primary indication for reconstructive hand surgery is refractory functional impairment, limiting activities of daily living.
- Total joint arthroplasty to replace the knee or hip should also be considered when pain cannot be controlled adequately with medications or when joint instability causes significant fall risk.

COMPLICATIONS

- RA patients are susceptible to **infections** owing to the immunosuppressive medications used for treatment.
- RA patients are at increased risk for **lymphoproliferative disorders, particularly lymphomas.**
- **Cervical instability** at the atlantoaxial articulation is a complication of long-standing, severe RA. Evaluation for cervical instability is particularly important in the perioperative setting, when extension of the neck for intubation may lead to cord compromise with resultant neurologic impairment. Radiographs of the cervical spine, including lateral flexion and extension views, should be taken.
- Rheumatoid **vasculitis** is usually associated with long-standing, severe, erosive RA. Mononeuritis multiplex and skin ulcers are common manifestations of rheumatoid vasculitis.
- There are data on the inflammatory state in RA being an independent risk factor for **cardiovascular disease.**

FOLLOW-UP

- The course of RA differs between patients. Whereas some patients may experience mild disease and have spontaneous remission, others may suffer a chronic course with intermittent disease flares and progressive joint destruction.
- Patients should be monitored on a frequent basis for disease progression or remission, response to therapy, and drug toxicities.
- Drug therapies should be adjusted to attain the minimal effective doses with an emphasis on limiting use of chronic steroids.
- Mortality rates are increased in RA patients because of cardiovascular disease; other comorbidities include infections, pulmonary and renal disease, and GI bleeding and drug toxicities.

PROGNOSIS

- The presence of erosions at baseline and high titers of RF and anti-CCP antibodies predict radiographic progression in RA.
- Female sex, smoking, extra-articular disease, functional limitations, a large number of tender and swollen joints, elevated ESR or CRP, and HLA-DRB1*0401/*0404 positivity are other poor prognostic factors.

REFERENCES

1. Gabriel SE, Michaud K. Epidemiological studies in incidence, prevalence, mortality, and comorbidity of the rheumatic diseases. *Arthritis Res Ther.* 2009;11(3):229.
2. van Vollenhoven RF. Sex differences in rheumatoid arthritis: more than meets the eye. *BMC Med.* 2009;7(1):12.
3. Kvien TK, Uhlig T, Ødegård S, et al. Epidemiological aspects of rheumatoid arthritis: the sex ratio. *Ann N Y Acad Sci.* 2006;1069(1):212–222.
4. Viatte S, Plant D, Han B, et al. Association of HLA-DRB1 haplotypes with rheumatoid arthritis severity, mortality, and treatment response. *JAMA.* 2015;313(16):1645–1656.
5. McInnes IB, Schett G. The pathogenesis of rheumatoid arthritis. *N Engl J Med.* 2011;365(23):2205–2219.
6. Aletaha D, Neogi T, Silman A, et al. 2010 rheumatoid arthritis classification criteria: An American College of Rheumatology/European League against Rheumatism collaborative initiative. *Arthritis Rheum.* 2010;62:2569–2581.
7. Nishimura K, Sugiyama D, Kogata Y, et al. Meta-analysis: diagnostic accuracy of anti-cyclic citrullinated peptide antibody and rheumatoid factor for rheumatoid arthritis. *Ann Intern Med.* 2007;146:797–808.
8. O'dell JR, Haire CE, Erikson N, et al. Treatment of rheumatoid arthritis with methotrexate alone, sulfasalazine and hydroxychloroquine, or a combination of all three medications. *N Engl J Med.* 1996;334(20):1287–1291.
9. Moreland LW, O'dell JR, Paulus HE, et al. A randomized comparative effectiveness study of oral triple therapy versus etanercept plus methotrexate in early aggressive rheumatoid arthritis: the treatment of Early Aggressive Rheumatoid Arthritis Trial. *Arthritis Rheum.* 2012;64(9):2824–2835.
10. O'dell JR, Mikuls TR, Taylor TH, et al. Therapies for active rheumatoid arthritis after methotrexate failure. *N Engl J Med.* 2013;369(4):307–318.
11. Goekoop-Ruiterman YP, de Vries-Bouwstra JK, Allaart CF, et al. Comparison of treatment strategies in early rheumatoid arthritis: a randomized trial. *Ann Intern Med.* 2007;146:406–415.
12. van Vollenhoven RF, Ernestam S, Geborek P, et al. Addition of infliximab compared with addition of sulfasalazine and hydroxychloroquine to methotrexate in patients with early rheumatoid arthritis (Swefot trial): 1-year results of a randomised trial. *Lancet.* 2009;374(9688):459–466.
13. van Vollenhoven RF, Geborek P, Forslind K, et al.; Swefot Study Group. Conventional combination treatment versus biological treatment in methotrexate-refractory early rheumatoid arthritis: 2 year follow-up of the randomised, non-blinded, parallel-group Swefot trial. *Lancet.* 2012;379(9827):1712–1720.

14. Emery P, Hammoudeh M, FitzGerald O, et al. Sustained remission with etanercept tapering in early rheumatoid arthritis. *N Engl J Med.* 2014;371(19):1781–1789.

15. Weinblatt ME, Keystone EC, Furst DE, et al. Adalimumab, a fully human anti–tumor necrosis factor α monoclonal antibody, for the treatment of rheumatoid arthritis in patients taking concomitant methotrexate: the ARMADA trial. *Arthritis Rheum.* 2003;48(1):35–45.

16. Breedveld FC, Weisman MH, Kavanaugh AF, et al. The PREMIER study: A multicenter, random-ized, double-blind clinical trial of combination therapy with adalimumab plus methotrexate versus methotrexate alone or adalimumab alone in patients with early, aggressive rheumatoid arthritis who had not had previous methotrexate treatment. *Arthritis Rheum.* 2006;54(1):26–37.

17. Smolen JS, Kay J, Doyle MK, et al. Golimumab in patients with active rheumatoid arthritis after treatment with tumour necrosis factor alpha inhibitors (GO-AFTER study): a multicentre, ran-domised, double-blind, placebo-controlled, phase III trial. *Lancet.* 2009;374(9685):210–221.

18. Smolen JS, Landewé RB, Mease PJ, et al. Efficacy and safety of certolizumab pegol plus methotrexate in active rheumatoid arthritis: the RAPID 2 study. A randomised controlled trial. *Ann Rheum Dis.* 2009;68(6):797–804.

19. Cohen S, Hurd E, Cush J, et al. Treatment of rheumatoid arthritis with anakinra, a recombi-nant human interleukin-1 receptor antagonist, in combination with methotrexate: results of a twenty-four-week, multicenter, randomized, double-blind, placebo-controlled trial. *Arthritis Rheum.* 2002;46(3):614–624.

20. Cohen SB, Emery P, Greenwald MW, et al. Rituximab for rheumatoid arthritis refractory to anti–tumor necrosis factor therapy: results of a multicenter, randomized, double-blind, placebo-controlled, phase III trial evaluating primary efficacy and safety at twenty-four weeks. *Arthritis Rheum.* 2006;54(9):2793–2806.

21. Porter D, Van Melckebeke J, Dale J, et al. Tumour necrosis factor inhibition versus rituximab for patients with rheumatoid arthritis who require biological treatment (ORBIT): an open-label, ran-domised controlled, non-inferiority, trial. *Lancet.* 2016;388(10041):239–247.

22. Schiff M, Keiserman M, Codding C, et al. Efficacy and safety of abatacept or infliximab versus placebo in ATTEST: a phase III, multi-center, randomized, double-blind, placebo-controlled study in patients with rheumatoid arthritis and an inadequate response to methotrexate. *Ann Rheum Dis.* 2008;67(8):1096–1103.

23. Schiff M, Weinblatt ME, Valente R, et al. Head-to-head comparison of subcutaneous abatacept ver-sus adalimumab for rheumatoid arthritis: two-year efficacy and safety findings from AMPLE trial. *Ann Rheum Dis.* 2014;73(1):86–94.

24. Maini RN, Taylor PC, Szechinski J, et al. Double-blind randomized controlled clinical trial of the interleukin-6 receptor antagonist, tocilizumab, in European patients with rheumatoid arthritis who had an incomplete response to methotrexate. *Arthritis Rheum.* 2006;54(9):2817–2829.

25. Emery P, Keystone E, Tony HP, et al. IL-6 receptor inhibition with tocilizumab improves treat-ment outcomes in patients with rheumatoid arthritis refractory to anti-tumour necrosis factor bi-ologicals: results from a 24-week multicentre randomised placebo-controlled trial. *Ann Rheum Dis.* 2008;67(11):1516–1523.

26. Genovese MC, Fleischmann R, Kivitz AJ, et al. Sarilumab plus methotrexate in patients with active rheumatoid arthritis and inadequate response to methotrexate: results of a phase III study. *Arthritis Rheumatol.* 2015;67(6):1424–1437.

27. Burmester GR, Lin Y, Patel R, et al. Efficacy and safety of sarilumab monotherapy versus adalim-umab monotherapy for the treatment of patients with active rheumatoid arthritis (MONARCH): a randomised, double-blind, parallel-group phase III trial. *Ann Rheum Dis.* 2017;76(5):840–847.

28. van Vollenhoven RF, Fleischmann R, Cohen S, et al. Tofacitinib or adalimumab versus placebo in rheumatoid arthritis. *N Engl J Med.* 2012;367(6):508–519.

29. Lee EB, Fleischmann R, Hall S, et al. Tofacitinib versus methotrexate in rheumatoid arthritis. *N Engl J Med.* 2014;370(25):2377–2386.

30. Genovese MC, Kremer J, Zamani O, et al. Baricitinib in patients with refractory rheumatoid arthritis. *N Engl J Med.* 2016;374(13):1243–1252.

31. Taylor PC, Keystone EC, van der Heijde D, et al. Baricitinib versus placebo or adalimumab in rheu-matoid arthritis. *N Engl J Med.* 2017;376(7):652–662.

Osteoarthritis

Michiko Inaba and Prabha Ranganathan

11

GENERAL PRINCIPLES

Definition

The major clinical symptoms of osteoarthritis (OA) are chronic pain, locomotor restriction, inactivity-related joint stiffness (<30 minutes), and, on radiographs, joint space narrowing.

OA has evolved from being considered a part of the natural aging process and non-inflammatory to now being considered the result of a complex interplay of mechanical, biochemical, genetic, and immunologic phenomena, with variable inflammation of the synovium, leading to degradation of the articular cartilage.

Classification

- **Primary or idiopathic:** The localized form affects one to two of these joint groups: distal interphalangeal (DIP), proximal interphalangeal (PIP), or carpometacarpal (CMC) joints of the hands; cervical and/or lumbar spine; knees, hips and first metatarsophalangeal (MTP) joints of the feet (Fig. 11-1). The generalized form involves three or more joint groups and is frequently associated with Heberden's nodes (bony enlargement of the DIP joints) or Bouchard's nodes (bony enlargement of the PIP joints).
- **Secondary:** This should be considered if a patient has an identifiable etiology for secondary OA, such as repeated trauma or surgery, obesity, congenital abnormalities, gout, rheumatoid arthritis, or diabetes.
- **Erosive OA:** Also known as inflammatory OA, it usually affects the DIP joints, PIP joints, and first CMC joints of the hands bilaterally, with negative rheumatoid factor (RF) and anti–cyclic citrullinated protein (CCP) antibodies.

Epidemiology

- OA is the most common joint disease, affecting 240 million people globally and more than 20 million people in the United States alone.
- The prevalence of OA increases with age and is 10% in men and 18% in women older than 60 years.
- The number of joint replacements done for OA is increasing by 10% each year, and it is estimated that 572,000 total hip replacements and 3,480,000 total knee replacements will be done for OA by 2030.
- It is estimated the social cost of OA could be between 0.25% and 0.50% of a country's gross domestic product (GDP).[1]

Etiology

The etiology of OA is multifactorial and includes factors such as joint injury, aging, obesity, heredity, and overuse.

Pathophysiology

- Chondrocytes are responsible for balancing the anabolic and catabolic processes in the joint.
- Biomechanical stressors trigger chondrocytes to release matrix metalloproteinases and to synthesize matrix proteins, including fibrillar type II collagen.

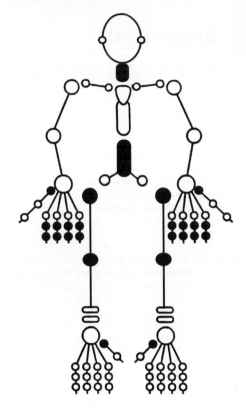

FIGURE 11-1. Distribution of osteoarthritis.

- The matrix metalloproteinases lead to cartilage degradation. Synthesis of matrix proteins leads to new bone growth, resulting in osteophyte formation.
- Inflammatory cytokines, notably interleukin (IL)-1β, tumor necrosis factor (TNF)-α, and IL-6 as well as number of other cytokines, produced by articular chondrocytes, drive catabolic pathways and perpetuate disease progression.[2]
- Over the years, this process of cartilage degradation and osteophyte formation results in loss of joint space (bone-on-bone) and, sometimes, even instability of the joint with use.

Risk Factors
- Risk factors for primary OA
  - **Age:** The prevalence of OA greatly increases with age.
  - **Gender:** Women suffer from OA more often than men.
  - **Obesity:** Increased stress on weight-bearing joints, such as the knees and hips, leads to OA. Obesity can affect non–weight-bearing joints, such as the first CMC joints, owing to adipokine-mediated inflammation.[3]
  - **High bone mass:** Women with osteoporosis are less likely to have OA.
  - **Mechanical factors:** Repetitive use of joints, malalignment of joints, lower limb length inequality, and joint laxity are all risk factors for OA.

- **Genetic:** Although typically thought to be a disease of people over the age of 50 years, animal models suggest that mutations in genes encoding for extracellular matrix proteins could lead to premature OA.
- Risk factors for secondary OA
  - **Injured or damaged joints:** This includes mechanical injuries as well as joint damage inflicted by inflammatory arthritis, such as rheumatoid arthritis (RA), psoriatic arthritis (PsA), and septic arthritis.
  - **Metabolic/infiltrative diseases:** Acromegaly, Paget's disease, Cushing's syndrome, crystalline arthropathies, ochronosis, hemochromatosis, Wilson's disease, and amyloidosis increase the risk of OA.
  - **Hemarthrosis:** Whether it is due to trauma, or disease states such as factor deficiencies or inhibitors, or anticoagulation, persistent or recurrent blood in the synovial fluid leads to cartilage destruction.
  - **Neuropathic joints:** The pattern of joints involved depends on the underlying disease state. Diabetic neuropathy tends to involve the foot and ankle; tabes dorsalis involves the hips, knees, and ankles; and syringomyelia tends to involve the shoulders and elbows.

DIAGNOSIS

- OA diagnosis is a clinical diagnosis based on the history and physical examination.
- If the clinical presentation is confusing, synovial fluid analysis, serum inflammatory markers, and joint radiographs can be used to assist in diagnosis.

Clinical Presentation

Unless there is a strong family history, the patient presents with pain, usually after the age of 40 years.

History

- Patients complain of pain or "locking" of the affected joints that is mechanical in nature and worsens with activity.
- As the disease progresses, stiffness can occur, but is typically less than 30 minutes in duration compared to the stiffness in RA that lasts more than 60 minutes. Stiffness can occur after a period of inactivity; this is called "gelling."

Physical Examination

- Examination of the suspected joint may demonstrate mild tenderness to palpation, usually without evidence of inflammation. Crepitus, bony enlargement, decreased range of motion, joint effusion, and osteophytes along the periphery of the joint may be detectable.
- The joints most commonly involved are the DIP, PIP, and first CMC joints of the hands, knees, hips, and spine. Secondary OA or another disease process should be considered if other joints are involved.

Diagnostic Criteria

- OA may be diagnosed confidently on clinical grounds alone if there is:
  - Persistent activity-related joint pain in one or more joints
  - Age greater than 45 years
  - Morning stiffness less than 30 minutes in duration[4]
- Listed here are the American College of Rheumatology (ACR) criteria for OA involving the hands, hips, and knees, but it is important to remember that these were created to meet eligibility for clinical trials and should be used more as guidelines rather than absolute criteria:

○ **Hand:** Hand pain or stiffness and at least three of the following: hard-tissue enlargement of more than one of the selected joints (second and third DIP or PIP; the first CMC joint of each hand), hard-tissue enlargement of more than one DIP joint, deformity of at least two or more of ten DIP joints, and fewer than three swollen metacarpophalangeal (MCP) joints

○ **Hip:** Hip pain and at least two of the following: erythrocyte sedimentation rate (ESR) <20 mm/hour, radiographic acetabular or femoral osteophytes, and radiographic joint space narrowing

○ **Knee:** Knee pain plus three of the following: ESR less than 20 mm/hour, age greater than 50, stiffness less than 30 minutes, crepitus, no palpable warmth, and bony hypertrophy

Differential Diagnosis

The following diagnoses must be considered when diagnosing OA: RA; seronegative spondyloarthropathies such as psoriatic arthritis, reactive arthritis, ankylosing spondylitis, and enteropathic arthritis; crystalline arthropathies; infectious arthritis, including bacterial and viral etiologies; paraneoplastic and neoplastic synovitis; hemarthrosis, periarticular bursitis, and tendinitis; and referred pain from a different joint.

Diagnostic Testing

Laboratories
- There are no laboratory tests to confirm the diagnosis of OA.
- Inflammatory makers (CRP, ESR) are normal or only minimally increased in OA, but they may be useful to exclude other diagnoses.

Imaging
- Plain radiography may be used to support the clinical diagnosis of OA, including osteophyte formation, joint space narrowing, subchondral sclerosis, and cysts. The Kellgren and Lawrence (KL) classification is a common method of classifying the severity of OA based on the presence of joint space narrowing and osteophytes. Please see Table 11-1.[5]
- Typical features seen on radiographs include joint space narrowing, subchondral sclerosis, osteophytes at the periphery of joints, and subchondral cysts. However, radiographic changes do not necessarily correlate with symptomatic disease.

Diagnostic Procedures
- If the patient has an effusion and the clinical picture is confusing and there is suspicion for coexisting crystal deposition disease or infection, joint aspiration is required.
- Synovial fluid is noninflammatory and has few WBCs (<2,000 WBCs/mL).

TABLE 11-1	THE KELLGREN AND LAWRENCE SYSTEM
Grade 0	No radiographic features of OA present
Grade 1	Doubtful joint space narrowing (JSN) and possible osteophytic lipping
Grade 2	Definite osteophytes and possible JSN on anteroposterior weight-bearing radiograph
Grade 3	Multiple osteophytes, definite JSN, sclerosis, possible bony deformity
Grade 4	Large osteophytes, marked JSN, severe sclerosis, and definite bony deformity

JSN, joint space narrowing; OA, osteoarthritis.

TREATMENT

Both Osteoarthritis Research Society International (OARSI) 2017 and the ACR 2012 recommendations use a combination of nonpharmacologic modalities and pharmacologic
agents in a stepwise manner.

Medications

Pharmacologic therapy is focused on symptom management because there are currently no
approved disease-modifying osteoarthritis drugs (DMOADs) available.

The main pharmacologic interventions in OA include acetaminophen, oral and topical nonsteroidal anti-inflammatory drugs (NSAIDs), topical capsaicin, duloxetine, and
intra-articular glucocorticoids.

- **Acetaminophen** was found to have a low efficacy in a recent meta-analysis, recommended as a short-term analgesic. A 2012 safety review indicated increased risk of
  adverse events associated with acetaminophen use, including gastrointestinal (GI)
  adverse events and multiorgan failure. Although Food and Drug Administration
  (FDA)-approved acetaminophen dose is up to 4 g/day, conservative dosing (2–3 g/day)
  is generally recommended.
- **NSAIDs:** No one NSAID has been proven to be more effective than another.
  - NSAIDs are often more effective than acetaminophen therapy, but their use in patients
    with comorbidities is limited by the increased risk of cardiovascular (CV), renal, and
    GI toxicity.
  - Cyclooxygenase-2 (COX-2) inhibitors were associated with a lower risk of GI ulcer
    complications compared with nonselective NSAIDs in a 2011 comparative effective-
    ness review.
  - Some data suggest that the CV safety of naproxen may be moderately superior to that
    of COX-2 selective NSAIDs.
- **Topical NSAIDs** are recommended over oral NSAIDs for mild OA of superficial joints
  (knee and hands).[6] The risk of GI toxicity is significantly lower with topical NSAIDs
  compared to oral NSAIDs (three-fold lower).[7]
- **Topical capsaicin**
  - Capsaicin is a substance derived from hot chili peppers that decreases pain through
    the depletion of substance P. 0.025% capsaicin cream applied four times a day over a
    6-week period was effective in decreasing pain from knee OA.
- **Duloxetine** is appropriate for patients with generalized OA with concomitant comorbid-
  ities that may contraindicate oral NSAID use, and for patients with knee OA who have
  not responded satisfactorily to other interventions.
- **Intra-articular glucocorticoid injections**
  - Two recent studies demonstrated clinically significant improvement in pain in the short
    term (4 weeks) with intra-articular steroids that were superior to intra-articular hyal-
    uronic acid.
  - The current recommendation is to repeat steroid injections no more frequently than
    every 3 months. However, a randomized clinical trial in 2017 showed cartilage volume
    loss in the knee after intra-articular injections with triamcinolone acetonide every 3
    months over 2 years sounding a note of caution with this approach.[8]

Other Nonpharmacologic Therapies

- Education on self-management, weight loss, and joint protection techniques
- Aerobic/or resistance land-based exercises, strength training, and aquatic exercises for
  knee and hip OA
- Assistive devices to help with patients' activities of daily living (ADLs)
- Instruction in the use of thermal modalities
- Splints for patients with hand OA, wedge insoles for foot, and knee OA

Surgical Management

- Arthroscopic irrigations have failed to demonstrate any benefit in knee and hip OA.
- Knee and hip arthroplasties (total joint replacement) have demonstrated improvement in pain and function in about 85% of patients receiving these surgeries.
- Prosthetic joints typically last 15 years.

Novel Therapies

- Tanezumab is a humanized monoclonal antibody against nerve growth factor (NGF). Elevated levels of NGF are seen in the synovial fluid of patients with inflammatory arthritis, and animal models have suggested a benefit in OA. A dramatic response was seen in phase II trials, but phase III trials for knee, hip, and shoulder OA were closed by the FDA because some patients developed bone necrosis. However, based on favorable reviews of nonclinical data by the FDA, phase III trials resumed in 2015, and this drug is currently under investigation again.[9]
- **Diacerein** is a novel drug with IL-1 inhibitory activity. In animal models, this drug leads to potent inhibition of metalloproteinases that are necessary for cartilage destruction. Several large, randomized controlled trials have been performed with conflicting results. Diacerein is currently available in many countries including France and Armenia but is not approved for use in the United States because of its significant side effects and the lack of concrete evidence.[10]

Other Interventions

Both ACR and OARSI do not recommend glucosamine or chondroitin because there is no good evidence for their benefits in OA.

REFERENCES

1. Puig-Junoy J, Ruiz Zamora A. Socio-economic costs of osteoarthritis: a systemic review of cost-of-illness studies. *Semin Arthritis Rheum.* 2015;44:531–541.
2. Sohn DH, Sokolove J, Sharpe O, et al. Plasma proteins present in osteoarthritic synovial fluid can stimulate cytokine production via Toll-like receptor 4. *Arthritis Res Ther.* 2012;14:R7.
3. Visser AW, Ioan-Facsinay A, de Mutsert R, et al. Adiposity and hand osteoarthritis: the Netherlands Epidemiology of Obesity study. *Arthritis Res Ther.* 2014;16:R19.
4. National Clinical Guideline Centre. *Osteoarthritis: The Care and Management of Osteoarthritis in Adults.* London, UK: National Institute for Health and Clinical Excellence; 2008.
5. Kellgren JH, Lawrence JS. Radiological assessment of osteoarthrosis. *Ann Rheum Dis.* 1957;16:494–501.
6. Tugwell PS, Wells GA, Shainhouse JZ. Equivalence study of a topical diclofenac solution (pennsaid) compared with oral diclofenac in symptomatic treatment of osteoarthritis of the knee: A randomized controlled trial. *J Rheumatol.* 2004;31(10):2002–2012.
7. Persson MSM, Stocks J, Walsh DA, et al. The relative efficacy of topical non-steroidal anti-inflammatory drugs and capsaicin in osteoarthritis: a network meta-analysis of randomised controlled trials. *Osteoarthritis Cartilage.* 2018;26:1575–1582.
8. McAlindon TE, LaValley MP, Harvey WF, et al. Effect of intra-articular triamcinolone vs saline on knee cartilage volume and pain in patients with knee osteoarthritis: A randomized clinical trial. *JAMA.* 2017;317:1967–1975.
9. Lane NE, Schnitzer TJ, Birbara CA, et al. Tanezumab for the treatment of pain from osteoarthritis of the knee. *N Engl J Med.* 2010;363:1521–1531.
10. Fidelix TA, Soares B, Maxwell LJ, et al. Diacerein for osteoarthritis. *Cochrane Database Syst Rev.* 2014;(2):CD005117.

Systemic Lupus Erythematosus

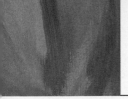

Iris Lee, Heather A. Jones, and
Alfred H. J. Kim

GENERAL PRINCIPLES

- Systemic lupus erythematosus (SLE) is a **chronic, systemic, inflammatory disease** characterized by **autoantibodies** (particularly antinuclear antibodies [ANAs]), **immune complex deposition**, and immune dysregulation.
- Affected organs include the skin, musculoskeletal system, nervous system, serous membranes, hematologic system, reproductive system, heart, lungs, kidneys, and gut.
- The symptoms can range from mild to life-threatening, and the pattern of symptoms experienced within the first several years of illness tends to predominate throughout the remainder of the disease.
- SLE mainly affects **women of childbearing age.**
- Criteria exist to assist in the classification of SLE, but SLE remains a challenging disease to diagnose because of the absence of pathognomonic signs, symptoms, or laboratory findings.

Definition

- The diagnosis of SLE requires the presence of **multiorgan disease** in the setting of immune dysfunction, specifically the presence of **autoantibodies**.
- Classification criteria for SLE have evolved over time—the criteria were recently revised by the American College of Rheumatology (ACR) and The European League Against Rheumatism (EULAR) in 2019. The 1997 ACR criteria are listed in Table 12-1. In addition, criteria generated from the Systemic Lupus International Collaborating Clinics (SLICC) are also available.[1] Although these can be helpful for diagnosis, they should not be strictly used for the diagnosis of SLE because the purpose of these criteria is to classify SLE for clinical research. In addition, they fail to highlight common nonspecific manifestations of SLE, such as Raynaud's phenomenon, lymphadenopathy, keratoconjunctivitis sicca (secondary Sjögren's syndrome), elevated erythrocyte sedimentation rate (ESR), and hypocomplementemia.

Classification

- There are systemic only forms of SLE, systemic plus cutaneous, and cutaneous limited forms. The cutaneous limited subtype portends a better prognosis.
  - Cutaneous manifestations of SLE include those findings that are considered specific to patients with SLE and those that are nonspecific and noted in higher frequency in this patient population.
  - SLE-specific cutaneous findings are then subcategorized as follows:
    - Acute cutaneous lupus erythematosus (ACLE)
    - Subacute cutaneous lupus erythematosus (SCLE)
    - Chronic cutaneous lupus erythematosus (CCLE) (including discoid lupus erythematosus [DLE])
  - **Drug-induced lupus (DIL):** DIL and drug-induced SCLE (DI-SCLE) both exist.

TABLE 12-1	AMERICAN COLLEGE OF RHEUMATOLOGY CRITERIA FOR DIAGNOSIS OF SYSTEMIC LUPUS ERYTHEMATOSUS (1997)
Criterion	**Definition**
Malar rash	Fixed erythema, flat or raised, over the malar eminences, tending to spare the nasolabial folds
Discoid rash	Erythematosus raised patches with adherent keratotic scaling and follicular plugging; atrophic scaring may occur in older lesions
Photosensitivity	Skin rash as a result of unusual reaction to sunlight, by patient history or physician observation
Oral ulcers	Oral or nasopharyngeal ulceration, usually painless, observed by a physician
Arthritis	Nonerosive arthritis involving ≥ 2 peripheral joints, characterized by tenderness, swelling, or effusion
Serositis	Pleuritis: Convincing history of pleuritic pain or rub heard by a physician or evidence of pleural effusion. Pericarditis: Documented by EKG, rub, or evidence of pericardial effusion
Renal disorder	Persistent proteinuria >0.5 g/day or >3+ if quantification not performed. Cellular casts: May be red cell, hemoglobin, granular, tubular, or mixed
Neurologic disorder	Seizures or psychosis: In the absence of offending drugs or known metabolic derangements (uremia, ketoacidosis, or electrolyte imbalance)
Hematologic disorder	Hemolytic anemia: With reticulocytosis or leukopenia <4,000/mm^3 total on two or more occasions or lymphopenia <1,500/mm^3 on two or more occasions or thrombocytopenia <100,000/mm^3 in the absence of offending drugs
Immunologic disorders	Positive antiphospholipid antibody Anti-dsDNA: Antibody to native DNA in abnormal titer Anti-Sm: Presence of antibody to Smith nuclear antigen False-positive serologic test for syphilis known to be positive for at least 6 months and confirmed by *Treponema pallidum* immobilization or fluorescent treponemal antibody absorption test
Antinuclear antibody	An abnormal titer of antinuclear antibody by immunofluorescence or an equivalent assay at any point in time in the absence of drugs known to be associated with "drug-induced lupus" syndrome

Four or more of the manifestations must be present, either serially or simultaneously, to establish a diagnosis of SLE. These criteria were developed for classifying SLE patients for study purposes. Virtually, all rheumatologists would argue that a negative ANA should exclude an SLE diagnosis.

dsDNA, double-stranded DNA; EKG, electrocardiogram; Sm, Smith.

Epidemiology

- Roughly 20 to 250 cases of SLE per 100,000 persons in the United States have been reported.[2]
- Prevalence and severity of the disease depend on **gender and race**.

○ **Gender:** In children, female-to-male ratio is 4:3. This ratio increases in adults to 9:1.[3]
○ **Race:** More prevalent in Asians, African Americans, African Caribbeans, and Hispanic Americans compared to Caucasians. Lupus is thought to be rare in Africa.[2]

Etiology

- The etiology of SLE is unknown.
- Multiple factors appear to play a role in disease susceptibility, including genetic, hormonal, immune, and environmental.
  ○ Genetic
    ▪ There is a high concordance of SLE between monozygotic twins (hazard ratio [HR] of 85.7). In addition, first-degree relatives have an HR of 10.3 in a Danish population.[4]
    ▪ Over 40 loci have been associated with SLE as identified by genome-wide association studies. They affect lymphocyte signaling, interferon (IFN) signaling, clearance of immune complexes, and products of apoptosis. Each gene contributes a relative risk of less than 2 and can be associated with multiple autoimmune diseases. These include:
      □ Deficiencies of the complement component C1q, C4A and C4B, and C2
      □ Three prime repair exonuclease 1 (TREX1) mutations (enzyme needed to degrade DNA)
      □ HLA-DR2 and HLA-DR3
      □ Genes involved with high levels or enhanced responsiveness to IFN-α (such as *STAT4, PTPN22,* and *IRF5*)[5,6]
    ▪ There is also dysregulation in epigenetic factors including DNA methylation and expression changes in various microRNAs (miRNAs).[5]
  ○ Hormonal
    ▪ The significant increase in risk seen in women strongly suggests a role of sex hormones in SLE; sex hormones are well-established regulators of the immune system, leading to the hypothesis that they play a role in SLE pathophysiology. Estrogen-containing contraceptives increase the risk of developing SLE (relative risk 1.5).[7]
    ▪ Postmenopausal administration of estrogen and early menarche (age ≤ 10 years) double the risk of SLE development.[8]
  ○ Immune
    ▪ Numerous abnormalities of the immune system have been observed in SLE patients, but the significance of these abnormalities remains unclear.
    ▪ Currently, it is believed that many of these abnormalities are due to the loss of tolerance to self-antigens.
  ○ **Environmental:** Several environmental factors are associated with triggering disease onset or worsening disease activity in SLE.
    ▪ Viruses activate the type 1 IFN pathway, an important antiviral immune mechanism. This is the same pathway thought to be critical in promoting SLE activity. Recurrent Epstein–Barr virus (EBV) and cytomegalovirus (CMV) infections have been associated with a higher risk of SLE development.
    ▪ Patients with SLE have higher serum levels of lipopolysaccharide, a cell wall component of Gram-negative bacteria.
    ▪ The microbiome seems to be implicated as well—women with SLE have a lower *Firmicutes* to *Bacteroidetes* ratio in their gut. In addition, recent data suggest *Enterococcus gallinarum* that have translocated through the gut epithelium may be associated with SLE.[9]
    ▪ Ultraviolet light exposure commonly triggers cutaneous manifestations of SLE, likely through the upregulation of IFN-κ.[10]
    ▪ Several drugs are associated with DIL (see Laboratories later).

Pathophysiology

- Many of the clinical manifestations of SLE are thought to be due to **the presence of autoantibodies and generation of immune complexes.**
- In renal disease, autoantibodies to nuclear antigens either deposit or form within mesangial, subendothelial, or subepithelial regions of the glomerulus. These immune complexes activate the complement system, leading to the inflammation and recruitment of inflammatory cells to the kidney. This cycle eventually leads to fibrinoid necrosis, scarring, and reduction in kidney function.

Risk Factors

Female gender, certain ethnicities, geographical location, ultraviolet exposure, and certain medications (Table 12-2) have been associated with increased SLE prevalence or severity of disease.

Prevention

Because the etiology of disease remains unknown, no primary preventative measures are known though patients are routinely advised to avoid sunlight and smoking.

TABLE 12-2	DRUGS ASSOCIATED WITH A DEFINITE, PROBABLE, OR POSSIBLE RISK OF DRUG-INDUCED LUPUS	
Definite	**Probable**	**Possible**
Procainamide[a]	Anticonvulsants	Gold salts
Hydralazine[a]	Phenytoin	Penicillin
Minocycline	Ethosuximide	Tetracycline
Diltiazem	Carbamazepine	Reserpine
Penicillamine[a]	Antithyroid drugs	Valproate
Isoniazid	Antimicrobial agents	Statins
Quinidine	Sulfonamides	Griseofulvin
Anti–TNF-α therapies	Rifampin	Gemfibrozil
Interferon-α	Nitrofurantoin	Valproate
Methyldopa	β-Blockers	Ophthalmic timolol
Chlorpromazine	Lithium	5-Aminosalicylate
Practolol	Captopril	
	Interferon-γ	
	Hydrochlorothiazide	
	Glyburide	
	Sulfasalazine	
	Terbinafine	
	Amiodarone	
	Ticlopidine	
	Docetaxel	

[a]Associated with high risk of inducing drug-induced lupus.
TNF, tumor necrosis factor.

Associated Conditions

- As the prototypical connective tissue disease, **SLE can overlap with signs and symptoms from other connective tissue diseases**. For example, SLE can overlap with rheumatoid arthritis ("rupus"), primary Sjögren's syndrome, Raynaud's disease, systemic sclerosis, or polymyositis/dermatomyositis.
- Non-Hodgkin's lymphoma (particularly diffuse large B cell) is associated with SLE.
- Many other conditions are associated with SLE (see Diagnosis).

DIAGNOSIS

The diagnosis of SLE remains one of the most challenging in medicine. No single sign, symptom, or laboratory value is pathognomonic for SLE.

Clinical Presentation

- SLE presents in a highly variable manner, both in terms of onset and in course.
- Many of the early symptoms are nonspecific (i.e., fatigue, malaise, arthralgias, and fever).
- Severe manifestations (i.e., nephritis) usually occur at the onset or early in the course of disease.
- Patient's complaints may be due to SLE, medication side effects, or unrelated intercurrent illnesses.
- **General signs and symptoms**
  - Virtually all SLE patients present with **fatigue**. This may be due to disease activity, but anemia, infection, medications, fibromyalgia, or poor sleep are other causes.
  - **Weight loss, lymphadenopathy, and fever** are also common in SLE. Weight loss usually precedes the diagnosis. All fevers must be evaluated for infection.
- **Musculoskeletal signs and symptoms**
  - **Arthralgias and arthritis** are the most common presenting symptoms in SLE.
    - Arthralgias may involve any joint, but symmetric involvement of the hands, wrists, and knees is most typically seen.
    - Arthritis tends to be **symmetric, migratory, and nonerosive**.
    - Although deformities are rare, most deformities associated with SLE are reversible. Both **reversible** "swan-neck" and "boutonniere" deformities (see Chapter 2) can be seen. **Jaccoud's arthropathy** occurs when there is reversible ulnar deviation and subluxation of the second to fifth metacarpophalangeal (MCP) joints.
  - Diffuse **myalgias** are also commonly seen, sometimes in association with **fibromyalgia** (see Chapter 53). **Myositis** is uncommon, but muscle inflammation otherwise typical of primary polymyositis/dermatomyositis may be associated with SLE. Myopathy induced from steroids or hydroxychloroquine (HCQ) can be seen (see Chapter 9).
  - **Osteoporosis** is common and worsens from steroids used to treat flares (see Chapter 52).
- **Mucocutaneous signs and symptoms**
  - Almost all patients have **photosensitivity**. Photosensitivity can take the form of **skin rash or blistering**, but more commonly, **extreme fatigue or malaise** occurs. Usually, symptoms occur **within minutes** of exposure to ultraviolet rays.
  - There are three subtypes of cutaneous lupus erythematosus: **ACLE, SCLE,** and **CCLE**. Each of these is associated with SLE to a different degree.
  - **ACLE is the most strongly associated with lupus.** More than 90% of patients with ACLE have SLE. The most common manifestation is the malar rash, which is present in 50% of patients with SLE.[11]
    - **Malar rash** (also known as a butterfly rash) is a fixed erythema, either flat or raised, over the malar eminences, **sparing the nasolabial folds**.
    - The differential diagnosis for malar rash includes acne rosacea, seborrheic dermatitis, polymorphous light eruption, and contact dermatitis.

- Half of SCLE patients have SLE, 10% of SLE patients have SCLE.[12]
  - Erythematous, papulosquamous, or annular lesions commonly occur on sun-exposed skin.
  - Photosensitivity is a prominent feature of SCLE.
  - Most patients with SCLE will have Sjögren's syndrome–related antigen A (SSA) antibody.
- **Discoid lupus** is the most common form of CCLE. The rash starts as erythematous papules or plaques that become infiltrated and have an adherent scale. Follicular plugging is prominent. The lesions expand, leaving **central hypopigmentation, atrophic scarring,** and permanent alopecia. They commonly occur on the scalp, along the hairline and within the conchal bowls.
  - Only 10% of these patients will develop SLE; however, the presence of disseminated DLE lesions, including those occurring below the head and neck area, is associated with increased likelihood of developing SLE.
  - In long-standing, untreated lesions in DLE, there is a risk of malignant transformation to **cutaneous squamous cell carcinoma.**
- **Oral and/or nasopharyngeal ulcers** are typically painless and occur on the hard palate.
- Nonspecific cutaneous eruptions are also very common in patients with SLE and include nonscarring alopecia, livedo reticularis, and vasculitis. Soft-tissue swelling and erythema can also occur in between the joints of fingers (compared to Gottron's papules seen in dermatomyositis; see Chapter 13).
- **Renal signs and symptoms**
  - Renal involvement occurs in **over 50% of SLE patients** and is a major cause of morbidity and mortality in SLE patients.[13]
    - Findings range from asymptomatic proteinuria to frank nephritic and nephrotic syndrome.
    - Pathologic abnormalities can be seen in patients without known renal disease (silent lupus nephritis).
  - The International Society of Nephrology/World Health Organization (ISN/WHO) criteria published in 2003 were based on **glomerular** findings in kidney biopsy. The most recent revision in 2018 eliminated several subcategories in favor of activity and chronicity scores (summarized in Tables 12-3 and 12-4).[14,15] In general, classes III and IV have more severe nephritis and are associated with poorer prognosis.

TABLE 12-3	INTERNATIONAL SOCIETY OF NEPHROLOGY/RENAL PATHOLOGY SOCIETY REVISED CLASSIFICATION OF LUPUS NEPHRITIS
Class I	Minimal mesangial lupus nephritis
Class II	Mesangial proliferative lupus nephritis
Class III	Focal lupus nephritis
Class IV	Diffuse lupus nephritis
Class V	Membranous lupus nephritis[a]
Class VI	Advanced sclerotic lupus nephritis

[a]Class V may occur in combination with class III or IV, in which case both will be diagnosed.

Adapted from: Barjema IM, Wilhelmus S, Alpers CE, et al. Revision of the International Society of Nephrology/Renal Pathology Society classification for lupus nephritis: clarification of definitions and modified National Institutes of Health activity and chronicity indices. *Kidney Int.* 2018;93(4):789–796.

TABLE 12-4 CLINICAL CORRELATES TO LUPUS NEPHRITIS CLASSES

| Class | Pattern | Site of Immune Complex Deposition | Clinical Clues[a] | | | | | |
			Urine Sediment	Proteinuria (24 hours)	Serum Creatinine	Blood Pressure	Anti-dsDNA	C3/C4
I	Normal	None	Bland	<200 mg	Normal	Normal	Absent	Normal
II	Mesangial	Mesangial only	RBC or bland	200–500 mg	Normal	Normal	Absent	Normal
III	Focal and segmental proliferative	Mesangial, subendothelial, and/or subepithelial	RBC, WBC	500–3,500 mg	Normal-to-mild elevation	Normal to elevated	Positive	Decreased
IV	Diffuse proliferative	Mesangial, subendothelial, and/or subepithelial	RBC, WBC, RBC casts	1,000–>3,500 mg	Normal to dialysis dependent	High	Positive to high titer	Decreased
V	Membranous	Mesangial, subepithelial	Bland	>3,000 mg	Normal-to-mild elevation	Normal	Absent to modest titer	Normal

[a]These are only guidelines, and parameters may vary, substantiating the need for biopsy when precise diagnosis is required.

dsDNA, double-stranded DNA; RBC, red blood cell; WBC, white blood cell.

Adapted from: Buyon JP. Systemic lupus erythematosus: A. Clinical and laboratory features. In: Klippel JH, Stone JH, Crofford LJ, et al., eds. *Primer on the Rheumatic Diseases.* 13th ed. New York, NY: Springer Science + Business Media; 2008:303–318.

- ○ Although the classification of lupus nephritis is based on glomerular involvement, other portions of the kidneys can be affected.
  - ■ **Tubulointerstitial nephritis** is often seen in lupus nephritis and is associated with progressive clinical course, including the development of worsening creatinine and hypertension.
  - ■ **Vascular disease** can present as immune complex deposition within the endothelium of the vessel, immunoglobulin microvascular casts, vasculitis, or a thrombotic microangiopathy similar to thrombotic thrombocytopenic purpura (TTP) or atypical hemolytic–uremic syndrome (aHUS). Necrotizing vasculopathy is a poor prognostic sign.
- ○ **Kidney biopsies** should be performed when renal functioning is worsening, abnormal urinary sediments are seen, or when the clinical picture is unclear. Other causes of worsening renal function in SLE patients include nonsteroidal anti-inflammatory drug (NSAID) toxicity, uncontrolled hypertension, and TTP.
- ○ End-stage renal disease due to long-standing lupus nephritis requires hemodialysis, and some patients may be suitable for transplantation. Recurrence of nephritis in allograft transplantation occurs in 3.8% to 44% of patients.[16]
- • **Gastrointestinal (GI) signs and symptoms**
  - ○ Common symptoms include anorexia, nausea, or vomiting.
  - ○ Most symptoms are from **medication side effects** rather than SLE itself.
    - ■ NSAIDs, azathioprine (AZA), and glucocorticoids are associated with **pancreatitis**.
    - ■ Abnormal hepatic function tests can be seen, particularly in the setting of concurrent NSAID use. Frank autoimmune hepatitis is rare in the setting of SLE.
  - ○ Abdominal pain has a wide range of etiologies.
    - ■ Infection, thrombosis (sometimes associated with antiphospholipid antibody syndrome [APLS]), medication side effects, appendicitis, peptic ulcer disease (from steroids or NSAIDs), and gastroenteritis are the most common causes. Consider CMV infection in patients on immunosuppression with abdominal pain and GI bleeding.
    - ■ Abdominal pain due to SLE is usually from **peritoneal inflammation**, though this is much less common than pleural inflammation.
    - ■ Less commonly, **mesenteric vasculitis** can occur. This can present with lower abdominal pain. Symptoms can be mild in nature because of the inflammatory blunting associated with immunosuppressive medications. However, these patients can rapidly deteriorate and end up with bowel infarction, perforation, and peritonitis.
    - ■ Abdominal computed tomography (CT) with arteriogram may be necessary to differentiate from more benign causes of abdominal pain. High-dose steroid use may mask serious abdominal conditions.
- • **Pulmonary signs and symptoms**
  - ○ **Pleuritic chest pain** is the most common pulmonary symptom. This may be due to costochondritis and can be distinguished from pleuritis by palpating the painful areas.
  - ○ The most common sign is **pleural effusion** and is usually associated with **pleuritis**.
    - ■ Most pleural effusions are asymptomatic.
    - ■ Pleural fluid is typically exudative with 3,000 to 5,000 white blood cells (WBC)/mm^3, normal glucose, decreased complement levels, and positive ANA.
  - ○ Pneumonitis, interstitial lung disease, pulmonary hypertension, and alveolar hemorrhage occur less commonly (<10%).
    - ■ **Acute pneumonitis** and **alveolar hemorrhage** can present identically. Fever, cough, dyspnea, pleurisy, and late inspiratory crackles occur in both settings. CT has a ground-glass appearance, which is a nonspecific finding. Bronchoscopy may be useful for directly observing blood on repeated bronchoalveolar lavage, associated with alveolar hemorrhage.

- The prevalence of **interstitial lung disease** is increased in those who were diagnosed with SLE as a child and now are in their 20s to 30s. These patients will have a restrictive pattern on pulmonary function testing (PFTs).
  - **Thromboembolic involvement** occurs in the setting of APLS (see Chapter 44).
  - **Shrinking lung syndrome** is rare and characterized by dyspnea, episodic pleuritic chest pain, and progressive reduction in lung volume in the absence of interstitial fibrosis or pleural disease on CT.
- **Cardiovascular signs and symptoms**
  - **Pericardial disease** is the most frequent cause of symptomatic cardiac disease.
    - Typically presents with positional substernal chest pain that may be associated with an audible rub on auscultation. Often co-presents with other serositis symptoms (pleuritic and pleural effusion)
    - Echocardiogram (EKG) usually reveals a pericardial effusion that is not hemodynamically compromising.
      - **Pericardial effusion** is one of the most common EKG findings and may occur in asymptomatic patients.
      - **Pericardial tamponade** most commonly occurs after prolonged periods of uncontrolled pericarditis; it is very unusual to be a presenting manifestation of SLE. When the effusion is severe, pericardiocentesis must be performed. Purulent, neoplastic, or tuberculous causes should be considered.
  - **Myocarditis** is an uncommon, asymptomatic manifestation usually seen with pericarditis.
    - Most typical presentation is a resting tachycardia out of proportion to temperature with nonspecific EKG findings and cardiomegaly.
    - Global hypokinesis on EKG is a common finding.
  - **Coronary artery disease (CAD)** is a common cardiac manifestation in SLE patients and most often due to **accelerated atherosclerosis**, not coronary artery vasculitis.
    - Young women have up to a 55-fold increase in the risk of CAD compared to their nonlupus cohort.[17]
    - Suspicion for CAD must be high in any SLE patient, even in young females.
  - **Systolic murmurs** are common, occurring in up to 40% of SLE patients.[18]
    - Functional murmurs can occur from anemia, fever, tachycardia, or cardiomegaly, but structural valvular disease is the most common. Valve thickening can be seen in 70% of patients on transesophageal echocardiogram (TEE).[19]
    - **Mitral valve involvement**, particularly mitral valve prolapse, is the most common valvular etiology of systolic murmur.
    - Valvular disease in SLE patients confers an increased risk of serious complications from cerebrovascular disease, peripheral embolism, heart failure, and infectious endocarditis.
    - A more extreme example of valvular disease is **Libman–Sacks endocarditis**.
      - Verrucous lesions are found near the edge of the mitral, aortic, or tricuspid valves and can lead to **regurgitation** in severe cases.
      - Lesions are usually asymptomatic but can break off producing **systemic emboli**.
      - These lesions are sterile, unlike in bacterial endocarditis. However, the risk of **infective endocarditis** is also increased.
      - The development of lesions does not correlate with disease activity.
  - **Raynaud's phenomenon** is common and manifests in the hands, feet, ears, nipples, or nose. Color changes can be induced by cold temperatures or stress. Two color changes (red, white, or blue) must be reported to confirm the diagnosis.
  - **Pediatric considerations:** In mothers with positive anti-SSA (Ro) antibodies, there is a 1% to 7.5% risk for the fetus to develop **neonatal lupus with congenital heart block**.[20]

- **Neuropsychiatric signs and symptoms**
  - The range of symptoms is extremely broad, encompassing subtle symptoms (i.e., poor concentration and emotional disturbance) to severe symptoms (i.e., stroke, seizures, and psychosis).
  - The ACR has defined central and peripheral manifestations (Table 12-5).[21]
    - Even with these criteria, it can be very difficult to determine whether the symptom is functional (i.e., from a psychological basis) or organic (i.e., from a central or peripheral source). If organic, one must determine whether the symptom is from SLE or another cause. Some believe that antineuronal antibodies may be able to distinguish SLE-derived disease.
    - From most to least common, symptoms include depression, cognitive disturbance, headache, mood disorder, cerebrovascular disease, seizure, polyneuropathy, anxiety, and psychosis.
    - Other signs and symptoms of SLE often accompany central nervous system (CNS) manifestations.
    - CNS lupus patients may have **antiribosomal P protein antibody**.
  - **Psychiatric**
    - A diagnosis of psychiatric disturbance from SLE is always one of exclusion. Infection, electrolyte abnormalities, renal failure, drug effects, mass lesions, arterial emboli, and primary psychiatric disorders must be ruled out. Depression is the most common psychiatric symptom seen in SLE patients.
    - Most acute psychiatric disturbances occur within the first 2 years of diagnosis.
    - **SLE-associated psychosis is a medical emergency** (see Chapter 7). Treatment with **antipsychotics and pulse-dose glucocorticoids** must be started as soon as possible to prevent permanent brain damage.

TABLE 12-5	ABRIDGED VERSION OF THE AMERICAN COLLEGE OF RHEUMATOLOGY DEFINITIONS FOR NEUROPSYCHIATRIC MANIFESTATIONS OF SYSTEMIC LUPUS ERYTHEMATOSUS

Central	Peripheral
Headache	Polyneuropathy
Cognitive dysfunction	Cranial neuropathy
Mood disorders	Mononeuropathy
Seizure disorders	Acute inflammatory demyelinating
Cerebrovascular disease	polyradiculoneuropathy
Anxiety disorder	Autonomic disorder
Acute confusional state	Myasthenia gravis
Psychosis	Plexopathy
Myelopathy	
Aseptic meningitis	
Movement disorder	
Demyelinating syndrome	

Adapted from: Sinclair KC, Miner JJ, Kim AHJ. Immunological mechanisms of neuropsychiatric lupus. *Curr Immunol Rev.* 2015;11:93–106.

□ Glucocorticoids are often associated with psychosis. Symptoms often correlate with initiation or dose increase of drug.

□ Nevertheless, given the significant impact SLE-associated psychosis has on long-term brain function, increasing the glucocorticoids dose is justified when in doubt.

■ **Cognitive defects** range from short-term or long-term memory difficulty, impaired judgment and abstract thinking, aphasia, apraxia, agnosia, and personality changes. Cognitive dysfunction has not been directly correlated with disease activity.

○ **Neurologic**

■ **Stroke** occurs in 3% to 20% of SLE patients.[22]

□ Hypertension, hyperlipidemia, and baseline disease activity are established risk factors.

□ Antiphospholipid antibodies are often present (see Chapter 44). Transient ischemic attacks and small recurrent strokes are most commonly seen in this cohort.

■ **Seizures** are observed in 6% to 51% of SLE patients.[23]

□ Both partial (both complex and focal) and generalized seizures occur.

□ Associated with antiphospholipid and anti-Smith (anti-Sm) antibodies

■ **Headaches,** both tension and migraine, commonly occur in SLE.

■ **Neuropathy** occurs in 10% to 15% of patients, usually due to a vasculopathy of the small vessels affecting peripheral nerves. Electromyographic and nerve conduction abnormalities can be seen, suggesting axonal degeneration.

□ **Sensory nerves** are more affected than motor nerves. Most commonly, bilateral asymmetric paresthesias or numbness occurs and is worse at night. **Small-fiber neuropathy** is underdiagnosed and causes painful symptoms in the absence of nerve conduction study changes.

□ Typically, symptoms are worse later in disease.

■ Uncommon manifestations include transverse myelitis, CNS vasculitis, reversible posterior leukoencephalopathy syndrome (RPLS), movement disorders (such as chorea or ataxia), cranial neuropathies, and aseptic meningitis.

□ **Transverse myelitis** is a medical emergency and requires immediate assessment. It presents with sudden onset of bowel and bladder incontinence along with lower extremity weakness that rapidly ascends, possibly with sensory loss (see Chapter 7). Cerebrospinal fluid (CSF) analysis reveals increased protein and pleocytosis. Urgent imaging with magnetic resonance imaging (MRI) is essential.

□ **CNS vasculitis** is an extremely rare manifestation of SLE. This entity presents with fever, severe headache, and confusion progressing rapidly to psychosis, seizures, and coma.

□ **RPLS** presents with seizures, altered mental status, vision changes, and headache. MRI can help differentiate this from CNS lupus by demonstrating vasogenic cerebral edema predominantly in the posterior cerebral hemisphere.

• **Hematologic signs and symptoms**

○ **Anemia** is the most common hematologic abnormality in SLE.

■ **Anemia of chronic disease (AOCD) is the most common etiology,** but autoimmune hemolytic anemia (AIHA), microangiopathic hemolytic anemia (MAHA), renal failure, and iron deficiency are also seen.

■ **Hemolytic anemias (HAs)** are characterized by low haptoglobin levels (which may be obscured by its increase as an acute-phase reactant), and elevated indirect bilirubin, reticulocyte count, and lactate dehydrogenase.

□ **Autoimmune HA (AIHA):** Peripheral smear with spherocytes, and positive Coombs test. A positive Coombs test can be seen in the absence of AIHA and vice versa.

□ **Microangiopathic HA (MAHA):** Peripheral smear with schistocytes. One must be vigilant to the features of TTP (see later).

- ○ **Leukopenia** is also common and correlates with disease activity.
  - ▪ **Neutropenia** may result from disease activity, medications (i.e., cyclophosphamide [CYC] or AZA), bone marrow dysfunction, or hypersplenism. Interestingly, CNS lupus has been associated with severe neutropenia.
  - ▪ **Lymphopenia**, particularly of T cells, is observed in over 50% of SLE patients.[24] Both SLE disease activity and steroid therapy can depress lymphocyte counts; therefore, it is important to consider what other manifestations are present to correctly assign causality.
  - ▪ Depressed eosinophil and basophil counts are typically associated with steroid therapy.
- ○ **Thrombocytopenia** has several potential causes, including iatrogenic (i.e., heparin). Mild thrombocytopenia (platelet counts between 100,000 and 150,000/µL) is seen in up to 50% of patients, with counts of less than 50,000/µL in only 10%.
  - ▪ **Idiopathic thrombocytopenic purpura (ITP)** is a major etiology, with antibody binding to platelets, followed by splenic phagocytosis causing immune-mediated destruction. ITP may be the first presenting sign of SLE in some patients.
  - ▪ **TTP** leads to platelet consumption and is a medical emergency (see Chapter 7).
    - □ Affected patients can have concurrent renal failure, MAHA, fever, and neurologic involvement.
    - □ Schistocytes on peripheral blood smear with an elevated lactate dehydrogenase (LDH), reduced haptoglobin, and elevated bilirubin will be seen.
    - □ Urgent plasmapheresis should be initiated.
    - □ Antibodies that inhibit ADAMTS13 are typically seen, but therapy should not be delayed until results of this specialized test are reported.
- ○ **Thrombocytosis** is infrequent and is associated with increased risk of thromboembolic disease, particularly in the setting of APLS or nephrotic syndrome (renal vein thrombosis).
- ○ **Pancytopenia** can be due to peripheral destruction or bone marrow failure.
  - ▪ Acute leukemia, large granular lymphocyte leukemia, myelodysplastic syndromes, overwhelming infection, and paroxysmal nocturnal hemoglobinuria (PNH) all can induce bone marrow failure with autoimmune features resembling SLE.
  - ▪ **Macrophage activation syndrome (MAS)** is a form of hemophagocytic lymphohistiocytosis (HLH) seen in connective tissue diseases.
    - □ **Marked cytopenias of two or three cell lines** are seen, with a reduction in ESR, elevations in prothrombin time (PT) and activated partial thromboplastin time (aPTT), hypertriglyceridemia, and hyperferritinemia.
    - □ Low or absent natural killer cell activity and elevations in soluble CD25 (interleukin [IL]-2 receptor) are typically seen.
    - □ Fever, weight loss, arthritis, and rash are common symptoms.
    - □ Bone marrow biopsy will reveal hemophagocytosis.
    - □ MAS responds well to immunosuppression.
- ○ APLS (see Chapter 44) is associated with an elevated aPTT, thrombocytopenia, **arterial and venous thrombosis**, and **fetal loss**. The presence of **lupus anticoagulant, anticardiolipin antibodies, or anti–β-2-glycoprotein-1 antibodies** (especially of the immunoglobulin M [IgM] and IgG subclasses) characterizes this syndrome.
- • **Ophthalmologic signs and symptoms**
  - ○ Dry eye (**keratoconjunctivitis sicca**) is the most common manifestation of the eye. Dry eye can be associated with Sjögren's syndrome (see Chapter 14).
  - ○ Anterior uveitis, keratitis, scleritis, and episcleritis present with photophobia and pain.
  - ○ Retinal vasculopathy is characterized by cotton-wool exudates and hemorrhages, similar to hypertensive or diabetic retinopathy. It is usually associated with CNS disease.
  - ○ The optic nerve and cranial nerves can also be affected, causing vision loss and double vision, respectively.

- Glucocorticoids may worsen or cause glaucoma and cataract formation. Patients need yearly screening by an ophthalmologist for plaquenil retinopathy (Bull's-eye maculopathy).

Diagnostic Criteria

- The ACR and EULAR revised SLE classification criteria in 2018 to establish the presence of SLE for clinical research, which are expected to be published in 2019 (1997 criteria in Table 12-1). These criteria are not to be used to strictly diagnose SLE. Nevertheless, they can assist the clinician in recognizing signs and symptoms observed in SLE.
- The diagnosis of SLE requires **multiorgan involvement with evidence of autoimmunity.**
- Symptoms are often vague at initial presentation, and the diagnosis may become more apparent over time.
- A thorough history and physical examination is necessary to confidently diagnose SLE because no single diagnostic test is pathognomonic. Lab tests and imaging should be based on findings from history and physical examination.

Differential Diagnosis

- The highly variable manifestations of SLE lead to a very broad differential diagnosis.
- Typically, infection, other connective tissue diseases, and other systemic conditions such as sarcoidosis, amyloidosis, and malignancies are considered.

Diagnostic Testing

SLE is one of the diseases where the diagnostic testing only supplements a careful history and physical examination. **There is no test that rules in SLE.**

Laboratories
- Comprehensive metabolic panel (CMP), complete blood count (CBC) with differential, ESR, C-reactive protein (CRP), and urinalysis (UA) provide diagnostically useful information and should be obtained for every suspected and established SLE patient. **Complement (C3 and C4) levels** can be beneficial in those patients whose complement levels correlate with disease activity (lower complement levels, higher disease activity). In addition, cell-bound complement split products (such as erythrocyte- or B-cell–bound C4d) has been shown to be helpful in subsets of patients with SLE.
- Autoantibodies are characteristic of SLE and represent autoreactivity to nuclear proteins and nucleic acids. As a result, these are usually the first diagnostic tests ordered (see Chapter 5).
  - **ANA is present in more than 99% of SLE patients,** meaning that its absence virtually rules out SLE.
    - Patients with SLE typically have ANA positivity in **significant titers** (>1:160). Suspicion of an autoimmune disorder should be elevated with titers of more than 1:640.
    - **The pattern of ANA reactivity has little diagnostic value** because recognition of patterns is dependent on the experience of the operator and serum dilution.
    - The false-positive rate in healthy people varies from 30% with titers of 1:40 (high sensitivity, low specificity) to 3% with titers of 1:320 (low sensitivity, high specificity).[25]
    - Among patients referred to a rheumatologist with a positive ANA (titer ≥ 1:40), only 19% were diagnosed with SLE.[26] Most of the ANA-positive patients without SLE had no underlying disease or had fibromyalgia-like manifestations.
    - Low-titer ANAs can be found in other autoimmune diseases, such as Sjögren's syndrome, scleroderma, juvenile idiopathic arthritis, rheumatoid arthritis, interstitial lung disease, primary autoimmune cholangitis, or autoimmune hepatitis or thyroiditis.

- Certain medications (Table 12-2) can induce ANA positivity and **DIL**, which includes **drug-induced SLE (DI-SLE), DI-SCLE, and tumor necrosis factor (TNF) inhibitor–induced SLE.**
  - □ **DI-SLE** has minimal cutaneous findings, largely systemic findings. Positive ANA, positive anti-histone Ab. Procainamide, hydralazine, isoniazid, chlorpromazine, phenytoin, quinidine, methyldopa, and minocycline have been linked to **DI-SLE.**
  - □ **DI-SCLE** has largely cutaneous findings. Positive SSA/Ro. Hydrochlorothiazide, terbinafine, diltiazem, taxanes, griseofulvin, and omeprazole have been known to cause DI-SCLE.
  - □ **TNF inhibitor–induced SLE** has both cutaneous and systemic findings. Positive ANA and positive double-stranded DNA (dsDNA) are observed. Anti-histone Ab may not be positive.
  ○ If a significant titer ANA (>1:160) is noted, speciation of the autoantibodies should be performed, including assays for **anti-dsDNA, anti-Sm, anti-SSA (Ro), anti-SSB (La), anti-RNP, antiphospholipid antibodies, and antiribosomal P protein antibodies.**
    - **Anti-dsDNA** and **anti-Sm** are highly specific for SLE. Anti-dsDNA antibodies may correlate with disease activity and nephritis. Unfortunately, they have poor sensitivity, with only about 30% of SLE patients showing positivity for these tests.
    - **Anti-RNP** can be found in SLE, mixed connective tissue disease, and scleroderma.
    - **Anti-SSA** and **anti-SSB** are associated with Sjögren's syndrome and neonatal lupus. Anti-SSA is seen with lymphopenia, photosensitivity, C2 deficiency, and SCLE.
    - **Antiribosomal P protein** is associated with CNS lupus.

Imaging
Decision to pursue imaging is dependent on the patient's symptoms and the test's diagnostic or prognostic value.

- For chest pain, consider EKG and/or chest radiograph or CT.
- For joint pain, consider plain radiographs of affected joints.
- For renal involvement, consider renal ultrasound to assess kidney size and rule out urinary tract obstruction.
- For abdominal pain, consider abdominal and pelvic CT and/or angiogram if vasculitis is suspected.
- For CNS manifestations, consider brain MRI.
- For peripheral neuropathies or weakness, consider nerve conduction studies with electromyography.

Diagnostic Procedures
As with imaging, decision to obtain fluid or tissue is dependent on the symptoms and the value to diagnosis or prognosis.

- For rash, consider skin biopsy.
- For renal involvement, consider kidney biopsy.
- For fluid associated with serositis (pleural effusion, pericardial effusion, or ascites), consider draining fluid.
- For cytopenias with suspected bone marrow involvement, consider bone marrow biopsy.
- For joint effusions, consider arthrocentesis.

TREATMENT

- **Treatment is based on the type and severity of clinical manifestations** (see Chapter 9).
- Symptoms that are mild and not organ- or life-threatening are typically treated with less potent immunosuppressive medications or nonpharmacologic therapies to minimize side effects.

- Conversely, **organ- or life-threatening disease requires maximal immunosuppression.**
  ○ These usually include **induction** and **maintenance** therapies.
  ○ Because SLE is a chronic, incurable condition characterized with flares, certain drugs are reserved for quickly resolving lupus flares and some are best for suppression of subsequent flares. Typically, drugs used for flares have side-effect profiles, preventing their long-term use.
  ○ The maintenance medications are used for cytotoxic- and steroid-sparing purposes and to suppress future flares. These medications do not rapidly resolve active flares.

Medications
Mild Disease
- Lifestyle modifications including **photoprotection** and smoking cessation as mentioned in the following are important.
- Mucocutaneous, musculoskeletal, hematologic (excluding HA and MAS), and serosal disease can usually be treated with less potent immunosuppressive therapies.
- **NSAIDs/cyclooxygenase (COX)-2 inhibitors** are used for the treatment of arthralgias, arthritis, fever, and mild serositis.
- **Aspirin** (see Chapter 44)
- **HCQ**
  ○ HCQ is an antimalarial drug. It is **very useful for mucocutaneous disease, arthritis, alopecia, and fatigue.** Because of its beneficial effect on lipid profiles, it may also help prevent CAD. **Daily dose of up to 5 mg/kg (200–400 mg/day) after meals is typical.**
  ○ Onset of action is very slow (about 6 weeks), and peak efficacy may not be reached for 4 months.
  ○ GI side effects, especially nausea, are the most common.
  ○ Regular ophthalmologic visits (yearly, starting after the first 5 years of treatment) depending on age, liver and kidney function, and dose) should occur because HCQ can cause macular toxicity, leading to blindness.[27]
  ○ Test for **glucose-6-phosphate deficiency** as these patients are at increased risk for hemolysis.
  ○ If there are no contraindications, almost all SLE patients are placed on HCQ therapy, regardless of the type of disease. There is solid evidence for a reduced frequency of flare if blood levels more than 1,000 ng/mL are achieved.[28]
- **Dapsone**
  ○ Dapsone is used for **cutaneous lupus** such as bullous lupus, subacute cutaneous lupus, and discoid lupus. Starting dose is 50 mg orally (PO) qday, with a typical dose of 100 mg PO qday.
  ○ Test for **glucose-6-phosphate deficiency** as these patients are at increased risk for hemolysis. Hemoglobin and reticulocyte count should be monitored during therapy.
- **Topical steroids**
  ○ Hydrocortisone can be used early in mild skin disease, but most require fluorinated preparations with increased potency. Do not use fluorinated steroids on the face.
  ○ Ointments are more effective than creams.
  ○ Scalp lesions should be treated with lotions, gels, or solutions.
- **Low-dose systemic glucocorticoids:** Doses of prednisone ≤10 mg PO daily are effective until a steroid-sparing agent (i.e., HCQ) can take effect.
- **Thalidomide**
  ○ Thalidomide is used as third- or fourth-line treatment in **cutaneous lupus**, with about a 90% response[29] rate depending on the subtype of cutaneous lupus according to a recent systematic review.
  ○ Its use is limited by high cost, teratogenicity, and adverse effects. Peripheral neuropathy is the most common side effect at 16%, with 4% of patients experiencing persistent symptoms after withdrawal of thalidomide.[29]

Moderate–Severe Disease

- **High-dose systemic glucocorticoids**
  - These are the most potent and fastest-acting class of immunosuppressive medications. They are used primarily for **induction** therapy.
  - **Pulse-dose glucocorticoids (methylprednisolone)**
    - Reserved for organ-threatening disease
    - Dosed 1 g intravenously (IV) daily for 3 days, followed by a taper with oral steroids (prednisone 1 mg/kg PO qday)
    - This approach is entirely empiric, with no clinical data supporting this dosing regimen; nevertheless, it is widely used.
  - **Oral glucocorticoids (prednisone)**
    - Used for moderately severe flares or tapering from pulse-dose steroids
    - Goal is to change to steroid-sparing therapies as quickly as possible to reduce the risk of the numerous side effects associated with steroids.
    - Every SLE patient on glucocorticoids should be considered for a steroid-sparing agent, especially once the acute flare has been controlled.
    - Osteoporosis prevention should be considered.
- **CYC**
  - CYC is reserved for **severe and life-threatening disease manifestations,** such as severe lupus nephritis, CNS lupus, APLS, or vasculitis.
  - It is considered **induction therapy,** but onset of action is somewhat longer than that for glucocorticoids, so it is often used concomitantly with high-dose steroids in induction therapy.
  - CYC can be delivered IV (monthly) or PO (daily).
    - In general, **IV CYC** has shown efficacy in inducing the remission of severe SLE manifestations, such as diffuse proliferative nephritis. This approach is more advantageous than daily PO CYC because the total dose of drug is less over a fixed period of time. This reduces the risk of severe side effects seen with CYC therapy. Concomitant use of 2-mercaptoethane sulfonate sodium (MESNA) may also reduce the risk of cystitis and bladder cancer. However, oral CYC is considered to be more potent.
    - High-dose IV CYC (National Institutes of Health protocol) has been traditionally used for severe disease. More recently, low-dose IV CYC protocol (Euro-Lupus protocol) has been increasingly used with equal efficacy for proliferative lupus nephritis.[30]
    - Check a CBC 8 to 10 days after IV CYC infusion to monitor for a dose-dependent nadir in leukocyte count. The target count should be 2.5 to 3.5/mm^3. Lymphopenia will be common, but **neutropenia should be avoided**.
  - Nausea, vomiting, alopecia, bone marrow suppression, infections, and bladder carcinoma are the most common adverse reactions.
- **Mycophenolate mofetil (MMF)**
  - MMF is typically used to prevent renal allograft rejection. Data suggest MMF noninferiority to IV CYC in short-term remission from lupus nephritis with a better safety profile.[31]
  - It may also be useful as a steroid-sparing agent.
  - Dosing ranges from 500 to 1,500 mg PO twice daily (bid). Most will see efficacy at 1,000 mg PO bid.
  - Side effects include GI upset, cytopenias, and increased risk of infections.
- **AZA**
  - AZA is used as a **steroid-sparing agent** and thus is considered a maintenance medication.
  - Starting dose is 1 mg/kg/day and is uptitrated to between 2 and 2.5 mg/kg/day.

- ○ **Thiopurine methyltransferase** (TPMT) inactivates AZA, so TPMT enzyme activity should be checked prior to use to prevent bone marrow toxicity. Even low doses of AZA can cause pancytopenia in individuals with low TPMT enzyme activity.
- ○ **Regularly monitor hepatic and renal function** as it is hepatically metabolized and renally excreted.
- ○ Be cautious with its use with allopurinol because acute pancytopenia can occur with concurrent use.
- ○ AZA can be used in pregnancy but does pass into breast milk and breastfeeding is not advised.
- **Methotrexate (MTX)**
  - ○ There are conflicting results regarding the use of MTX for SLE within the literature.
  - ○ It appears that MTX may be efficacious for **cutaneous and articular manifestations**, allowing for tapering of steroid. It is considered a steroid-sparing agent.
  - ○ It is usually dosed between 7.5 and 20 mg PO once weekly.
  - ○ Folic acid supplementation (1 mg PO qday) may be needed to abrogate some of the side effects of MTX, including alopecia, GI complaints, hepatic function test elevations, and mucositis.
  - ○ MTX should be discontinued 6 months prior to pregnancy for both males and females.
- **Cyclosporine**
  - ○ Cyclosporine is not commonly used for SLE but has been efficacious for moderate systemic manifestations of lupus as a steroid-sparing agent.
  - ○ Dosages range from 2.5 to 5 mg/kg/day.
  - ○ Side effects are dose dependent and reversible, including **hypertension, transaminitis** and **creatinine elevations,** GI complaints, tremor, and infections.
  - ○ Although effective for membranous glomerulonephritis, long-term treatment can induce interstitial fibrosis and tubular atrophy.
- **B-cell modulating agents are usually used in disease resistant to standard therapies**.
  - ○ **Belimumab** is a human monoclonal antibody against B-cell survival factor. It has been Food and Drug Administration (FDA) approved for use in SLE. It is typically used for active musculoskeletal or cutaneous disease.[32]
  - ○ **Rituximab** is a B-cell depleting chimeric monoclonal antibody. Use in patients unresponsive to standard therapy is controversial—small trials in SLE showed efficacy, but two randomized trials did not show benefit.[33] Nevertheless, many SLE experts believe this can be highly efficacious in certain SLE populations.
- **Other therapies** that have been utilized with varying success include IV immunoglobulin, plasmapheresis, and immunoablation with or without autologous stem cell transplantation.
- Drug development for SLE is advancing at a very rapid rate, with several candidate drugs demonstrating potential.

Other Medications
- **Bisphosphonates** should be started with long-term, high-dose prednisone use, or with evidence of osteopenia with an appropriate Fracture Risk Assessment Tool (FRAX) score. Treatment should last for 3 to 5 years.
- **Statins** should be used based on guidelines for the general population.

Lifestyle/Risk Modification

- Low-impact exercise (i.e., water aerobics) is extremely beneficial for SLE patients. This prevents deconditioning and weight gain.
- For patients with photosensitivity, **avoiding intense sun exposure** with routine sunscreen use (SPF > 50) and appropriate clothing is necessary.
- **Smoking cessation** is important because smoking is associated with higher disease activity and can reduce the efficacy of several medications. Strongly advise patients to stop smoking.

SPECIAL CONSIDERATIONS

- Although variable, SLE may significantly worsen during **pregnancy**.
- Best outcomes occur when the disease has been quiescent from 6 to 12 months prior to conception.
- Fetal loss is highest when high lupus activity occurs in the first or second trimester or when new-onset lupus nephritis occurs in the first trimester.
- Preeclampsia can mimic SLE flares (proteinuria, thrombocytopenia).
- Pregnant SLE patients should be followed closely by a rheumatologist and high-risk obstetrician.

REFERRAL

- It is appropriate to refer to a rheumatologist when you suspect that a patient has symptoms consistent with SLE and has a positive ANA.
- **Any patient with established SLE should see a rheumatologist for disease management and monitoring for side effects from immunosuppressive medications.**
- Ophthalmology referral for HCQ drug toxicity monitoring is required.
- For difficult skin manifestations from lupus, dermatology referral is highly recommended.

PATIENT EDUCATION

- At the time of initial diagnosis, patients are unfamiliar with the disease and its complexity. Consequently, education and counseling are important. Several foundations and organizations dedicated to patients with lupus have excellent resources for the newly diagnosed.
- Patients must be informed of the side effects associated with their specific immunosuppression regimen to avoid life-threatening complications.

MONITORING/FOLLOW-UP

- The goal during follow-up is to monitor for drug-induced toxicity, infection, and flares.
- A history and physical examination, along with laboratory testing, should be routinely done during the follow-up period.
  - When relapses occur, the history and physical findings will typically mimic the patient's initial presentation.
  - CMP, CBC, ESR, CRP, and UA with microscopic examination along with urinary protein-to-creatinine ratios should be obtained with each visit. In some patients, complement levels (C3 and C4) and anti-ds DNA titers parallel disease activity and may be useful in monitoring activity.
  - Lipid profiles and 25-hydroxyvitamin D levels should be checked annually.
  - Dual-emission x-ray absorptiometry (DEXA) scan should be obtained every 2 years.
  - Routine vaccinations with inactivated virus vaccines should be performed.

OUTCOME/PROGNOSIS

- SLE has a variable clinical course.
- Many patients relapse, requiring high-dose steroids or induction treatment with cytotoxic agents.
- Despite this, **the 5-year survival rate is more than 90%.** Likelihood of survival is highly dependent on organs involved. Best outcomes are associated with skin or musculoskeletal involvement only, whereas **kidney and CNS involvement confer the poorest prognoses.**
- Early in disease, the major cause of mortality is active disease or infection related to medications. Late in disease, SLE itself (i.e., end-stage renal disease), vascular disease, infections, non-Hodgkin's lymphoma, and lung cancer are the leading causes of death.

REFERENCES

1. Petri M, Orbai AM, Alarcon GS, et al. Derivation and validation of the Systemic Lupus International Collaborating Clinics classification criteria for systemic lupus erythematosus. *Arthritis Rheum.* 2012;64(8):2677–2686.
2. Rees F, Doherty M, Grainge MJ, et al. The worldwide incidence and prevalence of systemic lupus erythematosus: a systematic review of epidemiological studies. *Rheumatology (Oxford).* 2017;56(11):1945–1961.
3. Mina R, Brunner HI. Update on differences between childhood and adult-onset systemic lupus erythematosus. *Arthritis Res Ther.* 2013;15:218.
4. Ulff-Møller CJ, Simonsen J, Kyvik, KO, et al. Family history of systemic lupus erythematosus and risk of autoimmune disease: Nationwide Cohort Study in Denmark 1977–2013. *Rheumatology.* 2017;56:957–964.
5. Tsokos GC, Lo MS, Costa Reis P, et al. New insights into the immunopathogenesis of systemic lupus erythematosus. *Nat Rev Rheumatol.* 2016;12:716–730.
6. Bentham J, Morris DL, Graham DSC, et al. Genetic association analyses implicate aberrant regulation of innate and adaptive immunity genes in the pathogenesis of systemic lupus erythematosus. *Nat Genet.* 2015;47:1457–1464.
7. Bernier MO, Mikaeloff Y, Hudson M, et al. Combined oral contraceptive use and the risk of Systemic Lupus Erythematosus. *Arthritis Rheum.* 2009;61:476–781.
8. Cosenbader KH, Feskanich D, Stampfer MJ, et al. Reproductive and menopausal factors and risk of systemic lupus erythematosus in women. *Arthritis Rheum.* 2007;56:1251–1262.
9. Rosenbaum JT, Silverman GJ. The microbiome and systemic lupus erythematosus. *N Engl J Med.* 2018;378:2236–2237.
10. Sarkar MK, Hile GA, Tsoi LC, et al. Photosensitivity and type I IFN responses in cutaneous lupus are driven by epidermal-derived interferon kappa. *Ann Rhuem Dis.* 2018;77:1–12.
11. Watanabe T, Tsuchida T. Classification of lupus erythematosus based upon cutaneous manifestations. Dermatological, systemic and laboratory findings in 191 patients. *Dermatology.* 1995;190:277–283.
12. Sontheimer RD. Subacute cutaneous lupus erythematosus: 25-year evolution of a prototypic subset (subphenotype) of lupus erythematosus defined by characteristic cutaneous, pathological, immunological, and genetic findings. *Autoimmun Rev.* 2005;4:253–263.
13. Mok CC, Kwok RC, Yip PS. Effect of renal disease on the standardized mortality ratio and life expectancy of patients with systemic lupus erythematosus. *Arthritis Rheum.* 2013;65:2154–2160.
14. Barjema IM, Wilhelmus S, Alpers CE, et al. Revision of the International Society of Nephrology/Renal Pathology Society classification for lupus nephritis: clarification of definitions and modified National Institutes of Health activity and chronicity indices. *Kidney Int.* 2018;93(4):789–796.
15. Buyon JP. Systemic lupus erythematosus: A. Clinical and laboratory features. In: Klippel JH, Stone JH, Crofford LJ, et al., eds. *Primer on the Rheumatic Diseases.* 13th ed. New York, NY: Springer Science + Business Media; 2008:303–318.
16. Contreras G, Mattiazzi A, Guerra G. Recurrence of lupus nephritis after kidney transplantation. *J Am Soc Nephrol.* 2010;21:1200–1207.
17. Manzi S, Meilahn EN, Rairie JE, et al. Age-specific incidence rates of myocardial infarction and angina in women with systemic lupus erythematosus: comparison with the Framingham Study. *Am J Epidemiol.* 1997;145:408.
18. Mandell BF. Cardiovascular involvement in systemic lupus erythematosus. *Semin Arthritis Rheum.* 1987;17:126.
19. Roldan CA, Qualls CR, Sopko KS, et al. Transthoracic versus transesophageal echocardiography for detection of Libman-Sacks endocarditis: a randomized controlled study. *J Rheum.* 2008;35:224–229.
20. Buyon JP, Kim MY, Copel JA, et al. Anti-RO/SSA antibodies and congenital heart block: necessary but not sufficient. *Arthritis Rheum.* 2001;44:1723–1727.
21. Sinclair KC, Miner, JJ, Kim, AHJ. Immunological mechanisms of neuropsychiatric lupus. *Curr Immunol Rev.* 2015;11:93–106.
22. de Amorim LCD, Maia FM, Rodrigues CEM. Stroke in systemic lupus erythematosus and antiphospholipid syndrome: risk factors, clinical manifestations, neuroimaging, and treatment. *Lupus.* 2017;26:529–536.
23. Hanly JG, Urowitz MB, Su L, et al. Seizure disorders in systemic lupus erythematosus results from an international, prospective, inception cohort study. *Ann Rheum Dis.* 2012;71:1502–1509.
24. Fayyaz A, Ingoe A, Kurien BT, et al. Haematological manifestations of lupus. *Lupus Sci Med.* 2015;2:1–18.
25. Mosca M, Tani C, Bombardieri S. A case of undifferentiated connective tissue disease: is it a distinct clinical entity? *Nat Clin Pract Rheumatol.* 2008;4:328–332.

26. Shiel WC Jr, Jason M. The diagnostic associations of patients with antinuclear antibodies referred to a community rheumatologist. *J Rheumatol.* 1989;16:782–785.

27. Melles RB, Marmor MF. The risk of toxic retinopathy in patients on long-term hydroxychloroquine therapy. *JAMA Ophthalmol.* 2014;132:1453–1460.

28. Costedoat-Chalumeau N, Amoura Z, Hulot JS, et al. Low blood concentration of hydroxychloroquine is a marker for and predictor of disease exacerbations in patients with systemic lupus ERYTHE-MATOSUS. *Arthritis Rheum.* 2006;54:3284–3290.

29. Chasset F, Tounsi T, Cesbron E, et al. Efficacy and tolerance profile of thalidomide in cutaneous lupus erythematosus: a systematic review and meta-analysis. *J Am Acad Dermatol.* 2018;78:342–350.e4.

30. Houssiau FA, Vasconcelos C, D'Cruz D, et al. Immunosuppressive therapy in lupus nephritis: the Euro-Lupus Nephritis Trial, a randomized trial of low-dose versus high-dose intravenous cyclophosphamide. *Arthritis Rheum.* 2002;46:2121–2131.

31. Ginzler EM, Dooley MA, Aranow C, et al. Mycophenolate mofetil or intravenous cyclophosphamide for lupus nephritis. *N Engl J Med.* 2005;353:2219–2228.

32. Navarra SV, Guzman RM, Gallacher AE, et al. Efficacy and safety of belimumab in patients with active systemic lupus erythematosus: a randomised, placebo-controlled, phase 3 trial. *Lancet.* 2011;377(9767):721–731.

33. Merrill JT, Neuwelt CM, Wallace DJ, et al. Efficacy and safety of rituximab in moderately-to-severely active systemic lupus erythematosus: the randomized, double-blind, phase II/III systemic lupus erythematosus evaluation of rituximab trial. *Arthritis Rheum.* 2010;62:222–233.

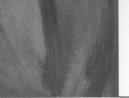

Inflammatory Myopathies

13

Shuang Song and Prabha Ranganathan

GENERAL PRINCIPLES

The inflammatory myopathies (IMs) are a heterogeneous group of disorders characterized by symmetric proximal muscle weakness caused by inflammation of the skeletal muscles (**myositis**).

Classification

Idiopathic inflammatory myopathies (IIMs) are classified into several subtypes: **dermatomyositis (DM)**, **polymyositis (PM)**, **immune-mediated necrotizing myopathy (IMNM)**, and **inclusion body myositis (IBM)**. The DM spectrum includes **clinically amyopathic dermatomyositis (CADM)**.[1]

Epidemiology

- IIMs are rare, with an estimated incidence of about 1 in 100,000 individuals per year. DM and PM are the most common subtypes.
- IIM can occur in any age group. The mean age at onset for PM is 50 to 60 years of age, but it can occur at a younger age. DM has a bimodal distribution: one peak at 5 to 15 years and the other at 30 to 60 years of age. IBM peaks after the age of 50 and is the most frequent acquired myopathy after age 50 years.
- Females are affected more often than males (3:1) in the both DM and PM cases, whereas IBM affects more men than women (3:1).
- African Americans are at increased risk for DM and PM.
- IMNM is very rare, and the estimated incidence is about two per million per year.[2]

Etiology

Etiology is unknown, but genetics, autoimmunity, and the environment may play important roles.

- **Genetic factors:** The strongest association is within the 8.1 ancestral haplotype (8.1 AH) of the *MHC* genes, where HLA-DRB1*03:01 and HLA-B*08:01 are independent risk alleles for IIM. Non-MHC loci of significant association, such as *PTPN22*, *STAT4*, *UBE2L3*, and *BLK*, overlap with risk variants for other autoimmune diseases.[3] A recent large study on IBM confirmed three HLA-DRB1 alleles, HLA-DRB1*03:01, DRB1*01:01, and DRB1*13:0, which were strongly associated with IBM.[4]
- **Autoimmunity:** Autoantibodies, including **myositis-specific autoantibodies (MSAs)** and **myositis-associated autoantibodies (MAAs)**, are present in 50% to 80% of patients with IIM, although whether they are pathogenic is controversial.
- **Environment:** Viral infections (e.g., influenza, HIV, human T-lymphotropic virus 1, hepatitis B and C viruses), bacterial infections, drugs, vaccinations, physical exertion, smoking, and ultraviolet light irradiation have all been implicated in causing muscle inflammation.[5]

Pathophysiology

- The exact mechanisms of pathogenesis are unknown.
- Autoantibodies are common in IIM. The pathogenicity of autoantibodies is unclear. Anti-histidyl-tRNA synthetase antibodies are the most frequent **MSAs** that target the protein synthesis pathway and are associated with antisynthetase syndrome. Others are directed against nuclear or other cytoplasmic components and are associated with distinct clinical subtypes, such as anti–Mi-2, MDA-5, signal recognition particle (SRP), and 3-hydroxy-3-methylglutaryl-coenzyme A reductase (HMGCR) (Table 13-1).[6] **MAAs** such as PM/Scl are often present in overlap syndromes (Table 13-2).[7]
- Complement activation occurs early in DM, leading to damage to capillaries, which may explain the perivascular distribution of CD4+ T cells and occasional B cells in the perimysium in DM. Type 1 interferons (IFNs) are often upregulated in DM.[8]
- Cytotoxic T lymphocytes directed against the muscle fibers are prominent in PM and IBM, which are characterized by predominant endomysial inflammatory aggregates of activated CD8+ T cells, macrophages, and few CD4+ T cells.[8]
- Overexpression of class I MHC is seen early in PM, IMNM, and IBM in non-necrotic muscle cells, preceding inflammatory cell infiltration possibly indicating activation of nuclear factor κB and endoplasmic reticulum (ER) stress response pathways.[8]

Associated Conditions

- IIM is associated with an increased risk of cancers within 3 to 5 years after its onset.[8]
- Relative risk for cancer is three- to six-fold in DM and about two-fold in PM. IMNM can also occur in association with cancer. IBM is not associated with an increased risk of malignancy.
- The types of cancers are similar to those seen in the normal populations, except for an increased incidence of ovarian cancer. The most common cancers are ovarian cancer, breast cancer, colon cancer, melanoma, nasopharyngeal cancer (in Asians), and non-Hodgkin's lymphoma.[8]
- Workup of myositis should include **age- and risk-appropriate cancer screening** and annual screening in the first 3 years after disease onset. When patients with IIM do not respond to therapies, more advanced testing for cancer should be considered.

DIAGNOSIS

- Diagnostic evaluation includes a detailed history, physical examination, laboratory testing for autoantibody profiles, imaging, histopathology, and electromyography (EMG), all of which will be described here.
- Extramuscular manifestations of IM described here can occur at any time and need monitoring.
- The 2017 American College of Rheumatology (ACR)/The European League Against Rheumatism (EULAR) classification criteria for IIM are a useful tool to aid IIM diagnosis.[1]

Clinical Presentation

- DM
  - Muscle weakness
    - Patients often present with subacute or insidious onset of proximal symmetric muscle weakness caused by muscle inflammation. The weakness is typically in the neck, shoulders, thighs, and pelvic area.
    - Dysphagia, dyspnea, gastroesophageal reflux disease (GERD), and urinary and rectal incontinence may occur because of striated muscle involvement.

TABLE 13-1	CLINICAL ASSOCIATIONS OF MYOSITIS-SPECIFIC AUTOANTIBODIES (MSA)		

Autoantigen		Frequency	Clinical Associations
ASA	Aminoacyl tRNA synthetases	Jo-1: 9%–24% adult PM/DM; non–Jo-1: <5% adult PM/DM	Myositis, rash, ILD (non–Jo-1 > Jo-1), mechanics hands, arthritis, Raynaud's phenomenon
SRP	Signal recognition particle	5% Caucasian adult PM/DM; 8%–13% Asian/African adult PM/DM	Highly elevated CK, severe weakness, necrotizing myopathy, dysphagia
HMGCR	3-Hydroxy-3-methylglutaryl-coenzyme A reductase	6% adult PM/DM	Highly elevated CK, necrotizing myopathy, associated with statin use
Mi-2	Nucleosome-remodeling deacetylase complex	9%–24% adult IIM	Rash
SAE	Small ubiquitin-like modifier activating enzyme	6%–8% Caucasian adult PM/DM; 2% Asian adult PM/DM	Rash
MDA-5	Melanoma differentiation-associated gene 5	10%–48% Asian adult DM; 0%–13% Caucasian adult DM	Rash, ILD, rapidly progressing ILD in Asian cohorts
NXP2	Nuclear matrix protein 2	1%–17% adult PM/DM	Rash, possible association with cancer in adults, calcinosis in juveniles
TIF1	Transcriptional intermediary factor 1	13%–31% adult PM/DM	Rash, strongly associated with cancer in adults
cN1A	Cytosolic 5'-nucleotidase 1A	0%–5% adult PM/DM; 33%–34% IBM	Mainly seen in IBM

CK, creatine kinase; DM, dermatomyositis; IIM, idiopathic inflammatory myopathies; ILD, interstitial lung disease; PM, polymyositis.

Adapted from: Betteridge Z, McHugh N. Myositis-specific autoantibodies: an important tool to support diagnosis of myositis. *J Intern Med*. 2016;280:8–23.

- Cutaneous manifestations
  - Gottron's papules are lilac-colored papules that occur on the extensor aspects of the metacarpophalangeal joints (MCPs), proximal interphalangeal joints (PIPs), wrists, elbows, or knees. Gottron's papules are pathognomonic of DM.

TABLE 13-2	CLINICAL ASSOCIATIONS OF MYOSITIS-ASSOCIATED AUTOANTIBODIES (MAA)	
Autoantigen		**Clinical Associations**
PM/Scl	Exosome protein complex (PM/Scl75/100)	Overlap PM/SSc
C1D	Exosome-associated protein	Overlap PM/SSc
U1-RNP	U1 small nuclear RNP	MCTD
Fibrillarin (U3-snRNP)	Fibrillarin	SSc
Ku	DNA-PK regulatory subunit	PM/SSc, potentially severe ILD
Ro52	Ro52/TRIM21	ILD, frequently coupled with other MSA
Ro60/SSA	Ro60/SSA	SS, SLE
La/SSB	SSB	SS, SLE

ILD, interstitial lung disease; MCTD, mixed connective tissue disease; PM, polymyositis; SLE, systemic lupus erythematosus; SS, Sjögren's syndrome; SSc, systemic sclerosis.

Adapted from: Palterer B, Vitiello G, Carraresi A, et al. Bench to bedside review of myositis auto-antibodies. *Clin Mol Allergy.* 2018;16.

- Gottron's sign refers to a macular rash (without papules) in the same distribution as Gottron's papules.
- Heliotrope rash is a purplish discoloration of the upper eyelids, often associated with periorbital edema.
- Photosensitive erythematous rash on the face, scalp, neck, anterior chest (V sign), and back and shoulders (shawl sign) is common but not specific for DM.
- **Calcinosis** (e.g., in the elbows or knees) is common in juvenile DM, but is occasionally seen in adult DM.
- **Mechanic's hands:** Dilated and irregular capillary loops at the nail folds, irregular and thickened cuticles, and darkened horizontal cracks across the lateral and palmar aspects of the fingers and hands lead to "mechanic's hands." This is often seen in the antisynthetase syndrome and less often in PM.
- Rash can precede muscle weakness by months or even years.
○ Lung disease
- Interstitial lung disease (ILD) is a major risk factor for morbidity and mortality.
- The most common type of ILD in DM is nonspecific interstitial pneumonia (NSIP), followed by cryptogenic organizing pneumonia. Usual interstitial pneumonia (UIP) is less common.
- Antisynthetase and anti–MDA-5 antibodies are strongly associated with ILD.
○ **Arthritis:** Mild joint pain and swelling is common in patients with DM. Arthritis is often symmetric and affects the small joints of the hands and feet. Antisynthetase autoantibodies, especially anti–Jo-1 antibodies, are frequently associated with arthritis.
○ Other systemic manifestations
- Cardiac involvement manifests as conduction abnormalities and arrhythmia.
- Gastrointestinal (GI) tract is often affected in DM. Weakness of the tongue, pharyngeal muscles, lower esophagus, and anal sphincter muscles can cause dysphagia, aspiration pneumonia, and incontinence.

- ○ **Malignancy:** DM is associated with the highest risk of cancer among IIMs. Anti-TIF1γ/α (anti-p155/p140) and anti-NXP2 (anti-MJ) confer the strongest risk of malignancy.[6]
- ○ Antisynthetase syndrome
  - ▪ A subset of patients with DM with antisynthetase autoantibodies have a clinically distinct group of features, often called antisynthetase syndrome.
  - ▪ These clinical features include myositis, ILD, Raynaud's phenomenon, nonerosive symmetric polyarthritis of the small joints, and mechanic's hands.[9]
  - ▪ Anti-Jo-1 is the most common antisynthetase antibody.
- ○ CADM
  - ▪ Patients with CADM have the characteristic cutaneous features of DM without muscle weakness. CADM is "provisional" after 6 months and "confirmed" after 2 years.
  - ▪ CADM comprises two subtypes, amyopathic dermatomyositis (AMD) and hypomyopathic dermatomyositis (HDM).
  - ▪ Extramuscular manifestations can develop in CADM, such as ILD.
  - ▪ Anti–MDA-5 is strongly associated with CADM and ILD.[10]
- ○ **Overlap syndromes:** DM and PM may overlap with other rheumatologic diseases, such as scleroderma, systemic lupus erythematosus (SLE), and mixed connective tissue disease. Certain MAAs are associated with overlap syndromes such as anti-PM/Scl, anti–U1-RNP, anti-Ku, anti-C1D, anti-Ro52, and anti–cN-1A.
- **PM**
  - ○ Muscle weakness in PM is similar to that in DM, but the characteristic cutaneous findings in DM are not seen in PM.
  - ○ Similar to DM, PM may be complicated by lung, cardiac, and GI tract involvement and joint pain.
  - ○ The risk of malignancy is increased in PM.
  - ○ Antisynthetase syndrome is seen in a subgroup of PM patients with antisynthetase antibodies.
  - ○ PM patients with certain MAAs may have overlap syndromes.
- **IMNM**
  - ○ IMNM is characterized by severe proximal weakness, myofiber necrosis with minimal inflammatory cell infiltrates on muscle biopsy, and infrequent extramuscular involvement.
  - ○ There are three subtypes of IMNM: anti-SRP myopathy (39%), anti-HMGCR myopathy (26%), and seronegative IMNM (35%).[11]
  - ○ Both anti-HMGCR and anti-SRP are strongly specific for IMNM.
  - ○ Anti-HMGCR myopathy is often associated with statin exposure.
  - ○ Anti-SRP myopathy patients have severe muscle weakness.
  - ○ Seronegative IMNM patients have the highest malignancy risk. Synchronous malignancy was diagnosed in 21.4% of seronegative IMNM and 11.5% of anti-HMGCR patients. This risk is higher compared to the general population. Anti-SRP IMNM is not associated with an increased incidence of malignancy.[11]
- **Sporadic IBM**
  - ○ IBM is the most common IIM in people aged 50 years or older.
  - ○ IBM is characterized by insidious onset of muscle weakness that is localized predominantly in the quadriceps muscles and finger flexors. Decreased grip strength or asymmetric foot drop along with asymmetric proximal muscle weakness are the most characteristic findings. Axial muscles in the back and neck may be affected. Dysphagia occurs in more than 50% of patients.
  - ○ Unlike DM or PM, IBM is not associated with ILD, cardiac involvement, or an increased risk of malignancy.
  - ○ Anti-cN1A is seen in 37% of IBM patients and, rarely, in DM or PM patients (<5%), but it is also observed frequently in Sjögren's syndrome (36%) and SLE (20%) patients.[12]

Differential Diagnosis

- **Neuromuscular diseases:** One of the first steps in diagnosing IIM is to exclude a neuropathy or neuromuscular disease (e.g., motor neuron diseases, myasthenia gravis, Lambert–Eaton myasthenic syndrome) being the cause of muscle weakness. EMG and muscle biopsies are the most useful tools for differentiation between neuromuscular diseases and IIMs.
- **Muscular dystrophies**
  - **Limb-girdle muscular dystrophies** (LGMDs) include a number of inherited disorders with progressive muscular dystrophy caused by genetic defects.[13]
  - The age at presentation is highly variable, and patients can present even late in adult life.
  - There is a preferential weakness and atrophy of the biceps muscle.
  - Creatine kinase (CK) levels can be dramatically elevated and cannot be used to differentiate between dystrophies and IIM.
  - Magnetic resonance imaging (MRI) is highly useful as in active IIM, there is edema on short tau inversion recovery (STIR) imaging indicative of inflammation whereas LGMD shows extensive fatty replacement, although edema can be seen in the early stages of LGMD.
  - Muscle biopsies may show inflammatory cell infiltrates in LGMD, but the inflammation is often limited to areas adjacent to necrotic fibers.
  - Diagnosis is made by genetic testing and immunohistochemical examination of muscle biopsy.
- **Metabolic myopathies**
  - These rare diseases of muscle energy metabolism may present with muscle weakness, elevated CK, and myopathic changes on EMG.[14]
  - Patients with glycogen metabolism abnormalities or with myoadenylate deaminase deficiency (the most common metabolic myopathy) have exercise intolerance and may be asymptomatic at rest.
  - The forearm ischemic exercise test is a useful screening test that involves checking ammonia and lactate levels before and after vigorous forearm exercise with a blood pressure cuff inflated above systolic pressure.
  - Metabolic myopathies should be suspected in patients who are young, have a family history of myopathy, or fail to respond to immunosuppressive therapy.
- **Mitochondrial myopathies**
  - Mitochondrial disorders can present with isolated proximal muscle weakness, but symptoms tend to be mild or exercise related.[15]
  - Checking lactate levels before and after vigorous exercise may be helpful in the diagnosis.
  - The classic hallmark of mitochondrial disease is subsarcolemmal and intermyofibrillar accumulations visualized on Gomori trichrome staining owing to compensatory proliferation of mitochondria, also known as "ragged red fibers."
  - Special mitochondrial stains that detect succinate dehydrogenase and Cox staining are helpful in diagnosis.
- **Drug- or toxin-induced myopathies**
  - Procainamide and penicillamine, among other drugs, can cause an immune-mediated myopathy.
  - Statins and other lipid-lowering agents may cause mitochondrial dysfunction and myopathy.
  - Chronic ethanol use is associated with painless proximal muscle weakness and atrophy with normal CK.
  - Zidovudine-induced myopathy can demonstrate inflammatory infiltrates on muscle biopsy much like IIM but is reversible over several months if the medication is stopped.

- **Endocrine myopathies**
  - **Glucocorticoid myopathy** is common and usually occurs after months of use; CK levels are normal. Similarly, Cushing's syndrome also manifests as muscle weakness and wasting.
  - **Hypothyroid and hyperthyroid myopathy** can present like PM with progressive symmetric proximal muscle weakness. Serum muscle enzymes, such as CK, aspartate aminotransferase (AST), and alanine aminotransferase (ALT), are often normal or low in hyperthyroidism and elevated in hypothyroidism.
- **Infectious myopathies**
  - HIV myopathy typically presents with a subacute onset and progresses slowly. Similar to IIM, muscle weakness is often proximal and symmetric.
  - Human T-lymphotropic virus 1 myopathy can mimic PM and IBM.
- **Parasitic myopathies:** Parasitic infections such as toxoplasmosis, malaria, echinococcosis, and trichinosis can cause myositis that manifests as myalgias and focal swelling of the muscles. A combination of muscle biopsy and serologic tests is often diagnostic.

Diagnostic Testing

Laboratories
- **Muscle enzymes** are typically elevated, including CK, lactate dehydrogenase (LDH), aldolase, AST, and ALT.
- CK level can be very high ($\geq$50 times the upper limit of normal) in IMNM, and normal or slightly elevated (up to 10 times the upper limit of normal) in IBM; DM and PM are in between.
- Testing of **autoantibodies**, especially MSAs, is important for diagnosis, classification, predicting additional clinical complications, and response to treatment (Tables 13-1 and 13-2).
- **Autoantibodies**
  - **MSAs** are detected primarily in patients with IIM (Table 13-1).[6,7]
    - Traditionally, **anti–Mi-2** is associated with the classic photosensitive rash of DM and predicts a good response to therapy. **Antisynthetase antibodies**, namely, anti-histidyl (Jo 1), anti-threonyl (PL-7), anti-alanyl (PL-12), anti-glycyl (EJ), anti-isoleucyl (OJ), anti-asparaginyl (KS), anti-phenylalanyl (ZO), and anti-tyrosyl (YRS/HA) tRNA synthetases, are strongly associated with the antisynthetase syndrome.
    - Newer MSAs are usually found in DM. **Anti-TIF1γ/α (anti-p155/p140) and anti-TIF1/β** are strongly associated with cancer-associated DM. They are both sensitive (78%) and specific (89%) as cancer markers in older patients with DM. **Anti-MJ/NXP-2** in DM has a positive association with ILD and malignancy. **Anti–MDA-5** seen in CADM is a marker of rapidly progressive ILD. Ulcerative cutaneous lesions, arthritis, abnormal liver functions, and elevated ferritin have been reported with positive anti–MDA-5.
    - **Anti-SRP** and **anti-HMGCR** are almost exclusively seen in PM and IMNM, but not in DM. **Anti-cN1A** is seen in approximately one-third of IBM patients and, rarely, in DM or PM patients.
  - **MAAs** and **antinuclear antibodies (ANAs)** are detected with other autoimmune diseases that may be associated with myositis (Table 13-2).[7]
    - MAA and ANA are present in 30% in adult DM and are more commonly present in juvenile DM (70%).
    - **Anti-Ro52** is frequently associated with other MSAs, such as antisynthetase antibodies, and more commonly found in adult patients with clinical features of DM (24%–35%). Anti-Ro/SSA antibodies seen in Sjögren's syndrome, and SLE are directed against both Ro52-kDa and Ro60-kDa antigens. Ro60 is localized to the nucleus and nucleolus, whereas Ro52 is localized to the cytoplasm.[16]

- **Anti-PM/Scl** is seen in patients with an overlap of myositis and limited scleroderma, often complicated by cardiac involvement and ILD. Anti-Ku and anti-C1D are associated with PM/Scl overlap syndrome. High-titer **anti–U1-RNP** is associated with mixed connective tissue disease.

Imaging

- **MRI** is the modality of choice because it detects inflammation, edema, fat infiltration, fibrosis, and calcification in the skeletal muscles. It also helps guide the site for muscle biopsy.
- **Radiographs and high-resolution computed tomography (CT)** of the lungs are needed to detect and follow ILD.

Diagnostic Procedures

- **EMG** can assist in diagnosis and differential diagnosis.
- EMG in IIM often shows characteristic active or chronic myopathic changes, although they are not specific to each subtype of IIM.[17]
  - Active myopathy is characterized by EMG findings of prominent muscle membrane irritability (fibrillations and positive sharp waves) and motor unit action potentials (MUAPs) that are small, short, polyphasic, and with early recruitment.
  - Chronic myopathy may not show muscle membrane irritability on EMG. A mixed pattern of small and long duration MUAPs may be seen.
- Needle insertion can damage muscle fibers for biopsy; hence, performing EMGs and muscle biopsies on the same side should be avoided.
- **Pulmonary function tests** are useful for initial assessment and monitoring of lung involvement. A restrictive ventilatory impairment is typical for ILD associated with IIM. In patients with a forced vital capacity (FVC) less than 70% or a decrease of more than 10% of FVC, pharmacologic therapy is often indicated.
- **Muscle biopsy** is very important for diagnosing IIM. Histopathology is the "gold standard" for the diagnosis of IIM.[8]
  - **DM:** Perivascular, perimysial, and perifascicular inflammatory infiltrates of mainly CD4+ T cells and B cells; necrotic fibers in "wedge-like" infarcts; perifascicular atrophy; reduced capillaries
  - **PM:** Endomysial infiltrates of CD8+ T lymphocytes with rare B cells; widespread expression of MHC class I antigens
  - **IBM:** CD8+ T cells invading healthy fibers; widespread expression of MHC class I antigens; autophagic vacuoles; congophilic amyloid deposits
  - **IMNM:** Scattered necrotic fibers with macrophages; CD8+ T cells; deposits of complement on capillaries; upregulation of MHC class I antigens in non-necrotic muscle fibers

TREATMENT

The treatment for DM, PM, and IMNM is discussed first. Inclusion body myopathy is discussed at the end of this section.

- **Glucocorticoids**
  - High-dose prednisone at 1 mg/kg orally (PO) daily is the recommended initial treatment, with an average dose of 60 mg, sometimes up to 80 mg daily. In patients with severe myositis or respiratory compromise due to ILD, intravenous (IV) methylprednisolone 1 g daily for 3 days is recommended.
  - High doses should be maintained for 4 to 6 weeks and then tapered with the goal of achieving a low daily dose of prednisone of 5 to 10 mg daily within 6 months.[18] The total duration of glucocorticoid therapy is typically approximately 1 year.

- Muscle enzymes begin to decline within a few weeks of treatment and often normalize in 2 to 3 months.
- **Traditional nonbiologic immunosuppressive agents**
  - **Methotrexate** (15–25 mg weekly) and **azathioprine** (2–3 mg/kg daily) are the first-line choices of steroid-sparing therapy. Either one is often used in combination with glucocorticoids as an initial therapy in myositis. They allow effective reduction of prednisone dose and superior long-term improvement, compared with glucocorticoids alone.[18]
  - **Mycophenolate mofetil** (MMF) may be used as a second-line therapy in patients who have failed methotrexate or azathioprine or in those with ILD.[18]
  - **Calcineurin inhibitors**, including cyclosporine and tacrolimus, target T cells. They are second-line therapy for myositis and myositis-associated ILD. They are generally reserved for patients with refractory myositis because of toxicities requiring drug-level monitoring.[19]
  - **Cyclophosphamide** is a third-line treatment and may be used in patients with severe myositis, rapidly progressive ILD, overlapping systemic vasculitis, or disease refractory to other agents. Bladder toxicity, cytopenias, and increased risk of malignancy are concerns with use of cyclophosphamide.
- **Biologic agents**
  - Rituximab depletes CD20+ B cells and is an effective treatment for myositis. A randomized controlled trial demonstrated that rituximab significantly improved myositis with a median time of 20 weeks, especially in patients with antisynthetase antibodies and anti–Mi-2 antibodies.[18]
  - Anti–tumor necrosis factor (TNF) therapies for myositis have shown mixed results.[18] They are not recommended in general but can be considered for refractory myositis.
  - Tocilizumab, an IL-6 receptor antagonist, has demonstrated effectiveness in myositis in a few case series.[18] Its efficacy in treating adults with refractory PM and DM is under further investigation.
  - Abatacept is a fully humanized fusion protein of cytotoxic T-lymphocyte antigen 4 (CTLA4) and the Fc portion of human immunoglobulin G1 (IgG1) that inhibits T-cell costimulation. Pilot studies show encouraging results of abatacept in treating PM and DM.[20]
  - Anakinra, a recombinant IL-1 receptor antagonist (IL-1Ra), showed beneficial effects in myositis in a recent study.[21]
- **Intravenous immunoglobulin (IVIG):** High-dose IVIG (2 g/kg over 2–5 consecutive days per month) has beneficial effects in IIM, although the precise mechanism of action is unknown. IVIG is usually combined with other immunosuppressive agents and not routinely used because of the high cost and long administration time.
- **Exercise:** Exercise/physical therapy is recommended in patients with both active and stable myositis to prevent muscle loss, atrophy, and joint contractures and preserve muscle function.
- **ILD**
  - High-dose PO or IV glucocorticoids are used as initial therapy. Glucocorticoids combined with azathioprine or MMF are the first-line therapy. Some case reports describe the effective use of IVIG in some patients with refractory myositis–associated ILD. Methotrexate should be used cautiously because of its potential to cause pneumonitis.
  - In severe cases, the initial therapy comprises IV glucocorticoids and rituximab or cyclophosphamide.[18]
  - Calcineurin inhibitors (tacrolimus or cyclosporine), especially tacrolimus, have demonstrated efficacy in treating myositis-associated ILD.
- **Inclusion body myopathy**
  - Immunosuppressive drugs such as glucocorticoids, azathioprine, or methotrexate are not effective in IBM.
  - IVIG can be considered in patients with dysphagia.[22]

OUTCOME/PROGNOSIS

- The severity of IIM is variable, ranging from easily treated mild weakness to life-threatening refractory disease.
- Clinical predictors of poor prognosis include older age, severe weakness at presentation, dysphagia, respiratory muscle weakness, extramuscular involvement of the heart and lungs, and concomitant malignancy.
- MSA and MAA profiles are very helpful in defining clinical phenotypes and prognosis. These are being used increasingly to guide management and to assess prognosis.

REFERENCES

1. Lundberg IE, Tjärnlund A, Bottai M, et al. 2017 European League Against Rheumatism/American College of Rheumatology classification criteria for adult and juvenile idiopathic inflammatory myopathies and their major subgroups. *Ann Rheum Dis.* 2017;76:1955–1964.
2. Basharat P, Christopher-Stine L. Immune-mediated necrotizing myopathy: update on diagnosis and management. *Curr Rheumatol Rep.* 2015;17:72.
3. Rothwell S, Lamb JA, Chinoy H. New developments in genetics of myositis. *Curr Opin Rheumatol.* 2016;28:651–656.
4. Rothwell S, Cooper RG, Lundberg IE, et al. Immune-array analysis in sporadic inclusion body myositis reveals HLA-DRB1 amino acid heterogeneity across the myositis spectrum. *Arthritis Rheumatol.* 2017;69:1090–1099.
5. Miller FW, Lamb JA, Schmidt J, et al. Risk factors and disease mechanisms in myositis. *Nat Rev Rheumatol.* 2018;14:255–268.
6. Betteridge Z, McHugh N. Myositis-specific autoantibodies: an important tool to support diagnosis of myositis. *J Intern Med.* 2016;280:8–23.
7. Palterer B, Vitiello G, Carraresi A, et al. Bench to bedside review of myositis autoantibodies. *Clin Mol Allergy.* 2018;16.
8. Dalakas MC. Inflammatory muscle diseases. *N Engl J Med.* 2015;372:1734–1747.
9. Mahler M, Miller FW, Fritzler MJ. Idiopathic inflammatory myopathies and the anti-synthetase syndrome: a comprehensive review. *Autoimmun Rev.* 2014;13:367–371.
10. Sato S, Hoshino K, Satoh T, et al. RNA helicase encoded by melanoma differentiation-associated gene 5 is a major autoantigen in patients with clinically amyopathic dermatomyositis: Association with rapidly progressive interstitial lung disease. *Arthritis Rheum.* 2009;60:2193–2200.
11. Allenbach Y, Mammen AL, Benveniste O, et al. 224th ENMC International Workshop:: Clinico-sero-pathological classification of immune-mediated necrotizing myopathies Zandvoort, The Netherlands, 14–16 October 2016. *Neuromuscul Disord.* 2018;28:87–99.
12. Herbert MK, Stammen-Vogelzangs J, Verbeek MM, et al. Disease specificity of autoantibodies to cytosolic 5'-nucleotidase 1A in sporadic inclusion body myositis versus known autoimmune diseases. *Ann Rheum Dis.* 2016;75:696–701.
13. Khadilkar SV, Patel BA, Lalkaka JA. Making sense of the clinical spectrum of limb girdle muscular dystrophies. *Pract Neurol.* 2018;18:201–210.
14. Lilleker JB, Keh YS, Roncaroli F, et al. Metabolic myopathies: a practical approach. *Pract Neurol.* 2018;18:14–26.
15. Pfeffer G, Chinnery PF. Diagnosis and treatment of mitochondrial myopathies. *Ann Med.* 2013;45:4–16.
16. Defendenti C, Atzeni F, Spina MF, et al. Clinical and laboratory aspects of Ro/SSA-52 autoantibodies. *Autoimmun Rev.* 2011;10:150–154.
17. Paganoni S, Amato A. Electrodiagnostic evaluation of myopathies. *Phys Med Rehabil Clin N Am.* 2013;24:193–207.
18. Oddis CV, Aggarwal R. Treatment in myositis. *Nat Rev Rheumatol.* 2018;14:279–289.
19. Sharma N, Putman MS, Vij R, et al. Myositis-associated interstitial lung disease: predictors of failure of conventional treatment and response to tacrolimus in a US cohort. *J Rheumatol.* 2017;44:1612–1618.
20. Tjärnlund A, Tang Q, Wick C, et al. Abatacept in the treatment of adult dermatomyositis and polymyositis: a randomised, phase IIb treatment delayed-start trial. *Ann Rheum Dis.* 2018;77:55–62.
21. Zong M, Dorph C, Dastmalchi M, et al. Anakinra treatment in patients with refractory inflammatory myopathies and possible predictive response biomarkers: a mechanistic study with 12 months follow-up. *Ann Rheum Dis.* 2014;73:913–920.
22. Schmidt K, Schmidt J. Inclusion body myositis: advancements in diagnosis, pathomechanisms, and treatment. *Curr Opin Rheumatol.* 2017;29:632–638.

Sjögren's Syndrome

14

Divya Jayakumar and Deepali Sen

GENERAL PRINCIPLES

- Sjögren's syndrome (SS) is one of the more prevalent autoimmune diseases, and its most common features are **dry eyes (keratoconjunctivitis sicca) and dry mouth (xerostomia).**
- Treatment should be aimed at symptomatic relief by keeping mucous membranes moist.

Definition

- SS is a chronic inflammatory disorder characterized by **lymphocytic infiltration and autoimmune destruction of exocrine glands.**
- The **salivary and lacrimal glands** are commonly affected, leading to symptoms of dry mouth (xerostomia) and dry eyes (keratoconjunctivitis sicca). There may also be nasal, external auditory canal and vaginal dryness.

Epidemiology

- Prevalence of SS is approximately 0.5 to 3 million persons in the United States. The incidence of primary SS in the general population is estimated to be 4 per 100,000 annually.
- SS most often occurs in women (female-to-male ratio, 20:1) in their fifth and sixth decades of life.[1]

Pathophysiology

- The primary pathologic mechanism of SS consists of focal infiltration of lymphocytes into glandular tissue.
- SS most commonly affects salivary and lacrimal glands but may occur in any exocrine glandular tissue.
- Antibodies against nuclear antigens **SSA/Ro and SSB/La** are commonly associated with SS, but it is not known if they are pathogenic.
- Although the exact pathophysiologic mechanisms of SS are not completely understood, several different hypotheses have been formulated.
  - A combination of genetic, hormonal, and environmental factors is thought to play a role in the initiation and progression of SS.[2]
  - Certain HLA-DR and HLA-DQ alleles are associated with SS.
  - Viral infections, including Epstein–Barr virus, retroviruses, and hepatitis C, might predispose patients to SS by indirectly altering immune response to favor autoimmune glandular destruction.
  - Glandular epithelial cells become activated and assist in the attraction of B cells, T cells, and dendritic cells to the exocrine glands and promote the release of inflammatory cytokines.[1]
  - The inflammation becomes chronic because of immune dysregulation, resulting in cell-mediated glandular destruction, leading to decreased exocrine secretions.
- Inadequate tearing in SS causes dryness and increased friction between mucosal surfaces. This results in distortion of epithelial cells during the blinking process, leading to **corneal irritation and abrasions.** A localized inflammatory response is precipitated. In addition, the loss of the nutritive effects of tears delays healing.

- Similar pathologic processes affect the oral cavity. Inflammatory destruction of salivary glands leads to quantitative and qualitative changes in saliva production. The normal bacterial flora is altered by changes in salivation, leading to an **increased frequency of dental caries, oral candidiasis, and periodontal diseases.**

Associated Conditions

- SS may occur as a primary disease.
- However, it **commonly occurs as a secondary disease in patients with other systemic autoimmune diseases** (e.g., rheumatoid arthritis [RA], systemic lupus erythematosus [SLE], scleroderma [SSc], mixed connective tissue disease [MCTD], inflammatory myopathies, and autoimmune liver and thyroid diseases).

DIAGNOSIS

Clinical Presentation

History

- Symptoms of SS develop insidiously, commonly over several years.
- Mucosal dehydration, manifested as **dry eyes and dry mouth,** is the most common complaint associated with SS.
- Symptoms of dry eyes include foreign-body sensation, itching, light sensitivity worse in the evening, and thick, crusting film present on awakening. Symptoms are commonly aggravated by airline travel, dry windy conditions, and use of contact lenses.
- Dry mouth often manifests as increased thirst and difficulty swallowing dry foods. Rapidly progressive dental caries, recurrent oral and gingival infections, and discomfort wearing dentures may all be associated with SS.
- **Additional features of exocrine gland dysfunction** include symptoms of dry skin (xerosis), vaginal dryness, upper airway dryness creating a dry cough, and recurrent upper respiratory infections.
- Extraglandular involvement of SS may also occur.
  - **Fatigue and arthralgias** (sometimes arthritis) are common complaints with SS.
  - **Skin lesions** include palpable purpura, urticaria, annular lesions, xerosis, and Raynaud's phenomenon.
  - **Patients can have** increased frequency of sinusitis, bronchitis, pneumonia, and pleural effusions. The most common pulmonary manifestation of SS is interstitial lung disease, specifically lymphocytic interstitial pneumonia (LIP). Patients with LIP should be checked for an underlying SS. **Cardiac involvement** may include pericardial effusions or autonomic dysfunction. Patients with primary SS have an increased risk of cardiovascular disease.
  - **Neurologic complications** may include cognitive dysfunction, demyelinating disease similar to multiple sclerosis, myasthenia gravis, and peripheral neuropathies.
  - **Renal involvement** may manifest as chronic interstitial nephritis and renal tubular acidosis. Membranoproliferative glomerulonephritis can rarely occur with SS.
  - **Gastrointestinal manifestations** include dysphagia, esophageal dysmotility, nausea, dyspepsia, atrophic gastritis, and hepatic abnormalities.

Physical Examination

- Salivary gland enlargement occurs in up to half of the affected patients.
- The glands are usually diffusely firm and nontender. Painful episodic swelling is common and may be either unilateral or bilateral. If the glands get swollen and painful after meals, salivary duct obstruction should be ruled out.

• A hard, nodular gland may suggest a neoplasm. This distinction is clinically significant because there is an **increased incidence of B-cell lymphomas** in salivary glands affected with SS. If the salivary glands are persistently enlarged, hard, or increasing in size, biopsy is recommended.

Diagnostic Criteria

In 2016, new classification criteria for SS were accepted by the American College of Rheumatology (ACR) and the European League Against Rheumatism (EULAR).

These criteria can be applied to patients with either ocular or oral dryness. A total score ≥ 4 is essential for classification of SS:

• Positive serum anti-SSA/Ro (3)
• Labial salivary gland biopsy exhibiting focal lymphocytic sialadenitis with a *focus score ≥ 1 foci/mm² (3)
• Ocular staining score ≥ 5 (or van Bijsterveld score ≥ 4) on at least one eye (1)
• Schirmer's test ≤ 5 mm/5 minutes (1)
• Unstimulated salivary flow rate ≤ 0.1 mL/min (1)

These criteria have a sensitivity of 96% and a specificity of 95%.[3]

Differential Diagnosis

The differential diagnosis of SS includes any disease process that leads to symptoms of dry eyes and dry mouth, including the following:

• **Infiltrative diseases** (e.g., sarcoidosis, amyloidosis, hemochromatosis, immunoglobulin G4 [IgG4]-related syndromes, lymphoma)
• **Infectious diseases** (e.g., viral infections [HIV, hepatitis B and C, mumps, influenza, Coxsackie A, cytomegalovirus], syphilis, trachoma, tuberculosis, bacterial infection)
• **Fat deposition** from diabetes, alcoholism, pancreatitis, cirrhosis, and hypertriglyceridemia
• **Anticholinergic side effects** from medicines (e.g., antidepressants, neuroleptics, antihypertensives, antihistamines, decongestants)
• **Endocrine dysfunction** including acromegaly and gonadal hypofunction

Diagnostic Testing

Laboratories

A general diagnostic workup for SS should include the following laboratory tests:

• Complete blood count (CBC), erythrocyte sedimentation rate (ESR) or C-reactive protein (CRP), rheumatoid factor (RF), antinuclear antibodies (ANAs), and serum protein electrophoresis
• ANA is positive in about 85% and RF is positive in up to 50% of SS patients.
• If the ANA is positive, obtain autoantibodies **SSA/Ro and SSB/La.** SSA/Ro is positive in about 50% and SSB/La in about 33% of patients. Isolated SSB positivity is rare.
• Patients may have mild anemia, cytopenias and increased ESR or CRP.
• Polyclonal hypergammaglobulinemia is common in SS, affecting up to 60% of patients. Monoclonal gammopathies may develop over time.

Diagnostic Procedures

• Functional studies may include **Schirmer's test** for tear secretion.
• Lissamine green or fluorescein dye staining with **slit-lamp examination** is used to detect damaged corneal epithelium. Rose bengal dye is no longer used because of toxic corneal effects.

- **Sialometry, sialography, or scintigraphy** can be performed to measure salivary gland function.
- **Ultrasonography and magnetic resonance imaging (MRI)** may help detect parenchymal abnormalities in salivary glands.
- The gold standard for the diagnosis of SS can be obtained by performing a **minor salivary gland biopsy**, most often obtained from minor salivary glands in the lower lip. Pathologic findings of **focal lymphocyte aggregates, plasma cells, and macrophages** support the diagnosis.
- **Focal lymphocytic sialadenitis** from the labial salivary gland biopsy records the **focus score**, which is the number of foci of lymphoid tissue normalized to 4 mm^2 surface area.

TREATMENT

- Most patients with SS can be managed with education and simple symptomatic relief measures designed to keep mucous membranes moist.
- For dry eyes, patients should use **artificial tears** on a regular basis. Numerous brands are available, and patients are encouraged to try various formulas to find the most suitable one. In general, preservative-free solutions are better tolerated.
  ○ Some patients may benefit from **punctal occlusion** to prolong the efficacy of artificial tears.
  ○ **Topical 0.05% cyclosporine** twice daily for patients with moderate-to-severe dry eye disease has been shown to give the best results in terms of symptomatic relief.[4,5]
  ○ In cases where ocular symptoms are severe and refractory, refer to an ophthalmologist for initiation of topical steroids or nonsteroidal anti-inflammatory drugs (NSAIDs) under their monitoring.
- For dry mouth, patients are encouraged to **drink water frequently.**
  ○ Stimulation of salivary glands with sugar-free gum or candy may also be useful.
  ○ Patients should avoid dry foods as well as alcohol and smoking.
  ○ Artificial saliva products are available.
  ○ Some patients may benefit from treatment with the **muscarinic agonists pilocarpine,** 5 mg orally (PO) four times a day (qid), or **cevimeline,** 30 mg PO three times a day (tid); however, many patients experience side effects of increased urination and defecation, sweating, abdominal cramping, and flushing.[4,6]
  ○ Patients with xerostomia are at increased risk of dental caries and should be followed closely by a dentist. **Topical fluoride treatments** may help prevent tooth decay. Meticulous daily dental hygiene is of utmost importance.
- Dry skin can be managed with moisturizing lotions.
- Vaginal dryness is improved with lubricants.
- Arthralgias and other musculoskeletal complaints are often remedied with NSAIDs.
- Symptoms of arthritis, myalgia, and fatigue may respond favorably to hydroxychloroquine, though there is no proven evidence.
- In those patients with severe progressive disease manifestations of vasculitis, nephritis, interstitial lung involvement, or neuropathy, a combination of steroids and immunosuppressive agents such as azathioprine, methotrexate, mycophenolate mofetil, and intravenous (IV) cyclophosphamide can be considered. Intravenous immunoglobulin (IVIG) may be beneficial in severe motor neuron involvement. Rituximab may also be considered in life-threatening circumstances.[4,7]

COMPLICATIONS

- Cryoglobulinemia can occur with SS and can present with cutaneous or renal vasculitis. Low complement levels can be seen in cryoglobulinemic vasculitis. Cryoglobulinemia may also indicate an underlying lymphoid malignancy.

- SS has been associated with the development of **lymphoma,** with a lifetime risk between 5% and 10%. This is thought to arise because of unregulated B- and T-cell stimulation. **Non-Hodgkin's lymphoma** is observed, of which marginal zone B-cell lymphoma is the most predominant type seen. Factors associated with an increased risk of lymphoma include lymphadenopathy, splenomegaly, low CD4 count, parotid gland enlargement, cryoglobulinemia, neutropenia, low complement levels, and purpura/vasculitis.[8-10] It is recommended that serum protein electrophoresis, serum cryoglobulin level, and serum complement level tests be done annually for these patients.

REFERRAL

Patients with sicca symptoms should be followed closely by a **rheumatologist** and should be referred to both a **dentist** and an **ophthalmologist,** given their increased risk of developing caries and corneal abrasions, respectively. ENT referral may be needed for salivary duct blockages and for salivary gland biopsy in suspected lymphoma.

PATIENT EDUCATION

- Patients with SS should be advised to keep mucous membranes moist for symptomatic relief.
- Encourage patients to avoid dry environments, wind, cigarette smoke, and medications with anticholinergic side effects.
- Humidifiers can counter low-humidity indoor environments, especially in winter months when centralized heating leads to dry air.

OUTCOME/PROGNOSIS

In patients with primary SS without transformation to lymphoma, there does not appear to be an increase in all-cause mortality when compared with the general population; those with lymphoma have a higher mortality rate.

REFERENCES

1. Alamanos Y, Tsifetaki N, Voulgari PV, et al. Epidemiology of primary Sjögren's syndrome in north-west Greece, 1982–2003. *Rheumatology (Oxford).* 2006;45:187–191.
2. Voulgarelis M, Tzioufas A. Pathogenetic mechanisms in the initiation and perpetuation of Sjögren's syndrome. *Nat Rev Rheumatol.* 2010;9:529–537.
3. Shiboski CH, Shiboski SC, Seror R, et al. 2016 American College of Rheumatology/European League Against Rheumatism Classification Criteria for Primary Sjogren's Syndrome: A Consensus and Data-Driven Methodology Involving Three International Patient Cohorts. *Arthritis Rheumatol.* 2017;69:35–45.
4. Ramos-Casals M, Tzioufas A, Stone J, et al. Treatment of primary Sjögren syndrome: a systematic review. *JAMA.* 2010;304:452–460.
5. Sall K, Stevenson OD, Mundorf TK, et al. Two multicenter, randomized studies of the efficacy and safety of cyclosporine ophthalmic emulsion in moderate to severe dry eye disease. CsA Phase 3 Study Group. *Ophthalmology.* 2000;107:631–639.
6. Petrone D, Condemi JJ, Fife R, et al. A double-blind, randomized, placebo-controlled study of cevimeline in Sjögren's syndrome patients with xerostomia and keratoconjunctivitis sicca. *Arthritis Rheum.* 2002;46:748–754.
7. Ramos-Casals M, Brito-Zerón P, Muñoz S, et al; BIOGEAS STUDY Group. A systematic review of the off-label use of biological therapies in systemic autoimmune diseases. *Medicine (Baltimore).* 2008;87:345–364.

8. Theander R, Henriksson G, Ljungberg O, et al. Lymphoma and other malignancies in primary Sjögren's syndrome: a cohort study on cancer incidence and lymphoma predictors. *Ann Rheum Dis.* 2006;65:796–803.

9. Baimpa E, Dahabreh IJ, Voulgarelis M, et al. Hematologic manifestations and predictors of lymphoma development in primary Sjögren syndrome: clinical and pathophysiologic aspects. *Medicine (Baltimore).* 2009;88:284–293.

10. Solans-Laqué R, López-Hernandez A, Angel Bosch-Gil J, et al. Risk, predictors, and clinical characteristics of lymphoma development in primary Sjögren's syndrome. *Semin Arthritis Rheum.* 2011;41:415–423.

Scleroderma

15

Jaime Flores-Ruiz and Deepali Sen

GENERAL PRINCIPLES

- Scleroderma is a connective tissue disease characterized by skin thickening and tightening. It is divided into two main forms: localized and systemic.
- **Localized scleroderma only involves the skin**, with some atrophy of the subcutaneous tissue underlying the lesions.
  - Localized scleroderma (morphea) includes circumscribed (few circles on the trunk or limbs), generalized (many circles on the trunk and limbs), linear (lines of involvement on the limbs), scleroderma en coup de sabre (linear disease affecting only one side of the face and scalp), mixed (combination of circumscribed and linear or generalized and linear), and pansclerotic (involvement of all of the skin).[1]
  - Patients with localized scleroderma are generally managed by dermatologists because they have no internal organ involvement.
  - They may have low-titer antinuclear antibody (ANA) tests.
- The rest of this chapter focuses on **systemic scleroderma, also known as systemic sclerosis (SSc)**.

Definition

SSc is a complex multiorgan disease thought to be the result of autoimmunity, inflammation, vasculopathy, and progressive fibrosis of the skin and visceral organs.

Classification

- SSc is divided further into **limited cutaneous disease (lcSSc, formerly known as CREST syndrome: calcinosis, Raynaud's phenomenon [RP], esophageal dysmotility, sclerodactyly, and telangiectasias), diffuse cutaneous disease (dcSSc)**, and **scleroderma sine scleroderma** on the basis of the extent of skin involvement.
- Skin involvement in lcSSc is limited to the face, the upper extremities distal to the elbows, and the lower extremities distal to the knees, whereas dcSSc involves skin proximal to the elbows and knees, including trunk. This distinction is important in its prognostic implications. The rare case with visceral organ involvement but no skin changes is known as scleroderma sine scleroderma.

Epidemiology

- Estimated annual incidence of SSc in the United States is 1.9 per 100,000. The prevalence rate is estimated at 28 per 100,000.[2]
- SSc is about three to five times more common in women than men, with decline of predominance after menopause. The most common age of onset is between 30 and 50 years.[3]
- Having a first degree relative with disease confers a relative risk of about 13, but rates between monozygotic and dizygotic twins are similar.
- Blacks have a higher incidence and have earlier disease onset than whites. Blacks are more likely to have diffuse cutaneous involvement with aggressive interstitial lung disease (ILD) and pulmonary hypertension (PAH).[3]

Etiology

Etiology is unknown, and there are no animal models that simulate all the features of SSc. It has been hypothesized that environmental or infection events in people who are genetically susceptible trigger a process of inflammation, vascular alterations, autoimmunity, and fibrosis.[4,5]

Pathophysiology

- There are four distinct but interrelated pathogenic processes of SSc: autoimmunity, inflammation, vasculopathy, and fibrosis.
- It is thought that **autoimmunity with vascular reactivity** precedes development of SSc, because patients usually have autoantibodies and RP prior to the development of other organ involvement. Autoantibodies against components of the extracellular matrix found in 50% of SSc patients can activate fibroblasts, induce collagen production, and prevent collagen degradation, resulting in tissue fibrosis.[6]
- Endothelial injury appears to occur early in the course of SSc, but the trigger for the damage has not been identified. Injury results in endothelial cells becoming activated, producing adhesion molecules and inflammatory cytokines, which can lead to endothelial damage, resulting in tissue hypoxemia.
- Hypoxemia stimulates production of angiogenesis factors such as vascular endothelial growth factor (VEGF), tumor (or transforming) growth factor (TGF)-β, and endothelin 1 (ET-1), resulting in vasoconstriction without angiogenesis in SSc patients.

DIAGNOSIS

Clinical Presentation

History

- Disease manifestations vary from limited skin involvement with minimal systemic involvement (lcSSc) to widespread skin involvement accompanied by internal organ involvement (dcSSc).
- **RP** is almost universally present in SSc. It is **usually the first manifestation of SSc** and may precede the development of other features by months to years. Patients report episodic, bilateral color changes precipitated by the cold or by emotional stress. Digits, nose, and ears turn white when vasospasm occurs as a result of sympathetic hyperactivation. As oxygen supply is depleted, they turn blue and, upon rewarming, become red as reperfusion occurs.
- **Skin changes** occur in three phases: edematous, fibrotic, and atrophic. Often, the first complaint specific for scleroderma is swelling or "puffiness" of the fingers or hands corresponding to the edematous phase. Patients may also complain of pruritus, dry skin, tightening, and decreased flexibility along with skin ulcerations.
- The extent of skin involvement often correlates with overall clinical course.
  - lcSSc typically begins with RP followed by thickening of skin of the fingers, progressing to hands and forearms with possible later features of pulmonary fibrosis and PAH.
  - dcSSc has a more rapid course, with skin changes occurring shortly after the development of RP, progressing over the first 1 to 5 years, and then stabilizing thereafter. Skin thickening moves up to proximal part of the extremities and trunk. Unfortunately, internal organ involvement in dcSSc often occurs in the first 2 years and does not parallel the skin findings.
- Other complaints depend on visceral organ involvement. **Gastrointestinal (GI) complaints are common**, with involvement anywhere along the alimentary tract. **Gastroesophageal reflux** (GERD) is the most common complaint. Patients may also note dry mouth, dysphagia, dyspepsia, nausea, early satiety, cramping abdominal pain, diarrhea, and weight loss. Intestinal pseudo-obstruction may occur secondary to hypomotility.

- With **pulmonary involvement**, patients may complain of dyspnea on exertion or nonproductive cough.
- Chest pain may occur due to esophagitis, pleurisy, pericarditis, costochondritis, coronary vasospasms, and fibrosis of the chest wall.
- **Musculoskeletal complaints** are nonspecific. Patients often experience generalized arthralgias with stiffness of the joints under the fibrotic skin.
- Fatigue and weight loss are common in dcSSc.

Physical Examination
- Affected skin is thickened and leathery or hidebound; **sclerodactyly** refers to such skin changes affecting the fingers. Fingertips can appear tapered from ischemic loss of the digital pulp.
- Because RP is a transient phenomenon, it is usually not seen on examination, but **fingertip ulcerations** resulting from chronic hypoxia can be seen. Examination of a patient's nailfold capillary bed can be beneficial for early diagnosis.
  - Using a handheld ophthalmoscope with power less than 20 diopters or a nailfold capillaroscopy, nailfold capillaries are visualized through a water-soluble gel.
  - In cases of secondary RP (associated with scleroderma or inflammatory myopathies), the examination reveals enlarged capillary loops, loss of normal capillary beds, and occasional capillary hemorrhages.
- A tight "purse-lip" appearance associated with **decreased oral aperture** is attributed to increased fibrotic activity within the perioral skin.
- **Telangiectasias** may be appreciated over the face, oropharyngeal mucosa, chest, and hands.
- Hyperpigmentary and hypopigmentary changes may lead to a "salt-and-pepper" appearance of the skin.
- Subcutaneous **calcinosis** (calcinosis cutis) can also be seen.
- Other findings depend on organ involvement.
  - Hypertension, acute-onset renal failure, and microangiopathic hemolytic anemia are seen in **scleroderma renal crisis (SRC)**, but a few patients with SRC are normotensive. dcSSc patients and those recently commenced on high-dose glucocorticoids are at highest risk of developing SRC.[7]
  - Crackles can be heard in patients with ILD (more common in dcSSc).
  - Signs of right heart failure can be seen in the setting of PAH (more common in lcSSc).
  - Arrhythmias from conduction system fibrosis, pericardial rubs from pericarditis, or signs of congestive heart failure from myocardial fibrosis can be seen with cardiac involvement.
  - When inflammation and fibrosis of tendon sheaths are significant, coarse friction rubs can be heard with joint movement.

Diagnostic Classification Criteria
- The American College of Rheumatology/European League Against Rheumatism classification criteria for SSc are presented in Table 15-1.[8]
- Although these diagnostic criteria have a sensitivity of 91% and specificity of 92%, the criteria are meant for inclusion of SSc patients in studies, not for SSc diagnosis. Nevertheless, the list of items in the classification criteria mimics the clinical diagnosis. The diagnosis of SSc could also include items not present in the classification criteria, such as tendon friction rubs, calcinosis, and dysphagia.[8]

Differential Diagnosis
- Skin thickening as that in scleroderma but with some distinguishing features can be seen in other disorders. Keep in mind that **patients with these other diseases do not have RP or digital ulcerations**.

TABLE 15-1	THE AMERICAN COLLEGE OF RHEUMATOLOGY/EUROPEAN LEAGUE AGAINST RHEUMATISM CRITERIA FOR THE CLASSIFICATION OF SSc

Item	Sub Item(s)	Weight/Score[a]
Skin thickening of the fingers of both hands extending proximal to the MCP joints *(sufficient criterion)*	–	9
Skin thickening of the fingers (only count the higher score)	Puffy fingers	2
	Sclerodactyly of the fingers (distal to the MCP joints but proximal to the PIP joints)	4
Fingertip lesions (only count the higher score)	Digital tip ulcers	2
	Fingertip pitting scars	3
Telangiectasia	–	2
Abnormal nailfold capillaries	–	2
PAH and/or ILD *(maximum score is 2)*	PAH	2
	ILD	2
RP	–	3
SSc-related autoantibodies *(maximum score is 3)*	Anticentromere	3
	Scl-70	3
	Anti-RNA polymerase III	3

[a]The total score is determined by adding the maximum weight/score in each category. Patients with a total score of greater than 9 are classified as having definite SSc.

ILD, interstitial lung disease; MCP, metacarpophalangeal; PAH, pulmonary hypertension; PIP, proximal interphalangeal joints; RP, Raynaud's phenomenon; SSc, systemic sclerosis.

Adapted from: van den Hoogen F, Khanna D, Fransen J, et al. 2013 classification criteria for systemic sclerosis: an American College of Rheumatology/European League against Rheumatism collaborative initiative. *Arthritis Rheum.* 2013;65(11):2737–2747.

- **Nephrogenic systemic fibrosis (NSF)**, affecting mostly dialysis patients, tends to affect lower extremities more than upper extremities and generally spares the hands.
- Three syndromes with **paraproteinemia** have scleroderma-like skin changes:
  ○ **Scleredema**, complication of long-standing diabetes or paraproteinemia, causes thickening of the skin in the neck, shoulder girdle, proximal upper extremities, and back and is characterized by mucin deposition on skin biopsy.
  ○ **Scleromyxedema**, which can involve the hands but also skin, tends to be more folded and pendulous rather than tight and thickened.
  ○ **POEMS** (polyneuropathy, organomegaly, endocrinopathy, monoclonal gammopathy, and scleroderma-like skin changes) **syndrome**
- **Eosinophilic fasciitis** can have a rapid onset of skin thickening, with early development of flexion contractures due to fascial thickening. Skin tends to be more puckered appearing, but a deep biopsy demonstrates eosinophilic infiltration, separating it from SSc. Eosinophilia is common, and eosinophilic infiltrates are usually seen on biopsy.
- Other conditions with scleroderma-like skin thickening include diabetic digital sclerosis, chronic graft-versus-host disease, vinyl chloride exposure, vibratory injury, bleomycin

toxicity, complex regional pain syndrome/reflex sympathetic dystrophy, amyloidosis, porphyria cutanea tarda, and carcinoid syndrome.
- Diseases with similar organ involvement include primary pulmonary hypertension, ILD, primary biliary cirrhosis, intestinal hypomotility, and collagenous colitis.
- Diseases that may present in a similar manner to scleroderma include systemic lupus erythematosus (SLE), mixed connective tissue disease (MCTD), rheumatoid arthritis (RA), and inflammatory myopathies.

Diagnostic Testing

Diagnosis is on the basis of clinical findings described earlier. The following can be helpful in making the diagnosis or in delineating the extent of organ involvement.

Laboratories
- Ninety-five percent of patients with SSc will have autoantibodies. The prevalence of ANA autoantibody is more than 90% in SSc patients. The **anticentromere** staining pattern of ANA is specific but not sensitive for lcSSc (93% specificity and 44% sensitivity). **Anti–Scl-70 (anti–topoisomerase-I)** antibodies are specific but not sensitive for dcSSc (82% specificity and 37% sensitivity) and are associated with the risk for ILD.[9]
- Less commonly assayed antibodies associated with scleroderma include **anti-RNA polymerase I, anti-RNA polymerase II, anti-RNA polymerase III and U3-ribonucleoprotein (RNP)**. Anti-RNA polymerase III is associated with rapidly progressing dcSSc, SRC, ILD, and cancer.[10] RNP is associated with risk for PAH. Anti–U1-RNP antibodies are found in MCTD, and anti–PM-Scl antibodies may be present in overlap syndromes.

Electrocardiography
Electrocardiography (ECG) findings are highly variable, depending on which area of the heart is involved and the extent of involvement.

Imaging
- Transthoracic echocardiogram (echo) can be used to evaluate for PAH or pericardial effusion.
- Patients with ILD will have interstitial infiltrates on high-resolution computed tomography (CT) and a restrictive pattern on pulmonary function testing.

Diagnostic Procedures
- Reflux, dysphagia, and odynophagia are frequent complaints related to esophageal dysmotility, which can be evaluated with barium esophagram or esophageal manometry.
- Patients with elevated pulmonary pressures on echo or those with dyspnea unexplained by other causes should undergo a right heart catheterization, as echocardiography can underestimate or overestimate pulmonary pressures in about 10% of patients.[11]

TREATMENT

SSc has the highest mortality rate among the connective tissue disorders. There is no treatment for the underlying disease process; hence, treatment is targeted at specific organ complications and/or patient symptoms.

Medications
- **Skin involvement:** No effective antifibrotic therapy has been discovered to date. In patient with dcSSc and visceral involvement, the immunosuppression treatment should be directed to the visceral disease.
  - Two randomized controlled trials (RCTs) showed that **methotrexate** improves skin thickening in early SSc.[12–14]
  - **Mycophenolate mofetil** (MMF) has shown benefit in recent onset skin involvement and stabilization of pulmonary function.[15–17]

- RCTs suggest that cyclophosphamide and tocilizumab benefit skin thickening and ILD.[18–20] Two RCTs on autologous nonmyeloablative hematopoietic stem cell transplant (HSCT) showed improvement in skin sclerosis and stabilization of pulmonary function compared with cyclophosphamide, and one RCT on myeloablative autologous HSCT showed benefits in survival compared to cyclophosphamide in patients with severe internal organ disease.[21–23] However, there are concerns about safety- and treatment-related mortality of HSCT, and careful selection is of key importance.
- **RP:** Nonpharmacologic measures for treating RP include smoking cessation and avoiding cold exposure.
  - **Dihydropyridine calcium-channel blockers** such as amlodipine, nifedipine, and felodipine have been shown to reduce the frequency and severity of RP.[14]
  - Other medications that have been shown to have efficacy in RP treatment are **phosphodiesterase inhibitors** (PDE-5) such as sildenafil. Also fluoxetine might be an option for RP attacks. In severe disease that failed oral therapy, intravenous prostacyclin analogs could be an option.[14] All of these agents are more effective in primary RP than in RP associated with scleroderma.
- **Digital ulcers:** Ulcers are extremely painful and, because they result from ischemia, are difficult to heal. Analgesics and local wound care can be helpful.
  - RCT demonstrated the benefit of **sildenafil** in preventing new ulcer formation and greater healing rate.[24]
  - **Bosentan** has been shown in two RCTs to reduce the development of new ulcers but without any effect on existing ulcers.[25,26]
  - **Intravenous iloprost** has been shown to help heal ulcers and prevent new ones; however, only epoprostenol is available in the United States, and it must be administered via a central line with close monitoring.[14]
  - Sympathectomies, sympathetic blocks, and intra-arterial injections of vasodilators have been reported to help, but responses have been inconsistent.
- **SRC:** Used to be the number one cause of death in SSc patients; however, this has changed with the advent of **angiotensin-converting enzyme (ACE) inhibitors.**[27]
  - Immediate treatment with ACE inhibitor should be started even in the setting of elevated creatinine.[14]
  - Glucocorticoids could increase the risk of SRC. Therefore, blood pressure and renal function should be monitored in patients with SSc treated with glucocorticoids.[14]
  - Patients with early, active, inflammatory diffuse scleroderma are at highest risk and should be educated about warning signs and encouraged to monitor their blood pressure on a weekly basis.
- **ILD:** The optimal treatment for SSc-ILD is not known.
  - One RCT showed that **cyclophosphamide** has modest benefit in forced vital capacity, fibrosis, and dyspnea.[18]
  - Other studies have shown some benefit with MMF.[16,17]
  - A small RCT demonstrated improvement in ILD with **rituximab.**[28]
  - RCTs showed stabilization of pulmonary function and benefits in survival in patients who underwent HSCT compared to those treated with cyclophosphamide.[14,21–23]
- **PAH:** PAH therapy is directed at altering pulmonary vascular tone and remodeling rather than treating SSc. Early treatment is associated with better outcomes and should be managed by an expert in PAH. Prostaglandins epoprostenol, treprostinil, and iloprost; endothelin-receptor antagonists bosentan, ambrisentan, and macitentan; and phosphodiesterase inhibitors sildenafil, tadalafil, and riociguat have shown benefit in the treatment of PAH.[14]
- **GI**
  - **GERD** symptoms should be treated with **proton pump inhibitors**, but it may be necessary to use up to three times the usual dose.[14]
  - **Esophageal strictures** are treated with dilatation when necessary.

○ **Gastric antral venous ectasia** is the most common cause of GI bleeding in scleroderma and can be treated with endoscopic laser photocoagulation.
○ **Prokinetic agents** such as metoclopramide can be used for aperistaltic symptoms.[14] Intestinal pseudo-obstruction can be managed with octreotide.
• **Small-bowel bacterial overgrowth** can be managed with alternating doses of rifaximin, ciprofloxacin, metronidazole, and amoxicillin-clavulanic acid.[14]

Other Nonpharmacologic Therapies
• Avoiding excess bathing and using proper moisturizing creams can aid in skin care.
• Aggressive occupational and physical therapy may be helpful early in the course of disease to minimize contractures.

Surgical Management
Postoperative healing can be difficult in SSc patients. However, digital ulcers can become infected and may need debridement. Amputations may be necessary for deeper infections.

SPECIAL CONSIDERATIONS

Patients with scleroderma are at increased risk for depression and despair. Support groups may be beneficial. Fear of losing functionality and of increasing pain is a common emotion but is amenable to intervention by early recognition, patient education, and encouragement.

OUTCOME/PROGNOSIS

• The diagnoses of dcSSc and lcSSc have different prognostic implications.
• dcSSc has widely variable but overall poor prognosis, with survival of 40% to 60% at 10 years from the onset of the first non-RP scleroderma sign or symptom.
• lcSSc has a relatively good prognosis, with survival greater than 70% at 10 years.
• Prognosis of scleroderma sine scleroderma is generally poor but difficult to estimate because it is so rare.
• Increase risk of malignancy compared to general population.
• Most patients with SSc die from pulmonary disease or from infectious complications.

REFERENCES

1. Fett NM. Morphea localized scleroderma. *JAMA Dermatol.* 2013;149(9):1124.
2. Chifflot H, Fautrel B, Sordet C, et al. Incidence and prevalence of systemic sclerosis: A systematic literature review. *Semin Arthritis Rheum.* 2008;37:223–235.
3. Mayes MD, Lacey JV, Beebe-Dimmer J, et al. Prevalence, incidence, survival, and disease characteristics of systemic sclerosis in a large US population. *Arthritis Rheum.* 2003;48(8):2246–2255.
4. Allanore Y, Simms R, Distler O, et al. Systemic sclerosis. *Nat Rev Dis Primers.* 2015;1:15002.
5. Katsumoto TR, Whitfield ML, Connolly MK. The pathogenesis of systemic sclerosis. *Ann Rev Pathol.* 2011;6:509–537.
6. Abraham DJ, Krieg T, Distler J, et al. Overview of pathogenesis of systemic sclerosis. *Rheumatology.* 2009;48:iii3–iii7.
7. Denton CP, Lapadula G, Mouthon L, et al. Renal complications and scleroderma renal crisis. *Rheumatology.* 2009;48:iii32–iii35.
8. van den Hoogen F, Khanna D, Fransen J, et al. 2013 classification criteria for systemic sclerosis: an American College of Rheumatology/European League against Rheumatism collaborative initiative. *Arthritis Rheum.* 2013;65(11):2737–2747.
9. Reveille JD, Solomon DH; American College of Rheumatology Ad Hoc Committee on Immunologic Testing Guidelines. Evidence-based guidelines for the use of immunologic tests: anticentromere, Scl-70, and nucleolar antibodies. *Arthritis Rheum.* 2003;49(3):399–412.

10. Lazzaroni MG, Cavazzana I, Colombo E, et al. Malignancies in patients with anti-RNA polymerase III antibodies and systemic sclerosis: analysis of the EULAR scleroderma trials and research cohort and possible recommendations for screening. *J Rheumatol.* 2017;44(5):639–647.

11. Matucci-Cerinic M, Steen V, Nash P. The complexity of managing systemic sclerosis: screening and diagnosis. *Rheumatology (Oxford).* 2009;48:iii8–iii13.

12. van den Hoogen FH, Boerbooms AT, Swaak AJ, et al. Comparison of methotrexate with placebo in the treatment of systemic sclerosis: a 24 week randomized double-blind trial, followed by a 24 week observational trial. *Rheumatology.* 1996;35(4):364–372.

13. Pope JE, Bellamy N, Seibold JR, et al. A randomized, controlled trial of methotrexate versus placebo in early diffuse scleroderma. *Arthritis Rheum.* 2001;44(6):1351–1358.

14. Kowal-Bielecka O, Fransen J, Avouac J, et al. Update of EULAR recommendations for the treatment of systemic sclerosis. *Ann Rheum Dis.* 2017;76(8):1327–1339.

15. Le EN, Wigley FM, Shah AA, et al. Long-term experience of mycophenolate mofetil for treatment of diffuse cutaneous systemic sclerosis. *Ann Rheum Dis.* 2011;70(6):1104–1107.

16. Mendoza FA, Nagle SJ, Lee JB, et al. A prospective observational study of mycophenolate mofetil treatment in progressive diffuse cutaneous systemic sclerosis of recent onset. *J Rheumatol.* 2012;39(6):1241–1247.

17. Tashkin DP, Roth MD, Clements PJ, et al. Mycophenolate mofetil versus oral cyclophosphamide in scleroderma-related interstitial lung disease (SLS II): a randomised controlled, double-blind, parallel group trial. *Lancet Respir Med.* 2016;4(9):708–719.

18. Tashkin DP, Elashoff R, Clements PJ, et al. Cyclophosphamide versus placebo in scleroderma lung disease. *N Engl J Med.* 2006;354(25):2655–2666.

19. Khanna D, Denton CP, Jahreis A, et al. Safety and efficacy of subcutaneous tocilizumab in adults with systemic sclerosis (faSScinate): a phase 2, randomised, controlled trial. *Lancet.* 2016;387:2630–2640.

20. Khanna D, Denton CP, Lin CJ, et al. Safety and efficacy of subcutaneous tocilizumab in systemic sclerosis: results from the open-label period of a phase II randomised controlled trial (faSScinate). *Ann Rheum Dis.* 2018;77(2):212–220.

21. Burt RK, Shah SJ, Dill K, et al. Autologous non-myeloablative haemopoietic stem-cell transplantation compared with pulse cyclophosphamide once per month for systemic sclerosis (ASSIST): an open-label, randomised phase 2 trial. *Lancet.* 2011;378(9790):498–506.

22. van Laar JM, Farge D, Sont JK, et al. Autologous hematopoietic stem cell transplantation vs intravenous pulse cyclophosphamide in diffuse cutaneous systemic sclerosis: a randomized clinical trial. *JAMA.* 2014;311(24):2490–2498.

23. Sullivan KM, Goldmuntz EA, Keyes-Elstein L, et al. Myeloablative autologous stem-cell transplantation for severe scleroderma. *N Engl J Med.* 2018;378(1):35–47.

24. Hachulla E, Hatron PY, Carpentier P, et al. Efficacy of sildenafil on ischaemic digital ulcer healing in systemic sclerosis: the placebo-controlled SEDUCE study. *Ann Rheum Dis.* 2016;75(6):1009–1015.

25. Korn JH, Mayes M, Matucci Cerinic M, et al. Digital ulcers in systemic sclerosis: prevention by treatment with bosentan, an oral endothelin receptor antagonist. *Arthritis Rheum.* 2004;50(12):3985–3993.

26. Matucci-Cerinic M, Denton CP, Furst DE, et al. Bosentan treatment of digital ulcers related to systemic sclerosis: results from the RAPIDS-2 randomised, double-blind, placebo-controlled trial. *Ann Rheum Dis.* 2011;70(1):32–38.

27. Penn H, Denton CP. Diagnosis, management and prevention of scleroderma renal disease. *Curr Opin Rheumatol.* 2008;1;20(6):692–696.

28. Daoussis D, Liossis SN, Tsamandas AC, et al. Experience with rituximab in scleroderma: results from a 1-year, proof-of-principle study. *Rheumatology.* 2009;49(2):271–280.

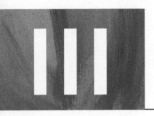

III Seronegative Spondyloarthropathies

Spondyloarthritis

16

Colin Diffie and Lisa A. Zickuhr

GENERAL PRINCIPLES

- The **spondyloarthritides** (SpAs) are a group of clinically related disorders known previously as the **seronegative spondyloarthropathies**. In contrast to rheumatoid arthritis (RA), they lack a positive rheumatoid factor and frequently affect the axial skeleton. These diseases are called spondyloarthritis (SpA) to reflect their inflammatory nature.
- SpA has an association with HLA-B27.
- These diseases are classified by their location (axial or peripheral) or by their subtype (e.g., psoriatic arthritis [PsA], reactive arthritis [ReA]).

Classification

- Common features include age of onset less than 45 years, **inflammatory back pain more than** 3 months, **enthesitis**, **dactylitis**, and a family history of SpA.
- Patients typically present with inflammatory back pain, but they may also have concomitant mechanical back pain from spinal ankylosis (Table 16-1).[1] Less frequently, patients with SpA describe their pain as purely mechanical without inflammatory features.
- Enthesitis is inflammation where tendons and ligaments insert into bone. Common sites include the Achilles tendon, plantar fascia, iliac crests, epicondyles, and tibial tuberosities.
- Traditional classification
  - The older classification scheme is based on the European Spondyloarthropathy Study Group (ESSG) and is used clinically and in ongoing research. This scheme differentiates the SpAs into **ankylosing spondylitis** (AS), **PsA**, **enteropathic arthritis**, **ReA**, and **undifferentiated spondyloarthritis** (USpA). Chapters 17 to 20 are organized using this nomenclature.
  - Although the names imply that these are different diseases, in clinical practice, the SpAs overlap significantly. Many patients have features of multiple types of SpA, such as a patient with AS who develops inflammatory bowel disease (IBD) or vice versa.
  - USpA describes patients who have features of SpA without AS, comorbid psoriasis or IBD, or a preceding infection that would account for the diagnosis of ReA.[2] For

TABLE 16-1	INFLAMMATORY VERSUS MECHANICAL BACK PAIN	
	Inflammatory Back Pain	**Mechanical Back Pain**
Age of onset	<45 years	Any age
Morning stiffness	>60 minutes	<30 minutes
Nocturnal pain	Frequent	Absent
Effect of exercise	Improvement	Exacerbation

Note that the sensitivity in patients with 2+ inflammatory back pain features is 70% to 80% for axial spondyloarthritis, but patients may present atypically.

Adapted from: Duba A, Matthew S. The seronegative spondyloarthropathies. *Primary Care.* 2018;45:271–287.

TABLE 16-2 · COMPARISON OF SPONDYLOARTHRITIDES BY TYPE

Type	HLA-B27+	Axial Involvement	Peripheral Involvement	Extra-articular Manifestations
Ankylosing Spondylitis	80%–95% of white, 50%–80% of nonwhite patients[5]	Universal. Bilateral sacroiliitis. Erosions, spinal fusion, **bamboo spine**	In up to 40%. Especially ankles, hips, knees	**Uveitis**[3] in 30%, psoriasis in 9%, IBD in 7%
Enteropathic Arthritis	30%. More frequent with axial disease[1]	10%–20% symptomatic. Asymptomatic disease in up to 40%[4]	Type 1: <5 joints Type 2: 5+ joints	**Crohn's, UC** Uveitis, pyoderma, erythema nodosum
Psoriatic Arthritis	10%–25%. Other *HLA* genes confer risk[5]	Rarely dominant. May have asymmetric SI involvement, "skip" syndesmophytes	Asymmetric oligoarthritis or symmetric polyarthritis common. **Pencil in cup. Dactylitis**	**Psoriasis. Nail pitting** or onycholysis Uveitis (7%)[1]
Reactive Arthritis	50%–80%[1]	Less prominent than peripheral disease	Asymmetric oligoarthritis, especially knees. Dactylitis	**Conjunctivitis, urethritis,** keratoderma blennorrhagica, circinate balanitis

IBD, inflammatory bowel disease; UC, ulcerative colitis.
See Chapters 17 to 20 for further discussion.

example, a patient with the HLA-B27 haplotype, uveitis, and an asymmetric oligoarthritis of the legs but without inflammatory back pain could be considered USpA (or peripheral SpA, as detailed later).
  ○ Table 16-2 compares these subtypes of SpA.[3–5]
• Classification by site of arthritis
  ○ The 2011 Assessment of SpondyloArthritis International Society (ASAS) criteria were devised to improve the sensitivity and specificity of identifying SpA earlier in disease onset.
  ○ Separate criteria exist for axial SpA (AxSpA) and peripheral SpA (see Table 16-3).[6,7]
  ○ Patients with axial disease are further subdivided into radiographic or nonradiographic SpA. Radiographic SpA is largely synonymous with AS (see Chapter 17). Nonradiographic SpA may represent an early form of AS.[5]

Epidemiology

• SpAs occur in about 1% to 1.6% of the general population.
• Of the subtypes of SpA, **AS and PsA are the most prevalent.**[1]
• The prevalence of HLA-B27 varies significantly between SpA subtypes, ranging from 30% to 95%.
• Most of the HLA-B27+ population do not have spondyloarthropathy. It is estimated that less than 5% develop disease, although this rate increases with a family history of SpA.[5]

TABLE 16-3	ASAS CLASSIFICATION CRITERIA FOR AXIAL AND PERIPHERAL SPONDYLOARTHRITIS		
Axial Spondyloarthritis		**Peripheral Spondyloarthritis**	
Inflammatory back pain ≥3 months, age at onset <45 years, AND either column here:		Arthritis, enthesitis, or dactylitis AND either column here:	
HLA-B27 AND ≥2 other SpA features: IBP Arthritis Enthesitis Uveitis Dactylitis Psoriasis IBD Good response to NSAIDs FHx HLA-B27 Elevated CRP	Sacroiliitis on imaging: Active inflammation on MRI OR Radiographic sacroiliitis (grade 2 if bilateral, grade 3 if unilateral) AND ≥1 other SpA feature	≥1 SpA feature: Uveitis Psoriasis IBD Preceding infection HLA-B27 Sacroiliitis on imaging	≥2 other SpA features: Arthritis Enthesitis Dactylitis IBP ever FHx of SpA

ASAS, Assessment of SpondyloArthritis International Society; CRP, C-reactive protein; FHx, family history; IBD, inflammatory bowel disease; IBP, inflammatory back pain; NSAIDs, nonsteroidal anti-inflammatory drugs; SpA, spondyloarthritis.

Adapted from: Rudwaleit M, van der Heijde D, Landewé R, et al. The development of Assessment of SpondyloArthritis international Society classification criteria for axial spondyloarthritis (part II): validation and final selection. *Ann Rheum Dis.* 2009;68:777–783.

DIAGNOSIS

- Diagnosis of SpA relies on clinical presentation and imaging.
- Classification criteria (Table 16-3) can guide the diagnosis of SpA, but they primarily exist to unify clinical studies. Individuals may be diagnosed or benefit from therapy despite failing to meet classification criteria.

Clinical Presentation

- Clinical manifestations include **inflammatory back pain, sacroiliitis, peripheral arthritis, enthesitis**, and **dactylitis**.
- Patients may have **extra-articular manifestations**. The most common ones are outlined in Table 16-2.
- Less common extra-articular manifestations include apical pulmonary fibrosis, oral ulcers, aortitis, aortic regurgitation, conduction abnormalities, pericarditis, immunoglobulin A (IgA) nephropathy, and secondary amyloidosis.
- The majority of patients present **before the age of 45**.
- Inflammatory back pain lasting longer than 3 months, positive magnetic resonance imaging (MRI) findings, and positive HLA-B27 status confer the highest likelihood ratios for disease.[5]

History

- History will often elicit symptoms of inflammatory back pain. In addition to the features listed in Table 16-1, patients may describe back pain that is insidious in onset, dull, and progresses. Patients may have **alternating buttock pain**. Pain is intermittent initially but may grow more persistent. It is exacerbated with rest, especially in the second half of the night, causing nocturnal awakenings.
- Additional articular symptoms include:
  - **Peripheral, asymmetric inflammatory arthritis**, usually in the lower limbs and affecting fewer than five joints
  - **Enthesitis**
  - **Dactylitis**, the "sausage digit," from tenosynovitis of the flexor tendons of the digits and synovitis in the joint spaces of the fingers and toes.
- Extra-articular symptoms may identify the subtype of SpA:
  - Current or prior scaling rash or nail pitting in PsA
  - Crampy abdominal pain, frequent diarrhea, mucus or blood in the stools from IBD in enteropathic arthritis
  - Infectious diarrhea, urethritis, cervicitis (often asymptomatic), or conjunctivitis within the past month for patients with ReA

Physical Examination

- Regardless of the subtype of SpA, a thorough musculoskeletal examination should be performed to assess for axial and peripheral disease.
- Axial disease deserves special attention when evaluating a suspected SpA patient, particularly range of motion.
  - One measure is the modified **Schober's test:** Make marks 10 cm above and 5 cm below the level of the sacral dimples (~L5). Next, have the patient maximally reach for the floor without bending his or her knees. The distance between these two marks should increase from 15 cm to ≥20 cm if normal spinal motion is present.
  - **Evaluate lateral rotation and lateral flexion** of the spine in both directions as well. Lateral rotation can be measured by the examiner standing behind the patient and placing examiner's hands on the patient's iliac crest, then having the patient laterally rotate the shoulders. The plane of the shoulders should normally reach a 45-degree angle with respect to the plane of the pelvis. For lateral flexion, ask the patient to stand upright and laterally flex to the floor. The distance from the middle fingertip to the floor can be measured and followed.

- The **occiput-to-wall distance** can be measured by having the patient stand with both heels and buttocks against the wall and measuring the gap between the occiput and the wall to evaluate for kyphosis and restricted cervical motion. The normal distance is zero,[8] and increasing distance indicates progression of cervical ankylosis.
- Evaluate **chest expansion** by measuring the circumference of the chest at the level of T4 at the end of both maximal inspiration and expiration. Expansion less than 2.5 cm is abnormal.
- **Peripheral joint findings** include swelling, effusions, erythema, reduced range of motion, and dactylitis.
- Patients may have gross deformities, such as digit telescoping in PsA mutilans (Chapter 18).
- Evaluate for tenderness in common sites of enthesitis, such as the Achilles insertion, plantar fascia, epicondyles, and tibial tuberosities. Gross inflammation can be seen.
- The **skin** should be assessed for evidence of psoriasis, including small patches in the umbilicus, hair, or gluteal fold that are commonly overlooked. Dermatology referral and skin biopsy may need to be considered.
- SpAs are systemic inflammatory disorders that can affect many organ systems. A thorough examination should be performed to evaluate for extra-articular manifestations.

Diagnostic Testing

Laboratories
- The acute-phase reactants such as erythrocyte sedimentation rate (ESR) and C-reactive protein (CRP) are poor markers of disease activity. They lack the sensitivity and specificity needed to indicate point-of-care disease activity by themselves.[5]
- HLA-B27 testing is included in the ASAS classification criteria. However, given that SpA occurs in less than 5% of HLA-B27 individuals, the positive predictive value for disease is relatively low without a compelling clinical picture.
- In general, HLA-B27 is predictive of axial involvement in a patient with SpA.[1]

Imaging
- **Plain radiography** of the sacroiliac (SI) joints and pelvis should be obtained in evaluation for AxSpA.
- Sacroiliitis may be present in any form of SpA without necessarily meeting criteria for AS.
  - Structural damage appears late in disease. Many patients with nonradiographic AxSpA go on to develop classical AS on radiography several years later.[5]
  - Affected peripheral joints should be imaged with plain x-rays to evaluate for erosions, secondary osteoarthritis, entheseal calcification, and osteitis.
- **MRI** is a valuable tool, especially for the assessment of early AxSpA. See Chapter 17, radiography section, for further details.
- MRI may also be beneficial in patients with peripheral arthritis whose radiographs are equivocal or nondiagnostic and in whom the results would alter management. It allows greater sensitivity for evaluation of occult erosions, synovitis, tenosynovitis, and effusions than x-ray imaging.

TREATMENT

Medications

- Pharmacologic treatment of SpA varies on the type and will be covered in greater detail in the corresponding chapters (Chapters 17–20).
- Most clinical trials evaluating the efficacy of pharmacologic treatment of SpA focus on AS or PsA. Few trials concentrate specifically on USpA.[2]
- For USpA, treatment is based on whether symptoms are predominantly axial (in which therapy will be most similar to that for AS) or peripheral (in which therapy is similar to PsA).[2]

Other Nonpharmacologic Therapies

- **Physical therapy and exercise** are mainstays for all SpAs.
- A combination of an exercise program with pharmacologic agents has been shown to be more effective than pharmacologic treatment alone.
- Exercises focusing on chest expansion and mobility are effective in improving functional outcomes in AS.[9]

COMPLICATIONS

- Complications of SpA result from long-standing inflammation affecting the target joint(s).
  - In the case of AxSpA, patients may develop fusion, or **ankylosis**, especially of the SI joint and spine. Fusion reduces the range of motion of the affected joint.
  - Lack of mobility in the thoracic spine leads to **decreased chest wall expansion**, which may cause restrictive lung disease.[5]
  - **Radiculopathies** can also result from ankylosis of the spine.
  - Inflammatory arthritis and enthesitis of peripheral joints may lead to joint erosions.
- **Extra-articular manifestations**[1] can cause other complications.
  - **Uveitis** can lead to glaucoma and vision loss.
  - Late **cardiac complications** include aortic dilation, aortic and mitral regurgitation, atrioventricular conduction blocks, and arrhythmias.
  - Patients with long-standing inflammatory conditions are at risk for development of secondary amyloidosis (see Chapter 48).[1]
- Pharmacologic treatments also have side effects that may lead to other complications. See Chapter 9 for further discussion.

REFERRAL

Patients with chronic back pain lasting longer than 3 months and one or more of the following should be referred to a rheumatologist[1]:

- Inflammatory back pain
- Inflammatory peripheral arthritis
- HLA-B27 positivity
- Sacroiliitis on imaging
- Failure to respond to conservative treatment

PATIENT EDUCATION

- Patients should be educated on the manifestations, complications, and therapeutic options of their disease.
- In addition, the benefits of exercise and physical therapy for improving functional status and limiting pain should be emphasized.[9]

REFERENCES

1. Duba A, Matthew S. The seronegative spondyloarthropathies. *Primary Care*. 2018;45:271–287.
2. Zochling J, Brandt J, Braun J. The current concept of spondyloarthritis with special emphasis on undifferentiated spondyloarthritis. *Rheumatology*. 2005; 44:1483.
3. Garrett S, Jenkinson T, Kennedy LG, et al. A new approach to defining disease status in ankylosing spondylitis: the Bath Ankylosing Spondylitis Disease Activity Index. *J Rheumatol*. 1994;21:2286–2291.
4. Stolwijk C, van Tubergen A, Castillo-Ortiz JD, et al. Prevalence of extra-articular manifestations in patients with ankylosing spondylitis: a systematic review and meta-analysis. *Ann Rheum Dis*. 2015;74:65–73.
5. Taurog JD, Chhabra A, Colbert RA. Ankylosing spondylitis and axial spondyloarthritis. *N Eng J Med*. 2016; 374:2563–2574.
6. Rudwaleit M, van der Heijde D, Landewé R, et al. The development of Assessment of SpondyloArthritis international Society classification criteria for axial spondyloarthritis (part II): validation and final selection. *Ann Rheum Dis*. 2009;68:777–783.
7. Rudwaleit M, van der Heijde D, Landewé R, et al. The Assessment of SpondyloArthritis international Society classification criteria for peripheral spondyloarthritis and for spondyloarthritis in general. *Ann Rheum Dis*. 2011;70:25–31.
8. Assassi S, Weisman MH, Lee M, et al. New population-based reference values for spinal mobility measures based on the 2009–2010 National Health and Nutrition Examination Survey. *Arthritis Rheum*. 2014;66:2628–2637.
9. Ortancil O, Sarikaya S, Sapmaz P, et al. The effect(s) of a six-week home-based exercise program on the respiratory muscle and functional status in ankylosing spondylitis. *J Clin Rheumatol*. 2009;15:68–70.

Ankylosing Spondylitis

17

Colin Diffie and Lisa A. Zickuhr

GENERAL PRINCIPLES

Ankylosing spondylitis (AS) belongs to a group of clinical disorders characterized by prominent involvement of the axial skeleton, known as the spondyloarthritides (SpAs).

Definition

- AS is an inflammatory arthritis causing back pain and progressive stiffness of the spine. Prominent sacroiliitis, fusion of the sacroiliac (SI) joints, and ankylosis of the spine distinguish it from other causes of SpA (i.e., psoriatic, enteric, and reactive arthritis).
- AS may also be associated with peripheral arthritis of the large joints and extra-articular manifestations involving the eyes, heart, lungs, skin, and bowels.
- Historically, AS was defined in patients presenting with inflammatory back pain and other axial features combined with evidence of sacroiliitis on imaging (see Table 17-1).[1]
- Recent classification criteria reorganize the SpAs into axial, peripheral, and nonradiographic axial SpA[2] (see Table 16-3). Under this updated nomenclature, AS is closest to axial spondyloarthritis (AxSpA), whereas nonradiographic AxSpA may represent an early form of AS.
- The recent classification criteria unite cohorts of patients for research. This chapter uses the term AS for educational purposes.

Epidemiology

- The prevalence of AS ranges from 0.9% to 1.4%, with a wide variation noted in different ethnic populations.[3]
- AS was originally thought to have a male predominance, with a historic ratio of 10:1. More recent studies suggest the ratio is 1:1, with women facing longer delays in diagnosis than men.[4]
- The age of onset is most often less than 45 years, with peak incidence between the ages of 20 and 30 years.
  - Interpretation of the **HLA-B27** test is not straightforward in the clinical setting. HLA-B27 is found in most patients with AS. This causes some practitioners to over-rely on the test for diagnosis. However, most patients with a positive HLA-B27 never develop AS, and some polymorphisms do not increase the risk of AS whatsoever.[5]
  - Less than 5% of people with the HLA-B27 allele develop SpA.
  - The prevalence of HLA-B27 in the North American population is 7% to 10%,[4] but 80% to 90% of white AS patients express HLA-B27.[5]
  - Its prevalence is not as high in nonwhite populations, making testing less useful in these populations.
  - Like all of the seronegative spondyloarthropathies, AS has a strong familial aggregation; however, HLA-B27 confers only about 30% of the genetic risk, suggesting other genes may also predispose to AS.
  - Because of this complexity, HLA-B27 must be interpreted in the appropriate clinical context.

TABLE 17-1	MODIFIED NEW YORK CRITERIA FOR ANKYLOSING SPONDYLITIS (1984)

At least one clinical criteria, plus radiographic criteria of grades 2–4 bilaterally or 3–4 unilaterally

Clinical Criteria	Radiographic Criteria
1. Low back pain and stiffness for more than 3 months, improved with exercise, not relieved with rest 2. Limitation of motion of the lumbar spine in both the sagittal and frontal planes 3. Limitation of chest expansion relative to normal values correlated for age and sex	Grade 0: Normal Grade 1: Suspicious changes Grade 2: Minimal abnormality: small localized erosion or sclerosis, without altered joint width Grade 3: Unequivocal abnormality: Moderate sacroiliitis with one or more of erosions, sclerosis, widening, or partial ankylosis Grade 4: Severe abnormality: total ankylosis.

Adapted from van der Linden S, Valkenburg HA, Cats A. Evaluation of diagnostic criteria for ankylosing spondylitis. A proposal for modification of the New York criteria. *Arthritis Rheum.* 1984;27:361–368.

Etiology

- The etiology of AS is incompletely understood, but evidence suggests that it is an immune-mediated response to an environmental trigger, possibly **enterobacterial pathogens.**[6]
- HLA-B27+ transgenic mice do not develop AS when raised in a germ-free environment. However, they will develop an AS-like disease when exposed to bacteria.[7]
- Patients with active AS have increased antibody titers to *Klebsiella* compared to controls.[6]
- Another theory includes dimerization of HLA-B27, a unique characteristic of this particular HLA allele. It is thought that dimerization causes an inflammatory response and production of interleukin (IL)-23.[5]
- GWAS studies have identified the IL-23 receptor as one polymorphism associated with AS.

Pathophysiology

- The hallmarks of AS are synovitis, enthesitis, and osteitis. Treatment targets in AS suggest a pivotal role of the IL-23/IL-17 and tumor necrosis factor (TNF)-α pathways. Serum concentrations of IL-23 are elevated in patients with AS.
- In mice, IL-23 increases T cells' expression of IL-17 within the entheses. This results in enthesitis and entheseal bone formation, and clinical features of AS.[8]
- TNF has widespread effects and plays multiple pathogenic roles in AS.
  - It stimulates the production of cell adhesion molecules and inflammatory cell recruitment.
  - It activates T cells and stimulates the production of other pro-inflammatory cytokines. Excess bone proliferation is likely mediated through the Wnt pathway, which stimulates osteogenesis.[9] In AS, the inhibitors of this pathway are downregulated. This is thought to play a role in formation of radiographic syndesmophytes.[10]

DIAGNOSIS

Clinical Presentation

- The key to diagnosing AS is having a high index of suspicion in young to middle-aged patients who complain of inflammatory-type back pain.
- Direct further history and physical examination at pursuing this diagnosis.
- Patients may have a family history of similar complaints or of other HLA-B27–related diseases.
- **Enthesitis** and the **distribution of affected joints** differentiate AS from rheumatoid arthritis (RA).
  - **Enthesitis** is inflammation of the entheses, where ligaments, tendons, and joint capsules attach to bone. It is a central feature of AS but not RA. This is what causes syndesmophytes to form in the axial skeleton. Peripheral examples include Achilles tendonitis, plantar fasciitis, and tennis or golfer's elbow.
  - Peripheral arthritis occurs in both AS and RA; however, the peripheral arthritis of AS predilects for large joints of the lower extremities, whereas RA favors small joints of the hand and wrists.
  - In general, men have more severe axial disease. Emerging data suggest women are more likely to have peripheral disease.[4]
- Patients may note a variety of **extra-articular manifestations** that may provide clues to their underlying diagnosis. The most common is anterior uveitis in up to 30%.[11] Less common manifestations include cardiac abnormalities (including conduction abnormalities, cardiomyopathy, or aortitis, leading to aortic regurgitation), pulmonary fibrosis, immunoglobulin A (IgA) nephropathy, and secondary (AA) amyloidosis. Patients may also go on to develop psoriasis (in 9%) or inflammatory bowel disease (IBD) (in 7%).
- Small, long-term prospective studies have shown that, in patients classified as nonradiographic AxSpA, 60% will go on to meet criteria for AS, with 40% having a relatively mild course without differentiating. Rarely, they may develop another defined type of SpA, such as PsA.[12]
- It is unclear whether treatment with anti-TNF therapy will prevent differentiation.

History

- Patients typically complain of **low back pain and stiffness**. The pain is inflammatory in nature (e.g., insidious onset without trauma, exacerbation of pain with rest, and improvement with activity). The pain may wake the patient at night. A warm shower, exercise, and anti-inflammatory drugs usually provide some relief.
- **Sacroiliitis,** a common initial feature, can present with buttock pain, typically alternating sides, and radiating down the thigh posteriorly.
- Symptoms progress gradually over a period of months to years and, over time, may lead to significant spinal deformities and loss of range of motion of the axial skeleton.
- Occasionally, **enthesitis, dactylitis, or oligoarticular arthritis** may be the presenting symptom.
- Patients may have a history of **uveitis**, causing blurry, painful vision, and photosensitivity.
- Patients should be queried regarding chest pain, palpitations, syncope, edema, or dyspnea to evaluate for cardiac and pulmonary involvement.
- Development of IBD-like symptoms should be investigated further with the help of a gastroenterologist.

Physical Examination

- Significant morbidity and physical disability result from flattening of the lumbar lordosis, kyphosis of the thoracic spine, flexion of the cervical spine, and flexion contractures in the pelvis and knee joints.
- The physical examination should include **evaluation of range of motion** of the spine.

- Measures may be done, including the Schober's test, measurement of lateral rotation and flexion, the occiput-to-wall distance, and of chest expansion. Serial performance of these measures may help track disease progression.
  - Please see Chapter 16, "Physical Examination," for detailed description of these maneuvers.
  - Clinical examination for **sacroiliitis** is variable and generally does not contribute to the diagnosis.
- Cardiac examination should evaluate for murmurs, such as the murmur of aortic regurgitation, and signs of heart failure. These features should raise concern for cardiac involvement and prompt referral to a cardiologist.
- Dry crackles may be auscultated in the upper lung fields from apical pulmonary fibrosis.
- A routine eye examination is generally inadequate for evaluation of suspected uveitis. Referral to an ophthalmologist should be done for slit-lamp evaluation.
- Patients may develop a psoriatic rash, nail pitting, or signs of IBD.

Diagnostic Testing
Laboratories
- Most laboratory tests for AS are nonspecific. Indicators of inflammation (e.g., elevated erythrocyte sedimentation rate [ESR] or C-reactive protein [CRP]) support the diagnosis but may not correlate with disease severity.
- Measurement of HLA-B27 may support the diagnosis and provide evidence of heritability.

Imaging
- **Sacroiliitis** in AS is typically bilateral and symmetric, as is the sacroiliitis associated with IBD. By contrast, sacroiliitis in psoriatic and reactive arthritis is often asymmetric.
  - On x-rays, the bones of the SI joint may appear radiodense because of sclerosis or have an irregular contour owing to SI joint erosions.
  - Advanced disease may lead to fusion of the SI joint with obliteration of the joint space.[1]
- In severe AS, radiographs of the spine may demonstrate ankylosis of the spine with **syndesmophytes** (osseous formations that attach to ligaments) and a **bamboo-spine** appearance. Spinal involvement in AS typically starts in the SI joints and ascends without "skip" areas, whereas discontinuous spinal involvement is more typical of psoriatic and reactive arthritis.
- **Radiographs** play an important role in the diagnosis of AS.
  - Anterior–posterior radiographs of the SI joints and other affected joints, including the spine or peripheral joints, are usually adequate and should be performed initially.
  - Additional findings, such as osteitis of the iliac crest or tuberosities from enthesitis, can be suggestive but are nondiagnostic of SpA.
- **Magnetic resonance imaging** (MRI) has a higher sensitivity and specificity for sacroiliitis, but is limited by cost. If the clinical suspicion for AxSpA is high and plain radiographs are negative or equivocal for sacroiliitis, an MRI of the SI joints should be pursued.
- Active sacroiliitis presents with bone marrow edema or osteitis on MRI. AS patients usually have two lesions in an individual MRI image or a single lesion present on two separate MRI images.[13]
- Other lesions, such as erosions, synovitis, or ankylosis, help support the diagnosis. Erosions are not seen in mechanical causes of sacroiliitis.[14]
- Over 20% of patients with mechanical low back pain and even some asymptomatic individuals can have bone marrow edema on MRI as well. Other causes of sacroiliitis on MRI include pregnancy and marathon running, where as many as 40% of patients will have false-positive MRI findings.[14] Therefore, MRI findings must be interpreted in the appropriate clinical context. Computed tomography (CT) is also sensitive for detection of sacroiliitis while offering the same degree of specificity. However, it does

involve more radiation than MRI, so it should probably be reserved for patients unable to undergo an MRI.

Differential Diagnosis

- The foremost differential of AS is mechanical back pain, which is common and may even coexist with AS. It also includes other seronegative spondyloarthritis (see Chapter 16), referred pain from intra-abdominal disease such as abdominal aortic aneurysm or gastrointestinal disease, or referred hip pain. Certain conditions such as osteitis condensans ilii and diffuse idiopathic skeletal hyperostosis (DISH) can be mistaken for AS.
- DISH is a type of noninflammatory back pain. An extreme form of osteoarthritis, DISH manifests with ossification of the anterior longitudinal ligaments and formation of bridging enthesophytes in the spine. The radiographic features can mimic those seen in AS, but DISH presents with large, bulky bridging enthesophytes that span at least four levels with nonerosive changes compared syndesmophytes in AS that occur contiguously within the spine and with erosive joint disease.

TREATMENT

- Treatment of AS is focused on providing symptomatic relief and returning patients to their best functional capacity, as well as preventing (as much as possible) the long-term consequences of spinal ankylosis, peripheral joint destruction, and extra-articular manifestations.
- A combination of medications, stretching, physical therapy, and/or surgical management is tailored to the individual patient to achieve these goals. Treatment with a combination of nonmedical and medical therapy is superior to medications alone.[15]

Medications

- A treat-to-target approach is recommended with the goal of disease **remission**, defined as the absence of clinical disease activity.[16] This target may be unfeasible in some patients with long-standing or refractory disease, in which case **minimal disease activity** is a reasonable alternative.
- Standardized measures should be routinely used, such as the Ankylosing Spondylitis Disease Activity Score (ASDAS) to trend disease activity.
- Treatment algorithms are similar in AS and nonradiographic AxSpA.
  - Nonsteroidal anti-inflammatory drugs (NSAIDs) are first-line therapy.[15]
  - Conventional synthetic disease-modifying antirheumatic drugs (csDMARDs) can treat peripheral arthritis in AS that does not respond to NSAIDs.[15]
  - A biologic disease-modifying antirheumatic drug (bDMARD) is indicated in patients with AxSpA who fail to achieve disease remission with NSAIDs alone.[15]
- Nonsteroidal anti-inflammatory drugs
  - The first-line therapy for patients with AS is NSAIDs to limit symptoms of inflammatory arthritis and back pain.
  - Classically, AS is treated with either indomethacin or naproxen, but patient satisfaction should dictate which NSAID works best.
  - For active disease, continuous NSAID therapy is recommended. NSAIDs can be taken on an as-needed basis in stable disease. Monitor NSAID-associated toxicities closely (see Chapter 9).
- Conventional synthetic disease-modifying antirheumatic drugs
  - Peripheral joint symptoms have been successfully treated with escalating doses of sulfasalazine.[17]

- At maximum tolerated doses, sulfasalazine improves peripheral joint symptoms but has limited effects on axial symptoms.
- Discontinue sulfasalazine if no response has been attained by 6 months or if severe toxicities occur.
- Monitor patients periodically (at least every 3 months) for leukopenia and neutropenia.
  ○ Traditional disease-modifying antirheumatic drugs (DMARDs) for RA, such as oral methotrexate and leflunomide, have been used for peripheral joint symptoms associated with AS.[15]
    - Methotrexate has conflicting data regarding its efficacy and is used infrequently.
    - Leflunomide also has not been shown to be effective in AS.
    - Evidence is conflicting as to whether oral DMARDs prevent TNF inhibitor drug discontinuation, as they do in RA. Therefore, no current recommendation exists to routinely place patients on oral DMARDs in addition to biologics.
- Anti-TNF agents
  ○ Significant symptomatic improvement has been demonstrated with the use of **anti-TNF agents** in AS.
  ○ Specifically, the anti-TNF agents **adalimumab, certolizumab, etanercept, golimumab**, and infliximab, are Food and Drug Administration (FDA)–approved for AS and have been shown to significantly limit disease activity and signs of inflammation in early AS.
    - Anti-TNF agents may reduce the radiographic progression of AS, especially when given within the first few years of the disease.[18,19]
    - There is no evidence to suggest superiority of one TNF inhibitor over another, except in patients with IBD or uveitis. In these patients, etanercept is avoided because of its inefficacy in IBD and its associated increased risk of uveitis flare in those with inflammatory eye disease.[15]
    - Currently, only adalimumab is approved for the treatment of noninfectious inflammatory uveitis by the FDA.
    - Biosimilars are biologic drugs shown to be similar but not identical to approved innovator drugs. Biosimilar drug CT-P13 demonstrated similar efficacy and safety to its innovator drug, infliximab, in the treatment of AS.[20] The FDA has approved its use in AS. Availability depends on local patent laws.
- Anti–IL-17A
  ○ **Secukinumab,** a soluble anti–IL-17A monoclonal antibody, reduces symptoms and slowed the rate of radiographic progression in patients with active AS.[21] It is FDA approved for the treatment of AxSpA.
    - Secukinumab does not reduce the rates of uveitis. There may be a mild steroid-sparing effect, although this requires further study.[22]
    - Potential side effects noted in trials include an approximately 1% per year risk of candidiasis and of IBD flare. Prior trials looking at secukinumab for the treatment of IBD have been stopped early for worse outcomes than placebo.[21]
  ○ Ixekizumab, another anti IL-17A antibody, is also currently FDA approved for the treatment of active AS.
- Other biologics: **Ustekinumab** is an antibody to the p40 subunit of IL-23 and IL-12. One small, open-label trial did have positive results for AS.[23] However, most subsequent trials have been terminated early, failing to meet their primary endpoints. Therefore, this therapy cannot be recommended for routine use in AS.
- Analgesics and glucocorticoids
  ○ Systemic glucocorticoids do not treat the axial disease of AS.[16] However, **local injections of steroids** may provide symptomatic relief to patients with otherwise poorly controlled joint pain. Either blind injections of SI joints or radiographically guided

injections can be used. In cases of enthesitis, tendon injections should be avoided because of the risk of tendon rupture.

○ Chronic usage of opiate therapy should be avoided because of the risk of tolerance and dependency.

Other Nonpharmacologic Therapies

• All patients diagnosed with AS should be referred for **physical therapy** for range of motion exercises and postural training.

○ Physical therapy can limit pain and improve functional status in most patients with AS.

○ Patients should be taught motion and flexibility exercises of the cervical, thoracic, and lumbar spine; stretching exercises for shortened muscles; and chest expansion exercises. Patients should be instructed to perform these exercises regularly at home.

• **Smoking cessation** should be encouraged in all patients with AS because smoking is a predictor of worse outcome.

Surgical Management

• Surgery may be beneficial for AS patients with significant morbidity from skeletal deformities.

○ **Total hip arthroplasty** can improve pain and decreased mobility resulting from damaged hip joints. This surgery may be performed at a younger age (40–60 years) than in osteoarthritis patients to improve mobility and quality of life in patients with AS.

○ **Spinal fusion** can be considered in patients with unstable vertebral articulations (including atlanto-axial subluxation).

○ **Spinal osteotomies** for severe kyphosis or fusion carry significant perioperative morbidity and mortality, with minimal improvement in symptoms. Therefore, routine performance is **not recommended**.[16]

• Anesthesiologists should be made aware of the AS diagnosis in an AS patient undergoing general anesthesia because intubation may be difficult.

COMPLICATIONS

Complications of AS are discussed in Chapter 16.

MONITORING/FOLLOW-UP

• Patients should be followed for development of worsened symptoms, physical deformity, and late complications (cardiovascular, pulmonary, and medication-related complications).

• Patients report of symptoms is sufficient to screen for the cardiopulmonary manifestations of AS. Screening echocardiograms and electrocardiograms (EKGs) are not recommended, though they are appropriate tests if patients develop corresponding symptoms.

• Osteoporosis is a common complication of AS. Recommendations do not specify when to begin screening for osteoporosis in AS patients. However, physicians should have a lower threshold for dual-energy x-ray absorptiometry (DEXA) screening in this population.

OUTCOME

• AS has not been associated with an increase in mortality but can produce significant morbidity if not recognized and treated appropriately.

• AS may progress to fusion of the entire axial skeleton at which point pain from spondyloarthritis itself frequently subsides. A complication of spinal fusion is **pseudoarthrosis** where a false "joint" is formed, frequently as a result of minor trauma. Clinical clues to pseudoarthrosis are increased local pain and enhanced spinal mobility. **Surgical referral is immediately recommended** because of possible spinal cord encroachment.

- Patients with nonradiographic AxSpA generally have better outcomes relative to their radiographic counterparts.[12]
- Most patients with AS have mild to moderately severe disease, usually characterized by a chronic relapsing and remitting course.[5]
- Severe AS occurs less commonly but produces significant morbidity related to axial skeletal fusion.
- One study has correlated seven **prognostic factors** with more severe disease.[24] The presence of hip arthritis was the most prognostic of a severe outcome. The other factors included ESR >30 mm/hour, dactylitis, oligoarthritis, decreased range of motion of the lumbar spine, limited efficacy of NSAIDs, and onset before age 16.

REFERENCES

1. Van der Linden S, Valkenburg HA, Cats A. Evaluation of diagnostic criteria for ankylosing spondylitis. A proposal for modification of the New York criteria. *Arthritis Rheum.* 1984;27:361–368.
2. Rudwaleit M, van der Heijde D, Landewé R, et al. The development of Assessment of Spondylo-Arthritis international Society classification criteria for axial spondyloarthritis (part II): Validation and final selection. *Ann Rheum Dis.* 2009;68:777–783.
3. Gremese E, Bernardi S, Bonazza S, et al. Body weight, gender and response to TNF-alpha blockers in axial spondyloarthritis. *Rheumatology.* 2014;53(5):875–881.
4. Duba A, Matthew S. The seronegative spondyloarthropathies. *Primary Care.* 2018;45:271–287.
5. Taurog JD, Chhabra A, Colbert RA. Ankylosing spondylitis and axial spondyloarthritis. *N Eng J Med.* 2016;374:2563–2574.
6. Rashid T, Wilson C, Ebringer A. The link between ankylosing spondylitis, Crohn's disease, Klebsiella, and starch consumption. *Clin Dev Immunol.* 2013; 2013:872632.
7. Sherlock JP, Joyce-Shaikh B, Turner SP, et al. IL-23 induces spondyloarthropathy by acting on ROR-γt⁺ CD3⁺CD4⁻CD8⁻ entheseal resident T cells. *Nature Med.* 2012;18:1069–1076.
8. Taurog J, Richardson J, Croft J, et al. The germfree state prevents development of gut and joint inflammatory disease in HLA-B27 transgenic rats. *J Exp Med.* 1994;180:2359–2364.
9. Smith JA. Update on ankylosing spondylitis: current concepts in pathogenesis. *Curr Allergy Asthma Rep.* 2015;15:489.
10. Heiland GR, Appel H, Poddubnyy D, et al. High level of functional dickkopf-1 predicts protection from syndesmophyte formation in patients with ankylosing spondylitis. *Ann Rheum Dis.* 2012;71:572–574.
11. Stolwijk C, van Tubergen A, Castillo-Ortiz JD, et al. Prevalence of extra-articular manifestations in patients with ankylosing spondylitis: a systematic review and meta-analysis. *Ann Rheum Dis.* 2015;74:65–73.
12. Zochling J, Brandt J, Braun J. The current concept of spondyloarthritis with special emphasis on undifferentiated spondyloarthritis. *Rheumatology.* 2005; 44:1483.
13. Lambert RG, Bakker PA, van der Heijde D, et al. Defining active sacroiliitis on MRI for classification of axial spondyloarthritis: update by the ASAS MRI working group. *Ann Rheum Dis.* 2016;75:1958–1963.
14. Weber U, Jurik AG, Zejden A, et al. Frequency and anatomic distribution of Magnetic resonance imaging features in the sacroiliac joints of young athletes: Exploring "Background Noise" toward a data-driven definition of sacroiliitis in early spondyloarthritis. *Arthritis Rheumatol.* 2018;70:736.
15. Van der Heijde D, Ramiro S, Landewé R, et al. 2016 update of the ASAS-EULAR management recommendations for axial spondyloarthritis. *Ann Rheum Dis.* 2017;76(6):978–991.
16. Smolen JS, Schöls M, Braun J, et al. Treating axial spondyloarthritis and peripheral spondyloarthritis, especially psoriatic arthritis, to target: 2017 update of recommendations by an international task force. *Ann Rheum Dis.* 2018;77:3–17.
17. Chen J, Liu C. Sulfasalazine for ankylosing spondylitis. *Cochrane Database Syst Rev.* 2005;2:CD004800.
18. Haroon N, Inman RD, Learch TJ, et al. The impact of TNF-inhibitors on radiographic progression in ankylosing spondylitis. *Arthritis Rheum.* 2013;65:2645–2654.
19. Van der Heijde D, Landewe R, Baraliakos X, et al. Radiographic findings following two years of infliximab therapy in patients with ankylosing spondylitis. *Arthritis Rheum.* 2008;58:3063–3070.

20. Yoo DH, Hrycaj P, Miranda P, et al. A randomised, double-blind, parallel-group study to demonstrate equivalence in efficacy and safety of CT-P13 compared with innovator infliximab when coadminis-tered with methotrexate in patients with active rheumatoid arthritis: the PLANETRA study. *Ann Rheum Dis.* 2013; 72:1613.

21. Braun J, Baraliakos X, Deodhar A et al. Effect of secukinumab on clinical and radiographic outcomes in ankylosing spondylitis: 2-year results from the randomized phase III MEASURE 1 study. *Ann Rheum Dis.* 2017;76:1070–1077.

22. Letko E, Yeh S, Foster CS, et al. Efficacy and safety of intravenous secukinumab in noninfectious uveitis requiring steroid-sparing immunosuppressive therapy. *Ophthalmology.* 2015;122:939–948.

23. Poddubnyy D, Hermann K, Callhoff J, et al. Ustekinumab for the treatment of patients with ac-tive ankylosing spondylitis: results of a 28-week, prospective, open-label, proof-of-concept study (TOPAS). *Ann Rheum Dis.* 2014;73:817–823.

24. Garrett S, Jenkinson T, Kennedy LG, et al. A new approach to defining disease status in an-kylosing spondylitis: the Bath Ankylosing Spondylitis Disease Activity Index. *J Rheumatol.* 1994;21:2286–2291.

Psoriatic Arthritis

18

Philip Chu and Deborah L. Parks

GENERAL PRINCIPLES

Definition

- Psoriatic arthritis (PsA) is an inflammatory arthritis that is associated with psoriasis. It is one of the five types of spondyloarthropathies (SpAs).
- The disease can range from asymptomatic to severely debilitating.

Classification

PsA can be classified by the pattern of arthritis,[1] and patients can have multiple combinations of disease features.
- **Symmetric polyarthritis:** Involvement of multiple joints in a symmetric pattern, resembling rheumatoid arthritis (RA)
- **Asymmetric oligoarthritis:** Affects four or fewer joints in an asymmetric distribution
- **Spondyloarthropathy or axial:** Includes sacroiliitis and spondylitis and may be difficult to distinguish from other spondyloarthritides, including reactive arthritis
- **Distal arthritis:** Involves the distal interphalangeal (DIP) joints of the hands or feet or both
- **Arthritis mutilans:** (Rare) Severe destructive arthritis with bone resorption, characterized by telescoping and flail digits

Epidemiology

- Consistent with the age of onset of SpA, PsA has a mean age of onset between 35 and 45 years.
- The overall prevalence of PsA in the United States is 0.25% and among patients with psoriasis is 30%. Caucasians are more commonly affected, and male-to-female ratio is 1:1.[2,3]

Pathophysiology

- As a member of the family of SpA, genetic, immunologic, and environmental factors are believed to have important roles in the development of the disease.
- PsA and psoriasis are associated with class I major histocompatibility complex (MHC) alleles. HLA-C*06 is associated with psoriasis. HLA-B*08, HLA-B*38, and HLA-B*39 have associations with PsA, HLA-B27 is associated with spondylitis.[2,4]
- Single-nucleotide polymorphisms in genes related to nuclear factor-κB signaling, interferon signaling, T-cell regulation, and the interleukin (IL)-23 pathway (IL-12B, IL-23R) suggest that genetic factors exert their effect through immune mechanisms.[2]
- CD8+ T cells, natural killer (NK) cells, and CD4+-type 17 helper (Th17) cells are important in the pathogenesis of PsA, with increased cells and cytokines at sites of disease.[2]
- Tumor necrosis factor (TNF)-α plays a role in cartilage degradation through matrix metalloproteinases and abnormal bone remodeling through osteoclast differentiation.[4]
- Environmental risk factors include obesity, infections, and localized trauma (Koebner's phenomenon).

Associated Conditions

PsA, like RA and other chronic inflammatory arthritides, is associated with increased risk of cardiovascular disease.[5]

DIAGNOSIS

Clinical Presentation

History

- Typical of SpA, patients with PsA classically present with **inflammatory arthritis** (symptoms of pain and stiffness in affected joints that is worsened with immobility and improved with activity and nonsteroidal anti-inflammatory drugs [NSAIDs]). The pattern of arthritis can be variable, as mentioned previously.
- Joint distribution tends to be **distal, asymmetric, involve all joints of the same digit** ("ray" distribution), and may have a purplish discoloration, unlike RA, which is characterized by proximal, symmetric, and affecting joints across multiple digits.[2]
- Manifestations of psoriasis precede arthritis by 10 years, but in 15% of cases, arthritis may precede skin disease or occur simultaneously.[2]
  - It is important to search thoroughly for psoriatic skin lesions in a patient with inflammatory arthritis symptoms, even if the patient does not complain of a rash. Conversely, patients with psoriasis should be questioned about joint pain, back pain, morning stiffness.
- The severity and activity of skin and arthritic disease are independent of each other.

Physical Examination

- The physical examination should evaluate for musculoskeletal system, integumentary system, and ocular manifestations of disease.
- **Musculoskeletal**
  - **Joint pain and effusions** are identified in one of the five distribution patterns noted earlier.
  - **Enthesitis** can be present and is typically manifested as pain in the heel and/or sole of the foot but can present elsewhere.
  - **Dactylitis** can be identified as inflammation at tendon insertions, along the tendon sheaths and in the joint spaces of the fingers and toes. It commonly causes the appearance of "sausage digits."
- **Integumentary**
  - The skin changes of psoriasis include **salmon-colored hyperkeratotic scaling plaques** commonly located on extensor surfaces. However, psoriasis can be present in the external auditory canal, umbilicus, intergluteal cleft, and axilla.
  - Typical **nail changes** include pitting, onycholysis, leukonychia, nail plate crumbling, oil-drop discoloration, nail bed hyperkeratosis, splinter hemorrhages, and red spots in the lunula.
  - Onycholysis is commonly mistaken for onychomycosis; therefore, it is important to examine nail scrapings for fungal elements and culture. **Nail changes can occur in up to 90% of patients with PsA.**[2]
- **Ocular:** As in other SpA, ocular inflammation, such as anterior uveitis (eye pain, redness, miosis, photophobia, blurred vision), may occur.

Diagnostic/Classification Criteria

The Classification Criteria for Psoriatic Arthritis (CASPAR) (Table 18-1) published in 2006 are the most widely used criteria.[6] The Assessment of SpondyloArthritis International Society (ASAS) has also developed classification criteria (refer to Chapter 16, Table 16-3)

TABLE 18-1	CLASSIFICATION OF PSORIATIC ARTHRITIS (CASPAR) CRITERIA

The presence of an inflammatory articular disease (joint, spine, or entheseal) plus ≥3 points from the following:
Evidence of psoriasis (one of the following)
Current psoriasis (2 points)
Personal history of psoriasis (1 point)
Family history of psoriasis (1 point)
Psoriatic nail dystrophy (1 point)
Negative test for rheumatoid factor (1 point)
Dactylitis (one of the following)
Current dactylitis (1 point)
History of dactylitis by a rheumatologist (1 point)
Radiological evidence of juxta-articular new bone formation

Adapted from: Taylor W, Gladman D, Helliwell P, et al. Classification criteria for PsA: Development of new criteria from a large international study. *Arthritis Rheum.* 2006;54:2665–2673.

for the broader diagnoses of spondyloarthritides: ankylosing spondylitis, PsA, inflammatory bowel disease (IBD)–related arthritis, and reactive arthritis.[7,8]

Differential Diagnosis

The differential diagnosis includes reactive arthritis, RA, ankylosing SpA, and gout.

Diagnostic Testing

Laboratories
- As with SpA in general, laboratory tests are not routinely useful in the diagnosis of PsA.
- Erythrocyte sedimentation rate (ESR) and C-reactive protein (CRP) are variably elevated and nonspecific.
- Anemia associated with chronic inflammation can occur but is also not specific.
- PsA usually occurs in the absence of rheumatoid factor (RF) or antinuclear antibodies (ANAs), but these tests may be positive in a small percentage of cases.
- Anti–cyclic citrullinated protein (anti-CCP) antibody can be present in patients with PsA and tends to be associated with a greater number of involved joints, with deformities and functional impairment of peripheral joints and with radiographic changes.[9]
- Hyperuricemia can be found in 20% of PsA patients and is due to increased epidermal cell turnover. It may be misleading, especially in PsA patients with monoarthritis.[4]

Imaging
- **Joint radiographs:** Classic findings include erosive changes and new bone growth in the distal joints, "pencil-in-cup" erosion, lysis of terminal phalanges, periostitis, and new bone growth at sites of enthesitis.
- **MRI:** As discussed in Chapter 17, MRI may be useful to identify early signs of disease: subclinical enthesitis, arthritis, and periarthritis. However, cost can preclude its routine use in diagnosis.
- **Ultrasound:** Power Doppler ultrasound is a low-cost, noninvasive imaging technique in evaluating enthesitis, synovitis, increased blood flow, and early erosive disease.[2]

TREATMENT

- The goals of treatment are to provide symptomatic relief of arthritis and skin disease, prevent structural damage, and preserve or restore functional capabilities.
- A **validated disease activity measure**, such as tender/swollen joint count, Disease Activity Index for Psoriatic Arthritis (DAPSA), or Psoriatic Disease Activity Score (PASDAS) should be used to assess whether the treatment regimen has **achieved target levels of disease activity** and whether the regimen should be continued or modified.
- Smoking cessation is important because smoking increases disease severity, decreases treatment response, and contributes to cardiovascular and pulmonary comorbidities.
- Physical activity and physical therapy are recommended, especially for patients with axial involvement.[10,11]
- Treatment by Domains of Psoriatic Arthritis: **Table 18-2** summarizes current therapies and treatment responses.[2]
- **Axial disease**
  - Nonsteroidal anti-inflammatory drugs (NSAIDs) are the first-line agents for treatment.
  - Initiation of **biologics** (such as **TNF-α, IL-17, or IL-12/IL-23 inhibitors**) is indicated in patients who have not responded to NSAIDs and physical therapy.
    - **TNF-α inhibitors** are usually chosen first because more experience is available.
    - There is no evidence that one **TNF-α inhibitor** is superior over another.
    - If no significant improvement is achieved within 3 to 6 months, one can switch to another **TNF-α inhibitor**, or switch to a different class of biologics (*IL-17, IL-12/IL-23 inhibitors*).
  - **Conventional synthetic disease-modifying antirheumatic drugs (csDMARDs)**, such as **methotrexate, leflunomide,** and **sulfasalazine**, are not effective for axial involvement.
  - Systemic glucocorticoid therapy is not recommended for axial disease.[10,11]
- **Peripheral arthritis**
  - **NSAIDs** are recommended for symptomatic management.
  - **csDMARDs (methotrexate, leflunomide, sulfasalazine)** are recommended, given low cost and universal access, although data on radiographic progression are lacking.
  - Glucocorticoids are conditionally recommended, either intra-articularly or systemically at the lowest doses required for efficacy and for short periods, because a withdrawal of systemic treatment can lead to a psoriasis flare.
  - **Biologics** should be initiated in patients who do not respond to **NSAIDs** and **csDMARDs.**
    - Early initiation of **biologics** can also be considered in patients with severe disease at the outset (increased levels of inflammatory markers, high joint counts with active disease). No evidence suggests that patients with peripheral arthritis benefit from continuing methotrexate therapy after starting a biologic.[10,11]
  - **Apremilast** is a newer, orally administered phosphodiesterase 4 inhibitor with moderate efficacy on cutaneous psoriasis and peripheral arthritis.
    - It has a favorable side-effect profile,[12] primarily with nausea and diarrhea, and serious adverse events are comparable to placebo.
    - Patients with multiple comorbidities (metabolic syndrome, infection risk) that preclude the use of **csDMARDs** or biologics may potentially benefit from apremilast. However, longer-term safety data are necessary to clarify its niche in PsA treatment.[10,11,15]
    - Apremilast should not be used on severe erosive disease, given lack of data on radiographic progression.[11]
  - **Abatacept** is a selective T-cell co-stimulation modulator, initially approved for RA and now approved for PsA. It can be given subcutaneously or intravenously. Although efficacious for treating arthritis, the effects on cutaneous psoriasis are mild.[12]

| TABLE 18-2 | EFFICACY OF DRUGS FOR THE TREATMENT OF PSORIATIC ARTHRITIS | | |

Drug	Joints	Skin	Structural Modification
NSAIDs	Mild response	No appreciable response	Not assessed
DMARDs			
Methotrexate	Mild response	Moderate response	Not assessed
Leflunomide	Mild response	Mild response	Not assessed
Sulfasalazine	No appreciable response	No appreciable response	Not assessed
Anti-TNF agents			
Adalimumab	Very good response	Moderate response	Moderate response
Certolizumab	Very good response	Moderate response	Moderate response
Etanercept	Very good response	Mild response	Moderate response
Golimumab	Very good response	Mild response	Moderate response
Infliximab	Very good response	Very good response	Moderate response
Anti–IL-17 agents			
Ixekizumab	Very good response	Very good response	Mild response
Secukinumab	Very good response	Very good response	Mild response
Anti–IL-12/IL-23 agent			
Ustekinumab	Very good response	Very good response	Mild response
PDE4 inhibitor			
Apremilast	Moderate response	Mild response	Not assessed
T-cell modulator			
Abatacept[12,13]	Very good response	Mild response	Moderate response
Janus kinase inhibitor			
Tofacitinib[14]	Very good response	Moderate response	Moderate response

IL, interleukin; PDE4, phosphodiesterase 4; TNF, tumor necrosis factor.

Modified from: Ritchlin CT, Colbert RA, Gladman DD. Psoriatic arthritis. *N Engl J Med.* 2017;376:957–970.

- ○ **Tofacitinib** is a newer, orally administered Janus kinase (JAK) inhibitor that was initially approved for RA and now approved for PsA, and has shown efficacy in patients who have failed csDMARDs and TNF-α inhibitor therapies.[14,16]
  - ▪ **Tofacitinib** may have higher risk of herpes zoster infections compared to other biologics.[17]
  - ▪ **Tofacitinib** should not be used in conjunction with other biologics due to infection risk.
- Enthesitis
  - ○ **NSAIDs** are first-line agents for the treatment of enthesitis based on expert opinion despite lack of randomized controlled trials. **Physical therapy** is recommended as well.
  - ○ **Biologics** (TNF-α, IL-17, IL-12/IL-23 inhibitors) and **apremilast** are effective for the treatment of enthesitis.
  - ○ **csDMARDs** are not effective for enthesitis.[10,11,18]
- Dactylitis
  - ○ **csDMARDs** are the first-line treatment of dactylitis.
  - ○ If symptoms are severe and affect multiple digits, **biologics** (TNF-α, IL-17, IL-12/IL-23 inhibitors) and **apremilast** are effective in dactylitis..
  - ○ Glucocorticoid injections can also be considered but lack randomized trial data.[10,11]
- Cutaneous psoriasis
  - ○ Topical agents such as emollients, glucocorticoids, vitamin D analogs, and calcineurin inhibitors are first-line treatment of mild psoriasis, followed by **phototherapy** and csDMARDs if insufficient clinical response.
  - ○ **Biologics** are recommended for those who do not respond to topical agents or unable to undergo phototherapy. Aggressive immunosuppression should not be utilized after phototherapy because the higher risk of melanoma and nonmelanoma skin cancers.[10,11]
- Nail psoriasis
  - ○ Similar to cutaneous psoriasis, nail psoriasis is managed with **topical glucocorticoids, vitamin D analogs,** and **calcineurin inhibitors**.
  - ○ Patients who are refractory to topical therapy or who have severe nail disease would benefit from **biologics, apremilast,** or **methotrexate**.[10,11]

Surgical Management

In severely disabled patients with significant joint deformities, surgery with joint replacements or arthroplasties may provide functional benefit and symptomatic relief.

REFERRAL

- As with all seronegative SpA, therapy should include consultation with physical and occupational therapists.
- Consultation with dermatologist is recommended to coordinate treatment and is especially useful in patients with severe skin involvement.

OUTCOME/PROGNOSIS

A poor prognosis is associated with an increased number of actively inflamed joints, elevated ESR, treatment failure, evidence of joint damage, decreased function as per the Health Assessment Questionnaire (HAQ), and reduced quality of life.

REFERENCES

1. Moll JM, Wright V. Psoriatic arthritis. *Sem Arthritis Rheum.* 1973;3:55–78.
2. Ritchlin CT, Colbert RA, Gladman DD. Psoriatic arthritis. *N Engl J Med.* 2017;376:957–970.
3. Villani AP, Rouzaud M, Sevrain M, et al. Prevalence of undiagnosed psoriatic arthritis among psoriasis patients: Systematic review and meta-analysis. *J Am Acad Dermatol.* 2015;73:242–248.
4. Cantini F, Niccoli L, Nannini C, et al. Psoriatic arthritis: a systematic review. *Int J Rheum Dis.* 2010;13:300–317.
5. Ahlehoff O, Gislason GH, Charlot M, et al. Psoriasis is associated with clinically significant cardiovascular risk: a Danish nationwide cohort study. *J Intern Med.* 2011;270:147–157.
6. Taylor W, Gladman D, Helliwell P, et al. Classification criteria for psoriatic arthritis: development of new criteria from a large international study. *Arthritis Rheum.* 2006;54:2665–2673.
7. Rudwaleit M, van der Heijde D, Landewe R, et al. The Assessment of SpondyloArthritis International Society classification criteria for peripheral spondyloarthritis and for spondyloarthritis in general. *Ann Rheum Dis.* 2011;70:25–31.
8. Rudwaleit M, van der Heijde D, Landewe R, et al. The development of Assessment of SpondyloArthritis international Society classification criteria for axial spondyloarthritis (part II): validation and final selection. *Ann Rheum Dis.* 2009;68:777–783.
9. Abdel Fattah NS, Hassan HE, Galal ZA, et al. Assessment of anti-cyclic citrullinated peptide in psoriatic arthritis. *BMC Res Notes.* 2009;2:44.
10. Wendling D, Lukas C, Prati C, et al. 2018 update of French Society for Rheumatology (SFR) recommendations about the everyday management of patients with spondyloarthritis. *Joint Bone Spine.* 2018;85:275–284.
11. Coates LC, Kavanaugh A, Mease PJ, et al. Group for research and assessment of psoriasis and psoriatic arthritis 2015 treatment recommendations for psoriatic arthritis. *Arthritis Rheumatol.* 2016;68:1060–1071.
12. Kawalec P, Holko P, Moćko P, et al. Comparative effectiveness of abatacept, apremilast, secukinumab and ustekinumab treatment of psoriatic arthritis: a systematic review and network meta-analysis. *Rheumatol Int.* 2018;38:189–201.
13. Mease PJ, Gottlieb AB, van der Heijde D, et al. Efficacy and safety of abatacept, a T-cell modulator, in a randomised, double-blind, placebo-controlled, phase III study in psoriatic arthritis. *Ann Rheum Dis.* 2017;76:1550.
14. Mease P, Hall S, FitzGerald O, et al. Tofacitinib or adalimumab versus placebo for psoriatic arthritis. *N Engl J Med.* 2017;377:1537–1550.
15. Yiu ZZ, Warren RB. Novel oral therapies for psoriasis and psoriatic arthritis. *Am J Clin Dermatol.* 2016;17:191–200.
16. Gladman D, Rigby W, Azevedo VF, et al. Tofacitinib for psoriatic arthritis in patients with an inadequate response to TNF inhibitors. *N Engl J Med.* 2017;377:1525–1536.
17. Curtis JR, Xie F, Yun H, et al. Real-world comparative risks of herpes virus infections in tofacitinib and biologic-treated patients with rheumatoid arthritis. *Ann Rheum Dis.* 2016;75:1843–1847.
18. Orbai AM, Weitz J, Siegel EL, et al. Systematic review of treatment effectiveness and outcome measures for enthesitis in psoriatic arthritis. *J Rheumatol.* 2014;41:2290–2294.

Reactive Arthritis

19

Iris Lee and María C. González-Mayda

GENERAL PRINCIPLES

Definition

- Reactive arthritis (ReA) belongs to the group of disorders known as spondyloarthropathies (SpA). Broadly, it is a syndrome of sterile, **inflammatory mono- or oligoarthritis** typically occurring in patients **days to weeks** after a **genitourinary (GU)** or **gastrointestinal (GI) infection.**
- It is distinguished from septic arthritis, which is caused by direct infection of the joint.
- ReA includes the syndrome formerly known as Reiter's syndrome (arthritis, uveitis, and conjunctivitis), an eponym that has fallen out of favor due to Hans Reiter's involvement in Nazi activities during World War II.[1]
- **Extra-articular manifestations** include urethritis, uveitis, oral ulcers, skin rashes, and nail changes.

Epidemiology

- While ReA appears to be **less common than the other SpA**, the precise prevalence and incidence of ReA are not well known partly because of the absence of well-accepted diagnostic criteria.[2,3] Thus, estimates of incidence have varied from 0.6 to 27/100,000.[4]
- A recent epidemiologic study showed an increase in nonchlamydial causes of ReA as well as increased progression to chronic disease.[4] Another showed a decreased incidence of ReA over time on the basis of coded diagnoses.[5]
- Typically, ReA affects the young and middle aged, probably influenced by infectious exposures.
- **ReA occurring after GU infections is generally more common in men,** while ReA occurring after GI infections affects men and women equally.[6]
- ReA tends to have a familial association, but appears to be less strongly **associated with HLA-B27** than ankylosing spondylitis.[7] The risk of developing ReA after an infection is about 1% to 4%, whereas in HLA-B27+ individuals, the risk is greater than 20%. The association of HLA-B27+ with ReA is stronger in more severe cases as well as the perpetuation of ReA into a chronic form.[8]

Etiology

While the arthritis in ReA is classically sterile (no organisms isolated), ReA classically follows GU or GI infections with *Chlamydia, Salmonella, Shigella* (especially *S. flexneri*), *Yersinia,* and *Campylobacter.*

- Antigenic RNA or DNA can be isolated from affected body fluid for years after the inciting infection.[8]
- Over time, there have been fewer cases of chlamydia causing ReA.[4,5]
- In addition to the classic triggers for ReA, numerous case reports also implicate other organisms, but they have not been studied systematically.

Pathophysiology

The pathogenesis of ReA is still poorly understood, but **strong clinical associations with certain bacterial infections and HLA-B27** implicate the immune system in pathogenesis, as discussed in Chapter 17. It is thought that CD4+ and CD8+ T cells cause both articular inflammation and an imbalance of Th2 cytokines.

DIAGNOSIS

Clinical Presentation

Clinical features of ReA after GI and GU infections are quite similar.

History
- Acute onset of asymmetric inflammatory oligoarthritis (<4 joints) with an additive or migratory course within 2 to 4 weeks of the initial infection is a common presentation.
- As the preceding infection may be clinically mild or occult, relying on symptoms of a triggering infection often results in underdiagnosis.

Physical Examination
- The joints most commonly affected include **knees, ankles, sacroiliac (SI) joints, lower lumbar spine, and feet.**
- **Enthesitis** is a hallmark feature, most commonly **Achilles tendonitis and plantar fasciitis,** often causing heel pain.
- **Dactylitis** ("sausage digits") may be seen.
- **Inflammatory low back pain** occurs, with symptoms consistent with sacroiliitis or spondylitis.
- Other symptoms associated with ReA include **conjunctivitis** and, in more severe instances, **anterior uveitis.**
- Mucosal features include **painless oral ulcers and sterile pyuria/dysuria** (seen in ReA following either GI or GU infections).
- Skin manifestations occur later and may include **circinate balanitis,** skin inflammation on the glans penis, and **keratoderma blennorrhagica,** hyperkeratotic pustular lesions found on the palms and soles that are histologically identical to pustular psoriasis.
- **Nail changes including pitting and onycholysis** can mimic psoriatic changes.
- On rare occasions, ReA can lead to **cardiac involvement,** including aortic insufficiency.

Diagnostic Criteria

- ReA is essentially a clinical diagnosis. Unlike other rheumatic disorders such as rheumatoid arthritis (RA) and SLE, there are no validated diagnostic criteria for ReA.[2,3] However, ReA is classified as one of the SpA, and there are now classification criteria for the SpA, including ReA, as discussed in Chapter 16.
- Except for the history of a preceding GI or GU infection, there are no clear clinical features that differentiate ReA from the other seronegative SpA. ReA can be distinguished from septic arthritis, which occurs in the setting of obvious, acute infection, and/or when organisms are cultured from the joint. ReA typically occurs sometime after the acute GI or GU infection has passed.
- ReA is considered chronic if symptoms persist for more than 6 months. It may have all of the features described in the acute phase, as well as chronic arthritis and enthesitis producing radiographic features described below.

Differential Diagnosis

Other disorders involving arthritis and the GI and/or GU tract should be considered. These include SpA associated with inflammatory bowel disease, gonococcal infection, Behçet's syndrome, and Whipple's disease.

Diagnostic Testing

Laboratories

- General markers of inflammation such as erythrocyte sedimentation rate (ESR) and C-reactive protein (CRP) may be elevated in ReA but are not useful diagnostically.
- **HLA-B27 has a limited positive predictive value and testing should not be used as a diagnostic tool** as discussed in Chapters 16 and 17.
- Serologic tests for organisms associated with ReA are usually not clinically useful because they have a high false-negative rate and, if positive, usually do not indicate recent infection. Joint aspirations for microbiologic culture should be negative; positive results indicate septic arthritis.
- Polymerase chain reaction (PCR) for microorganisms may be helpful for research studies but is generally not useful clinically.

Imaging

- Imaging studies may help exclude other diagnoses such as rheumatoid arthritis.
- **Sacroiliitis, syndesmophytes, periosteal new bone formation,** and **erosions** are often evident in chronic disease.
- Additional findings such as fluffy erosions at the calcaneus or pencil-in-cup erosions at the distal interphalangeal (DIP) joints support the diagnosis.
- **MRI or ultrasound of the sacroiliac joint** or other joints to detect earlier changes may be helpful but have not been studied in patients with ReA.

TREATMENT

- ReA is usually self-limited and abates spontaneously after several months. At an 8-year follow-up, patients with ReA were more likely to be able to perform at full work capacity than other inflammatory arthritides.[9]
- However, recurrent or chronic ReA can lead to significant joint destruction and disability.
- Disease activity is monitored primarily by clinical signs and symptoms. There are no set criteria for disease activity, but elevated ESR may respond to therapeutic intervention.

Medications

First Line

- In most cases of ReA, **nonsteroidal anti-inflammatory drugs (NSAIDs)** provide symptomatic relief for arthritis, but they are not efficacious for extra-articular manifestations.
- For limited joint involvement, circinate balanitis and keratoderma blennorrhagica, **intra-articular and topical steroids,** respectively, provide symptomatic short-term relief.

Second Line

- **Glucocorticoids generally should be avoided because they appear to be of limited benefit** and carry significant morbidity and toxicity.
- For more severe or relapsing and chronic disease states, use of steroid-sparing **disease-modifying antirheumatic drugs (DMARDs)** may be helpful.
- **Sulfasalazine (SSZ)** is the best studied DMARD for ReA with a modest, though significant, response rate of 62% for patients on 2,000 mg of SSZ per day versus 48% on placebo at 36 weeks in a Veterans Affairs Cooperative Study.[10] Similar responses were reported by others.[11] SSZ is generally considered to be helpful for peripheral arthritis but not axial disease.[12]
- Several **tumor necrosis factor alpha (TNF-α) receptor antagonists** have been approved by the Food and Drug Administration (FDA) for use in in ankylosing spondylitis. For ReA specifically, two open-label studies show benefit of etanercept[13,14] and other TNF blockers.[14]

- The use of **methotrexate, azathioprine, cyclosporine, tocilizumab,** and other agents in ReA has been used but not formally studied.
- Antibiotic therapy is controversial, and usage should follow standard infectious disease guidelines for the specific organism. For chronic ReA, it remains unclear if antibiotic therapy affects the outcomes of patients. Consequently, **routine antibiotic therapy is not generally recommended for chronic ReA.**

Other Nonpharmacologic Therapies

Physical therapy may be beneficial, especially to prevent contractures and muscle atrophy in patients with spinal involvement.

COMPLICATIONS

From 15% to 20% of patients develop chronic disease (see Monitoring/Follow-up).

REFERRALS

- Refer to a rheumatologist as soon as the diagnosis of ReA is suspected for prompt evaluation and initiation of treatment.
- Patients who develop eye redness associated with pain and/or photophobia should be referred to see an ophthalmologist immediately for evaluation of uveitis with a slit lamp exam.

MONITORING/FOLLOW-UP

Disease typically lasts 3 to 5 months, but 15% to 20% of patients may have chronic disease. Patients may also develop features of another class of spondyloarthritis. Treat these patients according to their presentation.

REFERENCES

1. Wallace DJ, Weisman MH. The physician Hans Reiter as prisoner of war in Nuremberg: a contextual review of his interrogations (1945–1947). *Semin Arthritis Rheum.* 2003;32:208–230.
2. Misra R, Gupta L. Time to revisit the concept of reactive arthritis. *Nat Rev Rheumatol.* 2017;13:327–328.
3. Townes JM. Reactive arthritis after enteric infections in the United States: the problem of definition. *Clin Infect Dis.* 2010;50:247–254.
4. Courcoul A, Brinster A, Decullier E, et al. A bicentre retrospective study of features and outcomes of patients with reactive arthritis. *Joint Bone Spine.* 2018;85:201–205.
5. Mason E, Wray L, Foster R, et al. Reactive arthritis at the Sydney Sexual Health Center 1992–2012: declining despite increasing chlamydia diagnosis. *Int J STD AIDS.* 2016;27:882–889.
6. Leirisalo M, Skylv G, Kousa M, et al. Follow-up study on patients with Reiter's disease and reactive arthritis, with special reference to HLA-B27. *Arthritis Rheum.* 1982;25:249–259.
7. Kaarela K, Jantti JK, Kotaniemi KM. Similarity between chronic reactive arthritis and ankylosing spondylitis. A 32–35-year follow-up study. *Clin Exp Rheumatol.* 2009;27:325–328.
8. Selmi C, Gershwin ME. Diagnosis and classification of reactive arthritis. *Autoimmun Rev.* 2014;13:546–549.
9. Kaarela K, Lehtinen K, Luukkainen R. Work capacity of patients with inflammatory joint diseases. An eight-year follow-up study. *Scand J Rheumatol.* 1987;16:403–406.
10. Clegg DO, Reda DJ, Weisman MH, et al. Comparison of sulfasalazine and placebo in the treatment of reactive arthritis (Reiter's syndrome). A Department of Veterans Affairs Cooperative Study. *Arthritis Rheum.* 1996;39:2021–2027.

11. Egsmose C, Hansen TM, Andersen LS, et al. Limited effect of sulphasalazine treatment in reactive arthritis. A randomised double blind placebo controlled trial. *Ann Rheum Dis.* 1997;56:32–36.
12. Clegg DO, Reda DJ, Abdellatif M. Comparison of sulfasalazine and placebo for the treatment of axial and peripheral articular manifestations of the seronegative spondyloarthropathies: a Department of Veterans Affairs cooperative study. *Arthritis Rheum.* 1999;42:2325–2329.
13. Flagg SD, Meador R, Hsia E, et al. Decreased pain and synovial inflammation after etanercept therapy in patients with reactive and undifferentiated arthritis: an open-label trial. *Arthritis Rheum.* 2005;53:613–617.
14. Meyer A, Chatelus E, Wendling D, et al. Safety and efficacy of anti-tumor necrosis factor alpha therapy in ten patients with recent-onset refractory reactive arthritis. *Arthritis Rheum.* 2011;63:1274–1280.

Enteropathic Arthritis

20

Shuang Song and Lisa A. Zickuhr

GENERAL PRINCIPLES

- Enteropathic arthritis is a form of spondyloarthritis (SpA). It is distinguished from the other types by its association with the **inflammatory bowel diseases (IBD)**: Crohn's disease **(CD)** and **ulcerative colitis (UC)**.
- This chapter will highlight the similar and unique features of enteropathic arthritis compared with the other forms of SpA.

Definition

Enteropathic arthritis is an SpA that presents as an extraintestinal manifestation of IBD.

Classification[1,2]

- **Peripheral arthritis**
  - **Type I is a pauciarticular arthritis** that affects the larger joints of the lower extremities in a migratory, asymmetric pattern. It is transient in duration and tends to correlate with IBD activity.
  - **Type II is a polyarticular arthritis** that occurs independently of the activity of bowel disease. Joint involvement is often symmetric, chronic, and includes the upper extremities.
- **Axial arthritis** is independent of the activity of bowel disease. Features can range from inflammatory back pain and sacroiliitis to ankylosis, mimicking ankylosing spondylitis (AS).
- **Enthesitis and dactylitis** can occur with all types.
- Arthralgias (noninflammatory joint pain) also commonly occur in patients with IBD; however, these are not part of the spectrum of enteropathic arthritis.

Epidemiology

- The reported prevalence of enteropathic arthritis varies widely among studies because of geographic and age-related heterogeneity.[3] Overall, in patients with IBD:
  - Peripheral arthritis is seen in 13%, with type I more prevalent than type II; and sacroiliitis in 10%, while about 3% will develop AS.
- Enthesitis is reported in 1% to 54% of IBD patients, and the estimates from Turkey (20%–54%) are considerably higher than those from other countries (1%–15%).
- Dactylitis is reported in up to 6% of IBD patients.
- Colonic involvement of IBD is a risk factor for enteropathic arthritis.[1]

Etiology

- As in other diseases, enteropathic arthritis likely occurs as a result of an environmental trigger in a genetically appropriate setting.
- An important environmental element appears to be a restricted and unbalanced gut microbiome.[4,5]
- Several candidate genes for IBD have been linked to the development of SpA.
  - HLA-B27 has the strongest association with SpA.[6,7] Mice transgenic for HLA-B27 and human β2-microglobulin develop sacroiliitis, peripheral arthritis, colitis, and

psoriasiform skin lesions. Disease, however, does not develop when mice are housed in germ-free conditions.[8]

○ SpA and IBD share many non-HLA genes.[6,7,9,10]

  ▪ Within the human genome, 65 genes are associated with both IBD and AS.

  ▪ Genes related to the dysregulation of IL-23R and IL-17 are associated with IBD and the other SpAs.

  ▪ Endoplasmic reticulum–associated protein 1 (ERAP1) and ERAP2 are thought to interact with HLA-B27 and alter the antigen-presentation pathway in both AS and IBD.

  ▪ Mutations in SEC16A, a gene encoding Sec16A, a scaffold protein important for coat protein complex II (COPII) formation and trafficking, are associated with IBD. In the presence of HLA-B27, these mutations are associated with axial SpA, suggesting SEC16A and HLA-B27 interact in the pathogenesis of axial SpA.

  ▪ The genetic similarities between enteropathic arthritis and AS may account for the clinical features shared between them. For example, the axial involvement of enteropathic arthritis resembles AS, whereas 7% of AS patients have comorbid IBD.[11]

Pathophysiology

Like other SpA, enteropathic arthritis is immune mediated. Gut dysbiosis, impaired gut mucosa barriers, proinflammatory cytokines, and dysregulated gastrointestinal (GI) lymphoid tissues upset the balance between inflammation and tolerance.[4-6] Tumor necrosis factor alpha (TNF-α) and the IL-23/IL-17 pathway play central roles in the pathogenesis of SpA (see Chapter 17 for further review).

Risk Factors

- No specific environmental risk factors have been identified for the development of enteropathic arthritis, other than the presence of IBD.
- Genetic risk factors include HLA-B27 as well as non-HLA genetic variants. However, the frequency of HLA-B27 in patients with IBD is only 30%, compared with 95% prevalence in patients with AS.[12]
- HLA-B27 positivity in IBD patients most strongly correlates with development of extraintestinal manifestations of axial SpA.[13]

DIAGNOSIS

- Diagnosis is based on a clinical presentation of SpA and a history of IBD.
- Classification criteria for SpA (Table 16-3) aid detection and diagnosis of SpA, and assist in differentiation from other types of arthritis.

Clinical Presentation

- Bowel pathology usually occurs before extraintestinal manifestations develop; however, **arthritis can sometimes be the presenting symptom of IBD.**
- As part of the spectrum of enteropathic arthritis, peripheral arthritis is typically **oligoarticular, migratory, and asymmetric, which generally affects the lower limbs.** The inflammation may lead to large joint effusions, especially in the knees.
- Other associated conditions include **uveitis, aortic regurgitation,** and skin manifestations. **Erythema nodosum and pyoderma gangrenosum** are associated with CD and UC, respectively.
- Uveitis occurring in enteropathic arthritis differs from that in AS. It is often posterior, bilateral, and chronic, whereas uveitis in AS is frequently anterior, unilateral, and acute in onset.[14]

History
- The patient may describe symptoms of inflammatory arthritis (morning stiffness lasting longer than 60 minutes, improvement of stiffness with activity, and/or joint swelling and warmth).
  ○ Peripheral joint involvement is most commonly asymmetric and affects the lower extremity joints (i.e., type I peripheral arthritis). However, it can also affect the hands in a symmetric, polyarticular pattern (i.e., type II peripheral arthritis).
  ○ Axial skeletal involvement may cause sacroiliitis, which can present with alternating buttock pain.
  ○ Enthesitis is more symptomatic in enteropathic arthritis than in AS.
  ○ Dactylitis is occasionally seen in enteropathic arthritis.
- One should assess for signs and symptoms of IBD in patients presenting with SpA who do not have a prior history of IBD. In those patients with an established diagnosis of IBD, disease activity should be assessed. Signs and symptoms include the following:
  ○ Frequent **diarrhea,** with or without hematochezia, mucus, steatorrhea, and malabsorption
  ○ **Crampy abdominal pain**
  ○ **Fistulas, abscesses, and aphthous ulcers**
  ○ Extraintestinal manifestations including **uveitis, pyoderma gangrenosum, and erythema nodosum**

Physical Examination
- The physical examination should evaluate for musculoskeletal and other extraintestinal manifestations of IBD.
- The musculoskeletal exam can be divided into axial and peripheral findings:
  ○ Examination of the axial skeleton may demonstrate **sacroiliac (SI) joint tenderness** and **decreased spinal mobility.**
  ○ Peripheral joint findings include **swelling, effusions, erythema, reduced range of motion, dactylitis, and enthesitis.**
- **Ocular redness, pain, and photosensitivity** raise suspicion for eye involvement. Referral to an ophthalmologist for evaluation of uveitis or scleritis may be required.
- Evaluation of the **skin** may reveal enterocutaneous fistulae, erythematous nodules, or ulcers. Dermatology referral and skin biopsy should be considered.
- Findings upon examination of the GI system may reveal aphthous ulcers, abdominal tenderness, rectal ulcers, and guaiac-positive stool.

Diagnostic Criteria
- No specific diagnostic criteria exist. Diagnosis is based on clinical suspicion and excluding other causes for symptoms.
- The Assessment of SpondyloArthritis International Society's (ASAS) classification criteria for axial and peripheral SpA (Table 16-3) are useful as general diagnostic guidelines.[15,16]
- Patients with enteropathic arthritis should meet the criteria for diagnosis of SpA and have active IBD or a history compatible with IBD. **Some patients may develop IBD after a diagnosis of undifferentiated SpA is made.**

Differential Diagnosis
- **Mechanical back pain** is the most common cause of lower back pain. Only 5% of patients seen in a primary care setting with chronic low back pain are diagnosed with SpA.[17]
- Other conditions may have similar clinical features involving bowel and joints, including reactive arthritis, Whipple's disease, Celiac disease, and Behçet's disease.
- In patients with established IBD presenting with monoarticular arthritis, **infectious arthritis** must be considered.

- **Arthralgias** (joint pain without inflammatory symptoms) may be found in patients with IBD. These are not part of the spectrum of enteropathic arthritis.

Diagnostic Testing

- Few diagnostic tests are of use for establishing a diagnosis of enteropathic arthritis.
- In patients with both SpA symptoms and diarrhea, abdominal pain, or weight loss, a GI referral to assess the possibility of IBD is indicated.
- Laboratory studies might be useful in diagnosing enteropathic arthritis.
- Imaging may demonstrate sacroiliitis or other inflammatory changes in the joint. In fact, MRI evidence of sacroiliitis is part of the current ASAS criteria for axial SpA.[15]

Laboratories
- Erythrocyte sedimentation rate (ESR) and C-reactive protein (CRP) may indicate a systemic inflammatory process. Unfortunately, these tests **rarely correlate with disease activity.**
- **HLA-B27 is positive in about 30% of patients** with enteropathic arthritis, 70% enteropathic axial SpA, and 90% idiopathic AS. Only 1% to 2% of people who carry HLA-B27 develop SpA. The recommendation of HLA-B27 testing is controversial. However, in both ASAS criteria for peripheral and axial SpA (2011 and 2009), HLA-B27 testing is included (Table 16-3).
- Calprotectin is an intestinal inflammatory marker that can assist the diagnosis of IBD. Recent studies indicated that fecal calprotectin may also be a disease activity biomarker for AS.[18]

Imaging
- **Plain radiography of the SI joints and spine** may demonstrate sacroiliitis, syndesmophytes, or ankylosis consistent with axial SpA (see Chapter 17).[5]
- **MRI of the spine** may demonstrate early inflammatory changes including bone marrow edema and fat infiltration, findings that define nonradiographic axial SpA (see Chapter 17).
- For peripheral joints, three modalities are used for imaging. Plain radiography may demonstrate **enthesitis and periosteal reaction.** Ultrasound and MRI may also be helpful in identifying subtle inflammatory changes within the joint and surrounding structures.

Diagnostic Procedures
- Gastroenterology referral and **endoscopy** should be considered in patients with a clinical presentation of SpA and bowel symptoms to evaluate for IBD if not already established.
- An **arthrocentesis** should be performed in any patient presenting with peripheral monoarticular arthritis with synovial fluid submitted for cell count and culture to evaluate for inflammation and rule out infectious arthritis.

TREATMENT

- Pharmacologic treatment of enteropathic arthritis depends on the presence of axial arthritis.
- **Often, control of IBD will result in control of enteropathic arthritis** and, therefore, should be the goal of therapy. However, when the arthritis is independent of bowel inflammation, additional therapy should be considered if joint symptoms persist despite IBD remission.
- The treat-to-target (T2T) strategy aiming at remission/inactive disease or low/minimal disease activity is recommended.[19]

Medications

The pharmacologic therapy of axial and peripheral enteropathic arthritis follows the general principles for treating axial and peripheral SpA (Chapter 17).

- **Nonsteroidal anti-inflammatory drugs (NSAIDs)**
  - **NSAIDs** are first-line therapy for the treatment of SpA. NSAIDs improve pain and stiffness but do not retard the radiographic progression of ankylosis. NSAIDs should be used with caution in enteropathic arthritis because they may trigger IBD flares.[20]
  - Brief courses (up to 2 weeks) of cyclooxygenase (COX)-2 inhibitors appear to be safe, but long-term data are lacking.
- **Conventional-synthetic disease-modifying antirheumatic drugs (csDMARDs)**, such as **sulfasalazine, methotrexate, leflunomide, and azathioprine**, are effective for peripheral arthritis.[21] They have no effect on axial arthritis.
  - **Sulfasalazine** is the preferred csDMARD. It is used for early disease of peripheral arthritis and mild to moderate IBD.
  - Immunosuppressive csDMARDs, namely, methotrexate, azathioprine, and leflunomide, may effectively treat IBD, peripheral enteropathic arthritis, and other extraintestinal manifestations of IBD, but not axial disease.
- **Biologic disease-modifying antirheumatic drugs (bDMARDs)**
  - Antitumor necrosis factor agents
    - **Antitumor necrosis factor (anti-TNF) agents** are highly effective in IBD and both peripheral and axial SpA.[21]
    - Adalimumab, certolizumab, golimumab, and infliximab are approved for use in IBD. While infliximab is the best studied, adalimumab and golimumab also show benefit in both axial and peripheral SpA.
    - Etanercept, however, is ineffective for the treatment of IBD.[22] It is also associated with an increased risk of uveitis in SpA patients.[23]
  - **IL-12/IL-23 inhibitor: Ustekinumab** has demonstrated efficacy in psoriatic arthritis (PsA) and in moderately to severely active CD refractory to anti-TNF therapy.[15,16] At the time of this writing, data supporting its use in enteropathic arthritis are lacking.
  - **IL-17 inhibitors** are effective for PsA and ankylosing SpA. However, a randomized, placebo-controlled trial in Crohn's patients demonstrated that the IL-17 inhibitor secukinumab increased the rates of disease flares and adverse events. Therefore, IL-17 inhibitors should be avoided in enteropathic arthritis.[24]
  - Anti-integrin therapy
    - **Vedolizumab** is approved for CD and UC. It is a humanized monoclonal antibody against α4β7 integrin and specifically targets the GI tract.
    - Preliminary data suggested that vedolizumab is effective for extraintestinal manifestations of IBD, including peripheral and axial SpA, but paradoxical skin lesions and arthritis may occur, highlighting the need for further investigation.[25,26]
  - Janus kinase (JAK) inhibitors (oral nonbiologic to targeted synthetic DMARDs)
    - **Tofacitinib** is approved for PsA. Recent studies demonstrated its efficacy in UC, but not in CD.[27]
    - Other JAK inhibitors are currently being studied in IBD and inflammatory arthritis.
  - **Glucocorticoids**
    - **Glucocorticoids, oral or intra-articular,** are useful in controlling bowel inflammation and may be useful for peripheral joint involvement. They are ineffective for the treatment of axial disease.
    - Glucocorticoids should be used at the lowest effective dose for the shortest period of time because of their extensive side-effect profile.

Other Nonpharmacologic Therapies

- **Physical therapy and exercise** are mainstays for all SpAs. An exercise program in combination with pharmacologic agents has been shown to be more effective than pharmacologic treatment alone.
- **Surgical management** is discussed in Chapter 17.

COMPLICATIONS

Complications of SpA depend on the type of arthritis.
- Type I arthritis is usually nondeforming.
- Type II arthritis can lead to joint erosions and/or ankylosis of an affected joint.
- Those with axial SpA may develop complications related to spinal fusion seen in ankylosis. See Chapter 16.

REFERRAL

- IBD patients with one or more of the following should be referred to a rheumatologist:
  - Inflammatory back pain
  - Sacroiliitis on imaging
  - Peripheral arthritis, enthesitis, or dactylitis
- Those patients who have inflammatory back pain or peripheral arthritis, enthesitis, or dactylitis with signs and symptoms suggestive of IBD should be referred to a gastroenterologist for further diagnostic testing.
- Ophthalmology referral is indicated for patients with light sensitivity and redness or pain in the eyes.

PATIENT EDUCATION

- Patients should be educated on the manifestations, complications, and therapeutic options of their disease.
- In addition, the benefits of exercise and physical therapy for improving functional status and limiting pain should be emphasized.

MONITORING/FOLLOW-UP

- Disease activity should be monitored based on bowel disease, morning stiffness, pain, physical exam, inflammatory markers, and imaging (when indicated).
- The recommended therapeutic target is clinical remission/inactive disease or alternatively low/minimal disease activity.[19]
  - The treatment-to-target (T2T) recommendations made by the 2017 task force prefer Ankylosing Spondylitis Disease Activity Score (ASDAS) as a measure for disease activity of axial SpA.
  - There is no specific recommendation for measuring disease activity in peripheral enteropathic arthritis. However, Disease Activity index for PSoriatic Arthritis (DAPSA) was originally derived and validated in reactive arthritis. Therefore, it could be used as a measure for peripheral enteropathic arthritis.
- The choice of the therapeutic target should take into account extra-articular manifestations, comorbidities, patient factors, and drug-related risks.

REFERENCES

1. Harbord M, Annese V, Vavricka SR, et al. The first European evidence-based consensus on extra-intestinal manifestations in inflammatory bowel disease. *J Crohns Colitis*. 2016;10:239–254.

2. Orchard TR, Wordsworth BP, Jewell DP. Peripheral arthropathies in inflammatory bowel disease: their articular distribution and natural history. *Gut*. 1998;42:387–391.

3. Karreman MC, Luime JJ, Hazes JMW, et al. The prevalence and incidence of axial and peripheral spondyloarthritis in inflammatory bowel disease: a systematic review and meta-analysis. *J Crohns Colitis*. 2017;11:631–642.

4. Breban M, Tap J, Leboime A, et al. Faecal microbiota study reveals specific dysbiosis in spondyloarthritis. *Ann Rheum Dis*. 2017;76:1614–1622.

5. Davis JC, Mease PJ. Insights into the pathology and treatment of spondyloarthritis: from the bench to the clinic. *Semin Arthritis Rheum*. 2008;38:83–100.

6. Asquith M, Rosenbaum JT. The interaction between host genetics and the microbiome in the pathogenesis of spondyloarthropathies. *Curr Opin Rheumatol*. 2016;28:405–412.

7. Ranganathan V, Gracey E, Brown MA, et al. Pathogenesis of ankylosing spondylitis–recent advances and future directions. *Nat Rev Rheumatol*. 2017;13:359–367.

8. Khare SD, Luthra HS, David CS. Spontaneous inflammatory arthritis in HLA-B27 transgenic mice lacking beta 2-microglobulin: a model of human spondyloarthropathies. *J Exp Med*. 1995;182:1153–1158.

9. O'Rielly DD, Uddin M, Codner D, et al. Private rare deletions in SEC16A and MAMDC4 may represent novel pathogenic variants in familial axial spondyloarthritis. *Ann Rheum Dis*. 2016;75:772–779.

10. Loft ND, Skov L, Rasmussen MK, et al. Genetic polymorphisms associated with development of psoriatic arthritis in patients with psoriasis. *PLoS One*. 2018;13.

11. Stolwijk C, van Tubergen A, Castillo-Ortiz JD, et al. Prevalence of extra-articular manifestations in patients with ankylosing spondylitis: a systematic review and meta-analysis. *Ann Rheum Dis*. 2015;74:65–73.

12. De Vos M. Joint involvement associated with inflammatory bowel disease. *Dig Dis*. 2009;27:511–515.

13. Arvikar SL, Fisher MC. Inflammatory bowel disease associated arthropathy. *Curr Rev Musculoskelet Med*. 2011;4:123–131.

14. Lyons JL, Rosenbaum JT. Uveitis associated with inflammatory bowel disease compared with uveitis associated with spondyloarthropathy. *Arch Ophthalmol*. 1997;115:61–64.

15. Rudwaleit M, van der Heijde D, Landewé R, et al. The development of Assessment of SpondyloArthritis international Society classification criteria for axial spondyloarthritis (part II): validation and final selection. *Ann Rheum Dis*. 2009;68:777–783.

16. Rudwaleit M, van der Heijde D, Landewé R, et al. The Assessment of SpondyloArthritis International Society classification criteria for peripheral spondyloarthritis and for spondyloarthritis in general. *Ann Rheum Dis*. 2011;70:25–31.

17. Reveille JD, Weisman MH. The epidemiology of back pain, axial spondyloarthritis and HLA-B27 in the United States. *Am J Med Sci*. 2013;345:431–436.

18. Duran A, Kobak S, Sen N, et al. Fecal calprotectin is associated with disease activity in patients with ankylosing spondylitis. *Bosn J Basic Med Sci*. 2016;16:71–74.

19. Smolen JS, Schöls M, Braun J, et al. Treating axial spondyloarthritis and peripheral spondyloarthritis, especially psoriatic arthritis, to target: 2017 update of recommendations by an international task force. *Ann Rheum Dis*. 2018;77:3–17.

20. Takeuchi K, Smale S, Premchand P, et al. Prevalence and mechanism of nonsteroidal anti-inflammatory drug-induced clinical relapse in patients with inflammatory bowel disease. *Clin Gastroenterol Hepatol*. 2006;4:196–202.

21. Peluso R, Manguso F, Vitiello M, et al. Management of arthropathy in inflammatory bowel diseases. *Ther Adv Chronic Dis*. 2015;6:65–77.

22. Braun J, Baraliakos X, Listing J, et al. Differences in the incidence of flares or new onset of inflammatory bowel diseases in patients with ankylosing spondylitis exposed to therapy with anti-tumor necrosis factor alpha agents. *Arthritis Rheum*. 2007;57:639–647.

23. Wendling D, Paccou J, Berthelot JM, et al. New onset of uveitis during anti-tumor necrosis factor treatment for rheumatic diseases. *Semin Arthritis Rheum*. 2011;41:503–510.

24. Hueber W, Sands BE, Lewitzky S, et al. Secukinumab, a human anti-IL-17A monoclonal antibody, for moderate to severe Crohn's disease: unexpected results of a randomised, double-blind placebo-controlled trial. *Gut.* 2012;61:1693–1700.
25. Fleisher M, Marsal J, Lee SD, et al. Effects of vedolizumab therapy on extra-intestinal manifestations in inflammatory bowel disease. *Dig Dis Sci.* 2018;63:825–833.
26. Tadbiri S, Peyrin-Biroulet L, Serrero M, et al. Impact of vedolizumab therapy on extra-intestinal manifestations in patients with inflammatory bowel disease: a multicentre cohort study nested in the OBSERV-IBD cohort. *Aliment Pharmacol Ther.* 2018;47:485–493.
27. Olivera P, Danese S, Peyrin-Biroulet L. JAK inhibition in inflammatory bowel disease. *Expert Rev Clin Immunol.* 2017;13:693–703.

IV

Crystalline Arthritides

Gout

21

Michiko Inaba and Amy M. Joseph

GENERAL PRINCIPLES

Definition

Gout is a type of inflammatory arthritis caused by the deposition of monosodium urate (MSU) crystals in the joints, soft tissues (termed *tophi*), or kidneys.

Classification

The natural history of gout classically has three stages:
- **Asymptomatic hyperuricemia** usually exists for years before the initial acute attack. Most patients with hyperuricemia do not develop gout.
- Those patients who go on to develop gout then enter the **acute intermittent gout** stage where they have acute attacks of arthritis followed by symptom-free intercritical periods. Over time, the attacks become more frequent and severe.
- **Chronic gouty arthritis** may then ensue in untreated patients, with persistent pain during the intercritical periods between acute attacks. Tophi (uric acid deposits) are often seen in articular, periarticular, bursal, bone, auricular, and cutaneous tissues. Patients may also develop gouty nephropathy in the kidneys and uric acid stones in any part of the urinary tract.

Epidemiology

- Gout is the most common form of inflammatory arthritis in men. In the United States, recently it has been estimated to affect 3.9% of adults.[1]
- Approximately 90% of gout occurs in men between the ages of 30 and 60.
- Gout is uncommon in premenopausal women, thought to be due to the uricosuric effects of estrogens.
- Gout and hyperuricemia are associated with several comorbid conditions including cardiovascular disease, hypertension, and chronic kidney disease.

Pathophysiology

- **Hyperuricemia** may be a primary disorder in the absence of conditions or medications that cause hyperuricemia, or secondary.
- Uric acid is normally produced in the liver in the purine metabolism pathway. Its immediate precursors are hypoxanthine and xanthine, which are converted by xanthine oxidase to uric acid.
- Normal uric acid levels reported by clinical laboratories may be misleading with respect to the pathophysiology of gout.
  ○ The upper limit of normal uric acid is often defined by laboratories as being 2 standard deviations above the mean of age-matched controls, which can be >8.5 mg/dL.

- However, uric acid levels >6.8 mg/dL in men and women exceed the solubility of uric acid at body temperature, leading to supersaturation in body fluids.
- Uric acid levels in children are typically low (<4.0 mg/dL), beginning to rise in males at the time of puberty.
- In postmenopausal women, uric acid levels approach those of men because of the loss of the uricosuric effects of estrogen.
- Two-thirds of uric acid is excreted by the kidney, with a small portion of uric acid excreted by the gastrointestinal (GI) tract.
- Primary hyperuricemia
  - Patients with a complete deficiency of hypoxanthine–guanine phosphoribosyl transferase (HGPRT) have X-linked **Lesch–Nyhan syndrome** with hyperuricemia, severe neurologic defects, gout, and uric acid stones.
  - Patients with a partial defect in HGPRT have Kelley–Seegmiller syndrome and classically present with early onset gout and/or uric acid nephrolithiasis without neurologic problems.
  - However, **most patients with primary hyperuricemia do not have an identifiable cause.**
- Secondary hyperuricemia
  - **Many medications, especially thiazide and loop diuretics, can cause hyperuricemia.**
  - Other medications that increase serum uric acid include cyclosporine, tacrolimus, low-dose aspirin, niacin, ethambutol, pyrazinamide, and L-dopa.
  - **Overproduction** of uric acid can occur with psoriasis, myeloproliferative disorders, multiple myeloma, hemoglobinopathies, and cytotoxic drugs.
  - **Underexcretion** of uric acid leading to hyperuricemia may occur in chronic renal disease, hypothyroidism, and lead poisoning. Around 90% of patients with hyperuricemia have decreased efficiency of renal uric acid excretion. The URAT1 uric acid transporter in the proximal tubule is responsible for the majority of renal reabsorption of uric acid.
- **Acute gout is an inflammatory response to monosodium urate (MSU) crystal deposition in the joint space.** This is more likely to happen in patients with high uric acid levels. It is not clear what initiates the inflammatory process because crystals can be present in the joint space during asymptomatic periods.
- MSU-induced inflammation appears to be a consequence of activation of the nucleotide-binding oligomerization domain (NOD)-like (NLR) family pyrin domain-containing 3 (NLRP3, also known as cryopyrin) inflammasome, proteolytic cleavage and activation of caspase-1, proteolytic cleavage and maturation of pro-interleukin (IL)-1β, and secretion of mature IL-1β.[2] This process is related to inflammation in diseases associated with gain of function mutations in NLRP3, including familial cold autoinflammatory syndrome, Muckle–Wells syndrome, and neonatal-onset multisystem inflammatory disease.

DIAGNOSIS

Clinical Presentation

- The sudden onset of **severe pain, erythema, swelling, and disability of typically a single joint** and tenosynovial inflammation characterizes an acute gout attack. The erythema and swelling may be accompanied by pruritus and low-grade fever. Inflammation often extends beyond the affected joint. Desquamation of the skin overlying the affected joint frequently occurs after the attack resolves.
- Typically, acute gout initially presents in men between the ages of 30 and 60 and in postmenopausal women. A much earlier age of onset should lead to an investigation for an inborn error of metabolism. Acute gout may be precipitated by alcohol binges, dehydration, recent trauma, surgery, and initiation of drugs that change uric acid levels.

- Early attacks of gout are typically **monoarticular and involve joints in the lower extremities.**
- The initial attack involves the metatarsophalangeal (MTP) joint of the great toe (**podagra**) in about 50% of cases, with about 90% of patient's ultimately experiencing podagra with recurrent attacks. Other common sites include the ankle, midfoot, knee, and wrist. Gout can affect any joint. The olecranon and prepatellar bursas are common sites for acute gouty bursitis.
- Acute attacks usually peak within the first 12 hours from onset, typically lasts 5 to 14 days, but a severe attack may last up to 3 weeks. Gouty attacks are self-limited and eventually resolve spontaneously.
- **Acute intermittent gout:** Between acute attacks, patients are asymptomatic for prolonged periods, termed *intercritical periods*. Without treatment, the typical patient can expect a recurrent attack within 2 years of the initial attack. However, some patients may not experience another attack. Over time, most patients' gout attacks become increasingly frequent and severe. Polyarticular attacks are more likely to occur, occurring overall around 20% of the time.
- **Chronic gouty arthritis:** Left untreated, the disease may progress to chronic gouty arthritis in approximately 12 years (range, 5–40 years).
- **Chronic tophaceous gout arthropathy (CTGA):** Characterized by the deposition of MSU in connective tissue as soft tissue masses known as *tophi*. Smaller tophi may cause joint erosions seen on radiographs, manifested as polyarticular deforming arthritis that particularly involves the hands. In some patients, this arthritis may be difficult to differentiate in clinical appearance from rheumatoid arthritis (RA).
- Tophi occur most commonly at the base of the great toe and in fingers, wrists, hands, olecranon bursas, and Achilles tendons. Higher uric acid levels are associated with more tophi. Complications of tophi include pain, deformity, joint destruction, and nerve compression.

Differential Diagnosis

- The differential diagnosis of an acute gout attack includes cellulitis, septic arthritis, and acute calcium pyrophosphate arthritis (pseudogout).
- Gout can **mimic cellulitis** in that the affected area is swollen, erythematous, and painful and may be accompanied by fever and leukocytosis.
  - If cellulitis is suspected, the joint should not be aspirated through the possibly infected overlying skin, to avoid seeding the joint.
  - It may be necessary to treat with antibiotics for 1 to 2 days while awaiting blood cultures and other clinical indications of infection before considering gout as a leading diagnosis.
- **Septic arthritis** must always be considered in a patient with acute monoarticular arthritis, especially when accompanied by fever and leukocytosis.
  - **Joint aspiration is critical to rule out bacterial infection;** treat suspicious cases with antibiotics as for cellulitis.
  - Gouty joints are more susceptible to bacterial infection, and the two conditions may occur simultaneously. The presence of crystals in synovial fluid does not preclude infection.
- **Pseudogout** should always be considered when entertaining the diagnosis of gout. It is most readily distinguished from gout by the presence of calcium pyrophosphate crystals in the joint and the absence of MSU crystals. Gout and pseudogout can coexist.
- Chronic gout may **mimic RA** because some chronic gout patients may display a symmetric polyarthritis. They may also develop tophi in sites where rheumatoid nodules typically occur. In contrast to RA, chronic gout typically presents at an older age and is seronegative. Radiographs may show changes typical of gout.

Diagnostic Testing

- **Hyperuricemia alone is not diagnostic for gout.** The diagnosis is based primarily on history, physical examination, and the presence of intracellular **MSU crystals** in synovial fluid or tophi.
- Although the presence of MSU crystals on synovial fluid analysis from an affected joint or bursa is the gold standard for making a diagnosis, the 2015 ACR/EULAR Gout Classification Criteria allow for the diagnosis to be made without synovial fluid analysis if the patient has a characteristic constellation of findings.[3]

Laboratories
- Patients with gout almost invariably have hyperuricemia, but **uric acid levels may be normal during an attack.**
- Attacks are also associated with an increased erythrocyte sedimentation rate (ESR), and C-reactive protein (CRP). The leukocyte count can be mildly elevated.
- None of these laboratory tests are helpful for distinguishing gout from other inflammatory arthritides.

Imaging
- **Joint radiographs** early in the course of the disease are normal, but as the disease progresses, **characteristic punched-out joint erosions with overhanging edges** ("rat-bite lesions") in the bone may be evident.
- **Magnetic resonance imaging** can detect bone erosions or evidence of synovial pannus in some patients with gout whose plain x-rays are normal, but these findings are not specific for gout.
- **Dual-energy computed tomography (DECT)** is a recently developed advanced imaging method that enables visualization and volume assessment of tophi.
- **Ultrasonography** is useful in detection of MSU crystal deposition in joints and monitoring therapy. In addition to being able to demonstrate effusions and bone erosions in gout, ultrasonography can detect crystal deposition on the cartilage surface (a linear density known as the *double contour sign*), crystal aggregates in synovial fluid (called the *snowstorm appearance*), and tophaceous deposits in joints and soft tissues.[4]

Diagnostic Procedures
- **Aspiration of the affected joint or bursa and synovial fluid analysis is the gold standard for diagnosing gout.** The synovial fluid analysis should include leukocyte count with differential cell count, Gram stain, and culture, along with examination for crystals under polarizing light microscopy.
- Monosodium urate crystals are needle shaped and demonstrate negative birefringence with polarized microscopy, meaning they appear yellow when parallel to the axis of the red compensator. Crystals can also be identified in the synovial fluid during the intercritical period in an asymptomatic patient but are usually not intracellular.
- Leukocyte counts are elevated in the joint fluid, usually 15,000/μL or higher with a predominance of neutrophils, although early in the course, leukocyte counts can be lower. Leukocyte count of greater than 50,000/μL should raise suspicion for a bacterial joint infection.

TREATMENT

First and foremost, one should treat an acute attack as early as possible. Consider the need for treating hyperuricemia later.
- **Acute gouty attack:** Medication choice is made based on patient comorbidities and preferences.

- Nonsteroidal anti-inflammatory drugs (NSAIDs) are considered first-line therapy, though contraindications may limit their use because the typical gout patient has co-morbid conditions.
  - Essentially any NSAID may be used.
  - NSAIDs are typically used at maximal anti-inflammatory doses with improvement in symptoms expected to begin within a few hours.
  - **Contraindications** include peptic ulcer disease, chronic kidney disease, cardiovascular disease, blood thinners, and drug allergy.
  - Commonly used NSAIDs are ibuprofen 800 mg three times per day, naproxen 500 mg twice per day, meloxicam 15 mg once daily, or indomethacin 50 mg three times per day.
  - The selective cyclooxygenase (COX)-2 inhibitor celecoxib may also be used in full dose with similar efficacy and lower GI toxicity, compared with the COX-nonspecific NSAIDs.
- **Colchicine** can be prescribed for some patients unable to take NSAIDs. It is most effective if started within the first 24 hours of onset of the attack.
  - Low-dose colchicine (1.2 mg, followed by 0.6 mg 1 hour later) is now recommended because it has been shown to be comparable in efficacy to high-dose colchicine with significantly lower toxicity.[5]
  - In patients with creatinine clearance of <30 mL/minute, colchicine dose adjustment is not required, but redosing within 2 weeks is not recommended.
  - Colchicine is generally avoided in hemodialysis patients with gout flares because it is not removed by dialysis.
  - **Intra-articular or systemic glucocorticoid** therapy can be used in some patients with contraindications to NSAID and colchicine usage. **Septic arthritis should be ruled out before initiating glucocorticoid therapy.**
  - Oral glucocorticoid therapy is reserved for patients who have failed or have a contraindication to NSAIDs or colchicine and are not appropriate for intra-articular glucocorticoids. A typical regimen of prednisone is started at 40 to 60 mg PO daily and tapered off over 2 weeks.
- **Adrenocorticotropic hormone (ACTH)** is an option in patients who cannot tolerate other recommended therapies. The dosage 40 to 80 IU in a single dose or every 12 hours for 1 to 2 days, SC or IM.
- **The IL-1 inhibitors anakinra, canakinumab, and rilonacept** block the pro-inflammatory cytokine IL-1β, which is produced as a result of the innate immune mechanisms activated by the inflammasome and plays a central role in the inflammation of acute gout flares. Although not Food and Drug Administration (FDA) approved for this indication, the IL-1 inhibitors may be considered for off-label use in acute gout when standard therapy is contraindicated or ineffective.
- **Prophylaxis of mobilization flares**
  - Prophylactic therapy may be given while initiating urate-lowering therapy, as changes in uric acid levels can precipitate acute attacks or mobilization flares.
  - Colchicine can be used to prevent mobilization flares in doses of 0.6 mg PO daily to twice a day in patients with normal renal and hepatic function. The dose must be reduced in patients with impaired kidney or liver function. Toxicity from colchicine overdose can include nausea and vomiting, diarrhea, demyelinating neuropathy, rhabdomyolysis, myocardial injury, cardiac arrhythmias, and fulminant hepatic failure.
  - **Low-dose daily NSAIDs** are alternative therapy for prevention of mobilization flares, for example, naproxen 220 mg PO twice a day. Patients with contraindications to NSAID use, such as peptic ulcer disease or chronic kidney disease, should avoid NSAIDs for prophylaxis.

- **Treatment of hyperuricemia**
  - **Asymptomatic hyperuricemia does not require treatment.**
    - Hyperuricemia is highly prevalent among hypertensive patients and those with chronic kidney disease.
    - The majority of patients with hyperuricemia will never develop gout.
    - Although hyperuricemia and gout are known to be associated with cardiovascular disease and premature mortality, it is not currently known whether treatment of hyperuricemia protects against those outcomes. So the current recommendation is to modify risk factors for gout and cardiovascular disease, but treatment of asymptomatic hyperuricemia is not indicated based on current knowledge.
  - Treatment of hyperuricemia in gout aims to reduce serum uric acid levels and prevent progression of disease to chronic gouty arthritis.
  - **Dietary treatment** of hyperuricemia includes achieving or maintaining healthy weight; avoiding organ meats, food and beverages containing high-fructose corn syrup; and limiting intake of beef, lamb, pork, seafood, and alcoholic beverages, especially beer.
  - **Avoiding medications that increase serum uric acid**, such as diuretics, especially thiazides, low-dose aspirin, and cyclosporine A, can be considered, taking into account the relative risks and benefits for the individual patient.
  - **Criteria for initiating pharmacologic urate-lowering therapy (ULT)** in patients with symptomatic gout include the following:
    - Tophaceous disease based on clinical exam or imaging study
    - Presence of erosions
    - Frequent attacks of acute gouty arthritis
    - Chronic kidney disease stage 2 or worse
    - Uric acid kidney stones
    - Gouty nephropathy
  - The goal of therapy is to achieve a serum uric acid level of less than 6 mg/dL.[6] When the uric acid level is <6.0 mg/dL, monosodium urate crystals are reabsorbed from the joint and soft-tissue tophi. The goal urate level <5.0 mg/dL is recommended in patients with tophi, as lower serum urate levels help to speed resolution of tophi.
  - Chronic ULT eventually leads to alleviation of the arthritis and prevents ongoing structural damage, although bony abnormalities and other structural defects are not reversed.
  - **Although it is best to avoid starting these agents during an acute attack,** in patients with contraindications to mobilization flare–preventing medications, ULT can be initiated once the acute inflammation has subsided while the patient is still being treated for the acute flare. Otherwise, ULT can be initiated at least 2 weeks after the attack subsides and while the patient has had at least 1 week of prophylactic therapy.
  - **If the patient is on an antihyperuricemic agent, do not discontinue it during an acute attack** because any alteration in serum uric acid levels may worsen or prolong attacks.
  - Continue ULT indefinitely. A common mistake is stopping treatment when uric acid level has normalized, which usually precipitates another attack.
  - **Xanthine oxidase inhibitors (XOIs)**
    - **Allopurinol is currently the preferred agent** for lowering uric acid levels in patients with arthritis and/or kidney involvement. It is especially useful in patients who overproduce uric acid and for tophaceous gout but is commonly used in uric acid underexcreters, who are the vast majority of gout patients.
    - It **decreases urate production** by inhibiting the final step of urate synthesis and thus decreases uric acid levels, facilitating tophus mobilization.
    - **Allopurinol may also precipitate acute attacks** when initiated or with dose changes; therefore, continue prophylactic colchicine or NSAIDs for 3 to 6 months after

achieving target serum uric acid level. More prolonged mobilization flare prophylaxis may be necessary in patients with tophi.

- The starting dose is 100 mg PO daily, with reduction to 50 mg daily for patients with stage 4 or higher chronic kidney disease (CKD). The dose is then titrated to goal uric acid level in 100 mg increments (or 50 mg increments in CKD) every 2 to 5 weeks.
- Allopurinol doses as high as 800 mg daily may be required to achieve serum uric acid goal.
- Allopurinol interacts with many medications, including amoxicillin, ampicillin, azathioprine, cyclosporine, mercaptopurine, and probenecid.
  □ The most common side effects of allopurinol are rash, diarrhea, nausea, and liver dysfunction. **If a rash develops, stop the allopurinol immediately.** The rash may herald a more severe but rare (<1 case per 1,000 patients treated) reaction especially in patients with renal insufficiency: exfoliative dermatitis, which can be accompanied by vasculitis, fever, hepatitis, eosinophilia, and acute interstitial nephritis. This **allopurinol hypersensitivity syndrome** carries up to a 25% mortality rate.[7]
  □ HLA-B*5801 screening should be considered in subpopulations (e.g., Koreans, Han Chinese, Thai, and possibly African Americans) prior to initiation of allopurinol because HLA-B*5801–positive subjects have a very high hazard ratio for severe allopurinol hypersensitivity reaction.
- ○ **Febuxostat** is another selective **inhibitor of xanthine oxidase.**
  - Febuxostat produces a dose-dependent decrease in serum urate levels. A daily dose of 40 mg produces a reduction that is roughly equivalent to that seen in patients who are treated with allopurinol 300 mg/day.[8] Febuxostat is started at 40 mg daily and can be increased to 80 mg daily if the goal uric acid is not achieved in 2 weeks on 40 mg.
  - It has high bioavailability, and less than 5% is excreted as unchanged drug in the urine. No dose reduction of febuxostat is recommended in CKD patients.
  - Febuxostat ULT is used for patients intolerant of other urate-lowering drugs and those in whom uric acid goals are not reached with other ULT.
  - Recent studies showed a trend toward greater frequency of adverse cardiovascular events and all-cause mortality in gout patients on febuxostat compared with those on allopurinol.[9]
- ○ Uricosuric agents
  - **Probenecid and lesinurad inhibit tubular reabsorption of urate.**
  - These agents are ineffective with renal impairment and are not recommended if the serum creatinine clearance is less than 50 mL/minute.
  - Uricosurics should not be used in patients with history of **uric acid kidney stones,** low urinary flow (<1 mL/minute), or baseline 24 hour urinary uric acid levels over 800 mg/24 hours.
  - Before initiating therapy, a 24-hour urine collection for creatinine and uric acid should be performed to determine whether the patient fits guidelines for use of uricosuric agents.
  - Probenecid is the first choice among uricosuric agents for ULT monotherapy.
  - Probenecid is started at 250 mg PO twice daily and titrated according to the serum urate concentration. The dose is typically raised every several weeks to a maintenance dose of 500 to 1,000 mg twice daily.
  - Lesinurad, an oral inhibitor of the urate-anion exchanger transporter 1 (URAT1), is used in combination with an XOI, in patients who have not reached goal uric acid level on xanthine oxidase inhibitor monotherapy.[10]
  - Patients on uricosurics should be advised to maintain a daily urine output >2 L to avoid precipitation of uric acid stones. To decrease this risk, alkalinizing agents

(potassium citrate) may be added. Alkalinization of urine with potassium citrate 10 mEq PO three times daily also helps reduce the risk of stones.

- Less potent uricosuric agents include the angiotensin 1 receptor antagonist losartan and the lipid-lowering agents atorvastatin and fenofibrate.
- Uricase
  - **Pegloticase** is a recombinant porcine PEGylated uricase developed for the treatment of refractory gout.
  - **Uricase** (urate oxidase) is the enzyme that catalyzes conversion of urate to the more soluble allantoin in most mammals, **but is absent in humans.**
  - Pegloticase is appropriate for patients with severe gout disease burden who are refractory to or are intolerant of standard ULT therapy.
  - Pegloticase is given as an intravenous infusion at a dose of 8 mg every 2 weeks.[11] Gout flare prophylaxis is recommended at least 1 week prior to the first infusion and continuing for at least 6 months. Side effects may include infusion reactions including anaphylaxis, development of low-titer antidrug antibodies, acute gout flares, nausea, and vomiting.
  - **Serum uric acid should be monitored prior to each infusion to confirm sustained urate-lowering efficacy** (serum urate <6 mg/dL) to ensure absence of the antibody formation toward pegloticase. **Pegloticase should be discontinued if serum uric acid level rises above 6 mg/dL.** Other ULT should not be prescribed while a patient is on pegloticase. Other ULT, however, is resumed if it is decided the patient will no longer receive pegloticase infusions.
  - **Pegloticase is contraindicated in glucose-6-phosphate dehydrogenase (G6PD) deficiency due to the risk of hemolysis and methemoglobinemia.**
- **Rasburicase** is used for the prevention of acute urate nephropathy from tumor lysis syndrome in patients with lymphoma and leukemia. However, it has not been well studied in gout, and rasburicase is thought to be more likely to cause anaphylaxis than the PEGylated drug.[12]

REFERENCES

1. Zhu Y, Pandya BJ, Choi HK. Prevalence of gout and hyperuricemia in the US general population: the National Health and Nutrition Examination Survey 2007–2008. *Arthritis Rheum.* 2011;63:3136–3141.
2. Mitroulis I, Kamba K, Ritis K. Neutrophils, IL-1β, and gout: is there a link? *Semin Immunopathol.* 2013; 35:501–512.
3. Neogi T, Jansen TL, Dalbeth N, et al. 2015 Gout Classification Criteria: an American College of Rheumatology/European League Against Rheumatism Collaborative Initiative. *Ann Rheum Dis.* 2015:74; 1789–1798.
4. Rheinboldt M, Scher C. Musculoskeletal ultrasonography in the diagnosis of acute crystalline synovitis. *Emerg Radiol.* 2016;23:623–632.
5. Terkeltaub RA, Furst DE, Bennett K, et al. High versus low dosing of oral colchicine for early acute gout flare: twenty-four-hour outcome of the first multicenter, randomized, double-blind, placebo-controlled, parallel-group, dose-comparison colchicine study. *Arthritis Rheum.* 2010;62:1060–1068.
6. Zhang W, Doherty M, Bardin T, et al. EULAR evidence based recommendations for gout. Part II: management. Report of a task force of the EULAR standing committee for international clinical studies including therapeutics (ESCISIT). *Ann Rheum Dis.* 2006;65:1312.
7. Gutiérrez-Macías A, Lizarralde-Palacios E, Martínez-Odriozola P, et al. Fatal allopurinol hypersensitivity syndrome after treatment of asymptomatic hyperuricaemia. *BMJ.* 2005;331:623–624.
8. Becker MA, Schumacher HR, Espinoza LR, et al. The urate-lowering efficacy and safety of febuxostat in the treatment of the hyperuricemia of gout: the CONFIRMS trial. *Arthritis Res Ther.* 2010;12:R63.
9. White WB, Saag KG, Becker MA, et al. Cardiovascular safety of febuxostat or allopurinol in patients with gout. *N Engl J Med.* 2018;378:1200–1210.

10. Bardin T, Keenan RT, Khanna PP, et al. Lesinurad in combination with allopurinol: a randomised, double-blind, placebo-controlled study in gout patients with inadequate response to standard of care (the multinational CLEAR 2 study). *Ann Rheum Dis*. 2016;76:811–820.

11. Sundy JS, Becker MA, Baraf HS, et al. Reduction of plasma urate levels following treatment with multiple doses of pegloticase (polyethylene glycol-conjugated uricase) in patients with treatment-failure gout: results of a phase II randomized study. *Arthritis Rheum*. 2008;58:2882–2891.

12. Richette P, Brière C, Hoenen-Clavert V, et al. Rasburicase for tophaceous gout not treatable with allopurinol: an exploratory study. *J Rheumatol*. 2007;34:2093–2098.

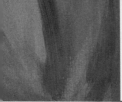

Calcium Pyrophosphate Dihydrate Crystal Deposition Disease

22

Michiko Inaba and Amy M. Joseph

GENERAL PRINCIPLES

Definition

- Calcium pyrophosphate deposition (CPPD) disease is characterized by an inflammatory reaction to calcium pyrophosphate (CPP) crystals in connective tissues.
- CPPD can affect ligaments, tendons, articular cartilage, and the synovium.
- It can have a clinical presentation that mimics other rheumatologic diseases such as gout, rheumatoid arthritis (RA), and osteoarthritis (OA).

Classification

- Asymptomatic CPPD
- OA with CPPD, previously referred to as "pseudo-OA," is seen in patients who have CPP crystals or chondrocalcinosis (CC) in joints affected by OA.
- Acute CPP crystal arthritis, formerly "pseudogout"
- Chronic CPP crystal inflammatory polyarthropathy, previously called "pseudo-RA"[1]

Epidemiology

- CPPD disease is primarily a **diagnosis of the elderly.**[2]
- **Radiographic evidence** of CPP deposition increases with age, reaching approximately 44% in those over age 84.[3]
- There is no male or female predominance overall, but some subclassifications have predilection toward females or males, as noted in this chapter.

Etiology

- The majority of cases of CPPD are **idiopathic.**
- Early onset CPPD disease is often related to the presence of risk factors or associated conditions.

Pathophysiology

- The pathologic formation of CPP crystals is believed to be secondary to **high levels of inorganic pyrophosphate** (PPi), which can precipitate with calcium to form crystals in the pericellular matrix of cartilage.
- Chondrocytes produce extracellular PPi, which combines with calcium ions to form CPP crystals in the extracellular matrix of cartilage. The crystals cause damage through inflammation mediated by the NALP3 inflammasome and by neutrophil extracellular traps, as well as through cartilage catabolism mediated by prostaglandins and matrix metalloproteinases, and by direct damage from crystal deposition in cartilage.[4]
- The crystal formation can be modulated by several factors including transforming growth factor beta (TGF-β), retinoic acid, nitric oxide, thyroid hormone, transglutaminase, and interleukin (IL)-1.

Risk Factors

- The largest risk factor for CPPD disease is age.
- **Joint trauma and/or surgery** have also been associated with an increased risk of developing CPPD disease.

Associated Conditions

- CC is frequently seen in joints affected by **OA**. Because both conditions frequently occur in the elderly, in some cases this may be concomitant presence of two commons diseases. However, given the fact that CPP crystals cause cartilage damage, in other cases the CPPD disease may be the cause of the OA in a particular joint.
- **Hypophosphatasia (low alkaline phosphatase activity)** is associated with CPPD disease because it results in increased PPi levels.
- **Hyperparathyroidism** is a risk factor for CPPD disease, presumably because of abnormal calcium metabolism.
- **Hemochromatosis** is associated with CPPD disease, especially the chronic inflammatory presentation affecting the second and third metacarpophalangeal joints (MCP) joints of the hands, possibly because iron inhibits degradation of pyrophosphates.
- **Hypomagnesemia** is also associated, which is why Gitelman syndrome is a risk factor for CPPD disease. Magnesium promotes CPP crystal solubility and is a cofactor for pyrophosphate degradation.[5,6]
- **Familial CPPD disease** has been linked in some affected families to mutations in the human homologue of the mouse progressive ankylosis (ANKH) gene. ANKH has been identified as a pyrophosphate regulator.
- CPPD disease has been reported to be associated with **bisphosphonates, joint injections of hyaluronate, loop diuretics, and parathyroidectomy.**[7–9]

Prevention

It has been hypothesized that an increase in dietary calcium could help in the prevention of CPPD.[10] However, there is currently no medication that reduces PPi levels to prevent CPPD disease, analogous to urate-lowering therapy in gout.

DIAGNOSIS

Clinical Presentation

- **Asymptomatic CPPD:** Patients who have CC, cartilage calcification, without CPPD disease are said to have asymptomatic CPPD.
- **CC** can be identified on radiographs of the wrist in the triangular fibrocartilage, the symphysis pubis, and the cartilage of the knee.
- Not all patients with CPPD disease have CC on x-ray, and not all patients with CC have CPPD disease.
- **Acute CPP crystal arthritis**
  - It manifests as severe **mono- or oligo-arthritis.**
  - Onset can be acute like gout, but can also be subacute, with more gradual onset than gout.
  - Acute CPPD arthritis is more likely than gout to affect upper extremity joints, especially involving the wrists, shoulders, and elbows.
  - Acute attacks can involve any joint but **most frequently affect the knee** (50% of cases).
  - It is more common in men.
  - Severe illness; joint trauma; surgery, especially parathyroidectomy and repair of hip fracture; or medications such as pamidronate and other bisphosphonates, and possibly loop diuretics and intra-articular hyaluronic acid may precipitate attacks.

- In addition to the acute warmth, swelling, and erythema of the joint and surrounding region, acute CPP crystal arthritis can be associated with fever, leukocytosis, and an increased erythrocyte sedimentation rate (ESR), resembling septic arthritis.
  - Unlike gout, acute attacks of CPP arthritis can last weeks to months.
- **OA with CPPD**
  - This presentation is more common in **women.**
  - It can present as **slowly progressive joint pain with cartilage damage affecting one or multiple joints.**
  - The patient's chronic disease course may be punctuated by acute attacks similar to gout.
  - **The knee is the most commonly affected joint,** but involvement of **joints that are not typically associated with OA** (e.g., wrists, shoulders, and ankles) is also frequently seen.
- **Chronic CPP crystal inflammatory arthritis**
  - This presentation affects less than 5% of patients with CPP crystal arthritis.
  - Chronic oligoarthritis or polyarthritis with superimposed flares of crystal inflammation is seen. Patients will typically present with **symmetric joint involvement and prominent systemic complaints** (e.g., morning stiffness and fatigue).
  - Involvement of the wrists along with the second and third MCP joints, resembling RA, is the most common presentation of arthritis associated with hereditary hemochromatosis.[11]
  - CPPD joints will exhibit **synovial thickening, local edema, flexion contractures, and decreased range of motion.**
- **"Pseudoneuropathic arthritis"**
  - Reports describe patients who present with a **severe destructive and painful monoarthritis,** which is not associated with neurologic abnormalities.
  - That is not included in European League Against Rheumatism (EULAR) 2011 terminology.
- **Spinal involvement**
  - CPP crystals can deposit in the intervertebral disks, facet joints, and ligaments of the spine.
  - The **crowned dens syndrome,** in which calcium deposits are seen on x-rays surrounding the odontoid process in the setting of intermittent neck pain, is caused by CPPD. Patients present with severe neck pain and stiffness, sometimes with jaw and shoulder pain, elevated ESR and C-reactive protein (CRP), and fever, mimicking polymyalgia rheumatica, giant cell arteritis, and even meningitis.[12]
  - **Cervical spine involvement** is believed to be an underrecognized etiology of acute neck pain.[13]
  - Cases of spinal cord compression secondary to CPP deposits have been reported, the majority in older women.

Diagnostic Criteria

- Diagnostic criteria for CPPD are presented in Table 22-1.[14]
- Definitive diagnosis of CPPD is by identification of CPP crystals in synovial fluid or biopsy tissue. Radiographic CC supports but does not confirm the diagnosis of CPPD, and its absence does not exclude it.[1]
  - CPP crystals can be rectangular, rhomboid-, or rod-shaped and of variable size.
  - They are weakly positively birefringent, that is, blue when parallel to the polarizer axis and yellow when perpendicular.

Differential Diagnosis

- Infection, RA, OA, neuropathic joint disease, trauma, other crystal-associated diseases (e.g., gout, basic calcium phosphate crystal deposition), and malignancy should be considered in the appropriate clinical setting.
- The presence of CPP crystals does not exclude the coexistence of the above diagnoses.

TABLE 22-1	DIAGNOSTIC CRITERIA FOR CALCIUM PYROPHOSPHATE DIHYDRATE DEPOSITION

Criteria

I Demonstration of CPPD crystals, obtained by biopsy, necropsy, or aspirated synovial fluid, by definite means (e.g., characteristic "fingerprint" by x-ray differentiation powder pattern or by chemical analysis).

IIa Identification of monoclinic or triclinic crystals showing a weak positive, or a lack of, birefringence by compensated polarized light microscopy.

IIb Presence of typical calcification on radiography.

IIIa Acute arthritis, especially the knee or other large joints.

IIIb Chronic arthritis, especially of knee, hip, wrist, carpus, elbow, shoulder, or metacarpophalangeal joint, particularly if accompanied by acute exacerbation; the chronic arthritis shows the following features helpful in differentiating it from OA.

1. Uncommon site of primary OA (e.g., wrist, metacarpophalangeal joints, elbow, or shoulder).
2. Radiographic appearance (e.g., radiocarpal or patellofemoral joint space narrowing, especially in isolation, femoral cortical erosion superior to the patella on the lateral view of the knee).
3. Subchondral cyst formation.
4. Severe progressive degeneration, with subchondral bony collapse (microfractures), and fragmentation of intra-articular radiodense body.
5. Variable and inconstant osteophyte formation.
6. Tendon calcification, especially of Achilles, triceps, and obturator tendons.
7. Involvement of axial skeleton and subchondral cyst of apophyseal and sacroiliac joints, multiple levels of disk calcification and vacuum phenomenon, and sacroiliac vacuum phenomenon.

Categories
Definitive: I OR IIa PLUS IIb
Probable: IIa OR IIb
Possible: IIIa OR IIIb

Diagnostic Testing

Laboratories
Screening for the metabolic diseases that are associated with CPPD arthritis, including hyperparathyroidism (calcium, phosphorous, PTH), hemochromatosis (iron, total iron-binding capacity, ferritin), hypophosphatasia (alkaline phosphatase), and hypomagnesemia, maybe appropriate after CPPD diagnosis, particularly in young patients or patients with severe arthritis.

Imaging
- Plain radiographs
  - **Chondrocalcinosis**
    - CC represents the accumulation of calcium salt in cartilaginous tissue, but can be found in the articular or periarticular regions. It can be seen on plain radiographs in the absence of an arthropathy.
    - It is classically seen on radiographs in fibrocartilage (knee menisci, triangular fibrocartilage of the wrist, symphysis pubis, glenohumeral joint) but may be seen in

hyaline and articular cartilage, as well as joint capsules and tendon insertion sites (Achilles, quadriceps).

- **Fibrocartilage calcifications** appear as shaggy and irregular radiodense areas that are typically in the center of the joint. **Hyaline cartilage calcifications** are seen as a parallel thin line in close proximity to the subchondral bone. **Synovial calcification** usually appears as an amorphous opacity in the joint margin. **Tendon calcifications** are thin and linear.
- **Radiographic calcification around the odontoid process is seen in the crowned dens syndrome.**
- **Hook-like osteophytes** can be seen. For example, they can be present on the metacarpal heads of MCP joints, especially in CPPD arthritis associated with hemochromatosis.
  - ○ Structural joint changes
    - CPPD arthritis can be associated with **subchondral sclerosis, subchondral cyst formation, and joint space narrowing.** Although the findings are also seen in OA, the location and the more fulminant course of CPPD arthritis may help differentiate the two diseases.
    - Unlike RA, CPPD **does not have typical bony erosions.**
- Ultrasound
  - ○ CPP crystals can be visualized as hyperechoic aggregates with a sparkling reflection.[15] Ultrasound can identify depositions in intra-articular cartilage, periarticular soft tissue, and tendons (close to the attachment).
  - ○ Ultrasonography has a sensitivity and specificity at least equal to that of plain radiography in identifying CPPD crystal calcifications.[16,17]
- Alternative imaging
  - ○ Calcifications can be visualized on computed tomography (CT), but it is not typically utilized in the assessment of an arthropathy. However, it is the preferred method of identifying calcium deposits in the upper cervical spine and craniovertebral junction in the crowned dens syndrome.
  - ○ Dual-energy computed tomography is currently a research tool and could play a role in knee and wrist CPPD.[18,19]
  - ○ Although MRI is often utilized to evaluate a painful joint, it can be difficult to visualize the calcifications of CPPD arthritis.

Diagnostic Procedures
- Arthrocentesis
  - ○ In an acute attack, the typical synovial **leukocytes** count is 15,000 to 30,000 cells/mm³, with a neutrophilic predominance.
  - ○ CPP crystals show **positive birefringence** that may vary in intensity (weak to none). They are smaller than urate crystals, frequently intracellular, vary in shape **from rods to rhomboids** (monoclinic or triclinic crystal structure) and are **usually more difficult to find** than urate crystals. In addition, they can be observed in the presence of urate crystals.
  - ○ CPP crystals can be visualized from joints aspirated between acute attacks.
  - ○ Even if crystals are seen, it is important to send synovial fluid for culture to **rule out coincident infection.**
- Paraffin-embedded tissue
  - ○ CPP crystals classically appear as amorphous basophilic to amphiphilic material that can be surrounded by foreign-body giant cell reaction.
  - ○ Nonaqueous alcoholic eosin staining allows for the observation of positive birefringence that may not be present on routine hematoxylin and eosin–stained slides.

TREATMENT

- 'Therapeutics are targeted at symptom control.[20]
- The basis for the majority of the treatment options comes from case reports and expert opinion.
- Treatment of associated conditions should be considered as appropriate, although it is not known whether this has a beneficial effect on the CPP arthritis.

Medications

- **Acute symptomatic treatment**
  - When no more than two joints are acutely inflamed and infection has been excluded, **intra-articular glucocorticoids** can be used.[20] Joint fluid aspiration and glucocorticoid injection usually provide relief within 8 to 24 hours.
  - **Nonsteroidal anti-inflammatory drugs (NSAIDs) in anti-inflammatory doses** are frequently utilized if they are tolerated and there are no contraindications.[20]
  - **Colchicine** is another option for acute cyclic citrullinated peptide (CCP) crystal arthritis in patients with normal renal and hepatic function but must be initiated early in the course of the attack. The recommended dose is no more than 1.8 mg in the first 24 hours, followed by 0.6 mg twice daily until symptoms improve or side effects develop.
  - **Oral glucocorticoids** are sometimes needed when NSAIDs and colchicine cannot be used but should be held until infection is excluded.
  - **Anakinra**, an IL-1 inhibitor, may also be utilized in acute attacks if no other options exist, at the dosage of 100 mg subcutaneously per day, or three times a week with hemodialysis treatment.[21,22] However, anakinra is not Food and Drug Administration (FDA) approved for this.
- **Treatment of chronic or recurrent symptoms**
  - Colchicine (0.6 mg daily or twice daily) may decrease the frequency of attacks.[23]
  - NSAIDs can be used in patients without contraindications, with proton-pump inhibitors for gastric protection in appropriate patients. This recommendation is based on data regarding management of gout and OA.[20]
  - Methotrexate (5–20 mg weekly) and hydroxychloroquine (200–400 mg daily) may be considered in resistant cases.[24-26] Although a recent study on methotrexate showed no effect on disease activity, it is possible that some individuals might benefit.[27]
  - Anakinra (100 mg SQ daily) has not been FDA approved for chronic CPP arthritis or for prevention of flares, but at least one case report supports its use.[28]

Nonpharmacologic Therapies

For acute CPP crystal arthritis, treatment should include ice or cool packs, temporary rest, and joint aspiration.

Surgical Management

- Surgical decompression is performed for CPPD causing compressive myelopathy.
- There are similar outcomes for knee and hip replacement in patients with CPPD disease as for those with OA.[29]

REFERENCES

1. Zhang W, Doherty M, Bardin T, et al. European League Against Rheumatism recommendations for calcium pyrophosphate deposition. Part I: terminology and diagnosis. *Ann Rheum Dis.* 2011;70(4):563–570.

2. Neame RL, Carr AJ, Muir K, et al. UK community prevalence of knee chondrocalcinosis: evidence that correlation with osteoarthritis is through a shared association with osteophyte. *Ann Rheum Dis.* 2003;62(6):513–518.

3. Wilkins ED, Dieppe PA, Maddison PE, et al. Osteoarthritis and articular chondrocalcinosis in the elderly. *Ann Rheum Dis.* 1983;42(3):280.

4. Rosenthal AK, Ryan LM. Calcium pyrophosphate deposition disease. *N Engl J Med.* 2016;374(26):2575–2584.

5. Kleiber Balderrama C, Rosenthal AK, Lans D, et al. Calcium pyrophosphate deposition disease and associated medical comorbidities: a National Cross-Sectional Study of US Veterans. *Arthritis Care Res.* 2017;69(9):1400–1406.

6. Richette P, Ayoub G, Lahalle S, et al. Hypomagnesemia associated with chondrocalcinosis: a cross-sectional study. *Arthritis Rheum.* 2007;57:1496–1501.

7. Doshi J, Wheatley H. Pseudogout: an unusual and forgotten metabolic sequela of parathyroidectomy. *Head Neck.* 2008;30:1650–1653.

8. Ali Y, Weinstein M, Jokl P. Acute pseudogout following intra-articular injection of high molecular weight hyaluronic acid. *Am J Med.* 1999;107:641–642.

9. Young-Min SA, Herbert L, Dick M, et al. Weekly alendronate-induced acute pseudogout. *Rheumatology.* 2005;44:131–132.

10. Zhang Y, Terkeltaub R, Nevitt M, et al. Lower prevalence of chondrocalcinosis in Chinese subjects in Beijing than in white subjects in the United States: The Beijing Osteoarthritis Study. *Arthritis Rheum.* 2006;54:3508–3512.

11. Dejaco C, Stadlmayr A, Duftner C, et al. Ultrasound verified inflammation and structural damage in patients with hereditary haemochromatosis-related arthropathy. *Arthritis Res Ther.* 2017;19(1):243.

12. Salaffi F, Carotti M, Guglielmi G, et al. The crowned dens syndrome as a cause of neck pain: clinical and computed tomography study in patients with calcium pyrophosphate dihydrate deposition disease. *Clin Exp Rheumatol.* 2008;26:1040–1046.

13. Sekijima Y, Yoshida T, Ikeda S. CPPD crystal deposition disease of the cervical spine: a common cause of acute neck pain encountered in the neurology department. *J Neurol Sci.* 2010;296:79–82.

14. Rosenthal AK, Ryan L. Calcium pyrophosphate crystal disease, pseudogout, and articular chondrocalcinosis. In: Koopman WJ, Moreland LW, eds. *Arthritis and Allied Conditions.* 15th ed. Philadelphia, PA: Lippincott Williams & Wilkins; 2005:2397–2416.

15. O'Neill J. Crystal related disease. In: O'Neill J, eds. *Essential Imaging in Rheumatology.* 1st ed. New York, NY: Springer; 2015:213–232.

16. Frediani B, Filippou G, Falsetti P, et al. Diagnosis of calcium pyrophosphate dihydrate crystal deposition disease: ultrasonographic criteria proposed. *Ann Rheum Dis.* 2005;64(4):638–640.

17. Zufferey P, Valcov R, Fabreguet I, et al. A prospective evaluation of ultrasound as a diagnostic tool in acute microcrystalline arthritis. *Arthritis Res Ther.* 2015;17(1):188.

18. Tanikawa H, Ogawa R, Okuma K, et al. Detection of calcium pyrophosphate dihydrate crystals in knee meniscus by dual-energy computed tomography. *J Orthop Surg Res.* 2018;13(1):73.

19. Ward IM, Scott JN, Mansfield LT, et al. Dual-energy computed tomography demonstrating destructive calcium pyrophosphate deposition disease of the distal radioulnar joint mimicking tophaceous gout. *J Clin Rheumatol.* 2015;21(6):314–317.

20. Zhang W, Doherty M, Pascual E, et al. EULAR recommendations for calcium pyrophosphate deposition. Part II: management. *Ann Rheum Dis.* 2011;70(4):571–575.

21. Announ N, Palmer G, Guerne PA, et al. Anakinra is a possible alternative in the treatment and prevention of acute attacks of pseudogout in end-stage renal failure. *Joint Bone Spine.* 2009;76(4):424–426.

22. McGonagle D, Tan AL, Madden J, et al. Successful treatment of resistant pseudogout with anakinra. *Arthritis Rheum.* 2008;58:631–633.

23. Das SK, Mishra K, Ramakrishnan S, et al. A randomized controlled trial to evaluate the slow-acting symptom modifying effects of a regimen containing colchicine in a subset of patients with osteoarthritis of the knee. *Osteoarthritis Cartilage.* 2002;10(4):247–252.

24. Chollet-Janin A, Finckh A, Dudler J, et al. Methotrexate as an alternative therapy for chronic calcium pyrophosphate deposition disease: An exploratory analysis. *Arthritis Rheum.* 2007;56:688–692.

25. Andres M, Sivera F, Pascual E. Methotrexate is an option for patients with refractory calcium pyrophosphate crystal arthritis. *J Clin Rheumatol.* 2012;18(5):234–236.

26. Rothschild B, Yakubov LE. Prospective 6-month, double-blind trial of hydroxychloroquine treatment of CPDD. *Compr Ther.* 1997;23:327–331.

27. Finckh A, Mc Carthy GM, Madigan A, et al. Methotrexate in chronic-recurrent calcium pyrophosphate deposition disease: no significant effect in a randomized crossover trial. *Arthritis Res Ther.* 2014;16(5):458.

28. Diamantopoulos AP, Brodin C, Hetland H, et al. Interleukin 1β blockade improves signs and symptoms of chronic calcium pyrophosphate crystal arthritis resistant to treatment. *J Clin Rheumatol.* 2012;18(6):310–311.

29. Kumar V, Pandit HG, Liddle AD, et al. Comparison of outcomes after UKA in patients with and without chondrocalcinosis: a matched cohort study. *Knee Surg Sports Traumatol Arthrosc.* 2017;25(1):319–324.

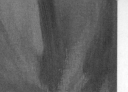

Basic Calcium Phosphate and Calcium Oxalate Crystal Associated Arthritis

Jaime Flores-Ruiz and Amy M. Joseph

23

Besides monosodium urate and calcium pyrophosphate (CPP) crystals, other crystals can be found in the synovial fluid of patients with arthritis. These include **basic calcium phosphate (BCP) crystals** and **calcium oxalate crystals.**

BASIC CALCIUM PHOSPHATE DEPOSITION DISEASE

GENERAL PRINCIPLES

Definition

- **BCP deposition disease** is characterized by an inflammatory reaction to BCP crystals in articular and periarticular connective tissues.
- Articular BCP crystal deposition is associated with osteoarthritis (OA) and destructive arthropathies that can be severe, whereas periarticular deposition is associated with self-limiting acute attacks lasting for several months.

Classification

BCP-associated musculoskeletal syndromes can be organized into **arthritis associated with BCP crystals** and **calcific periarthritis.**[1]

- Arthritis associated with BCP crystals includes OA with BCP crystals and destructive BCP crystal arthritis such as the Milwaukee shoulder syndrome.
- Calcific periarthritis is characterized by pain in the setting of deposition of crystals in tendons, bursae, and other soft tissues around joints.

Epidemiology

- OA with BCP crystals and destructive BCP crystal arthritis are associated with increasing age and occur predominantly in older women.[2,3]
- The prevalence of BCP crystals in synovial fluid in patients with knee OA is between 30% and 60%.[4] Importantly, studies have shown that BCP crystals are found in 100% of cartilage samples from patients with end-stage OA undergoing knee or hip replacement.[5,6]
- Calcific periarthritis affects all ages, but it is more common in middle-aged women.[7]

Etiology

- The etiology is unknown.
- BCP crystal formation appears to occur where joints or periarticular structures have been damaged by injury or inflammation.
- BCP crystals include carbonate-substituted hydroxyapatite, octacalcium phosphate, and tricalcium phosphate.

Pathophysiology

- The pathogenesis of BCP crystal formation is not well understood.
- Once the crystals have formed, they are thought to produce symptoms via three pathogenic mechanisms.[8,9]
  - BCP crystals can trigger an inflammatory cascade, possibly through innate immunity similar to the inflammation associated with gout and calcium pyrophosphate dihydrate (CPPD) arthropathy.
  - The crystals themselves can disrupt the mechanical function of the tissues in which they are deposited.
  - Crystals can trigger local cells to produce cytokines and other mediators that cause local damage in the absence of inflammation.

Risk Factors

- Trauma, overuse, and age have been associated with increased risk.
- Metabolic factors that increase calcium or phosphate levels predispose to BCP disease. Hypophosphatasia (low alkaline phosphatase activity), for example, causes hyperphosphatemia, which can be associated with calcific periarthritis.

Associated Conditions

- Articular BCP crystal deposition is more common in patients with severe **OA**. In patient with knee OA, BCP crystals are associated with more severe radiologic joint degeneration and larger joint effusions compared to joints without BCP crystals.[4]
- BCP crystal often coexist with **CPP crystals** in synovial fluid. This has been seen in patients with knee OA and Milwaukee shoulder syndrome.[3,10,11]

DIAGNOSIS

Clinical Presentation

- **BCP crystal arthritis**
  - BCP crystal arthropathy can range in severity from mild OA to destructive arthritis as exemplified by the Milwaukee shoulder syndrome, although this severe arthritis can also occur in the knees, hips, elbows, and ankles.[12]
  - The likelihood of a joint affected by OA containing BCP crystals increases as the severity of the OA increases.
  - Common symptoms of OA with BCP crystal arthropathy include **pain and subacute or chronic swelling without warmth** in one or more large joints. The **pain is worse with activity** and is not associated with prolonged morning stiffness.
  - The **Milwaukee shoulder syndrome** is the prototype of severe, destructive arthritis associated with BCP crystals, which can also occur in the knees, hips, ankles, and other joints.[13]
    - It occurs predominantly in elderly women (80%).
    - The dominant shoulder is usually affected, but it is often bilateral.
    - It typically presents as **insidious** shoulder pain and loss of function **over months or years,** with acute worsening of pain and large, often hemorrhagic, **glenohumeral joint effusions.**[14]
- **Calcific periarthritis**
  - The typical presentation is **acute onset of pain around a single joint lasting days to weeks.** There is pain at rest, worsened by movement.
  - The affected joint is sometimes warm, red, or swollen but without effusion.
  - The **shoulder is the most commonly affected joint,** especially in the **supraspinatus tendon,** but calcific periarthritis can occur around other joints and tendon insertion sites, **including the hand, foot, and spine.**

- ○ BCP podagra ("pseudo-pseudogout") can occur in young women.[15,16]
- ○ It is not known what triggers an acute attack.
- ○ Patients are most often in their 30s and 40s, but calcific periarthritis can occur at any age. Women are twice as likely as men to be affected.

Diagnostic Criteria

The diagnosis of BCP crystal–associated arthritis and calcific periarthritis is based on **clinical presentation and plain radiography.**
- • **Arthrocentesis** can be helpful in **BCP crystal–associated arthritis to exclude inflammation and other crystals as the cause.**
- • The presence of periarticular calcifications on plain radiographs of symptomatic areas confirms the diagnosis of calcific periarthritis in a patient whose history and examination are consistent with this diagnosis.[13]

Differential Diagnosis

- • Septic arthritis, rheumatoid arthritis, OA, neuropathic joint disease, trauma, other crystal-associated arthritis (e.g., gout, CPPD disease), rotator cuff arthropathy, malignancy, and hemochromatosis should be considered in the appropriate clinical setting.
- • The presence of BCP crystals does not exclude the coexistence of these diagnoses.

Diagnostic Testing

Laboratories
Erythrocyte sedimentation rate and C-reactive protein may be elevated in some patients with calcific periarthritis.

Imaging
- • Plain radiographs
  - ○ **BCP crystal arthritis:** Radiographic features of **BCP crystal arthritis are the same as those seen in OA**—joint space narrowing, subchondral sclerosis, subchondral cyst formation, altered bone contour, periarticular calcification, and soft-tissue swelling.
  - ○ **Milwaukee shoulder syndrome:** Radiographic features include **glenohumeral joint degeneration with sclerosis of the humeral head and sometimes erosions, soft-tissue calcification, upward subluxation reflecting rotator cuff tear, and soft-tissue swelling.**[13]
  - ○ **Calcific periarthritis**
    - ▪ This is identified on radiography as **localized periarticular calcification** overlying the tendons or bursae.[17]
    - ▪ Radiographically, the periarticular calcification usually resolves or markedly decreases within 2 to 3 weeks after the acute onset.[18]
- • Ultrasound
  - ○ Ultrasound can reveal effusions and tissue destruction in arthritis associated with BCP crystals.
  - ○ In calcific periarthritis, ultrasound demonstrates hyperechoic foci within the tendon, usually close to the tendon insertion. Ultrasound can also identify bursitis.[17]
- • Alternative imaging
  - ○ Calcifications can be visualized on a computed tomography scan, but it is not typically utilized in the assessment of BCP arthropathy.
  - ○ Although magnetic resonance imaging (MRI) is often utilized to evaluate a painful joint, it does not show calcium deposits well.[17] But in Milwaukee shoulder syndrome, MRI can demonstrate effusions, rotator cuff tears, glenohumeral joint narrowing, and subchondral bone destruction.[19,20]

Diagnostic Procedures

Arthrocentesis is the diagnostic procedure.

- **Synovial fluid analysis is important in the diagnosis of BCP crystal–associated arthritis.**
- The typical synovial leukocyte count is less than 1,000 cells/mm^3, with mononuclear cell predominance. Synovial fluid is often blood-tinged or hemorrhagic.
- **Polarized light microscopy is done to exclude monosodium urate and CPP crystals.** The BCP crystal size is below the limits of resolution of optic microscopy.[13]
- **Alizarin red S staining** of synovial fluid demonstrates **calcium-containing crystals** on light microcopy, but this is not universally available. The staining **does not discriminate between BCP and CPP crystals.**[21,22]
- High-resolution transmission electron microcopy (TEM), scanning electron microcopy (SEM), and Fourier-transform infrared spectroscopy (FTIR) are useful research tools but are not available for clinical use.[13]

TREATMENT

Treatment is targeted at symptom control.

Medications

- **OA with BCP crystals** is treated like OA without BCP, with acetaminophen, nonsteroidal anti-inflammatory drugs (NSAIDs), intra-articular glucocorticoids, and physical therapy (PT).
- **Milwaukee shoulder syndrome and other destructive BCP arthropathies**
  - There are no randomized, controlled trials of treatment for Milwaukee shoulder syndrome.
  - Analgesia with acetaminophen or NSAIDs is first-line therapy for Milwaukee shoulder syndrome.
  - Joint aspiration with glucocorticoid injection is beneficial for some patients.
- **Calcific periarthritis**
  - Usually, acute episodes are self-limiting. The goal is to decrease pain and inflammation and clear calcium deposits.[23]
  - Current treatment approaches include NSAIDs and intralesional glucocorticoids.[16]
  - A 3-day course of the IL-1 beta inhibitor anakinra was shown in a small open-label series to help patients refractory to standard treatment.[24]

Nonpharmacologic Therapies

- Patients who have OA with BCP crystal arthritis and Milwaukee shoulder syndrome benefit from PT, supervised exercise programs, and, if overweight, weight loss.
- Tidal irrigation followed by injection of intra-articular glucocorticoids and tranexamic acid could be considered in patients with Milwaukee shoulder syndrome refractory to medical treatment.[25]
- For acute calcific periarthritis, several nonpharmacologic modalities are recommended.
  - Heat, cold packs, and rest or immobilization can make patients more comfortable.
  - Barbotage, which is the needling of calcific lesions to help clear them, has been shown to be beneficial.
  - High-energy extracorporeal shock wave therapy can be used to help clear calcifications.[26]

Surgical Management

- Total joint arthroplasty provides symptomatic and functional improvement in patients with severe BCP arthritis.[13]
- Surgical removal of periarticular calcium deposits may be necessary in patients with refractory calcific periarthritis.

CALCIUM OXALATE CRYSTAL ARTHROPATHY

GENERAL PRINCIPLES

Definition

- Oxalate arthropathy is a rare crystal arthropathy seen in the setting of primary or secondary hyperoxaluria, a systemic condition characterized by high calcium oxalate levels resulting in deposition of calcium oxalate crystals in organs.
- Excess oxalate is renally cleared, which leads to kidney damage from oxalate crystals that precipitate in the kidneys. Progression of oxalate-induced kidney failure leads to even higher oxalate levels in the body.
- Calcium oxalate crystals deposit within bones, tendons, cartilage, and synovium, leading to oxalate arthropathy.
- Oxalate arthritis can be clinically indistinguishable from arthropathies caused by other crystals, such as uric acid, CPP, and BCP crystals.[27]
- Musculoskeletal manifestations include calcium oxalate osteopathy, acute and chronic arthropathy with chondrocalcinosis, synovial calcification, and bursitis.
- Extra-articular calcium oxalate crystal deposition causes cardiomyopathy, arrhythmias, valvulopathy, vascular calcifications leading to livedo reticularis and acrocyanosis, retinal deposits, neuropathy, myopathy, anemia, and skin calcification.[27]
- This section will focus on articular calcium oxalate in patients with hyperoxaluria.

Epidemiology

Calcium oxalate crystal deposition disease is seen in patients with primary and secondary hyperoxaluria.[28,29]

Etiology

- **Primary hyperoxaluria** (PH) is a consequence of one of several genetic disorders of oxalate metabolism.
- **Secondary hyperoxaluria**
  - Secondary hyperoxaluria occurs primarily in the setting of conditions of fat malabsorption, such as celiac disease, inflammatory bowel disease, short bowel syndrome, or chronic pancreatitis. Orlistat can also cause hyperoxaluria because of fat malabsorption.[30]
  - It can also occur with a large oxalate load, such as with ethylene glycol poisoning.[31]
  - Patients with end-stage renal disease on chronic dialysis can develop oxalate crystal deposition disease in rare instances. Increased intake of oxalate-rich foods or oxalate precursors, in the setting of decreased renal oxalate clearance, can also lead to hyperoxalemia.[32]

DIAGNOSIS

Clinical Presentation

- Patients often have a history of recurrent urolithiasis due to oxalate crystals.
- **Musculoskeletal manifestations of oxalate include arthritis, chondrocalcinosis, tenosynovitis, bursitis, and spinal stenosis.**
  - Oxalate arthritis is a rare form of arthritis.
  - Calcium oxalate crystals form in the joint space, triggering inflammatory arthritis that is very similar to other types of crystalline arthritis.
  - Metacarpophalangeal and proximal interphalangeal joints of the hands, elbows, knees, and ankles are frequently involved, often in a symmetrical pattern.[27]

- Patients with oxalate arthritis should be tested for underlying causes of oxalate excess, unless they are already known to have one.

Diagnostic Testing

Laboratories
- Synovial fluid analysis typically reveals calcium oxalate crystals, which are characteristically envelope-shaped, but they can sometimes be rod-shaped and positively birefringent, making them difficult to distinguish from CPP crystals.
- Calcium oxalate crystals stain with Alizarin red because of their calcium content, as do other calcium-containing crystals such as BCP crystals.

Imaging
Periarticular calcification and calcification of tendons and soft tissues can be seen on plain radiographs.

TREATMENT

- **Treatment of oxalate arthritis** is similar to treatment of other types of crystalline arthritis, with **colchicine, NSAIDs, and intra-articular glucocorticoids.** However, most patients have concomitant kidney failure, so colchicine and NSAIDs will be contraindicated.
- Treatment of the underlying disease process if possible, to reduce calcium oxalate levels, is the most important approach to treatment of the arthritis.
  - Hydration by intake of 3 L of fluid daily is helpful.
  - Inhibition of crystal formation with citrate, phosphorus, and magnesium can also help.
  - For patients with high oxalate from fat malabsorption, calcium supplements with meals can reduce oxalate absorption.
  - Patients with PH benefit from kidney transplant (PH2 and some PH1) or from combined liver–kidney transplant (PH1).

REFERENCES

1. Rosenthal AK. Basic calcium phosphate crystal-associated musculoskeletal syndromes: an update. *Curr Opin Rheumatol.* 2018;30(2):168–172.
2. Abhishek A, Doherty M. Epidemiology of calcium pyrophosphate crystal arthritis and basic calcium phosphate crystal arthropathy. *Rheum Dis Clin North Am.* 2014;40(2):177–191.
3. Halverson PB, Carrera GF, McCarty DJ. Milwaukee shoulder syndrome: fifteen additional cases and a description of contributing factors. *Arch Intern Med.* 1990;150(3):677–682.
4. Nalbant S, Martinez JA, Kitumnuaypong T, et al. Synovial fluid features and their relations to osteoarthritis severity: new findings from sequential studies. *Osteoarthritis Cartilage.* 2003;11(1):50–54.
5. Fuerst M, Bertrand J, Lammers L, et al. Calcification of articular cartilage in human osteoarthritis. *Arthritis Rheum.* 2009;60(9):2694–2703.
6. Fuerst M, Niggemeyer O, Lammers L, et al. Articular cartilage mineralization in osteoarthritis of the hip. *BMC Musculoskelet Disord.* 2009;10(1):166.
7. Louwerens JK, Sierevelt IN, van Hove RP, et al. Prevalence of calcific deposits within the rotator cuff tendons in adults with and without subacromial pain syndrome: clinical and radiologic analysis of 1219 patients. *J Shoulder Elbow Surgery.* 2015;24(10):1588–1593.
8. McCarthy GM, Dunne A. Calcium crystal deposition diseases—beyond gout. *Nat Rev Rheumatol.* 2018;14(10):592–602.
9. Stack J, McCarthy G. Basic calcium phosphate crystals and osteoarthritis pathogenesis: novel pathways and potential targets. *Curr Opin Rheumatol.* 2016;28(2):122–126.
10. Derfus BA, Kurian JB, Butler JJ, et al. The high prevalence of pathologic calcium crystals in pre-operative knees. *J Rheumatol.* 2002;29(3):570–574.
11. Halverson PB, McCarty DJ. Patterns of radiographic abnormalities associated with basic calcium phosphate and calcium pyrophosphate dihydrate crystal deposition in the knee. *Ann Rheum Dis.* 1986;45(7):603.

12. Dieppe PA, Doherty M, Macfarlane DG, et al. Apatite associated destructive arthritis. *Br J Rheumatol.* 1984;23(2):84–91.
13. Halvernes PB. Basic calcium phosphate crystal deposit disease and calcinosis. In: Koopman WJ, Moreland LW, eds. *Arthritis and Allied Conditions.* 15th ed. Philadelphia, PA: Lippincott Williams & Wilkins; 2005:2397–2416.
14. Campion GV, McCrae F, Alwan W, et al. Idiopathic destructive arthritis of the shoulder. *Semin Arthritis Rheum.* 1988;17(4):232–245.
15. Fam AG, Rubenstein J. Hydroxyapatite pseudopodagra: a syndrome of young women. *Arthritis Rheum.* 1989;32(6):741–747.
16. Hurt G, Baker CL. Calcific tendinitis of the shoulder. *Orthopedic Clin.* 2003;34(4):567–575.
17. O'Neill J. Crystal related disease. In: O'Neill J, eds. *Essential Imaging in Rheumatology.* 1st ed. New York, NY: Springer; 2015:213–232.
18. Doumas C, Vazirani RM, Clifford PD, et al. Acute calcific periarthritis of the hand and wrist: a series and review of the literature. *Emergency Radiol.* 2007;14(4):199–203.
19. Dewachter L, Aerts P, Crevits I, et al. Milwaukee shoulder syndrome. *JBR-BTR.* 2012;95(4):243–244.
20. Ersoy H, Pomeranz SJ. Milwaukee shoulder syndrome. *J Surg Orthop Adv.* 2017;26(1):54–57.
21. Paul H, Reginato AJ, Schumacher HR. Alizarin red S staining as a screening test to detect calcium compounds in synovial fluid. *Arthritis Rheum.* 1983;26(2):191–200.
22. Gordon C, Swan A, Dieppe P. Detection of crystals in synovial fluids by light microscopy: sensitivity and reliability. *Ann Rheum Dis.* 1989;48(9):737.
23. Rosenthal AK, Ryan LM. Nonpharmacologic and pharmacologic management of CPP crystal arthritis and BCP arthropathy and periarticular syndromes. *Rheum Dis Clin North Am.* 2014;40(2):343–356.
24. Zufferey P, So A. A pilot study of IL-1 inhibition in acute calcific periarthritis of the shoulder. *Ann Rheum Dis.* 2013;72(3):465.
25. Epis O, Caporali R, Scirè CA, et al. Efficacy of tidal irrigation in Milwaukee shoulder syndrome. *J Rheumatol.* 2007;34(7):1545–1550.
26. Louwerens JK, Veltman ES, van Noort A, et al. The effectiveness of high-energy extracorporeal shock-wave therapy versus ultrasound-guided needling versus arthroscopic surgery in the management of chronic calcific rotator cuff tendinopathy: a systematic review. *Arthroscopy.* 2016;32(1):165–175.
27. Lorenz EC, Michet CJ, Milliner DS, et al. Update on oxalate crystal disease. *Curr Rheumatol Rep.* 2013;15(7):340.
28. Watts RW. The clinical spectrum of the primary hyperoxalurias and their treatment. *J Nephrol.* 1998;11:4–7.
29. Hoffman GS, Schumacher HR, Paul H, et al. Calcium oxalate microcrystalline-associated arthritis in end-stage renal disease. *Ann Intern Med.* 1982;97(1):36–42.
30. Humayun Y, Ball KC, Lewin JR, et al. Acute oxalate nephropathy associated with orlistat. *J Nephropathol.* 2016;5(2):79–83.
31. Coqui JA, Reginato AJ. Calcium oxalate and or particular associated with arthritis. In: Koopman WJ, Moreland LW, eds. *Arthritis and Allied Conditions.* 15th ed. Philadelphia, PA: Lippincott Williams & Wilkins; 2005:2417–2438.
32. Maldonado I, Prasad V, Reginato AJ. Oxalate crystal deposition disease. *Curr Rheumatol Rep.* 2002;4:257.

V Vasculitides

Approach to Vasculitis

24

Anneliese M. Flynn and Jonathan J. Miner

GENERAL PRINCIPLES

- Vasculitis is **inflammation of the vessel wall.** It is an uncommon manifestation of a wide variety of autoimmune, infectious, malignant, and iatrogenic conditions.
- It is characterized by nonspecific signs and symptoms due to systemic inflammatory disease, but specific signs and symptoms depend on which vessels are involved.
- Damage to tissues occurs via ischemia or infarction secondary to a reduction in perfusion to tissue distal to the vasculitic lesion.
- The severity of symptoms ranges from a self-limited rash to life-threatening disease.

Definition

- Vasculitis is defined as inflammatory infiltration of vessel walls with damage to mural structures.
- **Vasculitis is a pathologic finding, not a diagnosis.** Efforts must be made to determine the cause.

Classification

Vasculitis can be divided into primary or secondary, on the basis of etiologies.

- **Primary vasculitis**
  - This typically refers to autoimmune causes.
  - Several classification schemes exist, but the most commonly used scheme was derived from the 1993 Chapel Hill Consensus Conference presented in Table 24-1.[1]
  - The Chapel Hill Consensus stratified the vasculitides by the size of vessel affected:
    - Large
    - Medium
    - Small
    - Often, a vasculitis will affect vessels of more than one size. These are classified on the basis of the size of the vessel the condition *primarily* affects.
  - Large-vessel vasculitides
    - Takayasu's arteritis (see Chapter 21)
      - **Granulomatous inflammation** affects primarily the **aorta and its main branches** and may involve all or just a portion of these vessels.
      - Separate classification criteria exist to aid diagnosis. Typically, this occurs in **young women from Far East Asia** (Japan) with pulseless disease in the upper extremities.
    - Giant cell arteritis (see Chapter 22)
      - **Granulomatous arteritis** occurs primarily in the **cranial branches of arteries arising from the aortic arch,** also affecting medium-sized vessels. Classically involves the **temporal artery.**
      - Associated with **polymyalgia rheumatica**
      - Separate classification criteria exist to aid diagnosis. Usually seen in patients **>50 years old, erythrocyte sedimentation rate (ESR) >50,** and is associated with headache and less commonly jaw or tongue claudication.
  - Medium-vessel vasculitides

TABLE 24-1	CLASSIFICATION OF VASCULITIS

Large vessel

Takayasu's arteritis
Giant cell arteritis

Medium vessel

Polyarteritis nodosa
Kawasaki disease
Primary angiitis of the central nervous system

Small vessel

Immune complex related
Hypersensitivity vasculitis[a]
Henoch–Schönlein purpura
Cryoglobulinemic vasculitis[b]
Connective tissue disease–associated vasculitis[c]

Pauci-immune
Granulomatosis with polyangiitis
Eosinophilic Granulomatous with Polyangiitis
Microscopic polyangiitis

---

[a]Most often caused by medications, infections, and malignancies.

[b]Most often associated with hepatitis B and C, Epstein–Barr virus, plasma cell dyscrasias, chronic inflammatory/autoimmune disorders, and lymphoproliferative malignancies.

[c]Most often associated with rheumatoid arthritis, systemic lupus erythematosus, and Sjögren's syndrome.

ANCA, antineutrophil cytoplasmic antibody.

Adapted from: Jennette JC, Falk RJ, Andrassy K, et al. Nomenclature of systemic vasculitides. Proposal of an international consensus conference. *Arthritis Rheum.* 1994;37:187–192.

- **Polyarteritis nodosa (PAN; see Chapter 23)**
  □ A **necrotizing systemic vasculitis** affecting both medium and **small muscular arteries,** without glomerulonephritis or vasculitis of the arterioles, capillaries, or venules
  □ Separate classification criteria exist to aid diagnosis. Although accounting for <10% of cases due to increased vaccination against hepatitis B, PAN is typically associated with hepatitis B. Clinically, **skin nodules, mononeuritis multiplex, orchitis, and mesenteric artery involvement are most common.**
- **Kawasaki disease**
  □ Primarily a medium-vessel vasculitis but can affect large and small vessels
  □ Separate classification criteria exist to aid diagnosis. Mostly seen in **children.** Predilection for **coronary arteries.** Occasionally associated with a **mucocutaneous lymph node syndrome**
- **Primary angiitis of the central nervous system:** a rare granulomatous vasculitis isolated to the medium and small arteries in the leptomeninges
- Small-vessel vasculitides: The small-vessel vasculitides are further **subdivided based on the presence or absence of immunoglobulins within the vessels.**
- **Presence of immune complexes in vessels** (immune complex related)

- **Henoch–Schönlein purpura (HSP,** see Chapter 27)
  - □ **Systemic** vasculitis where **IgA-containing immune complexes** deposit within tissues, such as the renal glomerulus, skin, and gut
  - □ Most common form of systemic vasculitis in children
  - □ Associated with arthralgias or arthritis, myalgias, and subcutaneous edema
  - □ Post-capillary venules are most affected.
- **Cryoglobulinemic vasculitis** (see Chapter 28)
  - □ Characterized by the presence of **cryoglobulins,** serum proteins that precipitate in the cold
  - □ Associated with **hepatitis B and C infection. Skin** (extremities) and **glomeruli** often involved
  - □ Affects arterioles, capillaries, and venules
- **Connective tissue disease–associated vasculitis**
  - □ Seen in small muscular arteries, arterioles, and venules
  - □ Typically associated with rheumatoid arthritis (see Chapter 10), systemic lupus erythematosus (SLE; see Chapter 12), and Sjögren's syndrome (see Chapter 37)
  - □ Behçet's syndrome (see Chapter 31), relapsing polychondritis (see Chapter 43), and inflammatory bowel disease also may present with a vasculitis in a similar vessel distribution to connective tissue diseases.
- ○ **Absence of immune complexes in vessels** (pauci-immune); these conditions are usually associated with antineutrophil cytoplasmic antibodies (ANCAs).
  - **Granulomatosis with polyangiitis,** also known as ANCA-associated granulomatous vasculitis (see Chapter 24)
    - □ Systemic vasculitis affecting small and medium arteries, along with arterioles and venules
    - □ **Lower respiratory tract chronic granulomatous vasculitic inflammation** is characteristic. Upper airways have chronic inflammation but typically without granulomatous inflammation.
    - □ Typically, patients start with sinus and upper airway symptoms, then symptoms of lower airway and kidney disease.
    - □ **Necrotizing, pauci-immune glomerulonephritis** seen in the kidneys
    - □ Associated with **anti-proteinase 3 (anti-PR3) antibody,** with a **cytoplasmic ANCA (c-ANCA)** staining pattern
  - **Eosinophilic Granulomatous with Polyangiitis** (see Chapter 25)
    - □ Also known as allergic granulomatosis and angiitis
    - □ Affects medium-size vessels
    - □ Classically affects **lung and skin arteries** but can be systemic
    - □ **Extravascular granulomatosis** is characteristic
    - □ Associated in approximately 50% of cases with **anti-myeloperoxidase (anti-MPO)** antibodies, yielding a **perinuclear ANCA (p-ANCA)** staining pattern
    - □ Separate classification criteria exist to aid diagnosis. Classic presentation is **older person with new onset, relatively refractory, and progressive asthma with eosinophilia.**
  - **Microscopic polyangiitis** (see Chapter 26)
    - □ Systemic vasculitis similar to granulomatosis with polyangiitis with the exception of absence of upper airway involvement, granulomatous inflammation, and serologic specificity
    - □ Associated with **anti-MPO** antibodies, yielding a positive p-**ANCA**
- **Secondary vasculitis**
  - ○ Usually refers to nonautoimmune causes of vasculitis
  - ○ **Medications, infections, and malignancies are the most common etiologies for secondary vasculitis.**

- ○ **Medications** typically cause hypersensitivity vasculitis manifested by skin involvement, specifically **leukocytoclastic vasculitis** (see Chapter 29). Separate classification criteria exist to aid diagnosis of hypersensitivity vasculitis.
- ○ **Viruses** associated with medium- and small-vessel vasculitis include hepatitis B, human immunodeficiency virus, cytomegalovirus, Epstein–Barr virus, and parvovirus B19.
  - ▪ Viral vasculitides often present similarly to PAN or microscopic polyangiitis.
  - ▪ It is important to differentiate between nonviral and viral vasculitis because treatment options differ significantly.
- ○ **Hematologic,** more so than solid malignancies can be associated with vasculitis.
  - ▪ Typically presents with palpable purpura
  - ▪ Hairy cell leukemia presents with a PAN-like picture or as a cutaneous vasculitis.
  - ▪ Lymphoproliferative disorders including myelodysplastic syndrome, Waldenström's macroglobulinemia, lymphocytic lymphoma, and chronic lymphocytic leukemia all can have associated vasculitis, with or without cryoglobulins.

Etiology

Multiple factors appear to play a role is disease susceptibility, including genetic, immune, and environmental. Much is yet to be learned about each.

Pathophysiology

- The mechanisms underlying the vasculitides remain poorly understood.
- Currently, it is believed that while immune complexes themselves are not innately pathogenic, their inflammatory potential can be augmented in the setting of increased antigen load, decreased clearance efficiency by the reticuloendothelial system (RES), or decreased solubility. The pathogenic immune complexes fix complement, leading to intense inflammation.
  - ○ Regarding immune complex solubility, when there are equal parts of antigen and antibody, large immune complexes form that are cleared by the RES without tissue damage.
  - ○ When an excess of antibody is present, small immune complexes are generated but remain soluble, and are not pathogenic.
  - ○ **When there is an excess of antigen, the immune complexes precipitate** and get trapped in capillaries or vessels damaged by turbulent blood flow. This leads to immune complex–mediated inflammation.
- Activating Fcγ receptors and the alternative pathway of complement are critical for ANCA-associated pauci-immune vasculitis induction. Activation of neutrophils and macrophages ensues, leading to endothelial injury.
- In giant cell arteritis, dendritic cells, T cells, and macrophages are strongly implicated in arterial wall destruction.
- Several models have been proposed to describe why vasculitic syndromes have a predilection for certain vessels[2]:
  - ○ Antigens distribute preferentially to tissues, thus inducing vasculitis in those vessels.
  - ○ Endothelial cells control the severity of inflammation at the vessel through expression of adhesion molecules and secretion of proteins, peptides, and hormones, which in turn control immune cell–blood vessel interactions.
  - ○ Nonendothelial cells modulate immune cell and/or endothelial cell behavior, modulating the level of inflammation.

DIAGNOSIS

- The diagnosis of vasculitis should be entertained whenever a patient with systemic symptoms has organ dysfunction.

- Characteristic symptoms are associated with the involvement of certain sized vessels. Thus, it is best to try to **assign the patient's signs and symptoms to a particular vessel size category,** then **determine what features of each disease within the category best fit the patient.**
- Use laboratory testing and diagnostic procedures to define the extent of disease or better elucidate any other characteristic features, particularly **biopsy of affected organs** because this typically yields the diagnosis.

Clinical Presentation

- Most common constitutional symptoms are fatigue, malaise, fever, and arthralgias.
- Several clinical features strongly suggest the presence of vasculitis:
  - **Purpura**
    - These are nonblanching skin lesions due to bleeding in the skin.
    - Those with isolated skin lesions are considered to have cutaneous leukocytoclastic vasculitis.
    - If the purpura is palpable and systemic involvement is seen, HSP or microscopic polyangiitis should be suspected.
  - **Mononeuritis multiplex**
    - This occurs when two or more nerves in separate parts of the body are damaged.
    - **"Foot-drop"** occurs because of damage to the sciatic or peroneal nerve; **"wrist-drop"** occurs because of damage to the radial nerve.
    - Of all the neurologic symptoms seen in vasculitis, mononeuritis multiplex is the most specific.
  - **Pulmonary–renal involvement**
    - Alveolar hemorrhage from capillaritis can cause **hemoptysis.** Hemoptysis can also be associated with a medium-sized vessel vasculitis due to a ruptured bronchial artery aneurysm.
    - Glomerulonephritis is associated with **red blood cell casts or dysmorphic red blood cells** in the urine.
    - While the ANCA-associated vasculitides can cause pulmonary–renal syndrome, anti-glomerular basement membrane syndrome, embolic disease, infection, and SLE should also be considered.

History

- Detailed history helps differentiate between primary and secondary causes of vasculitis.
- Ask about past history of:
  - Medications (hypersensitivity vasculitis)
  - Hepatitis B or C (PAN or cryoglobulinemia, respectively)
  - Connective tissue disease
  - Sexual history (HIV infection)
  - Illicit drug use (ergots, cocaine, or amphetamines)
- Certain age groups and gender are associated with specific vasculitides.
  - Granulomatosis with polyangiitis and PAN have mean age of onset between 45 and 50 years of age, whereas HSP and Takayasu's arteritis occur between 17 and 26 years of age within the adult population.
  - Giant cell arteritis affects an older population, with a mean age of onset of 69 years.
  - Takayasu's and giant cell arteritis occur predominantly in females.

Physical Examination

Certain clues are seen depending on vessel size (see Table 24-2).

TABLE 24-2	PHYSICAL EXAMINATION FEATURES OF VASCULITIS

Large vessel

Pulse deficits
Bruits

Medium vessel

Cutaneous nodules
Livedo reticularis
Digital infarction

Small vessel

Palpable purpura
Superficial ulcerations
Mononeuritis multiplex
Papulonecrotic lesions

Diagnostic Criteria

- The American College of Rheumatology has defined classification criteria for several of the vasculitides, including:
  - Takayasu's arteritis (see Chapter 21)
  - Giant cell arteritis (see Chapter 22)
  - PAN (see Chapter 23)
  - Kawasaki disease
  - Eosinophilic Granulomatous with Polyangiitis (see Chapter 25)
  - Hypersensitivity vasculitis (see Chapter 29)
- The remainder of the vasculitides do not have set criteria for diagnosis but are diagnosed clinically with the help of laboratory testing.

Differential Diagnosis

- Look for secondary causes of vasculitis when the patient does not appear to fit within any of the primary vasculitides.
- **Embolic disorders** (endocarditis, left atrial myxoma, cholesterol emboli) can mimic a small-vessel vasculitis.
- **Infections** such as sepsis, fungal infections (especially mycotic aneurysm with embolization), mycobacterial infections, rickettsial infections, and syphilis may mimic a small-vessel vasculitis.
- **SLE and amyloidosis,** in the absence of vasculitis, can present with vasculitis-type symptoms.
- **Ergots, cocaine, and amphetamines** can mimic medium- or small-vessel vasculitis.
- **Malignancies** seen with vasculitis-like symptoms include lymphomatoid granulomatosis, intravascular lymphoma, and angioimmunoblastic T-cell lymphoma.
- **Thrombocytopenia and myelodysplastic syndromes** can present with nonvasculitic purpura.

Diagnostic Testing

Laboratories
- Basic laboratory analysis should include:
  - Complete blood count with differential
  - Comprehensive metabolic panel (elevated creatinine)

- Muscle enzymes (creatine kinase, aldolase)
- ESR and C-reactive protein (CRP)
- Hepatitis and HIV serologies
- Urinalysis and urine toxicology screen
- More specific laboratory testing can include (see Chapter 5):
  - **Antinuclear antibodies** (ANA) if suspecting a connective tissue disease
  - **Complement** (low levels are seen in cryoglobulinemia, hypocomplementemic urticarial vasculitis, and the vasculitis associated with SLE)
  - Although not diagnostic, when **ANCA** is directed to PR3 by enzyme-linked immunosorbent assay (ELISA), strongly consider granulomatosis with polyangiitis. When directed to MPO, consider microscopic polyangiitis or Eosinophilic Granulomatous with Polyangiitis.

Imaging
- Decision to pursue imaging is dependent on the patient's symptom complex.
- Chest radiography may reveal pulmonary infiltration, including alveolar hemorrhage.
- Sinus computed tomography (CT) may reveal sinusitis in granulomatosis with polyangiitis.
- Echocardiogram should be done to rule out valve vegetations and atrial myxoma.
- Angiogram may reveal characteristic alternating dilatations and strictures in large- or medium-sized vasculitides—especially in PAN and temporal arteritis.

Diagnostic Procedures
- Usually, biopsy of affected tissue (e.g., skin, nerve, kidney, lungs) can reveal the pathologic findings of vasculitis.
- Delay in obtaining material from affected tissue is a common mistake in establishing a diagnosis in these conditions.

TREATMENT

- The goal of treatment is to first induce remission of disease, then maintain the patient on a less toxic immunosuppressant to prevent relapses.
- Treatment is based on the type and severity of clinical manifestations (see Chapter 9).
- In general, **immunosuppression** is the mainstay for treatment.

Medications
- **Glucocorticoids** are used in virtually all systemic vasculitis patients. Eosinophilic Granulomatous with Polyangiitis often undergoes remission with glucocorticoids alone.
- **Rituximab** is a B-cell depleting agent and is noninferior to cyclophosphamide for ANCA-associated vasculitis.[3] Rituximab has replaced cyclophosphamide as the first-line steroid-sparing agent due to the potential reduction in long-term side effects.
- **Cyclophosphamide** can also be utilized in combination with glucocorticoids for rapidly progressive vasculitides, such as the ANCA-associated conditions, especially in the setting of rituximab failure.
- **Methotrexate, azathioprine,** and **mycophenolate mofetil** have been used for less severe forms of vasculitis and also for maintenance therapy following rituximab.

COMPLICATIONS

- Inadequately treated or aggressive forms of vasculitis can lead to permanent end-organ damage and death.
- Relapse after induction treatment is unfortunately common, but re-treatment usually leads to a good response.

REFERRAL

- Referral to a rheumatologist should occur once a vasculitis is suspected to help confirm the diagnosis and direct the management of immunosuppression.
- Other specialists may be necessary depending on the severity of disease in a particular organ (such as nephrologists).

PATIENT EDUCATION

- Due to the relative infrequency of these syndromes, patient education is important to help the patient understand their disease and also to dispel inaccuracies found on the Internet.
- Patients must be informed of the side effects associated with their specific immunosuppressive regimen.

MONITORING/FOLLOW-UP

- The goal during follow-up is to slowly wean the level of immunosuppression to reduce potential drug-induced toxicity and monitor for flares and infections.
- Commonly, the procedures used to diagnose the patient are employed for monitoring, except for biopsy.
- A history and physical examination, along with laboratory testing, should be routinely done during the follow-up period.
  - When relapses occur, the history and physical findings will typically mimic the patient's initial presentation.
  - Routine vaccinations with killed vaccines should be done with every immunosuppressed patient.

OUTCOME/PROGNOSIS

- There is limited data regarding outcome.
- Most patients who are treated early and respond appropriately to treatment do not have significant reduction in survival.

REFERENCES

1. Jennette JC, Falk RJ, Andrassy K, et al. Nomenclature of systemic vasculitides. Proposal of an international consensus conference. *Arthritis Rheum.* 1994;37(2):187–192.
2. Deng J, Ma-Krupa W, Gewirtz AT, et al. Toll-like receptors 4 and 5 induce distinct types of vasculitis. *Circ Res.* 2009;104:488–495.
3. Stone JH, Merkel PA, Spiera R, et al. Rituximab versus cyclophosphamide for ANCA-associated vasculitis. *N Engl J Med.* 2010;363:221–232.

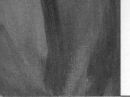

Takayasu's Arteritis

Can M. Sungur and Jonathan J. Miner

25

GENERAL PRINCIPLES

- A large vessel vasculitis classically affecting the aorta and its major branches
- The formal diagnosis of Takayasu's arteritis requires the presence of three out of six criteria listed in Table 25-1.[1]

Definition

- The Chapel Hill Consensus Conference defined Takayasu's arteritis (TA) as a rare **granulomatous inflammation of the aorta and its major branches.**[2]
- TA can also affect the pulmonary and coronary arteries.
- It is a chronic vasculitis characterized primarily by **stenotic** but also, less frequently, by aneurysmal lesions of the large arteries.

Epidemiology

- TA is most common in individuals of **Asian descent.** The incidence is highest in Japan, with 100 to 200 new cases per year. In the United States, the incidence is approximately 2.5 cases per million per year.
- TA characteristically affects **women** more than men, at approximately 10:1.
- Peak onset is in the **third decade.** Onset of the disease after age 40 is rare.

Pathophysiology

- The cause of TA is unknown.
- TA is a focal **panarteritis affecting large vessels and their major branches,** with subsequent stenosis and aneurysm formation. Approximately 98% of patients develop **stenoses. Aneurysms** are less common but may occur.

TABLE 25-1	AMERICAN COLLEGE OF RHEUMATOLOGY 1990 CRITERIA FOR TAKAYASU'S ARTERITIS

The presence of at least three of the following six are required:
- Age of onset before 40 years
- Claudication of extremities
- Decreased brachial artery pulse
- Blood pressure difference greater than 10 mm Hg
- Bruit over subclavian arteries or aorta
- Arteriogram abnormality

Adapted from: Arend WP, Michel BA, Bloch DA, et al. The American College of Rheumatology 1990 criteria for the classification of Takayasu Arteritis. *Arthritis Rheum.* 1990;33:1129–1134.

- On gross examination, the affected vessels are thick and rigid. The lumen is affected in a characteristic "skipped" fashion, with normal lumen alternating with stenoses or aneurysms.
- Microscopic examination of acute aortic inflammation reveals:
  - **Infiltration around the vasa vasorum** by lymphocytes and plasma cells.
  - Thickening of the adventitia is present along with leukocytic infiltration of the tunica media and intimal hyperplasia.[3]
  - **Granuloma formation and giant cells** are typically located in the media. Destruction and fibrosis of the media can lead to aneurysm formation.
  - **Intimal hyperplasia** due to myofibroblast proliferation leads to characteristic stenotic lesions.
- **Chronic inflammation** in TA is characterized by **fibrosis** of all the three vessel layers. Both acute and chronic inflammation are typically seen in the same patient at the same time, implying a **recurrent process.**
- The manifestations of TA are related either to the systemic effects of chronic inflammation or the effects of localized occlusion or aneurysm formation on organ function.

DIAGNOSIS

Clinical Presentation

- The clinical features of TA have been divided into **three monophasic stages.**
  - **Phase one** is the "prepulseless" inflammatory phase characterized by nonspecific **constitutional symptoms** such as fever, malaise, arthralgias, and weight loss.
  - **Phase two** is characterized by **vessel inflammation manifesting as vessel pain and tenderness.** This most commonly results in carotidynia (i.e., pain on palpation of the carotid artery).
  - **Phase three** is called the "burnt-out" or **fibrotic stage** and is characterized by arterial stenoses leading to **ischemic symptoms.**
- Disease presentation is variable. Only about half of the patients have constitutional symptoms, and many patients have both inflammatory and fibrotic manifestations at the same time. Monophasic disease may also occur.
- The classic presentation of TA is that of a young woman with signs and symptoms of abnormal cerebral or upper extremity blood flow.
- **Diagnosis prior to this stenotic phase of the disease is unlikely, given the nonspecific constitutional symptoms.**
- The signs and symptoms are dependent on the vessels affected.
  - **Subclavian** involvement occurs in over 90% of patients, resulting in arm claudication and pulselessness in about two-thirds.
  - **Aortic** involvement occurs in more than half of the patients and may result in signs and symptoms of aortic insufficiency, hypertension, and abdominal angina. **Hypertension** in this case is believed to be because of aortic stenosis resulting in decreased blood flow to the kidneys.
  - **Common carotid** involvement is also frequent and poses risk for visual defects, strokes, and transient ischemic attack (TIA).
  - The **renal arteries** are diseased in about one-third of the patients, typically leading to renovascular hypertension.
  - **Vertebral artery** involvement occurs at a similar rate and may trigger for dizziness and visual impairment.
- Other signs and symptoms include arrhythmia, ischemic chest pain, syncope, and visual loss. Last, congestive heart failure may occur and is typically related to the presence of hypertension.

- The average time between onset of symptoms and diagnosis is about 10 months.
- Common findings on physical examination include **pulselessness, unequal brachial blood pressures, subclavian/carotid bruits, and carotidynia.** These manifestations are attributed to ascending aorta and aortic arch involvement with resultant stenoses of their major branches and distal organ hypoperfusion.
- **Hypertension** may be noted as well and is often because of aortic or renal artery stenosis.

Diagnostic Criteria

- The American College of Rheumatology 1990 classification criteria for TA require that at least three of six criteria be met for diagnosis seen in Table 25-1 (sensitivity 90.5% and specificity 97.8%).[1]
- Criteria now show reduced sensitivity of 73.6% with unchanged specificity of 98.3%, with modern cohorts[4] prompting revision of criteria.
- Additional overlap has been identified with giant cell arteritis with involvement of thoracic vasculature.
- New classification criteria will incorporate modern imaging modalities, including MRI/ MRA, FDG-PET CT, and ultrasound.
- Current draft includes the following with sensitivity 94.52% and specificity 93.7%[5]:
  ○ Inclusion criteria (must have one of the following): diagnosis of vasculitis, age less than 60, or evidence of vasculitis on imaging.
  ○ Criteria are then based on a point system of findings that have to be greater than 5, including:
    ▪ **Clinical features:** female sex (+1), angina (+2), claudication (+2)
    ▪ **Vascular exam findings:** arterial bruit (+2), reduced pulses upper extremities (+2), reduced carotid pulse or tenderness (+2), systolic blood pressure difference in arms greater than 20 mm Hg (+1)
    ▪ **Imaging findings:** number of affected arteries (+1 for each up to +3), vasculitis affecting paired branch arteries (+1), abdominal aorta involved (+3)

Differential Diagnosis

The differential diagnosis of TA includes the **infectious aortitis** (e.g., tuberculous, mycotic, syphilitic aortitis), **Ehlers–Danlos syndrome, Marfan syndrome, seronegative spondyloarthropathies** with aortic root involvement, **giant cell arteritis, sarcoid vasculopathy,** and **fibromuscular dysplasia.**

Diagnostic Testing

Laboratories

- Lab data in TA are nonspecific. Anemia of chronic disease, mild to moderate thrombocytosis, hypergammaglobulinemia, and elevated erythrocyte sedimentation rate (ESR) are common.
- Elevations in C-reactive protein (CRP) and/or ESR may correlate with active disease but are not reliable in all patients.

Imaging
- Intra-arterial angiography has been the gold standard for detecting diseased vessels. However, it does not provide detail of the vessel wall but only the diameter of the lumen and pressure differences across stenotic lesions.
- MR and CT angiography are now available and can provide details about the vessel wall itself. Both modalities identify wall edema and vessel thickness. However, correlation between these wall changes and disease activity is not clear.

- Ultrasound can be used to evaluate for carotid and abdominal arterial disease.
- 18F-fluorodeoxyglucose PET scanning can detect glucose uptake in inflamed tissue and is being investigated as a technique to detect active arteritis. Also being studied is combining PET with CT scanning to help improve location of the inflammation.[3]

TREATMENT

Medications

- Medical treatment is used to treat the active inflammation in hopes of preventing the end-stage stenotic and aneurysmal arterial changes.
- Active inflammatory TA is treated initially with **oral glucocorticoids.**
  - The typical starting dose is 1 mg/kg/day of prednisone.
  - This dose may be continued for 1 to 3 months on the basis of symptoms and improvement, and then gradually tapered.
- If disease fails to improve or if the patient displays intolerance of the steroid dose, a **cytotoxic agent** is typically started.
- **Methotrexate** 0.3 mg/kg/week is the first choice, with an initial maximum dose of 15 mg/week that can be titrated up to 25 mg/week.
- Steroids are continued in addition to a cytotoxic agent.
- Approximately half of the patients will require a cytotoxic agent because of relapse or insufficient initial response to steroids.[2]
- If steroids cannot be tapered within 6 months or cannot be discontinued within 12 months of initiating a cytotoxic agent, the agent is considered a failure and is stopped.
- While results of methotrexate promoting remission have been promising, limited conclusions can be drawn because of the lack of randomized controlled studies.
- **Other cytotoxic agents** that have been used include **azathioprine, leflunomide, and mycophenolate mofetil.** Cyclophosphamide is usually only used after failure of all other therapies owing to toxicities including the long-term risk of hemorrhagic cystitis along with bladder and other malignancies.
- **Tocilizumab,** anti-IL-6 receptor monoclonal antibody, has been studied in refractory TA patients in a randomized control trial with reduction in relapses (p value 0.034) and improved time to relapse rates (p value 0.0596).[6]
- **Tumor necrosis factor (TNF)-α antagonists (infliximab and etanercept)** have been studied in an open label investigation in patients with relapsing disease and steroid toxicity with promising results.[7] Recent observational data showed longer sustained remission and less new lesions and complications when compared with DMARD and glucocorticoid-only-treated patients.[8]
- **Hypertension** is difficult to treat because ischemia may occur in vascular beds distal to stenotic lesions when blood pressure is lowered.
  - The risks of ischemia must be weighed against that of prolonged hypertension.
  - Furthermore, although limb blood pressure readings are useful in detecting occlusive disease and in monitoring the progression of stenoses and limb ischemia, they are inadequate in monitoring the treatment of hypertension.
  - Stenotic lesions may make peripheral blood pressure readings lower than that of central pressures.
  - β-blockers and angiotensin-converting enzyme (ACE) inhibitors are not contraindicated in TA.

Surgical Management

- **Bypass surgery** and **angioplasty** are used to treat the permanent arterial damage that results.
- The indications for surgery may include the following:

- ○ Hypertension associated with renal artery stenosis
- ○ Extremity ischemia that limits activities of daily living
- ○ Severe (>70%) stenosis of at least three cerebral vessels
- ○ Symptoms of cerebral ischemia
- ○ Moderate aortic regurgitation
- ○ Cardiac ischemia with proven coronary artery stenosis
- ○ An expanding aneurysm at risk of rupture also warrants surgical intervention.
- Angioplasty and endovascular stenting may also be used for stenosis. Most commonly, it is used for renal artery stenosis, although there is increasing experience with angioplasty and stenting of subclavian, coronary, and aortic stenoses.
- In one long-term cohort of 60 patients, 23 required 50 bypass procedures, while 11 required angioplasty. Autologous grafts fared better than synthetic bypass grafts.[9]
- Angioplasty appears to be complicated by restenosis much more frequently than bypass surgery.
- Success rates for revascularization procedures are highest in those patients who have inactive disease by histology at the time of operation.
- It is often very difficult to determine clinically whether disease is active, but systemic features (e.g., fever, myalgias, arthralgias), elevated ESR, features of vascular ischemia (e.g., claudication, pulse deficits, bruits, vascular pain, asymmetric blood pressure readings), and typical angiographic features are usually used as indicators. Unfortunately, patients often fail to meet these criteria of active disease despite pathologic specimens that demonstrate active inflammation. As mentioned previously, newer imaging modalities, such as CT and MR angiography, may give information about the vessel wall that correlates with active inflammation, but further study is needed.

MONITORING/FOLLOW-UP

- For most patients, TA is a chronic disease; few patients experience a monophasic course.
- The follow-up of patients who are in clinical remission has yet to be defined.
- Current markers of active disease are recognized as inadequate indicators of inflammation. Thus, when to start or taper treatment is a difficult decision.
- Monitoring disease via serial aortography is expensive and associated with risks, and the role of other imaging modalities has yet to be defined.
- Unfortunately, pathologic tissue is difficult to obtain and cannot be used for following disease activity.
- Reevaluate patients with recurring or relapsing signs and symptoms of systemic vascular inflammation as described earlier.

REFERENCES

1. Arend WP, Michel BA, Bloch DA, et al. The American College of Rheumatology 1990 criteria for the classification of Takayasu arteritis. *Arthritis Rheum.* 1990;33:1129–1134.
2. Jennette JC, Falk RJ, Andrassy K, et al. Nomenclature of systemic vasculitides. Proposal of an international consensus conference. *Arthritis Rheum.* 1994;37:187–192.
3. Mason JC. Takayasu arteritis—advances in diagnosis and management. *Nat Rev Rheumatol.* 2010;6:406–415.
4. Seeliger B, Sznajd J, Robson JC, et al. Are the 1990 American College of Rheumatology vasculitis classification criteria still valid? *Rheumatology.* 2017;56:1154–1161.
5. Luqmani R, Merkel P, Watts R. Diagnostic and classification criteria in vasculitis: Updated classification criteria for the large vessel vasculitis. Presented at: ACR 2018.
6. Nakaoka Y, Isobe M, Takei S, et al. Efficacy and safety of tocilizumab in patients with refractory Takayasu arteritis: results from a randomized, double-blind, placebo-controlled phase 3 trial in Japan (the TAKT study). *Ann Rheum Dis.* 2018;77:348–354.

7. Molloy ES, Langford CA, Clark TM, et al. Anti-tumour necrosis factor therapy in patients with refractory Takayasu arteritis: long-term follow-up. *Ann Rheum Dis.* 2008;67:1567–1569.
8. Gudbrandsson B, Molberg O, Palm O. TNF inhibitors appear to inhibit disease progression and improve outcome in Takayasu arteritis; an observational, population-based time trend study. *Arthritis Res Ther.* 2017;19:99.
9. Kerr GS, Hallahan CW, Giordano J, et al. Takayasu arteritis. *Ann Intern Med.* 1994;120:919–929.

Giant Cell Arteritis and Polymyalgia Rheumatica

26

Anneliese M. Flynn and Jonathan J. Miner

GIANT CELL ARTERITIS

GENERAL PRINCIPLES

- Giant cell arteritis (GCA, also known as temporal arteritis) is a **large- and medium-vessel vasculitis** affecting the **second- to fifth-order aortic branches**, often in the **extracranial vessels.**
  - ○ It is characterized by **granulomatous inflammation** in vessel walls.
  - ○ GCA is the **most common primary form of vasculitis among adults** in the United States and Europe, and occurs almost exclusively in older adults (>50 years).
- GCA presents with two major symptom complexes:
  - ○ **Vascular insufficiency** leading to impaired blood flow.
    - ▪ **Vision loss** from ischemic optic neuropathy is the most feared complication.
    - ▪ **Headache,** scalp tenderness, jaw claudication, or central nervous system (CNS) ischemia due to **cranial arteritis** can be seen.
    - ▪ **Large-vessel GCA** can lead to **arm claudication,** pulselessness, Raynaud's phenomenon, aortic aneurysm, or aortic insufficiency. All patients suspected of GCA should be screened for large vessel involvement.
  - ○ Signs of **systemic inflammation,** including malaise, fever, and weight loss are common.
- Patients with a reasonable suspicion of GCA should be **immediately started on high-dose oral or intravenous glucocorticoid therapy** to suppress the onset of GCA-related blindness. This will not interfere with temporal artery biopsy results if the biopsy is done within 10 to 14 days of glucocorticoid initiation. **Once visual compromise has started, recovery in the affected eye rarely occurs even with aggressive treatment.**

Definition

- GCA was defined by the Chapel Hill Consensus Conference as **granulomatous arteritis** of the aorta and its major branches, particularly the **extracranial branches of the carotid artery.**[1]
- Two forms of GCA have been identified, which are differentiated by the vascular bed involved.
  - ○ **Cranial arteritis** occurs when the extracranial branches of the carotid artery are involved. This manifests as headache, **jaw claudication,** and visual changes.
  - ○ **Large-vessel GCA** occurs when the carotid, subclavian, axillary, and other large vessels branching off the aorta are affected. Aortic arch syndrome (especially arm claudication) and aortitis can be seen.
  - ○ Typically, cranial arteritis and large-vessel GCA do not occur in the same patient.

Epidemiology

- GCA is seen almost exclusively in older individuals. **Mean age at diagnosis is >70 years.**
- Incidence is estimated to be 1:500 individuals >50 years of age.
- Women are affected two to three times more often than men.
- Forty to fifty percent of GCA patients have polymyalgia rheumatica (PMR).

Etiology

- The pathogenesis of GCA is unknown.
- Genetic factors have been correlated with GCA.
  - The presence of HLA-DR4 is significantly associated with GCA.
  - A polymorphism in the second hypervariable region of HLA-DRB1 (the region of HLA that binds to antigen) is associated with both GCA and PMR. This polymorphism is not seen in rheumatoid arthritis (RA) patients.[2]
- Infections may play an influential role in GCA development.
  - Cyclic (every 5–7 years) peaks of the incidence of GCA suggest that some triggering event such as infection may be important.[3]
  - Gamma-herpes virus infections in interferon-γ receptor–deficient mice promote a large-vessel vasculitis.[4]
  - An association with parvovirus B19 has also been proposed.[5]

Pathophysiology

- **Cell-mediated processes** appear to drive GCA pathology.
  - T cells in particular may play an important role because the majority of vessel-infiltrating lymphocytes are CD4 T cells.[6]
  - In addition to T cells, alterations of dendritic cell function have been identified.[7]
  - Macrophages play multiple roles, such as secretion of interleukin (IL)-1, IL-6, and transforming growth factor (TGF)-β; promoting oxidative damage; producing nitric oxide; and generating giant cells.[6]
  - Components of the humoral immune response appear to be less important. B cells are not found in GCA lesions, and hypergammaglobulinemia and autoantibodies are not found in patient sera.[6]
- Cytokines, particularly **IL-6**, play a role in disease activity.
  - IL-6 levels strongly correlate with disease activity.[8]
  - mRNA levels of interferon-γ (IFN-γ) and IL-1β within involved arteries correlate with ischemic symptoms (vision compromise or jaw claudication), whereas serum IL-2 levels associate with PMR.[9]
- The pathology within the vasculitic lesions of GCA explains the mechanism of vascular compromise.
  - The vasculitic lesion contains a mononuclear cell infiltrate comprising the T cells and macrophages that is present initially in the adventitia and subsequently in all layers of the arterial wall. As the inflammatory response progresses, the media of the arterial wall thins, while the intima becomes hyperplastic. This is the mechanism by which vascular compromise occurs, in addition to platelet aggregation.
  - The infiltrates may be granulomatous (particularly in the media), characterized by the presence of histiocytes and multinucleated giant cells.
    - **Although the presence of giant cells led to the naming of this disease, they are typically absent.**
    - When present, they are found close to the fragmented internal elastic lamina. This correlates with elevated platelet-derived growth factor (PDGF) levels and increased risk of ischemic complications.[10]
  - The presence of fibrinoid necrosis should suggest another type of vasculitic process.

Risk Factors

- Age is the greatest risk factor for GCA.
- Female gender is associated with GCA.
- Ethnicity is another risk factor for GCA development. Patients of Northern European descent are 2.5- to 4-fold more likely than Southern Europeans and 7.5- to 25-fold more likely than Hispanics and African-Americans to develop GCA.[11]

Prevention

No known preventive measures have been identified for GCA.

DIAGNOSIS

- It is rare to have GCA in individuals <50 years of age.
- **Headache is the most common presenting symptom for GCA, whereas jaw claudication highly predicts a positive temporal artery biopsy.**
- Anyone suspected to have GCA should be started on high-dose oral or intravenous glucocorticoid therapy, even if the temporal artery biopsy has not yet been performed.
- If the temporal artery biopsy is negative, but suspicion for GCA remains high, treat as if the patient has GCA and consider biopsy of the other temporal artery.
- GCA should also be considered in patients >50 years of age with fever of unknown origin.

Clinical Presentation

History
- In **GCA,** the onset of symptoms tends to be **gradual** rather than abrupt.
- **Cranial arteritis:** Eighty to ninety percent of all GCA cases present with cranial arteritis.
  - **Headache:** Over half of the patients will have a chief complaint of headache.
    - Characterized as throbbing, sharp, or dull
    - Located classically over the temporal regions but can be seen over the occipital or frontal lobes or can be generalized
  - **Temporal tenderness:** Individuals may also complain about temporal tenderness when wearing eyeglasses or lying on a pillow.
  - **Jaw claudication:** Fifty percent of patients will complain of fatigue or pain while eating, or trismus-like symptoms.
    - Patients may not recognize the significance of this, so they must be asked directly.
    - Symptoms are due to reduced blood flow through the extracranial branches of the carotid artery supplying the masseter or temporalis muscles.
    - A striking feature of GCA-associated jaw claudication is how quickly fatigue begins upon chewing and how disabling the pain can be.
    - Jaw claudication may be the most specific symptom for cranial arteritis. Fifty-four percent of those with jaw claudication had a positive temporal artery biopsy, whereas only 3% of those with a negative biopsy had jaw claudication.[12]
  - **Systemic complaints:**
    - Fifty percent will have low-grade fever (>37.7 °C), whereas 15% have fevers >39 °C.[13]
    - Fifteen percent of elderly patients with fever of unknown origin are diagnosed with GCA.[13]
    - Ten percent of patients will have constitutional symptoms or laboratory evidence of inflammation as the only symptoms/signs of GCA.[14]
  - **Visual complaints:** A wide variety of manifestations occur in GCA.
    - **Vision loss is sudden, painless, and usually permanent.**
    - **Amaurosis fugax** is a temporary monocular loss of vision caused by focal ophthalmic artery lesions. This leads to transient ischemia of the retina, choroid, or optic nerve, or a combination of the above. Patients will report **visual blurring** (associated with heat, exercise, or posture) and **diplopia.** If left untreated, the other eye will likely be affected in 1 to 2 weeks.
    - **Anterior ischemic optic neuropathy (AION)** may follow an episode of amaurosis fugax. It is due to compromise of blood flow through the posterior ciliary artery leading

to acute ischemia of the optic nerve head. Typically presenting unilaterally, the other eye can be affected within days or weeks if left untreated. **Although AION is the most common ocular presentation of GCA, only 5% of AION patients have GCA.**

- **Posterior ischemic optic neuropathy is a rare** (approximately 5%) etiology for the cause of blindness in GCA. This is due to compromised blood flow to the retrobulbar portion of the optic nerve.
- Despite effective therapy, vision loss occurs in one or both eyes in 15% to 20% of GCA patients. This is due, in part, to the fact that blindness may be the presenting symptom.
- **Diplopia** can occur not only from amaurosis fugax but also from ischemic injury to the oculomotor system or extraocular muscles, paresis of ocular motor nerves, and brainstem disease.
- **Bitemporal hemianopia** occurs when arteries supplying the optic chiasm are damaged.
- **Homonymous hemianopia** (vision defect involving either the two right or left halves of the visual field) results from damage to vessels feeding the retrochiasmal visual sensory pathways. In GCA, this most commonly occurs from lesions in the vertebrobasilar circulation, leading to occipital lobe infarction.
- **Visual hallucinations** can be induced by glucocorticoid-associated psychosis or from Charles Bonnet syndrome (the presence of visual hallucinations in psychologically normal patients due to vision loss from peripheral or central vision pathway lesions).
○ **Musculoskeletal complaints**
  - **PMR** (see later for symptoms) is observed in 40% to 50% of GCA patients, but only 15% of PMR patients have GCA. Five percent of patients considered to have isolated PMR will have a positive temporal artery biopsy.
  - **Peripheral synovitis and peripheral edema** of the distal extremities are also seen in a minority of GCA patients. These symptoms can mimic seronegative RA or remitting seronegative symmetrical synovitis with pitting edema (RS3PE) (see Differential Diagnosis).
○ **Neurologic complaints:** Neurologic manifestations occur in 20% to 30%.
  - **Transient ischemic attacks (TIAs) and strokes** are typically due to extradural internal carotid (less common) or vertebral artery (more common) vasculitic lesions. Aortic dissection can also compromise blood flow through these vessels leading to symptoms.
  - **Vertigo and hearing loss** can also occur with vertebral or carotid artery involvement.
  - **Intracranial vasculitis** is extremely rare (<1%).
- **Large-vessel GCA** represents 10% to 15% of all GCA cases and typically lacks cranial involvement. These patients are marginally younger (mean age = 66 years), have fewer complaints of headache, and are more likely to present with arm claudication. Fifty percent of these patients will have a negative temporal artery biopsy.
  ○ **Aortic arch syndrome:** Observed with involvement of the subclavian and axillary arteries.
    - **Arm claudication** is the most common symptom, seen in 51% of large-vessel GCA patients.
    - **Absent or asymmetric pulses and paresthesias** may also be seen.
  ○ **Aortitis**
    - Active aortitis was observed in 50% of GCA patients postmortem as well as at surgery, most commonly affects the **ascending aorta**, which can lead to dilatation of the aortic valve.
    - **Aneurysms** (particularly thoracic, can present similarly to Takayasu's arteritis [see Chapter 25]) and **dissections** (due to chronic aortitis) are the most significant complications.

○ There is a 17-fold increased incidence of thoracic aortic aneurysm development, which occurs in approximately 10% of GCA patients.[15]

○ Similarities between GCA and Takayasu's arteritis highlight the possibility that they are part of a spectrum of the same disease.

Physical Examination
- **GCA** patients are typically **chronically ill**-appearing, often with **fever.**
- **Temporal artery abnormalities:**
  ○ **Decreased or absent pulses:** If pulse was absent, likelihood ratio (LR) of a positive temporal artery biopsy was 2.7 over a patient without this finding.[16]
  ○ **Tender or thickened artery:** If the patient had a prominent or enlarged temporal artery, the LR = 4.3; if tender, LR = 2.6.[16]
  ○ Even in the absence of physical examination findings relative to the temporal artery, 33% will still have a positive temporal artery biopsy.[17]
- **Ophthalmologic findings**
  ○ May be normal in those with amaurosis fugax
  ○ Cotton-wool spots can be seen at areas of vascular lesions.
  ○ **Swollen pale optic disc with blurred margins** in those with acute vision loss from AION
  ○ Optic atrophy and pale, flat disc in those with permanent blindness from AION. These patients will also have a relative afferent pupillary defect (Marcus Gunn pupil manifested by positive swinging flashlight sign).
- **Cardiovascular findings**
  ○ **Bruits** may be heard on auscultation of supraclavicular, carotid, axillary, brachial, and femoral areas.
  ○ **Aortic regurgitation murmur** may indicate an ascending aortic aneurysm.
  ○ **Diminished pulses** in the extremities may be associated with asymmetric blood pressures in the affected extremities.
- **Musculoskeletal** (see Polymyalgia Rheumatica).

Diagnostic Criteria

- No true diagnostic criteria exist for GCA. The American College of Rheumatology (ACR) criteria, though, can influence the decision to proceed with subsequent temporal artery biopsy.
- The following clinical findings are effective in distinguishing GCA from other forms of vasculitis[18,19]:
  ○ Age ≥50 years at time of disease onset
  ○ Localized headache of new onset
  ○ Tenderness or decreased pulse of temporal artery
  ○ Erythrocyte sedimentation rate (ESR) >50 mm/h
  ○ Biopsy revealing necrotizing arteritis with a predominance of mononuclear cells or a granulomatous process with multinucleated giant cells
- If a patient has an existing diagnosis of vasculitis, the presence of three of these five criteria is associated with 94% sensitivity and 91% specificity for the diagnosis of GCA.[18]
- There is a 95% probability for a negative temporal artery biopsy with the following findings[20]:
  ○ ESR <40 mm/h
  ○ No jaw claudication
  ○ No temporal artery tenderness
  ○ Presence of synovitis

Differential Diagnosis

The differential diagnosis for GCA includes the following:
- Other large-vessel vasculitides (such as Takayasu's arteritis, which does not involve the temporal artery)

- Polyarteritis nodosa, granulomatosis with polyangiitis, or CNS vasculitis (if involving the temporal artery)
- Amyloidosis (presenting as jaw or arm claudication if vascular involvement of the temporal or subclavian artery occurs)
- Nonarteritic anterior ischemic optic neuropathy (NAAION) is associated with low inflammatory markers and hypertension, diabetes mellitus, and sildenafil use.

Diagnostic Testing

Laboratories
- No single laboratory test is pathognomonic for diagnosing GCA, but they can strongly suggest the presence of disease. Laboratory abnormalities resolve with glucocorticoid treatment.
- **Complete blood count (CBC): Normocytic anemia** is usually present at diagnosis of GCA. Interestingly, the white blood cell (WBC) count is generally normal despite systemic signs of inflammation.
- **Comprehensive metabolic panel (CMP): Transaminitis and an elevation in alkaline phosphatase** are seen in 25% to 35% of GCA patients; serum albumin levels are usually normal.[21]
- ESR and C-reactive protein (CRP)
  ○ **Significant elevations of ESR and CRP** values are characteristically seen in GCA.
  ○ In GCA, a normal ESR reduces the probability of a positive temporal artery biopsy by five-fold.[16] An ESR <40 mm/h correlates to fewer systemic systems but does not reduce the likelihood of visual loss in those with GCA.
  ○ In GCA, the CRP usually correlates with ESR values.
- **IL-6 concentrations closely correlate with clinical disease** in GCA and more strongly predict relapse than ESR. IL-6 testing is not yet widespread, and its clinical usefulness is unclear.[8]

Imaging
- **For GCA-associated cranial arteritis, imaging is typically not necessary.** Magnetic resonance angiography (MRA) has been utilized to identify areas of temporal artery inflammation, helping to guide temporal artery biopsy.
- **If large-vessel GCA is suspected, the study of choice is MRA.** Aortic, carotid, subclavian, and other large vessels can be visualized and assessed for the presence of vessel wall edema. Although MRA has been investigated in tracking disease activity and in the evaluation of response to treatment, vessel wall edema has not been always associated with disease activity or helpful in identifying new lesions. Therefore, its use should always be in conjunction with clinical findings in the setting of GCA.
- While currently investigational, the future use of positron emission tomography (PET) may be beneficial in the identification of large-vessel GCA.
- The role of conventional angiography has been limited with the use of MRA. It does play a role in those with large-vessel GCA in all four extremities where peripheral blood pressure measurements are unreliable. Aortography with central aortic pressure measurements may be useful in this setting.
- Ultrasound has shown mixed success in GCA, and its use in the diagnosis of GCA should be limited to medical centers with experience.

Diagnostic Procedures
- **Temporal artery biopsy** is the gold standard in establishing the diagnosis of GCA and should be done in all patients suspected to have GCA.
- Sensitivity of temporal artery biopsy is 94%.[18]
- The predictive value of a positive biopsy was significantly increased in patients with jaw claudication and higher yet with the addition of headache, scalp tenderness, or vision changes.[22]

- A 2-cm length of the temporal artery should be obtained unless the artery is visibly abnormal, where a smaller segment can yield the diagnosis. Complications are rare with this procedure.
- Full tissue processing should be performed, as there may be "skip" lesions.
- Controversy exists whether to obtain unilateral or bilateral temporal artery biopsy samples. Unilateral biopsy is usually sufficient to diagnose GCA, missing only 13% of cases compared with bilateral biopsies.[23,24]
- We suggest the following algorithm to decide on unilateral versus bilateral temporal artery biopsies (as proposed by the European League Against Rheumatism)[25]:
  - If an obvious temporal artery abnormality is present on examination, or headache is unilateral, biopsy of that vessel should be performed.
  - If there are no localizing hints, obtain a unilateral temporal artery biopsy.
  - If the unilateral biopsy result is negative, and clinical suspicion remains high, biopsy of the contralateral temporal artery should be considered.
  - Patient preference may play a role in the decision to obtain a simultaneous bilateral biopsy.
  - Regardless, **treatment for GCA should be initiated before the biopsy is scheduled.** The inflammatory infiltrate resolves slowly after starting prednisone, usually not resolving for weeks to months.
- Recognize that **negative biopsies do not exclude the possibility of large-vessel GCA** (look for arm claudication in those patients).
- **Biopsy of other vessels:** Temporal arteries are typically biopsied because they are easily accessible. If other vessels are abnormal (such as the facial or occipital arteries), then those can also be biopsied.

TREATMENT

The goal of treatment in GCA is to avoid AION. Unfortunately, once vision has been lost, the likelihood of significant visual improvement is small (<10%). **Thus, prevention of vision loss is of paramount importance.**
- Glucocorticoids
  - The standard of care is **glucocorticoids,** despite the lack of placebo-controlled studies. Their efficacy in GCA has been established through many years of use and the known consequences of untreated disease.
  - **Glucocorticoids must be started immediately once a patient is suspected to have GCA,** even before the diagnosis is confirmed. This is especially true if the patient has recent or potential vascular complications. **Nevertheless, temporal artery biopsies should be obtained as quickly as possible.**
  - The optimal initial dose is unclear, but virtually all cases should be started on a minimum of **prednisone 40 to 60 mg PO daily.**
  - Daily dosing is more efficacious than alternate-day dosing. Splitting a single daily dose into multiple doses during the day is no more effective than single daily dosing.
  - The use of **intravenous glucocorticoids** (15 mg/kg/day of methylprednisolone for three doses) was investigated in a small randomized, double-blind, placebo-controlled study, which concluded that those receiving IV methylprednisolone had[26]:
    - Higher rates of sustained remission following the discontinuation of glucocorticoid therapy.
    - Higher likelihood of achieving and maintaining low doses of prednisone (≤5 mg/day) at 9, 12, and 15 months following initial loading dose.
    - Lower median total glucocorticoid dose (excluding the initial loading dose).
    - Vision loss at diagnosis that did not improve significantly with parenteral glucocorticoids.

- In summary, although the use of parenteral glucocorticoids for those with visual dysfunction has not been rigorously tested, we believe that it is appropriate to use pulse-dose glucocorticoids for these patients.

- **Tocilizumab**
  - Tocilizumab, a humanized anti-IL-6 receptor monoclonal antibody, is the first-line steroid-sparing agent used to treat GCA.
  - A randomized, double-blind, placebo-controlled phase 3 trial showed tocilizumab (weekly or every other week) combined with prednisone resulted in higher rates of sustained glucocorticoid-free remission through 1 year of follow-up.[27]
  - Although tocilizumab is effective at increasing the rate of remission, the relapse rate on therapy is significant.
  - Diverticulitis is a contraindication to tocilizumab use, given the risk of intestinal perforation with the medication.
  - IL-6 plays an important role in the acute phase response. Therefore, CRP and ESR measurement cannot be used reliably to monitor disease activity in the setting of tocilizumab use.

- **Steroid taper**
  - **Patients should be maintained on the starting dose of glucocorticoids for at least 2 to 4 weeks or whenever disease activity resolves, whichever comes later.** A slow taper should follow this over the next 9 to 18 months.
  - Typically, patients will report resolution of symptoms 24 to 48 hours after treatment initiation (with the exception of vision loss from AION). Laboratory measures of inflammation will also begin to normalize during this time.
  - Tapering of prednisone should be done with the goal of avoiding flares.
  - **A reasonable initial goal for prednisone tapering is to reach 20 mg/day at 2 months of therapy.**
  - The tapering schedule will slow down after this. Usually, once 10 mg/day is reached, decrease the dose by 1 mg every month so that the full course of treatment is 9 to 12 months in total.
  - **If a patient flares during the tapering process, redosing with the initial starting dose should be done with a slower tapering schedule afterwards.**
  - Patients rarely flare at doses >15 mg/day but commonly do below this dose.

- **Aspirin:** The use of daily low-dose aspirin to reduce the risk of vision loss, TIA, and stroke has been recommended.[28] This benefit appears to be due to its antiplatelet effect.

- **Other medications**
  - Methotrexate (MTX)
    - Data from randomized trials on whether MTX can be used as a steroid-sparing agent show conflicting results.[29–31]
    - The use of MTX for GCA is not recommended at this time.

COMPLICATIONS

- Other than visual loss, no long-term complications typically occur directly from GCA as the disease is self-limited over months or years.
- Most complications occur as a result of prolonged glucocorticoid use and should be addressed as necessary. One should **anticipate side effects from prolonged use of prednisone therapy** (see Chapter 9).
  - Hyperglycemia, weight gain, infection, hypertension, and other side effects must be monitored.
  - Loss of bone integrity or frank **osteoporosis** can occur. Screening with bone density scans and prophylactic treatment with calcium, vitamin D, and an appropriate osteoporotic medication is recommended (see Chapter 52).

REFERRAL

- Those suspected with GCA should be immediately referred to a rheumatologist. If there is strong suspicion of disease or if there are visual symptoms, inpatient management with rheumatology consultation is warranted.
- Anyone requiring prolonged glucocorticoid use should be referred to a rheumatologist for medication toxicity monitoring.

PATIENT EDUCATION

- Patients must be informed of the side effects associated with prednisone and appropriately managed to avoid long-term complications.
- Recognition of symptoms of GCA must be emphasized to patients to aid in flare identification.

MONITORING/FOLLOW-UP

- **Monitoring for disease activity is challenging in GCA.** It can be difficult to assess the presence of flares in the setting of a prednisone taper.
- ESR and CRP can be used to monitor disease activity unless the patient is on tocilizumab, in which case the ESR and CRP become less reliable for disease activity monitoring.
- IL-6 may prove to be a more reliable measure of disease activity than ESR, although the clinical usefulness of this assay has not been thoroughly assessed.[8]

OUTCOME/PROGNOSIS

- Prognosis is typically very good in those with timely and appropriate treatment.
- Some may need lifelong low-dose glucocorticoid therapy for suppressing GCA disease activity.
- In those without visual compromise, new vision loss is uncommon once treatment has begun (<1%).
- In those with preexisting visual defects from GCA, the incidence of contralateral vision loss is estimated to be 13% over the next 5 years, even with appropriate treatment.[32] Age >80 years is the most significant risk factor for this outcome.
- Overall survival appears not to be affected in those with GCA.

POLYMYALGIA RHEUMATICA

GENERAL PRINCIPLES

- PMR is a musculoskeletal syndrome seen in individuals >**50 years of age** manifested by **symmetric pain and stiffness in the muscles of the neck, torso, shoulders, and hip girdle for at least 4 weeks.**
- It is associated with signs of systemic inflammation, elevated ESR and CRP, and anemia.
- PMR is closely related to GCA and is often considered a form of GCA that lacks fully developed vasculitis.
- PMR responds very well to low-dose oral glucocorticoid therapy.

Definition

PMR is a syndrome characterized by symmetric aching and morning stiffness of the shoulder and hip girdles, neck, and torso in individuals >50 years old with an ESR >50 mm/h.

Epidemiology

- PMR is seen almost exclusively in older individuals. **Mean age at diagnosis is >70 years.**
- Like GCA, it is rare to have PMR in individuals <50 years old.
- Women are affected—two to three times more often than men.
- Fifteen percent of PMR patients develop GCA.

Etiology

- The pathogenesis of PMR is unknown.
- Genetic factors have been correlated with PMR.
  - A polymorphism in the second hypervariable region of HLA-DRB1 (the region of HLA that binds to antigen) has been associated with PMR.[2]
  - Other genetic polymorphisms in intracellular adhesion molecule (ICAM)-1, TNF-α, vascular endothelial growth factor (VEGF), or carriage of certain alleles, such as the PI[A2] allele of the platelet glycoprotein IIIa gene, may also be associated with PMR.[33–36]

Pathophysiology

The pathophysiology of PMR is unknown.

Risk Factors

- Age is the greatest risk factor for PMR.
- Female gender is a risk factor for PMR.

Prevention

No known preventive measures have been identified for PMR.

DIAGNOSIS

Clinical Presentation

History
- **PMR** is characterized by the subacute or chronic onset of symmetric morning stiffness and achiness of the shoulder and hip girdles, neck, and torso.
- **Morning stiffness** and tenderness last >30 minutes, leading to difficulties in dressing or turning over in bed and may be due to bursitis and/or synovitis.
- Pain occurs in the **shoulders** more than in the hips or neck. It is worse with movement and can interfere with sleep. It may be associated with subjective weakness.
- Sleep is often disrupted.
- **Systemic symptoms** occur in up to 40% of patients and include malaise, depression, anorexia and weight loss, and fever (almost always low grade unless GCA is present).

Physical Examination
- **Pain** with active range of motion of the shoulders, neck, and hips
- **Tenderness to palpation of the shoulders**
- **Synovitis occurs** in the knees, wrists, and metacarpophalangeal (MCP) joints, and is typically mild, asymmetric, and nonerosive. It is also seen in 15% to 20% of GCA patients.
- **Tenosynovitis** and **peripheral edema** occur most commonly in the hands, wrists, ankles, and the dorsum of the feet, and are thought to represent regional tenosynovitis. Carpal tunnel syndrome is seen in 10% to 15% of patients.

Diagnostic Criteria

No diagnostic criteria exist for PMR, but the following have been suggested to strongly support the diagnosis[19]:
- Age > 50 years

- ESR > 40, or elevated CRP in the setting of normal ESR
- One month duration of morning stiffness >30 minutes and bilateral aching of the two of the following three areas: neck/torso, shoulders/proximal arms, and hip/proximal thighs.
- Prompt response (within 3 days) to low-dose glucocorticoid therapy (10–20 mg/day prednisone) has been suggested by some as another criterion.

Differential Diagnosis

- **Early seronegative RA** is the most common alternative diagnosis in patients presenting with symptoms consistent with PMR.
  - RA patients will have more swollen joints of the hands, wrists, and feet and usually only a partial response to low-dose prednisone compared with PMR patients. PMR patients will have complete resolution of any swollen joints and a more rapid decrease in acute phase reactants with low-dose prednisone than patients with RA.
  - Nevertheless, there is considerable symptom overlap between seronegative RA and PMR, making the diagnosis difficult at times.
- Other diagnoses mimicking PMR include:
  - Remitting seronegative symmetric synovitis with pitting edema (RS3PE)
  - Bursitis/tendinitis
  - Spondyloarthropathy
  - Calcium pyrophosphate deposition disease (CPPD)
  - Hypothyroidism
  - Fibromyalgia and depression
  - Malignancy (such as multiple myeloma)
  - Infective endocarditis
  - Inflammatory myopathy (pain is usually not a feature in myositis; creatine kinase is normal in PMR)
  - Parkinson disease
  - Hyperparathyroidism

Diagnostic Testing

Laboratories
- Similar to GCA, no single laboratory test independently diagnoses PMR but can strongly suggest the presence of disease. Laboratory abnormalities resolve with glucocorticoid treatment.
- **Normocytic anemia** is usually present at diagnosis. The WBC count is generally normal despite systemic signs of inflammation.
- **ESR and CRP are typically significantly elevated.**

Imaging
- For PMR, imaging is typically not required. Nevertheless, **MRI** and **ultrasound** have been shown to demonstrate inflammation of extra-articular synovial structures with tenosynovitis or shoulder bursitis with effusion.
- Plain films of the affected joints do not usually reveal abnormalities.

Diagnostic Procedures
No invasive diagnostic procedures aid in the diagnosis of PMR.

TREATMENT

- The goal of treatment is resolution of symptoms.
- **A prompt response (within 24–48 hours) to glucocorticoid therapy is highly characteristic of PMR.**

- **Prednisone**
  - Initial dosing of **prednisone 15 mg PO daily** is sufficient for most patients, but this may range from 10 to 20 mg/day.[37]
    - Symptom reduction should be evident within 3 days of treatment, often overnight.
    - **Maintain the initial dose of prednisone for 2 to 4 weeks.**
    - If symptoms are not well controlled, increase prednisone by 5 mg/day up to 30 mg/day.
    - **An alternative diagnosis should be entertained if little or no symptom relief is obtained with prednisone dose of 20 mg/day or higher.**
  - Generally, maintenance dosing and prednisone tapering protocols lack consensus. We recommend the following:
    - For those receiving ≥15 mg/day, reduce prednisone by 5 mg/day every 2 to 4 weeks to 15 mg/day.
    - For those receiving 10 to 15 mg/day, reduce by 2.5 mg/day every month.
    - For those receiving ≤10 mg/day, reduce by 1 mg/day every month.
    - **Flares typically occur if the tapering is too rapid.** Restart prednisone at approximately the last dose that achieved complete symptom control, and restart tapering at a slower rate (every 2–3 months).
    - If a flare occurs off prednisone, the patient may need to completely restart the initial dosing and tapering protocol.
    - Continue low-dose prednisone for at least 1 year to minimize the risk of relapse after discontinuation.
- **Other therapies**
  - MTX: Inconsistent results have been observed in those receiving MTX with prednisone compared with prednisone alone. Its use in PMR is typically not recommended.
  - **Tocilizumab:** Preliminary studies suggests tocilizumab may be effective as a steroid-sparing agent in the treatment of PMR.[38,39] Randomized controlled trials are needed to further evaluate this.
  - Nonsteroidal anti-inflammatory drugs (NSAIDs):
    - NSAIDs may be effective in some as glucocorticoid-sparing therapy, but drug-related side effects limit their use in this elderly patient population.
    - NSAIDs may be used as adjunct therapy with low-dose prednisone for osteoarthritis or tendinitis pain, but great care must be exercised to avoid gastrointestinal side effects. Concurrent proton-pump inhibitor (PPI) administration should be strongly encouraged.

COMPLICATIONS

- No long-term complications typically occur directly from GCA or PMR because the disease is self-limited over months or years.
- Most complications occur as a result of prolonged glucocorticoid use, and should be addressed as necessary. **One should anticipate side effects from prolonged use of prednisone therapy** (see Chapter 9).
  - Hyperglycemia, weight gain, infection, hypertension, and other side effects must be monitored.
  - Loss of bone integrity or frank **osteoporosis** can occur. Screening with bone density scans and prophylactic treatment with calcium, vitamin D, and an appropriate osteoporotic medication is recommended (see Chapter 52).

REFERRAL

Anyone requiring prolonged glucocorticoid use should be referred to a rheumatologist for medication toxicity monitoring.

PATIENT EDUCATION

- Patients must be informed of the side effects associated with prednisone and appropriately managed to avoid long-term complications.
- Recognition of symptoms of GCA must be emphasized to PMR patients.

MONITORING/FOLLOW-UP

- Monitoring for symptoms in PMR is the best method for picking up flares. Interpretation of ESR and CRP values must be done in the context of the patient's clinical presentation.
- **Those with PMR should be continuously monitored for symptoms of GCA.** In sum, 4.4% of those with "isolated" PMR had positive temporal artery biopsies.

OUTCOME/PROGNOSIS

- Overall survival appears not to be affected in those with PMR.
- Glucocorticoid therapy for PMR typically lasts for 2 to 3 years, but some may need long-term low-dose (<10 mg/day) treatment. Spontaneous relapse occurs in up to 25% of patients regardless of glucocorticoid dosing, particularly in the first 2 years.

REFERENCES

1. Jennette JC, Falk RJ, Andrassy K, et al. Nomenclature of systemic vasculitides. Proposal of an international consensus conference. *Arthritis Rheum.* 1994;37:187–192.
2. Weyand CM, Hunder NN, Hicok KC, et al. HLA-DRB1 alleles in polymyalgia rheumatica, giant cell arteritis, and rheumatoid arthritis. *Arthritis Rheum.* 1994;37:514–520.
3. Petursdottir V, Johansson H, Nordbord E, et al. The epidemiology of biopsy-positive giant cell arteritis: special reference to cyclic fluctuations. *Rheumatology (Oxford).* 1999;38:1208–1212.
4. Weck KE, Dal Canto AJ, Gould JD, et al. Murine gamma-herpesvirus 68 causes severe large-vessel arteritis in mice lacking interferon-gamma responsiveness: a new model for virus-induced vascular disease. *Nat Med.* 1997;3:1346–1353.
5. Gabriel SE, Espy M, Erdman DD, et al. The role of parvovirus B19 in the pathogenesis of giant cell arteritis: a preliminary evaluation. *Arthritis Rheum.* 1999;42:1255–1258.
6. Weyand CM, Goronzy JJ. Medium-and large-vessel vasculitis. *N Eng J Med.* 2003;349:160–169.
7. Ma-Krupa W, Jeon MS, Spoerl S, et al. Activation of arterial wall dendritic cells and breakdown of self-tolerance in giant cell arteritis. *J Exp Med.* 2004;199:173–183.
8. Roche NE, Fulbright JW, Wagner AD, et al. Correlation of interleukin-6 production and disease activity in polymyalgia rheumatica and giant cell arteritis. *Arthritis Rheum.* 1993;36:1286–1294.
9. Weyand CM, Tetzlaff N, Björnsson J, et al. Disease patterns and tissue cytokine profiles in giant cell arteritis. *Arthritis Rheum.* 1997;40:19–26.
10. Kaiser M, Weyand CM, Björnsson J, et al. Platelet-derived growth factor, intimal hyperplasia, and ischemic complications in giant cell arteritis. *Arthritis Rheum.* 1998;41:623–633.
11. Hunder GG. Giant cell arteritis and polymyalgia rheumatica. *Med Clin North Am.* 1997;81:195–219.
12. Hall S, Persellin S, Lie JT, et al. The therapeutic impact of temporal artery biopsy. *Lancet.* 1983;2:1217–1220.
13. Calamia KT, Hunder GG. Giant cell arteritis (temporal arteritis) presenting as fever of undetermined origin. *Arthritis Rheum.* 1981;24:1414–1418.
14. Gonzalez-Fay MA, Barros S, Lopez-Diaz ME, et al. Giant cell arteritis: disease patterns of clinical presentation in a series of 240 patients. *Medicine (Baltimore).* 2005;84:269–276.
15. Evans JM, O'Fallon WM, Hender GG. Increased incidence of aortic aneurysm and dissection in giant cell (temporal) arteritis. A population-based study. *Ann Intern Med.* 1995;122:202–207.
16. Smetana GW, Shmerling RH. Does this patient have temporal arteritis? *JAMA.* 2002; 287:92–101.
17. Manna R, Cristiano G, Todaro L, et al. Microscopic haematuria: a diagnostic aid in giant-cell arteritis? *Lancet.* 1997;350:1121.
18. Hunder GG, Bloch DA, Michel BA, et al. The American College of Rheumatology 1990 criteria for the classification of giant cell arteritis. *Arthritis Rheum.* 1990;33:1122–1128.

19. Salvarani C, Cantini F, Hunder GG. Polymyalgia rheumatica and giant-cell arteritis. *Lancet.* 2008;372:234–245.

20. Gabriel SE, O'Fallon WM, Achkar AA, et al. The use of clinical characteristics to predict the results of temporal artery biopsy among patients with suspected giant cell arteritis. *J Rheumatol.* 1995;22:93–96.

21. Hazleman B. Laboratory investigations useful in the evaluation of polymyalgia rheumatica (PMR) and giant cell arteritis (GCA). *Clin Exp Rheumatol.* 2000;18:S29–S31.

22. Younge BR, Cook BE Jr, Bartley GB, et al. Initiation of glucocorticoid therapy: before or after temporal artery biopsy? *Mayo Clin Proc.* 2004;79:483–491.

23. Pless M, Rizzo JF 3rd, Lamkin JC, et al. Concordance of bilateral temporal artery biopsy in giant cell arteritis. *J Neuroophthalmol.* 2000;20:216–218.

24. Breuer GS, Nesher G, Nesher R. Rate of discordant findings in bilateral temporal artery biopsy to diagnose giant cell arteritis. *J Rheumatol.* 2009;36:794–796.

25. Mukhtyar C, Guillevin L, Cid MC, et al. EULAR recommendations for the management of large vessel vasculitis. *Ann Rheum Dis.* 2009;68:318–323.

26. Mazlumzadeh M, Hunder GG, Easley KA, et al. Treatment of giant cell arteritis using induction therapy with high-dose glucocorticoids: a double-blind, placebo-controlled, randomized prospective clinical trial. *Arthritis Rheum.* 2006;54:3310–3318.

27. Stone JH, Tuckwell K, Dimonaco S, et al. Trial of Tocilizumab in Giant-Cell Arteritis. *N Engl J Med.* 2017;377:317–328

28. Lee MS, Smith SD, Galor A, et al. Antiplatelet and anticoagulant therapy in patients with giant cell arteritis. *Arthritis Rheum.* 2006;54:3306–3309.

29. Jover JA, Hernández-Garcia C, Morado IC, et al. Combined treatment of giant-cell arteritis with methotrexate and prednisone. A randomized, double-blind, placebo-controlled trial. *Ann Intern Med.* 2001;134:106–114.

30. Spiera RF, Mitnick HJ, Kupersmith M, et al. A prospective, double-blind, randomized, placebo controlled trial of methotrexate in the treatment of giant cell arteritis (GCA). *Clin Exp Rheumatol.* 2001;19:495–501.

31. Hoffman GS, Cid MD, Hellmann DB, et al. A multicenter, randomized, double-blind, placebo-controlled trial of adjuvant methotrexate treatment for giant cell arteritis. *Arthritis Rheum.* 2002;46:1309–1318.

32. Aiello PD, Trautmann JC, McPhee TJ, et al. Visual prognosis in giant cell arteritis. *Ophthalmology.* 1993;100:550–555.

33. Salvarani C, Casali B, Boiardi L, et al. Intercellular adhesion molecule 1 gene polymorphisms in polymyalgia rheumatica/giant cell arteritis: association with disease risk and severity. *J Rheumatol.* 2000;27:1215–1221.

34. Mattey DL, Hajeer AH, Dababneh A, et al. Association of giant cell arteritis and polymyalgia rheumatica with different tumor necrosis factor microsatellite polymorphisms. *Arthritis Rheum.* 2000;43:1749–1755.

35. Meliconi R, Pulsatelli L, Dolzani P, et al. Vascular endothelial growth factor production in polymyalgia rheumatica. *Arthritis Rheum.* 2000;43:2472–2480.

36. Salvarani D, Casali B, Farnetti E, et al. PlA1/A2 polymorphism of the platelet glycoprotein receptor IIIA and risk of cranial ischemic complications in giant cell arteritis. *Arthritis Rheum.* 2007;56:3502–3508.

37. Dasgupta B, Borg FA, Hassan N, et al. BSR and BHPR guidelines for the management of polymyalgia rheumatica. *Rheumatology (Oxford).* 2010;49:186–190.

38. Lally L, Forbess L, Hatzis C, et al. Brief Report: a prospective open-label phase IIa trial of tocilizumab in the treatment of polymyalgia rheumatica. *Arthritis Rheum.* 2016;68:2550–2554.

39. Devauchelle-Pensec V, Berthelot JM, Cornec D, et al. Efficacy of first-line tocilizumab therapy in early polymyalgia rheumatic: a prospective longitudinal study. *Ann Rheum Dis.* 2016;75:1506–1510.

Polyarteritis Nodosa — 27

Can M. Sungur and Jonathan J. Miner

GENERAL PRINCIPLES

- A formal diagnosis of polyarteritis nodosa (PAN) requires the presence of 3 of the 10 criteria listed in Table 27-1. Of these, a biopsy or angiogram demonstrating vasculitis of small- to medium-sized vessels particularly helps solidify the diagnosis.
- Mesenteric and renal angiography is sensitive and specific for PAN with gastrointestinal (GI) and kidney involvement.
- Classic PAN spares the lungs and glomeruli.

Definition

Defined by the Chapel Hill Consensus Conference as a necrotizing inflammation of medium- or small-sized arteries, without glomerulonephritis or vasculitis of the arterioles, capillaries, or venules.[1]

Epidemiology

- Affects men more frequently than women, between the ages of 40 and 60 years, with peak around 50 years of age.
- Classic PAN is rare with an estimated annual incidence rate of 2.0 to 9.0 per million.

Etiology

- Most cases of PAN are idiopathic.
- A minority of cases are caused by the **hepatitis B virus** (HBV). The prevalence rates of PAN are higher in populations with endemic HBV infection. Consequently, the widespread use of HBV vaccines has decreased the rate of HBV-related PAN.
- PAN has also been linked to other viral infections, especially **HIV and hepatitis C virus** (HCV).
  - In a cohort of 161 patients with HCV-related vasculitis, 31 of them (19.3%) were classified as having PAN.[2]
  - HCV-PAN was associated with a more acute and severe clinical presentation as well as a higher rate of clinical remission when compared to HCV-related mixed cryoglobulinemia (HCV-MC).
  - When compared to HBV-PAN, HCV-PAN was seen more frequently in an older female population, with a higher prevalence of skin involvement and relapse rate, and a worse prognosis.
- Myelodysplastic syndrome (MDS), chronic myelomonocytic leukemia, and hairy cell leukemia have been linked to PAN.

Pathophysiology

- The mechanism of PAN is not well understood but typically involves circulating foreign antigens, antibodies, Fc receptors, and complement.
- It appears to cause immune complex–mediated damage to vessel walls.
- In patients with HBV-related PAN, hepatitis B surface antigen–antibody interaction triggers activation of the complement cascade and Fcγ receptors.

TABLE 27-1	AMERICAN COLLEGE OF RHEUMATOLOGY 1990 CRITERIA FOR POLYARTERITIS NODOSA

The presence of at least 3 of the following 10 is required:
- Unintentional weight loss >4 kg since the start of illness
- Livedo reticularis
- Testicular pain or tenderness not due to infection, trauma, or other causes
- Diffuse myalgias, weakness, or leg tenderness
- Mononeuropathy or polyneuropathy
- Diastolic blood pressure > 90 mm Hg
- Blood urea nitrogen >40 mg/dL or creatinine >1.5 mg/dL, not due to dehydration, medications, or obstruction
- Hepatitis B virus infection
- Abnormal angiogram showing aneurysms or occlusions of visceral arteries, not due to atherosclerosis, fibromuscular dysplasia, or noninflammatory disease
- Biopsy of small- or medium-sized vessels demonstrating an artery containing polymorphonuclear leukocytes and mononuclear leukocytes in the vessel wall

Adapted from: Lightfoot RW Jr, Michel BA, Bloch DA, et al. The American College of Rheumatology 1990 criteria for the classification of polyarteritis nodosa. *Arthritis Rheum.* 1990;33:1088–1093.

- The clinical symptoms of PAN result from systemic manifestations secondary to the release of cytokines as well as from local inflammation and vessel damage.
- The pathologic lesion is a **focal segmental necrotizing vasculitis of medium- and small-sized arteries**. This inflammation commonly leads to disruption of the elastic lamina of the vessel wall with subsequent weakening and formation of **microaneurysms**, endothelial dysfunction, thrombosis, and stenosis.

DIAGNOSIS

Clinical Presentation
- The presentation of PAN may be nonspecific.
- Most of the patients develop **systemic symptoms of inflammation** (e.g., malaise, arthralgias, myalgias, fever, and/or weight loss) along with localized signs and symptoms of vasculitis (e.g., peripheral neuropathy and GI, testicular and/or cutaneous manifestations).
- Most patients present with acute illness and severe manifestations.
- HBV-related PAN
  - Patients tend to be less than 40 years old and have a more acute and fulminant form of PAN than those with PAN without HBV.
  - Malignant hypertension (HTN), renal infarction, and orchitis are more common in HBV-related PAN.
  - PAN tends to precede hepatitis, which is usually clinically silent at the time of the vasculitis.
  - Seroconversion often leads to remission of PAN.
- Limited forms of PAN
  - **Cutaneous PAN** (CPAN) refers to a chronic cutaneous vasculitis of medium-sized vessels with histologic features similar to PAN but without systemic vascular involvement.
    - These patients also usually present with extracutaneous manifestations, which include myalgias, arthralgias, malaise, fever, and neuropathy.

- Clinical manifestations of CPAN include **livedo reticularis, tender subcutaneous nodules, ulcers, and necrosis.**
- A workup to exclude systemic involvement is required before the diagnosis of CPAN can be made.
- Treatment ranges from nonsteroidal anti-inflammatory drugs (NSAIDs) and colchicine to steroids and other immunosuppressive agents, depending on the severity of symptoms.
- Its course tends to be chronic with remissions and relapses. Overall, it has a favorable prognosis and, **rarely, converts into systemic PAN.**
  - Rarely, microaneurysms and stenoses **limited to single organs without systemic involvement** occur.[3]

History
- Given the systemic involvement in PAN, a thorough history and a detailed review of systems are indicated.
- **Skin:** Inquire about the appearance of tender, erythematous nodules, bullous or vesicular lesions, ulcerations, and/or digital ischemia/gangrene.
- **Musculoskeletal:** Inquire about myalgias, muscle weakness, and claudication.
- **Cardiovascular:** Inquire about HTN, chest pain, and dyspnea on exertion as microaneurysm and thrombi formation as well as myocardial ischemia and coronary dissection may occur secondary to PAN.
- **GI:** Inquire about abdominal pain, especially after a meal; nausea; vomiting; diarrhea; and melena.
  - Pain may be intermittent or continuous. This may be indicative of mesenteric vasculitis with subsequent bowel wall ischemia, ulceration, and/or perforation.
  - The most commonly involved portion is the small bowel.
- **Kidney:** Renal ischemia secondary to vasculitis of the medium-sized muscular arteries leads to **HTN** through the activation of the renin–angiotensin system.
  - Hematuria has been reported; however, red blood cell (RBC) casts and other signs of glomerulonephritis are not common in PAN.
  - Their presence along with pulmonary symptoms such as hemoptysis merits consideration of a vasculitis, affecting primarily the smaller vessels such as microscopic polyangiitis (MPA) or granulomatosis with polyangiitis (GPA).
- **Neurologic:** The most common symptom is **mononeuritis multiplex,** present in more than 70% of patients, which may be the presenting symptom.
  - Characterized by an asymmetric sensory and motor peripheral neuropathy caused by ischemia and inflammation to the vasa nervorum supplying the affected nerve
  - The lower limbs, especially the sciatic nerve and its peroneal and tibial branches, are most commonly affected.
  - Hypoesthesia or hyperesthesia and pain are present in the areas of motor deficits.
  - The motor deficits may be abrupt and may precede the sensory symptoms.
  - Cranial nerve and central nervous system (CNS) involvement are rare but may include cranial nerve palsies and hemorrhagic or ischemic strokes.
- **Acute inflammatory orchitis:** PAN should be considered in the differential diagnosis.

Physical Examination
- A thorough physical examination is necessary to determine which organs are involved and the extent of vascular lesions.
- It is also important to seek the presence of additional disease processes that may be mimicking PAN.
- **Skin:** Cutaneous manifestations of classic PAN are uncommon and variable. They include palpable purpura, which is usually papular/petechial and sometimes bullous or vesicular, livedo reticularis, tender subcutaneous nodules, and distal gangrene.

- **GI:** The stool should be checked for occult blood.
- **Renal:** New-onset HTN may be indicative of renal involvement.
- **Neurologic:** Test especially for motor weakness and sensory deficits.

Diagnostic Criteria

- The diagnosis of PAN is based on the presence of systemic features as well as either an abnormal angiogram demonstrating the presence of aneurysms or thrombosis and/or a biopsy showing vasculitic involvement of the small- or medium-sized vessels.
- The American College of Rheumatology criteria are presented in Table 27-1.[4]

Differential Diagnosis

Multiple conditions can mimic PAN, which is why a broad differential must be considered and evaluated during your workup. These include the following:
- **Viral infections** such as hepatitis B and C, HIV, cytomegalovirus (CMV), parvovirus B19, and human T-cell lymphotropic virus 1 (HTLV-1)
- **Connective tissue diseases** (e.g., systemic lupus erythematosus, rheumatoid arthritis, Sjögren's syndrome, mixed connective tissue disease, systemic sclerosis) may present like PAN, with a vasculitis secondary to the connective tissue disease.
- **Bacterial endocarditis, cholesterol embolization, sepsis, and malignancy** should also be excluded.
- **Antineutrophil cytoplasmic antibody (ANCA)–associated vasculitides** such as MPA may have signs and symptoms similar to PAN, but are distinguished by small-sized vessel vasculitis in the pulmonary and renal vasculature, normal visceral angiography, presence of ANCA, and the greater tendency to relapse (see Chapter 30).
- PAN has been associated with MDS, chronic myelomonocytic leukemia, and hairy cell leukemia. The course of MDS tends to be more severe if associated with PAN.

Diagnostic Testing

Laboratories
- Erythrocyte sedimentation rate (ESR) greater than 50 mm/hour and an elevated C-reactive protein (CRP) greater than 10 mg/L
- Leukocytosis
- Hypereosinophilia (seen in 10%–30% of patients)
- Normocytic normochromic anemia of chronic inflammation
- Mild renal insufficiency, HTN, non-nephrotic range proteinuria, and mild hematuria. **Active urinary sediment is not a feature of PAN.**
- Check hepatitis serologies and investigate other causes of PAN as appropriate.
- Positive tests for ANCA are uncommon with PAN (<30%).

Imaging
- **Visceral angiography** may be useful to demonstrate **microaneurysms and stenoses in small-to medium-sized vessels**, usually in the renal, mesenteric, and/or hepatic arterial systems.
- Angiography may also be helpful, before hepatic or renal biopsies, to identify microaneurysms and minimize the risk of visceral bleeding.
- **Coronary angiography** can also reveal microaneurysms in the coronary arteries.
- In patients with coronary arteritis, a spiral computed tomography (CT) scan as well as cardiac magnetic resonance imaging (MRI) scans may better visualize aneurysms and myocardial ischemia.[5]

Diagnostic Procedures
- Seek biopsies of the affected organ, if possible.
- Although the skin is not routinely involved in PAN, a biopsy is indicated if lesions are present.

- Full-thickness skin biopsy is recommended because it requires tissue as deep as the subcutaneous fat to capture the small- and medium-sized muscular-walled arteries involved in PAN.
- Another potential site to biopsy is the sural nerve, especially if a lower extremity neuropathy is present.
- A muscle biopsy of the gastrocnemius muscle should be done concurrently because it increases the yield of finding vessel involvement with PAN if the sural nerve biopsy is negative.

TREATMENT

- Depends on the presence of HBV as well as the assessment of disease activity
- The French Cooperative Study Group (FCSG) for PAN devised a **five-factor score for determining prognosis.**[6]
- **The five parameters predicting higher mortality are as follows:**
  - Proteinuria greater than 1 g/day
  - Serum creatinine greater than 1.58 mg/dL (140 μmol/L)
  - Cardiomyopathy
  - GI involvement
  - CNS involvement

Medications

First Line
- First-line treatment includes **oral or (IV) intravenous glucocorticoids.**
- PAN without HBV and with none of the abovementioned five factors at the time of diagnosis can be treated with **oral prednisone** (1 mg/kg/day is a commonly used starting dose).
- **Pulse IV methylprednisolone** (1 g daily for 3–5 days) is usually employed if there are severe, life-threatening manifestations of vasculitis.
- The addition of immunosuppressants, such as cyclophosphamide, methotrexate, mycophenolate, or azathioprine, has prolonged the survival of patients with PAN.
  - **Pulse cyclophosphamide**, in addition to glucocorticoids, induces remission with fewer side effects in patients without poor prognostic factors, than oral cyclophosphamide.
  - Treat patients with a factor score 1 or above with pulse IV methylprednisolone (1,000 mg/day for 3–5 days) followed by oral prednisone (1 mg/kg/day) and pulse IV cyclophosphamide 0.5 to 2.5 g every week to every month depending on the patient's condition, renal function, response to previous therapy, and hematologic data.
  - Reserve oral cyclophosphamide for patients failing IV cyclophosphamide or for those with fulminant manifestations.
  - Taper prednisone slowly after the patient's clinical status improves and the ESR returns to normal, usually in approximately 1 month. The dose may be dropped by about 25% every 2 to 4 weeks.
  - IV cyclophosphamide therapy should in most cases not exceed 1 year when combined with glucocorticoids.
  - Rituximab given as 2 doses of 1 g separated by 2 weeks every 6 months is another option in resistant PAN cases in patients without hepatitis B. It has not been formally studied in PAN, but various case studies and initial studies done in ANCA-associated vasculitis support the use of rituximab.[7]
  - Patients receiving cyclophosphamide or rituximab should receive prophylaxis for *Pneumocystis jirovecii* pneumonia with oral trimethoprim 160 mg/sulfamethoxazole 800 mg, three times per week.
  - Once remission has been achieved with steroids and IV cyclophosphamide or rituximab, use azathioprine or methotrexate for 12 to 18 months for maintenance therapy.[8]

Second Line
- Consider **plasma exchange** in refractory cases.
- Management of HBV-related PAN involves treatment of both vasculitis and HBV infection.
  - Use steroids in the first few weeks to control the vasculitis, then stop them abruptly to enhance viral clearance and increase the rate of seroconversion of HBV e antigen to HBV e antibody. Continued use of steroids and other immunosuppressants jeopardizes viral clearance and promotes chronic infection.[9,10]
  - Standard anti-HBV agents (e.g., interferon-α 2b, lamivudine) are used in conjunction.
  - If seroconversion occurs, remission can be obtained and relapses are rare.

Other Nonpharmacologic Therapies

In patients with PAN associated with HBV infection, plasma exchange has been used after glucocorticoids are withdrawn to control the symptoms.[10]

Recurrent Disease

Mild recurrences can be treated with glucocorticoids, but moderate-to-severe recurrences will require reinitiation of remission-induction treatment as discussed earlier (combined glucocorticoids and IV cyclophosphamide or rituximab).

COMPLICATIONS

Complications of PAN vary and depend on which organ systems are involved as well as how much damage has occurred before treatment.

MONITORING/FOLLOW-UP

- Follow-up involves clinical and laboratory assessment of disease status and monitoring of medication side effects and toxicities.
- In patients with HBV-related PAN, consultation with a hepatologist is strongly advised.

OUTCOME/PROGNOSIS

- PAN tends to be monophasic.
- Prognosis depends on the number of five-factor score risk factors present.[6]
  - Patients with no risk factors have 88% 5-year survival rate.
  - Patients with one risk factor have 74% 5-year survival rate.
  - Patients with 2 and above risk factors have 54% 5-year survival rate.

REFERENCES

1. Jennette JC, Falk RJ, Andrassy K, et al. Nomenclature of systemic vasculitides: Proposal of an international consensus conference. *Arthritis Rheum.* 1994;37:187–192.
2. Saadoun D, Terrier B, Semoun O, et al. Hepatitis C virus-associated polyarteritis nodosa. *Arthritis Care Res (Hoboken).* 2011;63:427–435.
3. Maillard-Lefebvre H, Launay D, Mouquet F, et al. Polyarteritis nodosa-related coronary aneurysms. *J Rheumatol.* 2008;35:933–934.
4. Lightfoot RW Jr, Michel BA, Bloch DA, et al. The American College of Rheumatology 1990 criteria for the classification of polyarteritis nodosa. *Arthritis Rheum.* 1990;33:1088–1093.
5. Kobayashi H, Yokoe I, Hattan N, et al. Cardiac magnetic resonance imaging in polyarteritis nodosa. *J Rheumatol.* 2010;37:2427–2429.
6. Guillevin L, Lhote F, Gayraud M, et al. Prognostic factors in polyarteritis nodosa and Churg–Strauss syndrome: A prospective study in 342 patients. *Medicine (Baltimore).* 1996;75:17–28.

7. Silva L, Miranda K, Guedes A, et al. Rituximab as an alternative for patients with severe systemic vasculitis refractory to conventional therapy: Report of seven cases and literature review. *Rev Bras Reumatol.* 2015;55:531–535.

8. Guillevin L, Pagnoux C. Therapeutic strategies for systemic necrotizing vasculitides. *Allergol Int.* 2007;56:105–111.

9. Guillevin L, Lhote F. Treatment of polyarteritis nodosa and microscopic polyangiitis. *Arthritis Rheum.* 1998;41:2100–2105.

10. Guillevin L, Mahr A, Cohen P, et al. Short-term corticosteroids then lamivudine and plasma exchanges to treat hepatitis B virus-related polyarteritis nodosa. *Arthritis Rheum.* 2004;51:482–487.

Granulomatosis with Polyangiitis

28

Anneliese M. Flynn and Jonathan J. Miner

GENERAL PRINCIPLES

- Granulomatosis with polyangiitis (GPA) is a systemic vasculitis usually associated with **antineutrophil cytoplasmic antibodies (ANCAs)**.
- GPA most often affects the **respiratory tract and the kidney**.
- Treatment involves immunosuppression and is individually tailored primarily on the basis of severity of end-organ involvement.

Definition

GPA, also known as ANCA-associated granulomatous vasculitis, was defined by the Chapel Hill Consensus Conference as a granulomatous inflammation involving the respiratory tract and vasculitis affecting small- to medium-sized vessels, commonly with a necrotizing glomerulonephritis.[1]

Classification

- The European League Against Rheumatism (EULAR) recommends classification based on disease severity.[2]
- **Localized:** Upper and/or lower respiratory tract disease, without any other systemic involvement or constitutional symptoms
- **Early systemic:** Without organ-threatening or life-threatening disease
- **Generalized:** Renal or other organ-threatening disease, serum creatinine less than 5.6 mg/dL
- **Severe:** Renal or other vital organ failure, serum creatinine ≥5.6 mg/dL
- **Refractory:** Progressive disease unresponsive to glucocorticoids alone (common) and cyclophosphamide (uncommon)

Epidemiology

- GPA affects both men and women equally. GPA affects mostly Caucasians. The peak age of onset is in the range of 65 to 74, though there is wide variation.
- The prevalence has been estimated to be about 10 to 20 cases per million, although this may underestimate the true prevalence. Milder and more limited forms are being recognized with the availability of ANCA testing.
- The incidence is estimated to be about 3 to 14 cases per million.

Pathophysiology

- **ANCA is positive in GPA about 80% to 90% of the time.** The cytoplasmic ANCA (c-ANCA) in GPA has been identified as an **antibody to proteinase-3** (anti-PR3), a cytoplasmic glycoprotein present in active form in monocytes and endothelial cells and in the azurophilic granules of neutrophils. PR3 is involved in neutrophil migration and cytokine modulation.
- The role of c-ANCA in the pathogenesis of GPA is controversial. Although animal studies show that serum anti-PR3 antibodies result in lesions similar to those found in GPA, antibodies to PR-3 are not present in all cases.
- **GPA is a pauci-immune syndrome** in which immune complex deposition and complement activation are not prominent features.

DIAGNOSIS

Clinical Presentation

- **Initial phase**
  - The initial phase is characterized by chronic inflammation, usually in the upper airways. Sinusitis develops as the initial symptom in more than 50% of patients and develops in more than 85% of patients at some time during the course of illness. Other nasal symptoms include sinus obstruction, mucosal swelling, hearing loss, ulcers, septal perforation, epistaxis, serosanguinous discharge, and saddle-nose deformity. Sinusitis is commonly progressive and refractory to the usual therapies and severe. Sinus biopsies rarely show granulomatous inflammation.
  - Granulomatous inflammation may occur in the oral cavity, retrobulbar space, and trachea, especially if mass-type lesions are present.
  - Laryngotracheal disease can be asymptomatic or present as hoarseness, stridor, or acute airway obstruction. Subglottic stenosis occurs in approximately 15% of adults and 50% of children.
  - Myalgias and arthralgias are common presenting symptoms.
- **Generalized phase**
  - The generalized phase is characterized by **systemic signs and symptoms of small-vessel vasculitis. Fever and weight loss are common.**
  - **Pulmonary disease** is a cardinal feature. Cough, hemoptysis, and pleuritis are common. Pulmonary hemorrhage, infiltrates, cavities, nodules, pleural effusions, and mediastinal lymphadenopathy may be present.
  - **Renal disease develops in approximately 80% of patients, usually after other manifestations.** The disease progression can be rapid once glomerulonephritis develops.
  - GPA may affect any segment of the urinary tract. Hematuria without red blood cell (RBC) casts usually indicates nonrenal urinary tract involvement.
  - Although most patients experience **arthralgias,** some patients exhibit **migratory polyarthritis**.
    - The pattern of joint involvement is variable and may be monoarticular, oligoarticular, or polyarticular.
    - Presentation with symmetric polyarthritis can be mistaken for rheumatoid arthritis (RA), especially if a positive value for rheumatoid factor (RF) is obtained.
    - Low titers of RF are seen in 20% to 40% of patients with GPA.
  - **Neurologic disease** develops in approximately 50% of patients but is rarely a presenting feature.
  - **Mononeuritis multiplex and symmetric polyneuropathy** are the most common patterns.
  - **Cranial neuropathies** also occur, with II (optic neuritis), VI, and VII being the most common.
- **Common gastrointestinal (GI) manifestations** are abdominal pain, diarrhea, and bleeding from ulcerations in both the small and large intestines.
- **Cutaneous manifestations** are typical of the small-vessel vasculitis and include palpable purpura, ulcers, subcutaneous nodules, papules, and vesicles. They tend to parallel disease activity.
- GPA can also have **ocular manifestations,** including keratoconjunctivitis, scleritis, episcleritis, pseudotumor of the orbit, conjunctivitis, and uveitis.

Diagnostic Criteria

The American College of Rheumatology 1990 classification criteria for GPA are presented in Table 28-1.[3]

TABLE 28-1	AMERICAN COLLEGE OF RHEUMATOLOGY 1990 CRITERIA FOR GRANULOMATOSIS WITH POLYANGIITIS

The presence of at least two of the following four is required:
- Nasal or oral inflammation (painful or painless ulcers, purulent or bloody nasal discharge)
- Abnormal chest radiograph (nodules, fixed infiltrates, or cavities)
- Hematuria or red blood cell casts in urine sediment
- Pathologic evidence of granulomas, leukocytoclastic vasculitis, and necrosis

Adapted from: Leavitt RY, Fauci AS, Bloch DA, et al. The American College of Rheumatology 1990 criteria for the classification of Wegener's granulomatosis. *Arthritis Rheum.* 1990;33:1101–1107.

Differential Diagnosis

- **Cocaine,** especially when inhaled with the adulterant **levamisole,** can induce pseudovasculitis with nasal and upper airway lesions that are similar to GPA. ANCAs reacting with human neutrophil clastase (HNE) have been reported to distinguish the cocaine-related syndrome from a true autoimmune vasculitis.[4]
- The differential diagnosis of GPA should be considered carefully. Inappropriate diagnosis of GPA and subsequent **treatment with potent immunosuppression may prove fatal if the underlying disease is infectious.** Conditions to be considered include the following:
  - Granulomatous diseases (tuberculosis, histoplasmosis, blastomycosis, coccidioidomycosis, sarcoidosis)
  - Neoplastic diseases (lymphomas, head and neck malignancies, metastatic adenocarcinoma)
  - Connective tissue diseases (systemic lupus erythematosus, relapsing polychondritis, antiphospholipid antibody syndrome, scleroderma, mixed connective tissue disease, Still's disease)
  - Small-vessel vasculitides
  - Goodpasture's disease

Diagnostic Testing

Laboratories
- The presence of **c-ANCA and, more specifically, anti-PR3 antibodies,** supports the diagnosis, although c-ANCA may be negative in earlier and less fulminant forms of GPA.
- **Elevated serum creatinine and blood urea nitrate (BUN)** indicate renal impairment.
- Urinalysis may show hematuria, and microscopy may reveal RBC casts, indicating glomerulonephritis.
- Markers of inflammation, including elevated **erythrocyte sedimentation rate (ESR), C-reactive protein (CRP),** leukocytosis, and thrombocytosis, are commonly present in GPA.
- **Anemia of chronic disease** is common in GPA.
- Leukopenia and thrombocytopenia are rarely present in untreated GPA and should prompt a search for other disorders.
- Complement levels are typically normal or slightly elevated.

Imaging
- **Chest imaging**
  - Perform chest radiography on all patients suspected of having GPA; asymptomatic patients may have significant radiologic abnormalities.
  - Use chest computed tomography (CT) scans in patients with hemoptysis with clear plain films because early pulmonary hemorrhage, small areas of cavitation, nodules, and interstitial disease may not be visible on plain films. Chest CT should be considered in patients with abnormal plain films to further define the extent of disease.[3]
- **Sinus imaging:** Sinus CT scans are superior to plain sinus films to define the extent of disease.

Diagnostic Procedures
- **Pulmonary function tests** with flow volume loops may be useful to define irreversible extrathoracic or intrathoracic obstruction caused by airway inflammation, leading to tracheal stenosis or collapse.
- **Bronchoscopy** is useful when pulmonary hemorrhage is present or suspected. Transbronchial biopsy, bronchoalveolar lavage, and endoscopic inspection of lesions detected on imaging may be useful in helping to establish the diagnosis of GPA and also in ruling out infectious mimics.
- The yield of **tissue diagnosis** for GPA depends on the biopsy site, specimen size, and the manner in which the tissue is collected.
  - **Open lung biopsies** with adequate tissue are most often diagnostic, showing the hallmark features of **vasculitis, necrosis, and granulomatous inflammation**. The yield of open lung biopsy is highest when larger samples are obtained and is frequently diagnostic, especially if lesions are radiographically evident.
  - **Transbronchial biopsies are rarely diagnostic;** however, when used in combination with bronchoalveolar lavage and cultures, they are useful for ruling out infections that mimic or complicate GPA.
  - **Renal biopsy** shows **pauci-immune glomerulonephritis** with occasional medium-vessel vasculitis and, rarely, granulomatous changes. Immunofluorescence studies are negative or weakly positive for antibody and complement deposition. **Of note,** a focal segmental glomerulosclerosis (FSGS)/chronic scarring pattern can be seen later in the disease course on renal biopsy.
  - **Upper airway biopsies**, especially sinus biopsies, tend to show chronic, nonspecific inflammation and are rarely diagnostic. Most specimens are compatible with but not diagnostic of GPA because they show acute and chronic inflammation.

TREATMENT

- Base the treatment plan on the objective presence of activity, its site, and severity.
- Lung, kidney, neurologic, and vision-threatening ocular diseases usually merit high-dose glucocorticoids and immunosuppressants.
- **Glucocorticoids alone are inadequate in systemic disease, especially in patients with renal involvement.**

Medications
- **Induction therapy**
  - Intravenous (IV) methylprednisolone (1,000 mg) may be used for the first 3 days in cases of immediately life-threatening fulminant disease (e.g., pulmonary hemorrhage or rapidly progressive glomerulonephritis), followed by **oral prednisone,** 1 mg/kg daily dose with a prolonged taper.

- ○ **Rituximab,** 375 mg/m² weekly for 4 weeks, with glucocorticoids has been shown to be noninferior to cyclophosphamide and may be superior in preventing relapse. Rituximab has a less toxic side-effect profile compared to cyclophosphamide.[5]
- ○ Monthly IV cyclophosphamide, 15 mg/kg, has less toxicity compared to daily oral cyclophosphamide but may have a higher rate of relapse. IV cyclophosphamide 500 to 750 mg/m² every 4 weeks is an alternative option for dosing.
- ○ MESNA may be given with oral cyclophosphamide to reduce bladder toxicity.
- ○ Oral cyclophosphamide, approximately 2 mg/kg, is sometimes used in severe disease.
- **Maintenance therapy**
  - ○ Once a remission has been achieved, continue steroid taper and switch to maintenance rituximab 500 mg administered at days 0 and 14, then 500 mg every 6 months at months 6, 12, and 18.[6]
  - ○ **Azathioprine,** 2 mg/kg, is an alternative for maintenance therapy.[7]
  - ○ **Methotrexate** and **mycophenolate mofetil** are also alternatives for maintenance therapy. Methotrexate should not be used in patients with impaired renal function.
  - ○ **Trimethoprim/sulfamethoxazole** (TMP/SMX), 160 mg/800 mg three times a week, for *Pneumocystis jirovecii* pneumonia (PCP) prophylaxis should be considered in patients on immunosuppressants.
- **Limited upper airway involvement**
  - ○ Local therapy with nasal irrigation and nasal steroids may be given.
  - ○ TMP/SMX may also be effective.
  - ○ Subglottic stenosis is treated with mechanical dilatation and intratracheal injection of a long-acting steroid.
- IV immunoglobulin and plasmapheresis are generally not thought to be effective, though plasma exchange is sometimes used for severe pulmonary hemorrhage, renal vasculitis, or concomitant anti–glomerular basement membrane (GBM) disease.
- The recent PEXIVAS trial showed that plasmapheresis does not reduce the risk of end-stage renal disease or death in patients with ANCA vasculitis.[8]

MONITORING/FOLLOW-UP

- Follow-up should include laboratory and radiographic studies of the upper airway and lung and renal function.
- ANCA and anti-PR3 antibody levels correlate roughly with disease activity in large groups of patients, but direct studies of organ function should be the primary guide to therapy.[9]
- TMP/SMX, 160 mg/800 mg twice daily (bid), for 24 months during remission has been shown to prevent relapses.
- Monitoring for toxicity of treatment modalities and opportunistic infections should be done.
- Patients with GPA are at a high risk for deep vein thrombosis.

OUTCOME/PROGNOSIS

- There is considerable variability, mostly depending on the presentation. GPA limited to the upper airways has a better prognosis and higher response rate to treatment than generalized and severe GPA.
- **Alveolar hemorrhage and severe renal failure portend the worst prognosis.**
- **Relapse occurs in as many as 50% of patients.**
- Untreated patients have a survival rate of only 20% at 2 years. However, the 2-year survival rate for treated patients is about 90%.
- Morbidity of treated GPA is related to irreversible organ damage, treatment toxicity, and opportunistic infections.

REFERENCES

1. Jennette JC, Falk RJ, Andrassy K, et al. Nomenclature of systemic vasculitides. Proposal of an international consensus conference. *Arthritis Rheum.* 1994;37:187–192.
2. Mukhtyar C, Guillevin L, Cid MC, et al. EULAR recommendations for the management of primary small and medium vessel vasculitis. *Ann Rheum Dis.* 2009;68:310–317.
3. Leavitt RY, Fauci AS, Bloch DA, et al. The American College of Rheumatology 1990 criteria for the classification of Wegener's granulomatosis. *Arthritis Rheum.* 1990;33:1101–1107.
4. Walsh NM, Green PJ, Burlingame RW, et al. Cocaine-related retiform purpura: Evidence to incriminate the adulterant, levamisole. *J Cutan Pathol.* 2010;37:1212–1219.
5. Stone JH, Merkel PA, Spiera R, et al. Rituximab versus cyclophosphamide for ANCA-associated vasculitis. *N Engl J Med.* 2010;363:221–232.
6. Guillevin L, Pagnoux C, Karras C, et al. Rituximab versus azathioprine for maintenance in ANCA-associated vasculitis. *N Engl J Med.* 2014;371:1771–1780.
7. Jayne D, Rasmussen N, Andrassy K, et al. A randomized trial of maintenance therapy for vasculitis associated with antineutrophil cytoplasmic autoantibodies. *N Engl J Med.* 2003;349:36–44.
8. Walsh M, Merkel P, Jayne D. The effects of plasma exchange and reduced-dose glucocorticoids during remission-induction for treatment of severe ANCA-associated vasculitis. *Arthritis Rheum.* 2018;70(suppl 10).
9. Finkielman JD, Merkel PA, Schroeder D, et al. Antiproteinase 3 antineutrophil cytoplasmic antibodies and disease activity in Wegener granulomatosis. *Ann Intern Med.* 2007;147:611–619.

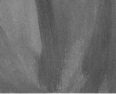

Eosinophilic Granulomatosis with Polyangiitis

29

Can M. Sungur and Jonathan J. Miner

GENERAL PRINCIPLES

- Previously known as Churg–Strauss syndrome (CSS)
- Involves small- and medium-size vessels and associated with eosinophilia and asthma
- Formal diagnosis outlined in section "Diagnostic Criteria"

Definition

The Chapel Hill Consensus Conference defines **eosinophilic granulomatosis with polyangiitis (EGPA)**, which was previously known as **Churg–Strauss Syndrome (CSS)**, as an eosinophil-rich, granulomatous inflammation involving the respiratory tract and necrotizing vasculitis affecting small- to medium-sized vessels associated with **asthma and peripheral eosinophilia**.

Epidemiology

- EGPA is a rare disease, with an annual incidence of approximately 2.4 cases per million.
- EGPA affects both men and women equally.
- The asthma associated with EGPA usually begins in the fourth or fifth decade but can occur at any age.

Pathophysiology

- The two diagnostic lesions are **arterial and venous vasculitis** and **extravascular necrotizing granulomas,** usually with eosinophilic infiltration of tissue. These findings coexist temporally only in few patients.
- The signs and symptoms of EGPA are caused by the effects these lesions have on the involved organ system at a given time and by the systemic effects of inflammation.
- The most commonly affected organ systems (in decreasing order) are pulmonary, neurologic, cutaneous, otorhinolaryngeal, musculoskeletal, gastrointestinal (GI), cardiac, and renal.
- **Antineutrophil cytoplasmic antibody (ANCA)**, in particular, the perinuclear **anti-myeloperoxidase (anti-MPO) variant**, has been associated with EGPA in 40% to 60% of patients, but its role in pathogenesis is not well understood.

Risk Factors

- An association with leukotriene modifiers (zafirlukast and montelukast) has been recognized in patients with steroid-dependent asthma who were tapered from glucocorticoids after initiation of the leukotriene modifier.
- Most of these patients had milder airway obstruction and a greater incidence of acute dilated cardiomyopathy than other patients with EGPA.
- It is unclear whether the leukotriene modifiers induced the disease or the steroid tapering led to expression of the disease in patients with preexisting EGPA. The latter seems more likely.[1]

DIAGNOSIS

Clinical Presentation

- **There are three phases** of EGPA.
  - The first is a **prodrome** beginning in childhood and lasting up to 30 years, characterized by **allergic rhinitis, sinusitis, and nasal polyposis. Asthma** develops later in life at an average age of 35 years. The asthma is usually severe and requires systemic glucocorticoids.
  - The second phase is characterized by **peripheral blood and tissue eosinophilia.** Löffler's syndrome (transient, acute, pulmonary eosinophilic infiltrates), chronic eosinophilic pneumonia, and eosinophilic gastroenteritis are common. The pulmonary infiltrates tend to be peripheral, patchy, parenchymal, migratory, and transient and may be associated with eosinophilic pulmonary effusions. However, these are neither sensitive nor specific pulmonary patterns.
  - The third phase is characterized by **small-vessel vasculitis**, with a mean time of onset of 3 years after the development of asthma. The symptoms are usually nonspecific, representing constitutional manifestations of systemic inflammation (e.g., myalgias, arthralgias, fatigue, and weight loss). Asthma usually worsens during this phase.
- **Organ system involvement**
  - **Pulmonary manifestations** include **asthma, which is present in over 95% of patients with EGPA.** Asthma is usually difficult to treat and requires glucocorticoids. It usually develops years before other organ involvement. Later on, eosinophilic pulmonary infiltrates, effusions, and, rarely, pulmonary hemorrhage may develop.[2]
  - **Cutaneous signs** are similar to those of other vasculitides and include palpable purpura of the lower extremities, subcutaneous nodules of the scalp and lower extremities, livedo reticularis, and infarction.
  - **Neurologic manifestations** are similar to those of polyarteritis nodosa (PAN), with **mononeuritis multiplex** in about two-thirds of cases. Distal, usually symmetric, **peripheral neuropathies** are also common. Cranial nerve palsies are less common, with ischemic optic neuritis being the most common. Cerebral infarctions are rare.
  - **Cardiac disease is the most common cause of death. Eosinophilic myocarditis and coronary vasculitis** are the most frequent cardiac lesions and can lead to severe heart failure or myocardial infarction (MI). Pericardial effusions are also common, but only occasionally lead to hemodynamic compromise. Endomyocardial fibrosis is rare.
  - **GI tract manifestations** account for a substantial number of deaths and include tissue eosinophilic infiltration and/or mesenteric vasculitis with resultant ischemia, infarction, and perforation.
  - **Renal involvement tends to be mild.** The most common manifestations are hematuria, albuminuria, and focal segmental necrotizing glomerulonephritis, although severe necrotizing glomerulonephritis has been described.

Diagnostic Criteria

The American College of Rheumatology 1990 criteria for EGPA are presented in Table 29-1.[3]

Differential Diagnosis

The differential diagnosis includes PAN, microscopic polyangiitis (MPA), granulomatosis with polyangiitis (GPA), chronic eosinophilic pneumonia, and idiopathic hypereosinophilic syndrome (IHS).

- **PAN** usually spares the glomeruli and lungs, demonstrates arterial microaneurysms and stenoses, and tends to be ANCA negative.
- **MPA** causes necrotizing vasculitis of arterioles, venules, and capillaries without granulomas. It often involves the glomeruli and lungs.

TABLE 29-1	THE AMERICAN COLLEGE OF RHEUMATOLOGY 1990 CRITERIA FOR EOSINOPHILIC GRANULOMATOSIS WITH POLYANGIITIS

The presence of at least four of the following six is required:
- Asthma
- Eosinophilia > 10%
- Mononeuropathy or polyneuropathy attributable to a systemic vasculitis
- Migratory or transient infiltrates on chest radiography
- Paranasal sinus abnormality (acute or chronic paranasal pain or radiographic opacification of paranasal sinuses)
- Extravascular eosinophils on biopsy

Adapted from: Masi AT, Hunder GC, Lie JT. The American College of Rheumatology 1990 criteria for the classification of Churg-Strauss syndrome (allergic granulomatosis and angiitis). *Arthritis Rheum*. 1990;33:1094–1100.

- The key clinical, laboratory, and histologic findings usually make the distinction between **GPA** and EGPA straightforward.
- **Chronic eosinophilic pneumonia** commonly has no extrapulmonary findings, affects women, and has no granulomatous or vasculitic component.
- **IHS** typically has endomyocardial fibrosis and no vasculitic, granulomatous, asthmatic, or allergic component. IHS responds poorly to systemic steroids.

Diagnostic Testing

A patient with late-onset and worsening asthma, peripheral eosinophilia, and transient migratory lung infiltrates should raise suspicion for EGPA.
- Laboratory data supporting EGPA include **peripheral eosinophilia** (usually 5,000–9,000 eosinophils/μL), elevated erythrocyte sedimentation rate (ESR), thrombocytosis, and **elevated immunoglobulin E (IgE)** levels.
- A positive **p-ANCA**, specifically **anti-MPO** antibody, supports the diagnosis, but its absence does not rule out EGPA.
- Urine protein and plasma creatinine and assessment of cardiac function provide prognostic information.

Diagnostic Procedures

- Biopsies of skin, nerve, or lung lesions may be highly suggestive.
- They may be nonspecific or helpful in sorting through the differential diagnosis.

TREATMENT

- Initial therapy to induce remission of EGPA includes the following options:
  - The response to **oral prednisone**, 1 mg/kg daily, is dramatic. Within 1 month, most patients are clinically improved and have a decreasing if not normal eosinophil count and ESR. Steroids should be tapered once the ESR has normalized.
  - **Pulse IV methylprednisolone**, 1,000 mg daily for 3 days, is used for life-threatening disease.
  - Studies suggest that combined therapy with **cyclophosphamide** (usually 0.6 g/m^2 monthly IV doses with adjustments based on laboratory response or 2 mg/kg everyday orally [PO] doses) has increased efficacy in those patients who have signs and symptoms of severe or life-threatening disease. IV cyclophosphamide is preferred for initial therapy, with oral administration reserved for severe disease or relapses.

○ Anti–interleukin 5 (anti–IL-5) antibodies such as mepolizumab and IL-5 receptor antibodies such as benralizumab are being studied for EGPA. They have previously been used in patients with severe asthma and eosinophilia. IL-5 is produced by eosinophils and potentially mediates the disease manifestations of EGPA. Mepolizumab has been approved for EGPA at 300 mg every 4 weeks in addition to glucocorticoid therapy in patients not controlled with glucocorticoids alone. A randomized clinical trial showed a higher proportion of patients achieving remission and longer sustained periods of remission reducing overall glucocorticoid use.[4]

○ Anti-IgE therapy with omalizumab has been beneficial for EGPA with primarily asthma and sinonasal disease. A retrospective series showed omalizumab reduced prednisone use and increased achievement of remission in refractory or relapsing EGPA.[5]

○ For milder disease, **methotrexate or azathioprine** may be used in combination with glucocorticoids to induce disease remission.

• **Long-term therapy** to maintain remission and allow reduction of glucocorticoid dose is often used in patients with EGPA.

○ Usually, **azathioprine, leflunomide, or methotrexate** is employed after induction of remission (6–12 months) or in patients who are in remission but require more than 10 to 20 mg of prednisone.

○ Methotrexate is used more cautiously because it can cause hypersensitivity pneumonitis that is difficult to distinguish from a reoccurrence of EGPA.[6]

• Mycophenolate mofetil, rituximab, hydroxyurea, intravenous immunoglobulin (IVIG), and plasma exchange have also been used for the treatment of steroid-resistant EGPA.[7–10]

COMPLICATIONS

• Complications of treatment are usually from opportunistic infections or related to long-term use of glucocorticoids.

• Patients receiving cyclophosphamide should receive prophylaxis for *Pneumocystis jirovecii* pneumonia with oral trimethoprim 160 mg/sulfamethoxazole 800 mg, three times per week.

• When cyclophosphamide is administered IV, mercaptoethane sulfonate (MESNA) should be given to reduce the risk of drug-induced cystitis (dosing of MESNA is the same as that of cyclophosphamide). Half of the dose is administered prior to the cyclophosphamide infusion, and the other half is infused 2 hours following the cyclophosphamide infusion.

• Glucocorticoids should be weaned as quickly as appropriate, and patients should be evaluated for osteoporosis, diabetes, and hypertension and warned about weight gain.

MONITORING/FOLLOW-UP

• Follow-up involves clinical and laboratory assessment of disease status and monitoring of medication side effects and toxicities.

• Perform frequent eosinophil counts, as increases in counts tend to precede flares of EGPA.

OUTCOME/PROGNOSIS

• With the use of steroids and immunosuppressants, remission rates have been more than 75%.

• Factors associated with lower 5-year survival rates include proteinuria more than 1 g/day, creatinine more than 1.6 mg/dL, cardiomyopathy, and GI tract or central nervous system (CNS) involvement.

REFERENCES

1. Weller PF, Plaut M, Taggart V, et al. The relationship of asthma therapy and Churg-Strauss syndrome: NIH workshop summary report. *J Allergy Clin Immunol.* 2001;108:175–183.
2. Lhote FC, Guillevin L. Polyarteritis nodosa, microscopic polyangiitis, and Churg-Strauss syndrome. Clinical aspects and treatment. *Rheum Dis Clin North Am.* 1995;21:911–947.
3. Masi AT, Hunder GC, Lie JT, et al. The American College of Rheumatology 1990 criteria for the classification of Churg-Strauss syndrome (allergic granulomatosis and angiitis). *Arthritis Rheum.* 1990;33:1094–1100.
4. Wechsler M, Akuthota P, Jayne D, et al. Mepolizumab or placebo for eosinophilic granulomatosis with polyangiitis. *N Engl J Med.* 2017;376:1921–1932
5. Jachiet M, Samson M, Cottin V, et al. Anti-IgE monoclonal antibody (omalizumab) in refractory and relapsing eosinophilic granulomatosis with polyangiitis (Churg-Strauss): Data on seventeen patients. *Arthritis Rheumatol.* 2016;68:2274–2282
6. De Groot K, Rasmussen N, Bacon PA, et al. Randomized trial of cyclophosphamide versus methotrexate for induction of remission in early systemic antineutrophil cytoplasmic antibody-associated vasculitis. *Arthritis Rheum.* 2005;52:2461–2469.
7. Assaf C, Mewis G, Orfanos CE, et al. Churg-Strauss syndrome: Successful treatment with mycophenolate mofetil. *Br J Dermatol.* 2004;150:598–600.
8. Jones RB, Ferraro AJ, Chaudhry AN, et al. A multicenter survey of rituximab therapy for refractory antineutrophil cytoplasmic antibody-associated vasculitis. *Arthritis Rheum.* 2009;60:2156–2168.
9. Lee RU, Stevenson DD. Hydroxyurea in the treatment of Churg-Strauss syndrome. *J Allergy Clin Immunol.* 2009;124:1110–1111.
10. Guiellevin L, Cevallos R, Durand-Gasselin B, et al. Treatment of glomerulonephritis in microscopic polyangiitis and Churg-Strauss syndrome. Indications of plasma exchanges, meta-analysis of 2 randomized studies on 140 patients, 32 with glomerulonephritis. *Ann Med Interne (Paris).* 1997;148:198–204.

Microscopic Polyangiitis

30

Anneliese M. Flynn and Jonathan J. Miner

GENERAL PRINCIPLES

Microscopic polyangiitis (MPA) is a **small-vessel vasculitis** initially deemed a microscopic form of polyarteritis nodosa (microscopic PAN) because of its clinical similarity to PAN, with the additional involvement of arterioles, capillaries, and venules giving rise to glomerulonephritis.[1,2] However, unlike PAN, MPA is not associated with hepatitis B.

Definition

- MPA is defined by the Chapel Hill Consensus Conference as a necrotizing vasculitis with few or no immune deposits (**pauci-immune**) affecting **small vessels such as capillaries, arterioles, and venules**. Medium-sized vessels may also be involved. This may result in **necrotizing glomerulonephritis and pulmonary capillaritis.**[1]
- Involvement of small-sized vessels distinguishes MPA from PAN.

Classification

MPA is classified as a small-vessel vasculitis. See Chapter 24 for further review of the classification of vasculitides.

Epidemiology

- The incidence of MPA in Europe is 2 to 11 cases per million. MPA is two to three times more frequent than granulomatosis with polyangiitis (GPA) in Southern Europe, whereas in Northern Europe, GPA is more prevalent.
- In Asia, there is a much greater incidence of MPA compared to GPA. Kuwait has the greatest incidence at 24 cases per million. The prevalence in other non-Caucasian populations is less well defined.
- The mean age is 50 to 70 years.

Etiology

- The etiology of MPA is not well established. Several environmental triggers have been implicated, but these do not explain the majority of cases.
- **Infections**
  - Some individuals with glomerulonephritis secondary to MPA have antibodies directed to human lysosomal membrane protein 2 (LAMP-2). The epitope recognized by anti–LAMP-2 antibodies is homologous to type 1 fimbrial adhesin (FimH), an adhesion protein produced by gram-negative bacteria. Rats immunized with FimH produce anti-LAMP antibodies and develop crescentic glomerulonephritis.[3]
  - Parvovirus B19 infection may induce antineutrophil cytoplasmic antibodies (ANCAs), but these are typically transient.[4]

- **Drugs**
  - Medications including hydralazine, minocycline, tumor necrosis factor (TNF) antagonists, penicillamine, sulfasalazine, and propylthiouracil (PTU) have been associated with anti-myeloperoxidase (MPO)–ANCA seropositivity and clinical vasculitis.
  - **PTU-induced MPA is the most recognized form of drug-induced vasculitis.** One-fifth of patients taking PTU will develop ANCA seropositivity, and of these, about one-fourth will develop overt vasculitis. Both the ANCA seropositivity and clinical vasculitis resolve with cessation of PTU.
- **Silica**
  - About 20% to 40% of patients with ANCA-associated vasculitis have been exposed to silica, and about 20% of perinuclear (p)-ANCA–positive individuals have been exposed to silica.
  - The odds ratio for the risk of association of silica exposure with vasculitis ranges from 2 to 14.[5]

Pathophysiology

- ANCA may be involved in the pathogenesis of MPA in a two-step process:
  - Low levels of inflammatory cytokines such as interleukin (IL)-1 and TNF-α prime neutrophils to express MPO on their surface.
  - Antibodies to MPO–ANCA bind neutrophils via the surface MPO antigen and/or Fc receptors. Neutrophils become activated, causing the release of reactive oxygen species and lytic enzymes.
- This process only occurs if neutrophils are attached to a surface such as a vessel wall.
- This model fails to address patients with MPA who are ANCA negative.

Risk Factors

- Environmental risk factors such as infections and silica exposure as mentioned previously have been suggested.
- Drugs such as hydralazine, minocycline, TNF antagonists, penicillamine, sulfasalazine, and PTU can induce MPA, but the risk is low.
- Genetic risk factors have not been identified.

DIAGNOSIS

Diagnosis is based on clinical, serologic, and pathologic findings.[2]

Clinical Presentation

- The most common manifestations of MPA are constitutional, renal, pulmonary, gastrointestinal (GI), cutaneous, musculoskeletal, and neurologic. Onset may be acute or indolent.
- **Constitutional symptoms** (e.g., weakness, weight loss, fevers, malaise, arthralgias) are present in more than 70% of patients.
- **Renal involvement** occurs in more than 80% and can range from asymptomatic active urinary sediment to end-stage renal failure requiring hemodialysis.
- **Pulmonary manifestations** occur in 25% to 55% of patients and include cough, dyspnea, hemoptysis, and pleuritic chest pain. **Pulmonary hemorrhage** occurs in approximately 25% of patients and may be due to either capillaritis or bronchial arteritis, interstitial fibrosis may also occur.
- **Cutaneous manifestations** occur in 30% to 60% of patients. **Palpable purpura** is the most common finding, but livedo reticularis, nodules, urticaria, and ulcers from skin necrosis may also be seen.
- **Abdominal pain** (30%–60%) and GI bleeding (20%–30%) may be present; however, severe hemorrhage, ulcerations, ischemia, and perforation are less likely to occur in MPA than in PAN.

- One-third to two-thirds of patients will have **neurologic manifestations,** such as **peripheral neuropathy and mononeuritis multiplex** and, less commonly, central nervous system (CNS) manifestations of pachymeningitis and cerebral infarctions (hemorrhagic or ischemic).

Differential Diagnosis

- Both small- and medium-size vessel vasculitides are included in the differential diagnosis of MPA.[1]
  - **Pauci-immune immunofluorescence on histology** differentiates MPA from the immune-complex–mediated small-vessel vasculitides, cryoglobulinemic vasculitis, and Henoch–Schönlein purpura.
  - Lack of granulomas on histopathology distinguishes MPA from GPA.
  - The presence of asthma and eosinophilia suggests EGPA.
- Distinguishing between MPA and PAN can be difficult. Table 30-1 compares these two diseases.[6]
  - Involvement of capillaries, arterioles, and venules distinguishes MPA from PAN.
  - **An association with ANCA is seen with MPA, but not with PAN. PAN is associated with hepatitis B, whereas MPA is not.**
- Other conditions to consider include Goodpasture's syndrome and vasculitis associated with other connective tissue diseases (e.g., systemic lupus erythematosus and rheumatoid arthritis).

TABLE 30-1	DISTINGUISHING FEATURES OF PAN AND MPA	
Manifestation	**PAN**	**MPA**
Vasculitis	Necrotizing, affects medium- and small-sized arteries, may sometimes involve arterioles, rarely granulomatous	Necrotizing, affects small vessels, may sometimes involve small- and medium-sized arteries, no granulomas
Renal	Renal vasculitis with renovascular hypertension, renal infarcts, and microaneurysms; no glomerulonephritis or RPGN	Glomerulonephritis including RPGN very common
Pulmonary	No alveolar hemorrhage	Alveolar hemorrhage common
Peripheral neuropathy	Present in 50%–80%	Present in 10%–50%
Relapses	Rare	Frequent
Lab data	ANCA positive in <20% of patients, association with HBV, mesenteric angiography commonly illustrates microaneurysms and stenoses	ANCA positive in 50%–80% of patients, no association with HBV, normal mesenteric angiography

ANCA, antineutrophil cytoplasmic antibody; HBV, hepatitis B virus; MPA, microscopic polyangiitis; PAN, polyarteritis nodosa; RPGN, rapidly progressive glomerulonephritis.

Adapted from: Guillevin L, Lhote F. Distinguishing polyarteritis nodosa from microscopic polyangiitis and implications for treatment. *Curr Opin Rheumatol.* 1995;7:20–24.

Diagnostic Testing

The diagnostic workup of MPA includes assessment of renal, pulmonary, and nerve function (e.g., serum creatinine, urinalysis, spirometry, chest radiography, nerve conduction studies).

Laboratories
- Common laboratory findings include elevated erythrocyte sedimentation rate (ESR) and C-reactive protein (CRP), leukocytosis, thrombocytosis, and normochromic normocytic anemia of chronic inflammation.
- Evaluation of renal function may reveal an elevated blood urea nitrogen (BUN) and creatinine and an **active urinary sediment** (proteinuria, hematuria, red blood cell [RBC] casts, and leukocyturia).
- C3 and C4 levels are normal or elevated.
- ANCA testing, either by indirect immunofluorescence or enzyme-linked immunosorbent assay (ELISA) for specific antigens (i.e., proteinase 3 [PR3] and MPO) is not uniformly standardized; therefore, diagnostic performance will vary by laboratory.
  - ANCA is present in about 75% of patients, usually p-ANCA/anti-MPO.[7]
  - ANCA positivity should be confirmed with ELISA testing for anti-MPO and anti-PR3 antibodies.[8]
  - In the appropriate clinical setting, p-ANCA has 98% specificity for MPA.[9]
  - The sensitivity of anti-MPO antibodies ranges broadly, depending on the kit used and the cutoff value selected.[9]
- Low-titer rheumatoid factor (RF) and antinuclear antibodies (ANAs) may also be present.

Imaging
- **Chest radiography** should be performed to evaluate for pulmonary manifestations. Patchy diffuse opacities are found in the setting of alveolar hemorrhage.
- **Computed tomography (CT) of the chest** demonstrates ground-glass opacifications in the setting of alveolar hemorrhage, and septal thickening and honeycombing may be present with interstitial fibrosis.
- **Mesenteric angiography** may be performed if necessary to differentiate PAN from MPA.
- Other organ-specific imaging may be required for evaluation of complications.

Diagnostic Procedures
- Almost all patients need **renal biopsies.**
  - **Focal segmental glomerulonephritis** is found in nearly 100% of patients with renal disease.
  - Glomerular crescents, fibrinoid necrosis, interstitial nephritis, and tubular atrophy may also be observed.
  - **The immunofluorescence pattern is pauci-immune**, with minimal immunoglobulin and complement deposition in the glomeruli.
- **Bronchoscopy with transbronchial biopsy and bronchoalveolar lavage** (BAL) is useful in demonstrating capillaritis and ruling out infectious causes of pulmonary hemorrhage.
  - BAL fluid is usually grossly hemorrhagic, and histology demonstrates hemosiderin-laden macrophages.
  - Biopsy of tissue in hemorrhagic areas can demonstrate necrotizing alveolar capillaritis with pauci-immune immunofluorescence. Other histologic patterns may demonstrate intra-alveolar and interstitial RBCs, fibrinoid necrosis, and intra-alveolar hemosiderosis.
- **Cutaneous biopsies** demonstrate **leukocytoclastic vasculitis.** Again, immunofluorescence demonstrates a pauci-immune pattern.

- **Nerve conduction velocity** (NCV) studies can identify peripheral neuropathies manifested as acute axonopathy, and **sural nerve biopsy** demonstrates necrotizing vasculitis in nearly 80% of patients with abnormal NCV studies.

TREATMENT

- Treatment is divided into two phases: induction and maintenance of remission.
  - **Glucocorticoids** are given at **induction,** and a prolonged taper is prescribed.
  - **Induction** of remission is established with **cyclophosphamide or rituximab,** whereas **maintenance** therapy is provided with **azathioprine or methotrexate.**
- Supportive measures with hemodialysis and mechanical ventilation may be required.
- Plasmapheresis may be considered in refractory cases.

Medications

- **Induction therapy**
  - **Intravenous (IV) methylprednisolone** (1,000 mg) may be used for the first 3 days in cases of immediately life-threatening fulminant disease (e.g., pulmonary hemorrhage or rapidly progressive glomerulonephritis), followed by oral prednisone, 1 mg/kg daily with a prolonged taper.
  - **Rituximab,** 375 mg/m² weekly for 4 weeks, with glucocorticoids has been shown to be noninferior to cyclophosphamide and may be superior in preventing relapse. Rituximab has a less toxic side-effect profile compared to cyclophosphamide.[10]
  - Monthly IV **cyclophosphamide** 15 mg/kg has less toxic complications compared to daily oral cyclophosphamide but may have a higher rate of relapse. IV cyclophosphamide 500 to 750 mg/m² every 4 weeks is an alternative option for dosing. MESNA should be given with IV cyclophosphamide to reduce bladder toxicity.
  - Oral cyclophosphamide, approximately 2 mg/kg, is also used.
- **Maintenance therapy**
  - Once remission has been achieved, continue steroid taper and switch to maintenance **rituximab** 1,000 mg administered at days 0 and 14 to prevent relapses.[11]
  - **Azathioprine,** 2 mg/kg orally (PO) daily, is an alternative for maintenance therapy.[12] Azathioprine is prescribed to complete a total of 18 months of therapy (from induction).
  - **Methotrexate** and **mycophenolate mofetil** could also be considered for maintenance therapy. Methotrexate should not be used with impaired renal function.
  - **Trimethoprim/sulfamethoxazole** (TMP/SMX), 160 mg/800 mg three times a week, for *Pneumocystis jirovecii* pneumonia (PCP) prophylaxis should be considered while on immunosuppression.
  - IV immunoglobulin and plasmapheresis are generally not effective, though plasma exchange is sometimes used for severe pulmonary hemorrhage, renal vasculitis, or concomitant anti–glomerular basement membrane (GBM) disease.
  - The recent PEXIVAS trial showed that plasmapheresis did not reduce the risk of end-stage renal disease or death in patients with ANCA vasculitis.[13]

COMPLICATIONS

- MPA can lead to end-organ failure. Complications depend on the organ(s) affected. Most common complications are respiratory and renal failure, which may need supportive care.
- Treatment-related toxicities may occur, and patients should be carefully monitored for these.

REFERRAL

- Patients should be referred to a rheumatologist for diagnosis, treatment, and management of MPA.
- Referral to other specialists should be considered based on specific organ involvement (e.g., nephrologist for renal disease).

PATIENT EDUCATION

Patients should be educated on the disease manifestations, complications, and treatment options for their disease.

MONITORING/FOLLOW-UP

- Follow-up involves the clinical and laboratory assessment of disease activity (complete blood count, renal function, urinary sediment, and acute-phase reactants) as well as monitoring of medication toxicities.
- Patients in remission should be monitored at least every 3 to 6 months for relapse.
- There is controversy as to whether ANCA levels are useful in monitoring disease activity. It is not recommended. More important are the assessments for end-organ damage.

OUTCOME/PROGNOSIS

- About 20% of patients progress to end-stage renal failure. A normal serum creatinine at diagnosis carries a more favorable prognosis.[2]
- Alveolar hemorrhage and pulmonary fibrosis carry a poor prognosis; patients are nine times more likely to die. In addition, higher relapse rates occur in those with pulmonary disease.

REFERENCES

1. Jennette JC, Falk RJ, Andrassy K, et al. Nomenclature of systemic vasculitides. Proposal of an international consensus conference. *Arthritis Rheum.* 1994;37:187–192.
2. Chung SA, Seo P. Microscopic polyangiitis. *Rheum Dis Clin North Am.* 2010;36:545–558.
3. Kain R, Exner M, Randes R, et al. Molecular mimicry in pauci-immune focal necrotizing glomerulonephritis. *Nat Med.* 2008;14:1088–1096.
4. Hermann J, Demel U, Stunzner D, et al. Clinical interpretation of antineutrophil cytoplasmic antibodies: Parvovirus B19 infection as a pitfall. *Ann Rheum Dis.* 2005;64:641–643.
5. Hogan SL, Satterly KK, Dooley MA, et al. Silica exposure in anti-neutrophil cytoplasmic autoantibody-associated glomerulonephritis and lupus nephritis. *J Am Soc Nephrol.* 2001;12:134–142.
6. Guillevin L, Lhote F. Distinguishing polyarteritis nodosa from microscopic polyangiitis and implications for treatment. *Curr Opin Rheumatol.* 1995;7:20–24.
7. Guillevin L, Durand-Gasselin B, Cevallos R, et al. Microscopic polyangiitis: Clinical and laboratory findings in eight-five patients. *Arthritis Rheum.* 1999;42:421–430.
8. Savige J, Gillis D, Benson E, et al. International consensus statement on testing and reporting of antineutrophil cytoplasmic antibodies (ANCA). *Am J Clin Pathol.* 1999;111:507–513.
9. Holle JU, Hellmich B, Backes M, et al. Variation in performance characteristics of commercial enzyme immunoassay kits for detection of antineutrophil cytoplasmic antibodies: What is the optimal cut off? *Ann Rheum Dis.* 2005;64:1773–1779.
10. Stone JH, Merkel PA, Spiera R, et al. Rituximab versus cyclophosphamide for ANCA-associated vasculitis. *N Engl J Med.* 2010;363:221–232.
11. Guillevin L, Pagnoux C, Karras C, et al. Rituximab versus azathioprine for maintenance in ANCA-associated vasculitis. *N Engl J Med.* 2014;371:1771–1780.
12. Jayne D, Rasmussen N, Andrassy K, et al. A randomized trial of maintenance therapy for vasculitis associated with antineutrophil cytoplasmic autoantibodies. *N Engl J Med.* 2003;349:36–44.
13. Walsh M, Merkel P, Jayne D. The effects of plasma exchange and reduced-dose glucocorticoids during remission-induction for treatment of severe ANCA-associated vasculitis. *Arthritis Rheum.* 2018;70(suppl 10).

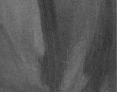

Immunoglobulin A Vasculitis (Henoch–Schönlein Purpura)

31

Can M. Sungur and Jonathan J. Miner

GENERAL PRINCIPLES

- Formerly called Henoch–Schönlein purpura
- Vasculitis that affects small vessels and is typically preceded by infection (commonly respiratory)
- Involves immunoglobulin A (IgA) deposition

Definition

Immunoglobulin A vasculitis (IgA vasculitis) was formerly known as Henoch–Schönlein purpura (HSP) and is defined as a **vasculitis with IgA-dominant immune deposits affecting small vessels**, including capillaries, venules, and arterioles (Chapel Hill Consensus Conference).[1]

Epidemiology

- The annual incidence is 14 cases per 100,000 people.
- Although IgA vasculitis can be seen at any age, the majority of patients are children less than 10 years of age. The mean age at presentation is 6 years.
- IgA vasculitis is slightly more common in males.
- IgA vasculitis presents most commonly in the fall and winter months, often after a respiratory infection.

Etiology

- Although many cases of IgA vasculitis follow respiratory infections, it may also be associated with the administration of drugs and vaccines. No single dominant etiologic agent has been identified.
- There may be genetic susceptibility with particular human leukocyte antigen (HLA) alleles.[2]

Pathophysiology

- IgA vasculitis is characterized by the deposition of IgA-dominant immune complexes in the walls of arterioles, capillaries, and postcapillary venules with resultant complement activation and **leukocytoclastic vasculitis.**
  - Skin and gastrointestinal (GI) manifestations are a direct result of **immune-complex–driven inflammation,** leading to tissue damage and extravasation of blood cells.
  - Renal biopsies demonstrate glomerulonephritis with prominent mesangial immune complex deposition.
- Aberrant glycosylation in the hinge region of the IgA1 subtype may play a role in pathogenesis.[3]

Associated Conditions

IgA vasculitis clinical picture develops in about 3% to 7% of patients with familial Mediterranean fever.[4,5]

DIAGNOSIS

Clinical Presentation

- IgA vasculitis primarily affects the **skin, kidneys, and GI tract.**
- It is often associated with **arthralgias and arthritis.**
- Occasionally, it affects the pulmonary vasculature, resulting in pulmonary capillaritis and **alveolar hemorrhage.**
- Coronary vessel vasculitis and neurologic sequelae are rare.
- There are two main distinctions between children and adults who present with IgA vasculitis.[6]
  - **Intussusception** is rare in adults.
  - Adults have a higher risk of developing **severe renal disease.**

History

- The typical presentation of IgA vasculitis is a child with **colicky abdominal pain** associated with **nausea** and **vomiting** as well as **lower extremity arthritis.** The skin lesions may also be early manifestations.
- The initial presentation is often followed by **bloody diarrhea and palpable purpura,** affecting predominantly the lower extremities and buttocks.
- Boys may present with **orchitis.**
- Rare presentations occur with headache or seizures.
- Symptoms of HSP are usually preceded by an **upper respiratory tract infection** (e.g., fever, rhinorrhea, cough).

Physical Examination

- **Palpable purpura**
  - In children, purpura may be preceded by a transient urticaria, angioedema, and maculopapular rash.
  - The purpura tends to occur in crops in regions on the **legs and buttocks.** However, purpura can present in other areas of the body and often presents before other manifestations of IgA vasculitis.
  - Individual lesions are 2 to 10 mm in diameter, typically last several days and resolve more quickly with bed rest.
- **Arthritis**
  - Arthritis is the second most common manifestation of IgA vasculitis and presents in 75% of patients.
  - The **knees, ankles, and feet** are typically involved.
  - While joints are usually warm and painful, joint effusions are not consistently present.
- **Gastrointestinal**
  - Abdominal pain, nausea, and vomiting
  - **Guaiac-positive stool** is seen in about half of the patients, but hemorrhage is rare.
- **Genitourinary:** Pain, tenderness, and swelling of the **testicle and/or scrotum** are less common manifestations of HSP.
- **Neurologic:** Rare reports of focal neurologic deficits, ataxia, and central and peripheral neuropathy.

Diagnostic Criteria

- The American College of Rheumatology 1990 criteria for the classification of IgA vasculitis are presented in Table 31-1.[7]
- In 2006, the European League against Rheumatism and Pediatric Rheumatology European Society published new criteria for pediatric IgA vasculitis, and these are presented in Table 31-2.[8]
- For typical presentations of IgA vasculitis in children, it is necessary to **exclude sepsis, thrombocytopenia, and clotting disorders.**
- In adults, further studies are needed to rule out other causes of small-vessel vasculitis.

TABLE 31-1	THE AMERICAN COLLEGE OF RHEUMATOLOGY 1990 CRITERIA FOR THE CLASSIFICATION OF IMMUNOGLOBULIN A VASCULITIS

The presence of at least two of the following four is required:
- Palpable purpura, not related to thrombocytopenia
- Age ≤ 20 years
- Bowel angina, defined as either diffuse abdominal pain that is worsened by meals or the diagnosis of bowel ischemia, usually with bloody diarrhea
- Histologic changes showing granulocytes in the walls of arterioles or venules

Adapted from: Mills JA, Michel BA, Bloch DA, et al. The American College of Rheumatology 1990 criteria for the classification of Henoch–Schönlein purpura. *Arthritis Rheum.* 1990;33:1114–1121.

TABLE 31-2	2006 EUROPEAN LEAGUE AGAINST RHEUMATISM AND PEDIATRIC RHEUMATOLOGY EUROPEAN SOCIETY CLASSIFICATION CRITERIA FOR IMMUNOGLOBULIN A VASCULITIS

Palpable purpura with at least one of the following:
- Diffuse abdominal pain
- Biopsy with predominant IgA
- Acute arthritis/arthralgias
- Hematuria or proteinuria

Adapted from: Ozen S, Ruperto N, Dillon MJ, et al. EULAR/PReS endorsed consensus criteria for the classification of childhood vasculitides. *Ann Rheum Dis.* 2006;65:936–941.

Differential Diagnosis

The differential diagnosis includes other causes of small-vessel vasculitis (granulomatosis with polyangiitis, microscopic polyangiitis, cryoglobulinemic vasculitis, and leukocytoclastic angiitis), polyarteritis nodosa (in cases of unusually chronic or severe IgA vasculitis), systemic lupus erythematosus, thrombotic thrombocytopenic purpura/hemolytic–uremic syndrome, exanthematous drug eruption, purpura fulminans, and septic vasculitis.

Diagnostic Testing

Laboratories
- **Urinalysis:** The most common renal manifestation is microscopic hematuria, but up to one-third of patients with nephritis have gross hematuria.
- Serum **creatinine** should be checked.
- Erythrocyte sedimentation rate (ESR) may be elevated.
- Complete blood count should be checked for possible leukocytosis and to ensure a normal platelet count.
- Coagulation studies to **rule out coagulopathies**.
- **Antinuclear antibodies** (ANAs) and **antineutrophil cytoplasmic antibody** (ANCA)
- **Immunoglobulins: IgA may be elevated** in up to 72% of children with HSP.[9]

Imaging
- **Abdominal plain films**
  - May have dilated loops of bowel
  - Can be used in combination with chest radiography to evaluate for perforation
- **Abdominal ultrasound:** A more effective means of identifying ileoileal intussusception
- **Doppler flow and/or radionuclide studies:** utilized in patients presenting with scrotal pain
- **Head computed tomography/magnetic resonance imaging (CT/MRI):** Utilized in rare cases of neurologic presentation to evaluate intracerebral hemorrhage

Diagnostic Procedures
- Renal biopsy
  - In children, renal biopsy is recommended when there is impaired renal function or marked proteinuria because histologic lesions are prognostic indicators.
  - **In adults, a biopsy may be needed to rule out other causes of small-vessel vasculitis.**
  - Mild disease often demonstrates **focal mesangial proliferation with IgA-dominant immune complex deposition and C3 deposits in the mesangial matrix.**
  - In patients with more severe renal disease, such as nephrotic range proteinuria, there is likely to be marked **cellular proliferation and crescentic glomerulonephritis.**
- Skin biopsy
  - In adults, a skin biopsy may be needed to confirm the diagnosis of IgA vasculitis.
  - Biopsies will demonstrate small-vessel **leukocytoclastic vasculitis**, most prominent in the postcapillary venules.
  - Immunofluorescence studies show **IgA-dominant immune complex deposition in combination with C3 deposits.**

TREATMENT

Most patients completely recover without specific therapy.

Medications

- **Angiotensin-converting enzyme (ACE) inhibitors** should be considered in cases of proteinuria or as a first-line agent in patients with hypertension.
- Nonsteroidal anti-inflammatory drugs (NSAIDs) are generally sufficient to relieve arthralgias and arthritis, but are often avoided because of side effects.
- **Glucocorticoids**
  - May be used for severe joint pain
  - May be used in severe abdominal pain, especially when intussusception is suspected
  - **Do not have a role in the treatment of purpura** because there is no decrease in the duration of the skin lesion or frequency of recurrences
  - **Do not appear to have a role in preventing nephritis**[10]
- Several treatment regimens for renal disease have been suggested, including glucocorticoids, azathioprine, cyclophosphamide, cyclosporine, mycophenolate mofetil, plasmapheresis, intravenous (IV) immunoglobulin, and rituximab.

Surgical Management

Those patients that progress to end-stage renal disease (ESRD) are candidates for a renal transplant, although the disease can reoccur following transplant.

COMPLICATIONS

GI involvement has the potential for serious complications including **intussusception** (typically ileoileal), **infarction, massive hemorrhage, and perforation.**

MONITORING/FOLLOW-UP

• In patients with mild renal disease, measurement of blood pressure, serum creatinine, and urinalysis should be obtained at least weekly while the disease is clinically active and once a month for 3 months when the disease remits.

• Females who were diagnosed with IgA vasculitis in childhood are at increased risk of proteinuria and hypertension during pregnancy and need to be carefully monitored during this time.

OUTCOME/PROGNOSIS

• IgA vasculitis resolves within 2 to 4 weeks in over 80% of childhood cases.

• Children generally have milder disease and are less likely to have nephritis.

• IgA vasculitis **is more severe and prolonged in adults**, with renal failure and nephritis occurring more frequently.

• **Recurrence of symptoms occurs in one-third** of patients; resolution in these patients often occurs within 4 months.

• Approximately 30% to 50% of patients with nephritis have persistent urinary abnormalities after long-term follow-up.

• Long-term prognosis of IgA vasculitis depends on the severity of renal impairment. Only 1% of patients develop ESRD.

  ○ Patients with gross hematuria, nephrotic syndrome, or hypertension are more likely to progress to ESRD.

  ○ If a renal biopsy has crescents involving more than 50% of the glomeruli, there is an increased rate of chronic renal failure and ESRD.

REFERENCES

1. Jennette JC, Falk RJ, Andrassy K, et al. Nomenclature of systemic vasculitides. Proposal of an international consensus conference. *Arthritis Rheum.* 1994;37:187–192.

2. Soylemezoglu O, Peru H, Gonen S, et al. HLA-DRB1 alleles and Henoch–Schönlein purpura: Susceptibility and severity of disease. *J Rheumatol.* 2008;35:1165–1168.

3. Novak J, Moldoveanu Z, Yanagihara T, et al. IgA nephropathy and Henoch–Schoenlein purpura nephritis: Aberrant glycosylation of IgA1, formation of IgA1-containing immune complexes, and activation of mesangial cells. *Contrib Nephrol.* 2007;157:134–138.

4. Ozodogan H, Arisoy N, Kasapçapur O, et al. Vasculitis in familial Mediterranean fever. *J Rheumatol.* 1997;24:323–327.

5. Aksu K, Keser G. Coexistence of vasculitides with familial Mediterranean fever. *Rheumatol Int.* 2011;31:1263–1274.

6. Pillebout E, Thervet E, Hill G, et al. Henoch–Schönlein purpura in adults: Outcome and prognostic factors. *J Am Soc Nephrol.* 2002;13:1271–1278.

7. Mills JA, Michel BA, Bloch DA, et al. The American College of Rheumatology 1990 criteria for the classification of Henoch–Schönlein purpura. *Arthritis Rheum.* 1990;33:1114–1121.

8. Ozen S, Ruperto N, Dillon MJ, et al. EULAR/PReS endorsed consensus criteria for the classification of childhood vasculitides. *Ann Rheum Dis.* 2006;65:936–941.

9. Fretzayas A, Sionti I, Moustaki M, et al. Clinical impact of altered immunoglobulin levels in Henoch–Schönlein purpura. *Pediatr Int.* 2009;51:381–384.

10. Chartapisak W, Opastiraku S, Willis NS, et al. Prevention and treatment of renal disease in Henoch–Schönlein purpura: A systematic review. *Arch Dis Child.* 2009;94:132–137.

Cryoglobulinemia and Cryoglobulinemic Vasculitis

32

Roseanne F. Zhao and Jonathan J. Miner

GENERAL PRINCIPLES

Definition

- Cryoglobulins are serum immunoglobulins that undergo reversible precipitation below normal body temperatures and redissolve on warming to 37°C.
- This phenomenon was first described in 1933 by Wintrobe and Bruell.[1] The terms "cryoglobulin" and "cryoprecipitation" were later coined by Lerner and Watson[2] in 1947 after these proteins had been identified in various diseases.
- Cryoglobulinemia refers to the presence of circulating cryoglobulins.
- Cryoglobulinemic vasculitis (CV) is defined as a vasculitis secondary to deposition and precipitation of cryoglobulin immune complexes in small- to medium-sized vessels such as arterioles, venules, and capillaries.[3,4]
- An important caveat is that **cryoglobulinemia is not always symptomatic and may not necessarily progress to CV.**
- Symptomatic cryoglobulinemia is a **heterogeneous disease in both etiology and clinical manifestations** that depend on the type of cryoglobulin involved. Symptoms range from purpura, skin ulcers, and retinal hemorrhage to arthralgias, glomerulonephritis, and peripheral neuropathy.
- The classic clinical triad of purpura, arthralgias, and asthenia that was described by Meltzer et al.[5] in 1966 is seen in about 30% of patients with mixed cryoglobulinemia (MC).

Classification

- Cryoglobulinemia is commonly classified according to Brouet et al.[6] based on immunoglobulin composition.
  - **Type I: isolated monoclonal immunoglobulins**
    - Usually immunoglobulin M (IgM) or IgG, rarely IgA or free immunoglobulin light chains
    - Develops in the setting of monoclonal gammopathies[7,8]:
      - Forty percent of patients have monoclonal gammopathy of unknown significance (MGUS).
      - Sixty percent of patients have an overt B-cell malignancy, including multiple myeloma, Waldenström's macroglobulinemia, chronic lymphocytic leukemia (CLL), and B-cell non–Hodgkin's lymphomas.
    - Serum levels are often high (5–30 mg/mL) and usually readily precipitate in cold. Cryoglobulin levels are not significantly different between MGUS and B-cell malignancies.
  - **Type II: immune complexes of polyclonal or monoclonal IgM rheumatoid factor (IgM-RF) directed against polyclonal IgG**
    - Most are IgM–IgG, although IgG–IgG and IgG–IgA can occur.
    - Associated with hepatitis C virus (HCV) infection in 80% to 90% of patients. Other causes include chronic HIV and hepatitis B virus (HBV) infections, connective

tissue diseases (e.g., rheumatoid arthritis [RA], systemic lupus erythematosus [SLE], Sjögren's syndrome, systemic sclerosis), and lymphoproliferative disorders.[9]
- Serum levels are usually high, with 40% of patients having levels greater than 5 mg/mL.
  - **Type III: polyclonal IgM-RF directed against polyclonal IgG**
    - These are consistently heterogeneous (always polyclonal).
    - More difficult to detect because they precipitate slowly and tend to be present in much smaller quantities (50–1,000 μg/dL).
    - Most result from a B-cell lymphoproliferative disorder in the setting of chronic infection or autoimmunity. It is associated with HCV to a lesser extent compared to type II cryoglobulins.
  - **Type II/III: oligoclonal IgM or mixed monoclonal/polyclonal IgM directed against polyclonal IgG.** May represent a transition from type III to type II cryoglobulinemia.
- **Types II and III are considered MC** because they contain a mixture of IgM and IgG.
- Essential MC refers to cases with no identifiable cause.

Epidemiology

- The laboratory assessment of cryoglobulinemia is not standardized and requires expertise beyond the ability of most labs. Improper handling of samples can lead to false negatives. Consequently, the actual prevalence may be underestimated.
- The prevalence of "essential" MC is reported to be approximately 1 in 100,000; however, **very few cases are truly "essential"** (no identifiable cause).
- Female-to-male ratio is 3:1.
- **MC is associated with chronic infection or inflammation.**
  - Forty percent to 60% of patients with HCV infection (as high as 65% in HIV/HCV coinfection) have MC, but only 15% to 20% are symptomatic and 5% develop CV.[10–12] However, this variation may be because of lead time bias, population selection, and high rate of false negatives on laboratory testing.
  - Fifteen percent to 20% of HIV patients have MC.
  - Ten percent of SLE patients have MC.[13]
  - Five percent to 20% of Sjögren's syndrome patients have type II cryoglobulinemia, which is a key prognostic factor in this disease resulting from its association with development of vasculitis, B-cell lymphoma, and poor prognosis.[14]
  - Cryoglobulinemia is associated with a **35-fold higher risk of non-Hodgkin's lymphoma.**[15] Risk increases with cryoglobulin levels.
  - Chronic HCV infection (>15 years) increases risk for developing B-cell non-Hodgkin's lymphoma.[16]
  - However, patients with non-HCV MC vasculitis have even higher risk for lymphoma as well as increased frequencies of renal involvement and worse prognosis.[9]

Associated Conditions

- Infections
  - **Viral:** hepatitis A virus (HAV), HBV, HCV, HIV, Epstein–Barr virus (EBV), cytomegalovirus (CMV), adenovirus, and parvovirus B19
  - **Bacterial:** syphilis, leprosy, Q-fever, brucellosis, streptococcal infection, infectious endocarditis, and Lyme disease
  - **Fungal:** coccidioidomycosis and candidiasis
  - **Parasitic:** leishmaniasis, toxoplasmosis, echinococcosis, malaria, schistosomiasis, and trypanosomiasis
- Hematologic/oncologic
  - Lymphoproliferative disorders
  - B-cell non-Hodgkin's lymphoma (marginal zone, follicular, diffuse large B-cell lymphomas)

- ○ Chronic myelogenous leukemia, CLL and hairy cell leukemia
- ○ Multiple myeloma
- ○ Waldenström's macroglobulinemia
- ○ MGUS
- ○ Myelodysplastic syndrome and myeloproliferative diseases
- ○ Castleman's disease
- ○ Thrombotic thrombocytopenic purpura
- **Autoimmune diseases**
- ○ Sjögren's syndrome
- ○ RA
- ○ SLE
- ○ Systemic sclerosis
- ○ Giant cell arteritis
- ○ Inflammatory bowel disease
- ○ Sarcoidosis
- ○ Dermatomyositis/polymyositis
- ○ Autoimmune thyroiditis

Pathophysiology

- The role of specific pathogen and host factors in the pathogenesis of cryoglobulinemia is largely unknown.
- **Lymphoproliferation, either primary or secondary to chronic immune stimulation, leads to the production of monoclonal, oligoclonal, or polyclonal cryoglobulins.**
- Clinical and histologic features indicate vascular deposits of cryoglobulins, leading to cold induced symptoms of vascular insufficiency secondary to occlusion of various small vessels.
- Circulating immune complexes may be present in both serum and occluded blood vessel walls.
- **Mechanisms of cryoprecipitation differ between type I versus types II and III cryoglobulinemia.**[12]
  - ○ **Type I**: Monoclonal cryoglobulins crystallize and aggregate at either low temperatures and/or high concentrations, resulting in occlusive disease with minimal inflammation. High concentrations of cryoglobulins (usually IgM isotype and when M-protein >4 g/dL) may also cause hyperviscosity syndrome. Vasculitis may occasionally be seen.
  - ○ **Types II and III**: Immune complexes form between IgM-RF and polyclonal IgG, which can then fix complement, resulting in recruitment of inflammatory cells and tissue injury including vasculitis and glomerulonephritis.
- **Low serum C4 is a signature of type II MC** and implicates classic pathway activation.
- HCV-related cryoglobulinemia results from chronic viral stimulation of B cells, leading to a lymphoproliferative disorder that may evolve into a B-cell non-Hodgkin's lymphoma.
  - ○ HCV infects hepatocytes and B cells via a transmembrane entry receptor (CD81) that forms a complex with CD21 and CD19, which, in conjunction with BCR stimulation by HCV antigen, stimulates the polyclonal expansion of B cells (type III).
  - ○ This initial phase is more frequently associated with asymptomatic cryoglobulinemia.
  - ○ Chronic stimulation by HCV leads to production of autoantibodies that can result in sicca syndrome, thyroiditis, diabetes, pulmonary fibrosis, and cytopenias.
  - ○ Chronic HCV infection increases the risk for genetic mutations, resulting in resistance to apoptosis and oligoclonal lymphoproliferation (type II and/or III).
  - ○ Clonal B cells with hypermutated immunoglobulin and proto-oncogenes emerge and produce monoclonal IgM (type II). Monoclonal RFs that bear the Wa cross-idiotype are responsible for most cases of CV in patients with HCV infection.
  - ○ These cryoglobulins bind to polyclonal IgG directed against HCV to form immune complexes, which can bind to endothelial cells of blood vessels via C1q, leading to CV.

○ Vasculitic lesions in different organs with HCV may vary. For example, although complexes of HCV RNA, monoclonal IgM-RF, IgG, and complement components are detected in skin, demonstration of HCV proteins in kidneys remains difficult.
- Cryoglobulinemic neuropathy may be caused by vasculitis of vasa nervorum as well as immunologically mediated demyelination, hyperviscosity, and microvascular occlusion.
- Vasculitis of intramuscular or cerebral arteries may cause paresis or plegia, strokes, or a diffuse encephalopathy.

DIAGNOSIS

Diagnosis of cryoglobulinemia is based on characteristic clinical signs and symptoms in the setting of laboratory finding of serum cryoglobulins. The history and physical examination should be aimed at identifying the underlying disease.

Diagnostic Criteria
- The American College of Rheumatology does not have a set of criteria.
- The *Gruppo Italiano di Studio delle Crioglobulinemie* published a system for defining and characterizing the cryoglobulinemic syndrome[17]; this is presented in Table 32-1.

Clinical Features

The prevalence of different clinical manifestations in type I and type II/III MC is presented in Table 32-2.[18]
- **Type I cryoglobulinemia**
  - ○ Type I tends to cause **signs of peripheral vascular occlusion and hyperviscosity**, though it may be associated with some small-vessel vasculitis features such as purpura, neuropathy, and glomerulonephritis.
  - ○ Hematologic abnormalities may be present depending on the underlying disease.
  - ○ High cryocrit and cryoglobulins may only be a casual finding.
- **Types II and III MC**
  - ○ Immune complex disorder more often associated with constitutional symptoms (such as fever, weakness, and anorexia) compared to type I cryoglobulinemia
  - ○ MC syndrome is characterized by Meltzer's triad of **purpura, weakness, and arthralgias** in about one-third of patients.

TABLE 32-1	PROPOSED SYSTEM FOR DEFINING AND CHARACTERIZING THE CRYOGLOBULINEMIC SYNDROME

- Cryocrit >1% for at least 6 months
- At least two of the following: purpura, arthralgia, and weakness
- C4 < 8 mg/dL
- Positive rheumatoid factor (monoclonal or polyclonal)
- Secondary, if associated with connective tissue diseases, chronic liver diseases, lymphoproliferative diseases, and infections
- Essential, if without an identifiable underlying cause
- Assess the extent of the vasculitis: hepatic/renal involvement, neuropathies
- Identification of microlymphoma-like nodules in the bone marrow

Adapted from: Invernizzi F, Pietrogrande M, Sagramoso B. Classification of the cryoglobulinemic syndrome. *Clin Exp Rheumatol.* 1995;13:S123–S128.

TABLE 32-2	CLINICAL MANIFESTATIONS OF CRYOGLOBULINEMIA	
	Type I	Type II/III
Hyperviscosity syndrome	Occasionally, usually in IgM isotype and when M-protein >4 g/dL	Rarely, never in type III
Purpura	70%	90%
Skin ulcers	30%	15%
Glomerulonephritis	30%	30%
Peripheral neuropathy	30%	30%
Arthralgia	30%	25%–40%
Cardiac, pulmonary, gastrointestinal, or central nervous system involvement	Almost never	5%

Adapted from: Muchtar E, Magen H, Gertz MA. How I treat cryoglobulinemia. *Blood.* 2017;129:289–298.

IgM, immunoglobulin M.

○ **Multisystem organ involvement,** including chronic hepatitis, membranoproliferative glomerulonephritis (MPGN), and peripheral neuropathy, due to leukocytoclastic vasculitis of small- and medium-sized vessels, is frequently observed.
- **CV in chronic HCV infection**
  ○ The natural history and prognosis of MC vasculitis are variable and highly dependent on renal involvement and overall extent of vasculitic lesions.
  ○ CV is usually associated with advanced age, longer duration of HCV infection, type II MC, high serum MC levels, and clonal B-cell expansion in both the blood and the liver.
  ○ Poor prognostic factors include age greater than 60 years at diagnosis and renal involvement.
  ○ Historically, the overall 5-year survival after the diagnosis of vasculitis ranged from 50% to 90% in cases with renal involvement. Even in the absence of significant renal failure, increased mortality from liver involvement, cardiovascular disease, infection, and lymphoma has been reported.
  ○ HCV is now curable with direct-acting antiviral therapy, with improvement in vasculitis and glomerulonephritis.
    ▪ However, some patients may have persistence or relapse of CV despite achieving and maintaining a sustained viral response (SVR),[19,20] though it should be noted that SVR does not always indicate complete HCV eradication.
    ▪ Although the majority of patients have decreased cryoglobulin levels with SVR, about 50% of these patients still have cryoglobulins.[21–23]
    ▪ Clonal cryoglobulin-producing B cells in HCV-infected patients persist after SVR.[24]
  ○ It is not yet completely clear how treatment with antiviral therapies for HCV affects the long-term disease course of cryoglobulinemia and CV.
- **Liver disease**
  ○ Usually related to HCV, characterized by diffuse lymphoid infiltration of liver (lupoid hepatitis)
  ○ Levels of cryoglobulins typically decrease as cirrhosis progresses.

- ○ Autoimmune hepatitis may share a number of extrahepatic features including leukocytoclastic vasculitis, hypocomplementemia, glomerulonephritis, and anti–smooth muscle antibodies, further confounding the diagnosis.
- **Renal disease**
  - ○ Most common in type II cryoglobulinemia, observed in 30% to 60% of MC and portending a poor prognosis
  - ○ Renal impairment occurs in 30% of patients and may lead to **non-nephrotic range proteinuria, microscopic hematuria, elevated creatinine (Cr), and/or hypertension.** This rarely presents as an acute nephritis/nephritic syndrome.
  - ○ **Type I MPGN** accounts for 80% of type II cryoglobulinemic nephropathy. There is thickening of glomerular basement membrane (GBM) and cellular proliferation on biopsy.
  - ○ Distinguishing histologic features in cryoglobulinemic MPGN
    - ▪ Marked influx of circulating macrophages
    - ▪ Intraluminal thrombi of precipitated cryoglobulins
    - ▪ Fingerprint subendothelial deposits by electron microscopy
    - ▪ IgM deposition in capillary loops by immunofluorescence
  - ○ Less common presentations:
    - ▪ Mild mesangial membranous nephropathy
    - ▪ Tubulointerstitial nephritis
    - ▪ Acute vasculitis of small- and medium-sized renal vessels
    - ▪ Thrombotic microangiopathy
    - ▪ Occasionally oliguria and rapidly progressive acute renal failure is seen.
  - ○ HCV RNA can be detected in the kidney of patients with HCV-associated MC.
- **Hyperviscosity syndrome:** This may manifest as headache, confusion, blurred vision, sudden deafness, oronasal bleeding, and heart failure.
- **Arthralgias/arthritis**
  - ○ Affects small **distal joints.** An **oligoarticular and nonerosive** pattern is usually seen in MC.
  - ○ Often sensitive to low doses of steroids, with or without hydroxychloroquine
  - ○ In HCV-associated MC, an erosive symmetrical polyarthritis may rarely develop.
  - ○ An **overlap syndrome of RA and MC must be considered.**
  - ○ Anti–cyclic citrullinated protein (CCP) antibodies may be a useful diagnostic tool as it is not increased in MC while RF positivity is seen in 30% to 70% of patients with HCV.[25–28]
- **Cutaneous manifestations**
  - ○ Often confined to acral sites (distal limbs, ears, nose). Manifestations include Raynaud's phenomenon, purpura, acrocyanosis, livedo reticularis, dystrophic manifestation, ulcers, and digital gangrene.
  - ○ **Purpura** is the main manifestation of CV. Seventy percent of patients have this cutaneous finding, which may be transient or may progress to **ulcers and gangrene.**
  - ○ Palpable purpura is usually found in the lower extremities.
- **Symmetric peripheral neuropathy**
  - ○ Symmetric peripheral neuropathy is the most common neurologic manifestation.
  - ○ It is more frequent in type III cryoglobulinemia.
  - ○ It may have an acute or subacute presentation, usually accompanied by cutaneous disease.
  - ○ It is typically a **sensory axonal neuropathy in a glove and stocking pattern.**
  - ○ Symmetric or asymmetric motor and/or sensory polyneuropathy is common.
  - ○ Mononeuritis multiplex may also be seen.
  - ○ Causes of neuropathy
    - ▪ Vasculitis of vasa nervosum

- Hyperviscosity with occlusion of microcirculation
- Immune-mediated demyelination
- Painful peripheral neuropathy (predominant sensory > motor involvement) is seen in 19% to 44% of patients and typically occurs in the lower extremities.
- **Rare findings**
  - Lymphadenopathy
  - Mesenteric vasculitis
  - Subclinical pulmonary fibrosis
  - Coronary vasculitis
  - Pulmonary vasculitis, pleurisy, dyspnea, cough, and hemoptysis are often overlooked.

Diagnostic Testing

Laboratories
- Cryoglobulins are heterogeneous in composition, thermal properties, and efficiency of complement activation.
- False-negative results may occur if samples are not handled properly owing to cold precipitation of cryoglobulins prior to serum extraction.
- A negative test should not exclude the disease; if clinical suspicion remains high, the test should be repeated.
- Detection of cryoglobulins
  - Sample collection is a critical step. Samples should be collected in warm tubes without anticoagulants to increase diagnostic yield.
  - Blood should be transferred and centrifuged at $37^{\circ C}$.
  - After serum extraction, samples should be stored for at least 7 days at $4^{\circ}C$. Precipitation usually occurs within hours in type I but may take longer time for MC.
  - If a cryoprecipitate is present, a small sample should be warmed to test for resolubility and rule out false positives because of cryofibrinogen or heparin-precipitable proteins.
  - The **cryocrit** can be quantified as the volume of packed cryoglobulins as a percentage of total serum volume.
    - It is higher in type I (can be >50%) and lowest in type III (typically <5%).
    - It does not necessarily correlate with severity, disease activity or manifestations, or treatment response.
  - Immunoglobulin levels can also be quantified.
  - Precipitates should be washed in cold buffer and then redissolved in warm buffer prior to electrophoresis and immunofixation at $37^{\circ C}$ to characterize the cryoglobulin components. Immunoblotting and two-dimensional (2D) polyacrylamide gel electrophoresis may also be used.
- **RF** and **complement studies** (**C3, C4**, and **CH50**) should also be performed.
  - Increased RF activity and hypocomplementemia (low C4 with normal/slightly low C3) are seen primarily in MC but may also occur in type I.
  - Total hemolytic complement, CH_{50}, may be zero because of cold activation (complement activation may occur after the sample is obtained).
- Tests for both HCV antibody and HCV RNA should be done, even if hepatic enzymes are normal.
  - HCV genotyping should be performed for positive test results.
  - A negative HCV test may rarely be because of HCV RNA concentrated in circulating cryoglobulin immune complexes. If clinical suspicion is high, the test may be performed on cryoprecipitates.
- Additional labs include complete blood cell count, serum chemistries, liver function studies, urinalysis, and either a urine protein-to-Cr ratio or 24-hour urine protein collection.
- Serum viscosity may be helpful in the setting of corresponding symptoms; symptoms rarely appear below 4.0 cP (normal ≤ 1.5 cP).

- Serum protein electrophoresis, serum free light chains, and urine protein electrophoresis may be performed if there is concern for an underlying monoclonal gammopathy.
- Other lab findings include elevated erythrocyte sedimentation rate (ESR), which may occur because of Rouleaux formation.

Diagnostic Procedures
- Renal biopsy is recommended if kidney involvement is suspected.[29]
  - **Light microscopy:** most commonly has morphologic aspects of MPGN, including mesangial proliferation and diffuse endocapillary hypercellularity; refractive thrombi in capillaries ("cryoplugs") that are strongly periodic acid–Schiff stain (PAS) positive; leukocytoclastic vasculitis of interlobular arteries and afferent arterioles; and fibrinoid necrosis with neutrophils and monocytes/macrophages.
  - **Immunofluorescence:** mesangial, subendothelial capillary wall or glomerular intracapillary deposits of IgG and IgM (may show clonal light-chain staining, usually κ); prominent staining for C3; variable staining for C4 and C1q
  - **Electron microscopy:** mesangial, subendothelial, and intracapillary immune deposits; extensive foot process effacement; double contour GBM secondary to new formation beneath subendothelial deposits. Deposits have a fibrillary or microtubular substructure.
- Biopsy of skin lesions may show leukocytoclastic vasculitis and fibrinoid necrosis of capillary walls.

TREATMENT

- Most patients with cryoglobulinemia remain asymptomatic and can simply be monitored.
- Treatment is primarily aimed at targeting the underlying disease process when possible.
- Patients with mild-to-moderate disease, such as arthralgias, asthenia, nondebilitating neuropathy, and skin lesions, may be treated with low-dose prednisone and colchicine.
- Moderate-to-severe diseases, including glomerulonephritis, cutaneous vasculitis, and progressive neuropathy, are treated with immunosuppressive therapy.
  - **First line:** glucocorticoids plus either rituximab or cyclophosphamide
  - **Second line:** plasma exchange, azathioprine, or mycophenolate mofetil (no controlled studies)
  - **Other options:** Methotrexate, cyclosporine A, melphalan and prednisone, or fludarabine
- Life-threatening manifestations including rapidly progressing glomerulonephritis, sensorimotor neuropathy, and extensive or visceral vasculitis (gastrointestinal [GI] ischemia, pulmonary hemorrhage) should be treated with plasma exchange and pulse steroids plus either rituximab or cyclophosphamide.
- Symptomatic hyperviscosity syndrome should be treated with urgent plasma exchange or plasmapheresis to remove cryoglobulins from circulation.
- **Monoclonal gammopathies:** B-cell malignancies should be treated in collaboration with an oncologist. There is limited evidence regarding the best approach to treatment.[7,8,18]
  - Multiple myeloma
    - A lenalidomide-/pomalidomide-based regimen may be considered in patients with neuropathy.
    - A bortezomib-based regimen may be considered for patients with renal failure.
    - Immunotherapy may be considered, but no data are available on its use in cryoglobulinemia.
    - Autologous stem cell transplant may be considered.
  - Waldenström's macroglobulinemia
    - Bortezomib as first-line therapy; can consider ibrutinib but no data are available on its use in cryoglobulinemia.

- Rituximab may be added after initial response is achieved but should not be started as first-line therapy because of the risk for IgM flare and hyperviscosity syndrome.
- If patients continue to have high IgM levels (≥4 g/dL), plasma exchange can be initiated to prevent an IgM flare.
  - MGUS
    - May consider single-agent prednisone, but many patients may require additional therapy.
    - Rituximab should be limited to patients with CD20+ B-cell clones or IgM isotype.
  - Owing to the risk of myelodysplasia and a secondary acute myeloid leukemia,[30] cytotoxic agents are not preferred.
- **HCV-associated MC:** Owing to the complexity of etiopathogenesis, **the treatment of HCV-associated MC is particularly challenging.**
  - Three important factors should be considered: HCV infection, the presence of an autoimmune disorder, and possible neoplastic associations.
  - The most effective treatment for HCV MC is **eradication of the underlying HCV infection** (i.e., removal of the antigen driving the process).
    - New highly potent direct-acting antiviral therapies induce SVR in more than 90% of patients.
    - Patients should be treated in collaboration with infectious disease physicians and hepatologists, following guidelines from the American Association for the Study of Liver Diseases and the Infectious Diseases Society of America.[31]
  - The symptoms of MC, CV, and evidence of B-cell lymphoproliferative disorders improve in patients with SVR. However, persistence or relapse of CV in patients with SVR may occur sporadically or in the setting of infection or associated malignancies.
  - Combination treatment with rituximab, in conjunction with direct-acting antiviral therapies, may help provide long-term remission.[32–34]
- **Non–HCV-associated MC**
  - Immunosuppression alone may lead to worsening of the underlying infectious disease and resistant cryoglobulinemia.
  - The underlying infection should be treated if possible, and immunosuppression may be added in cases of refractory MC.

Medications

- **Cyclophosphamide**
  - Cyclophosphamide is typically used in severe cases and remains the first-line cytotoxic agent.
  - For severe life-threatening disease, use daily oral cyclophosphamide with pulse steroids and plasmapheresis (doses similar to those used for Granulomatosis with Polyangiitis).
  - Severe but non–life-threatening disease may be treated with monthly pulse intravenous (IV) cyclophosphamide along with oral prednisone.
  - Once remission of severe disease is achieved, employ daily oral prednisone with weekly oral methotrexate or azathioprine.
  - Treatment of underlying causes is essential in preventing relapse.
- **Rituximab**
  - Systemic B-cell depletion with rituximab, a chimeric monoclonal antibody against CD20 antigen, has been utilized successfully in the treatment of MC.
    - Type I cryoglobulinemia appears to have a lower response rate than MC.
    - Neuropathy and renal involvement were more resistant to treatment, whereas skin and joint disease responded quickly.
  - Side effects include infection, serum sickness, thrombosis of retinal arteries, and development of cold agglutinin disease.

○ Recent treatment guidelines for MC syndrome in HCV-infected patients suggest that HCV viral load and liver function be carefully monitored in patients receiving rituximab and that antiviral prophylaxis should be given to HBV carriers.
- **Colchicine**
  ○ The rationale underlying the use of colchicine (0.6 mg twice daily [bid]) to treat MC is based on the drug's activity in reducing immunoglobulin secretion.
  ○ In a small open study, it had favorable effects on purpura, weakness, and leg ulcers.[35] Minor GI side effects are common at this dose.

Other Nonpharmacologic Therapies

- **Plasmapheresis** should be reserved for life-threatening forms of disease, including vasculitis, glomerulonephritis, severe central nervous system disease, malignant hypertension, vascular insufficiency with distal necrosis, and hyperviscosity syndrome.
- Concomitant immunosuppressive therapy must be instituted to prevent rebound antibody formation and relapse of disease after withdrawal of plasmapheresis. A protocol typically includes methylprednisolone 1 g daily for 3 days followed by oral prednisone and cyclophosphamide (doses similar to those used for treatment of Granulomatosis with Polyangiitis).
- Plasmapheresis, exchanging one plasma volume three times weekly for 2 to 3 weeks is generally used. Replacement fluid can be 5% albumin, which must be warmed to prevent precipitation of cryoglobulins.
- Optimal methods for assessment of efficacy are not clear as cryocrit may not correlate with disease intensity. Clinical examination is used to guide further therapy. Skin, arthritic, and renal manifestations can improve rapidly, whereas cryoglobulinemic neuropathy does not remit in short-term therapy.[36]

REFERENCES

1. Wintrobe MB. Hyperproteinemia associated with multiple myeloma, with report of case in which extraordinary hyperproteinemia was associated with thrombosis of retinal veins and symptoms suggesting Raynaud's disease. *Bull Johns Hopkins Hosp.* 1933;52:156–165.
2. Lerner AB, Watson CJ. Studies of cryoglobulins; unusual purpura associated with the presence of a high concentration of cryoglobulin (cold precipitable serum globulin). *Am J Med Sci.* 1947;214:410–415.
3. Jennette JC, Falk RJ, Andrassy K, et al. Nomenclature of systemic vasculitides. Proposal of an international consensus conference. *Arthritis Rheum.* 1994;37:187–192.
4. Jennette JC, Falk RJ, Bacon PA, et al. 2012 revised International Chapel Hill Consensus Conference Nomenclature of Vasculitides. *Arthritis Rheum.* 2013;65:1–11.
5. Meltzer M, Franklin EC, Elias K, et al. Cryoglobulinemia–A clinical and laboratory study. II. Cryoglobulins with rheumatoid factor activity. *Am J Med.* 1966;40:837–856.
6. Brouet JC, Clauvel JP, Danon F, et al. Biologic and clinical significance of cryoglobulins. A report of 86 cases. *Am J Med.* 1974;57:775–788.
7. Terrier B, Karras A, Kahn JE, et al. The spectrum of type I cryoglobulinemia vasculitis: New insights based on 64 cases. *Medicine (Baltimore).* 2013;92:61–68.
8. Harel S, Mohr M, Jahn I, et al. Clinico-biological characteristics and treatment of type I monoclonal cryoglobulinaemia: A study of 64 cases. *Br J Haematol.* 2015;168:671–678.
9. Saadoun D, Sellam J, Ghillani-Dalbin P, et al. Increased risks of lymphoma and death among patients with non–hepatitis C virus–related mixed cryoglobulinemia. *Arch Intern Med.* 2006;166:2101–2108.
10. Horcajada JP, García-Bengoechea M, Cilla G, et al. Mixed cryoglobulinaemia in patients with chronic hepatitis C infection: Prevalence, significance and relationship with different viral genotypes. *Ann Med.* 1999;31:352–358.
11. Cicardi M, Cesana B, Del Ninno E, et al. Prevalence and risk factors for the presence of serum cryoglobulins in patients with chronic hepatitis C. *J Viral Hepat.* 2000;7:138–143.
12. Roccatello D, Saadoun D, Ramos-Casals M, et al. Cryoglobulinaemia. *Nat Rev Dis Primers.* 2018;4:11.

13. García-Carrasco M, Ramos-Casals M, Cervera R, et al. Cryoglobulinemia in systemic lupus erythematosus: Prevalence and clinical characteristics in a series of 122 patients. *Semin Arthritis Rheum.* 2001;30:366.

14. Tzioufas AG, Manoussakis MN, Costello R, et al. Cryoglobulinemia in autoimmune rheumatic diseases. Evidence of circulating monoclonal cryoglobulins in patients with primary Sjögren's syndrome. *Arthritis Rheum.* 1986;29:1098–1104.

15. Monti G, Pioltelli P, Saccardo F, et al. Lymphomas in a multicenter case file of patients with hepatitis C virus–related symptomatic mixed cryoglobulinemias. *Arch Intern Med.* 2005;165:101–105.

16. De Sanjose, S, Benavente Y, Vajdic CM, et al. Hepatitis C and non-Hodgkin lymphoma among 4784 cases and 6269 controls from the International Lymphoma Epidemiology Consortium. *Clin Gastroenterol Hepatol.* 2008;6:451–458.

17. Invernizzi F, Pietrogrande M, Sagramoso B. Classification of the cryoglobulinemic syndrome. *Clin Exp Rheumatol.* 1995;13:S123–S128.

18. Muchtar E, Magen H, Gertz MA. How I treat cryoglobulinemia. *Blood.* 2017;129:289–298.

19. Landau DA, Saadoun D, Halfon P, et al. Relapse of hepatitis C virus-associated mixed cryoglobulinemia vasculitis in patients with sustained viral response. *Arthritis Rheum.* 2008;58:604–611.

20. Sollima S, Milazzo L, Peri AM, et al. Persistent mixed cryoglobulinaemia vasculitis despite hepatitis C virus eradication after interferon-free antiviral therapy. *Rheumatology (Oxford).* 2016;55:2084–2085.

21. Saadoun D, Pol S, Ferfar Y, et al. Efficacy and safety of sofosbuvir plus daclatasvir for treatment of HCV-associated cryoglobulinemia vasculitis. *Gastroenterology.* 2017;153:49–52.

22. Sise ME, Bloom AK, Wisocky J, et al. Treatment of hepatitis C virus-associated mixed cryoglobulinemia with direct-acting antiviral agents. *Hepatology.* 2016;63:408–417.

23. Gragnani L, Visentini M, Fognani E, et al. Prospective study of guideline-tailored therapy with direct-acting antivirals for hepatitis C virus-associated mixed cryoglobulinemia. *Hepatology.* 2016;64:1473–1482.

24. Del Padre M, Todi L, Mitrevski M, et al. Reversion of anergy signatures in clonal CD21^{low} B cells of mixed cryoglobulinemia after clearance of HCV viremia. *Blood.* 2017;130:35–38.

25. Wener MH, Hutchinson K, Morishima C, et al. Absence of antibodies to cyclic citrullinated peptide in sera of patients with hepatitis C virus infection and cryoglobulinemia. *Arthritis Rheum.* 2004;50:2305–2308.

26. Siloși I, Boldeanu L, Biciușcă V, et al. Serum biomarkers for discrimination between hepatitis C-related arthropathy and early rheumatoid arthritis. *Int J Mol Sci.* 2017;18(6):E1304.

27. Liu FC, Chao YC, Hou TY, et al. Usefulness of anti-CCP antibodies in patients with hepatitis C virus infection with or without arthritis, rheumatoid factor, or cryoglobulinemia. *Clin Rheumatol.* 2008;27:463–467.

28. Jayakumar D, Huang X, Eisen S, et al. The predictive utility of anti-cyclic citrullinated peptide antibodies to diagnose rheumatoid arthritis in patients with hepatitis C and polyarthralgias [abstract]. *Arthritis Rheumatol.* 2018;70(suppl 10).

29. Fogo AB, Lusco MA, Najafian B, et al. AJKD atlas of renal pathology: Cryoglobulinemic glomerulonephritis. *Am J Kidney Dis.* 2016;67:e5–e7.

30. Bhatia, S. Therapy-related myelodysplasia and acute myeloid leukemia. *Semin Oncol.* 2013;40:666–675.

31. The American Association for the Study of Liver Diseases and the Infectious Diseases Society of America. HCV guidance: Recommendations for testing, managing, and treating hepatitis C. www .hcvguidelines.org. 2014–2018.

32. Roccatello D, Sciascia S, Rossi D, et al. The challenge of treating hepatitis C virus-associated cryoglobulinemic vasculitis in the era of anti-CD20 monoclonal antibodies and direct antiviral agents. *Oncotarget.* 2017;8:41764–41777.

33. Wink F, Houtmann P, Jansen T. Rituximab in cryoglobulinaemic vasculitis, evidence for its effectivity: A case report and review of literature. *Clin Rheumatol.* 2011;30:293–300.

34. Terrier B, Launay D, Kaplanski G, et al. Safety and efficacy of rituximab in nonviral cryoglobulinemia vasculitis: Data from the French Autoimmunity and Rituximab registry. *Arthritis Care Res (Hoboken).* 2010;62:1787–1795.

35. Monti G, Saccardo F, Rinaldi G, et al. Colchicine in the treatment of mixed cryoglobulinemia. *Clin Exp Rheumatol.* 1995;13:S197–S199.

36. Foessel L, Besancenot J, Bertrand M, et al. Clinical spectrum, treatment and outcome of patients with type II mixed cryoglobulinemia without evidence of hepatitis C infection. *J Rheumatol.* 2011;38:1–8.

Cutaneous Vasculitis

Roseanne F. Zhao and Jonathan J. Miner

GENERAL PRINCIPLES

Definitions

- Cutaneous vasculitis is a **small-vessel vasculitis affecting the skin.** However, small-vessel vasculitis is often not specific to just the small vessels, and there **may be involvement of the medium-sized vessels.**
- There are multiple different names for cutaneous vasculitis, which leads to confusion. **Leukocytoclastic vasculitis** (LCV) is often used to refer to cutaneous vasculitis. However, it is a pathologic term and refers to the nuclear "dust" because of degranulation of neutrophils seen under light microscopy. **Leukocytoclasia is nonspecific,** and LCV may be seen with multiple types of cutaneous vasculitides.
- **Necrotizing vasculitis is synonymous with LCV.**
- **Cutaneous leukocytoclastic angiitis (CLA)** refers to isolated cutaneous vasculitis without systemic vasculitis or glomerulonephritis. It has also been referred to as **primary cutaneous small-vessel vasculitis (PCSVV)**[1] or **single-organ cutaneous small-vessel vasculitis (SoCSVV).**[2]
- **Hypersensitivity vasculitis** is a cutaneous vasculitis of the small vessels (arterioles and venules) secondary to an immune response to an exogenous substance. However, there is often no clear evidence of an ongoing immune response or an inciting agent. CLA may be the preferred term over hypersensitivity vasculitis.
- **Lymphocytic vasculitis** is also a cutaneous vasculitis but is different histologically from LCV as it features a lymphocytic infiltrate. It is more commonly observed with vasculitis because of connective tissue disorders and Behçet's disease.

Etiology

- There are multiple causes of cutaneous vasculitis (Table 33-1).
- **One-third of cases are idiopathic.**
- The most common causes of cutaneous vasculitis are **drug induced** and **infection.**[3] Typically it does not involve other organs and presents as CLA.
- **Urticarial vasculitis** results in an urticarial-like rash that lasts longer than 24 to 48 hours. The lesions may progress to a purpuric stage with postinflammatory hyperpigmentation after resolution. There are two types of urticarial vasculitis: the **normocomplementemic form** and the **hypocomplementemic form.**
  - The latter is often associated with systemic lupus erythematosus (SLE)[4] and B-cell lymphoma.
  - Immunoglobulin E (IgE)-mediated disease should be considered in the normocomplementemic form.
- **Congenital immunodeficiencies,** including Wiskott–Aldrich syndrome, DADA2 (deficiency of adenosine deaminase 2), SAVI (STING-associated vasculitis of infancy), phosphoglucomutase 3 (PGM3) deficiency, and monogenic complement defects, may also present with LCV.
- **Viral infections,** including both hepatitis B and C as well as human immunodeficiency virus (HIV), have also been linked to vasculitis. In the case of hepatitis C virus (HCV),

mixed cryoglobulins (Types II and III) deposit in the small and medium vessels, leading to inflammation.
- **Connective tissue diseases** may present with cutaneous vasculitis. These include SLE, Sjögren's syndrome, and rheumatoid arthritis (RA) (rheumatoid vasculitis). The resulting vasculitis can also be lymphocytic.
- There are multiple **systemic vasculitides** that present with cutaneous involvement. These include all three of the antineutrophil cytoplasmic antibody (ANCA)-associated vasculitides, Behçet's disease, Henoch–Schönlein purpura (HSP), polyarteritis nodosa (PAN), and cutaneous PAN (vasculitic changes as with PAN but limited to the skin). As mentioned, hypocomplementemic urticarial vasculitis is often associated with SLE.
- **Erythema elevatum diutinum** is a specific form of chronic cutaneous vasculitis typified by papules and nodules on the extensor surfaces of the extremities. The cause, though unknown, is presumed to be immune complex related. Early lesions show LCV. Many potential associations have been made including infections and various rheumatologic disorders.[5]
- **Lymphoma, leukemia,** and even **solid tumors** have been associated with cutaneous vasculitis. However, malignancy accounts for less than 5% of cases.
- **Hypercoagulable states,** though not an inflammatory process, may appear on physical examination of the skin like a vasculitis because of the ischemia and damage to the vessel.

Pathophysiology

- The pathophysiology of cutaneous vasculitis depends on the etiology. Mechanisms include immune deposition, as well as neutrophil- and lymphocyte-mediated disease.
- Certain infections cause direct invasion of blood vessels (e.g., *Neisseria, Rickettsia*) or may induce immune complex deposition (e.g., hepatitis B virus infection).
- Other vasculitides may also be immune complex mediated (drug-induced or rheumatoid vasculitis) or because of Ig deposition (e.g., IgA in HSP). ANCA-associated vasculitis may involve the skin in addition to other organs, but the role of these antibodies in these cases is unclear.
- The size of the vessel involved dictates the clinical findings. With small-vessel vasculitis, **palpable purpura** is common but **nonpalpable purpura, urticaria, pustules, vesicles, superficial ulcerations, and splinter hemorrhages** all occur.
- When medium-sized vessels are involved, skin changes include **nodules, livedo reticularis, digital infarctions, ulcers, and papulonecrotic lesions.** These differences reflect the greater area of ischemia due to obstruction of a larger blood vessel.
- The majority of cutaneous vasculitis is classified as small vessel.
- Common types of medium-sized vasculitides include PAN, cutaneous PAN, rheumatoid vasculitis, and Buerger's disease.

DIAGNOSIS

The approach to vasculitis of the skin is to answer the following questions:
- Are the skin findings because of vasculitis?
- What is the etiology?
- Are other organ systems involved?

Clinical Presentation

History
- Cutaneous vasculitis usually appears suddenly and the lesions are often painless. In contrast, urticarial vasculitic lesions are often painful and burning rather than pruritic-like allergic urticaria. Myalgias or arthralgias may accompany the skin lesions.

- A history of a connective tissue disease (e.g., RA, SLE, Sjögren's syndrome) is important, as are symptoms of an underlying systemic disease (e.g., fever, night sweats, weight loss, hematuria, pulmonary issues, abdominal pain, joint pain, focal or generalized weakness).
- Cutaneous vasculitis is often the first sign of a serious illness.
- Examine the medication list for possible etiologic agents because **drugs are the most common cause.** Drug-induced vasculitis usually develops 7 to 21 days after starting a drug. Almost any drug can cause a vasculitic reaction, and the most common ones are listed in Table 33-1. Drug reactions typically resolve spontaneously upon discontinuing the medication.
- Hypocomplementemic urticarial vasculitis syndrome is characterized by urticaria for at least 6 months, along with LCV, angioedema, uveitis or episcleritis, glomerulonephritis, arthritis/arthralgia, and recurrent abdominal pain.
- B-cell lymphomas are less likely to be the underlying cause for symptoms less than 6 months.

Physical Examination

Palpable purpura is the classic lesion of cutaneous vasculitis. Nonpalpable purpura, nodules, urticaria, vesicles, and shallow or deep ulcerations are also seen, sometimes in combination.

TABLE 33-1 CAUSES OF CUTANEOUS VASCULITIS SYNDROMES

Cutaneous leukocytoclastic angiitis:
Usually idiopathic or drug induced

Drugs (most common cause):
Penicillins, sulfonamides, allopurinol, thiazides, quinolones, propylthiouracil, hydantoins, nonsteroidal anti-inflammatory drugs, and many others

Infections:
Bacterial: *Streptococcus, Neisseria, Chlamydia, Staphylococcus*, endocarditis
Viral: Hepatitis C (through type II and III cryoglobulins), HIV

Erythema elevatum diutinum:
Many potential associations including infections (e.g., *Streptococcus*, HIV), rheumatologic conditions (e.g., rheumatoid arthritis, relapsing polychondritis), and inflammatory bowel disease

Congenital immunodeficiencies:
Wiskott–Aldrich syndrome, DADA2 (deficiency of adenosine deaminase 2), SAVI (STING-associated vasculitis of infancy), phosphoglucomutase 3 (PGM3) deficiency, monogenic complement defects (including complement factor I deficiency, C4 deficiency, C3 gain-of-function), and others

Connective tissue diseases:
Rheumatoid arthritis, systemic lupus erythematosus, Sjögren's syndrome

Systemic vasculitides:
Henoch–Schönlein purpura, polyarteritis nodosa (classic and cutaneous), urticarial vasculitis, Behçet's disease, cryoglobulinemia (type II and III), granulomatous polyangiitis, eosinophilic granulomatosis with polyangiitis, microscopic polyangiitis

Malignancy:
Lymphoma, leukemia, solid tumors (e.g., lung, colon, breast, renal, prostate)

Inflammatory bowel disease

Idiopathic

TABLE 33-2	AMERICAN COLLEGE OF RHEUMATOLOGY 1990 CRITERIA FOR HYPERSENSITIVITY VASCULITIS

At least three of the following five should be present:
- Age >16 years
- Use of a possibly causative drug related temporally to symptoms
- Palpable purpura
- Maculopapular rash
- Biopsy demonstrating granulocytes around the arteriole or venule

Adapted from: Calabrese LH, Michel BA, Bloch DA, et al. The American College of Rheumatology 1990 criteria for the classification of hypersensitivity vasculitis. *Arthritis Rheum.* 1990; 33:1108–1113.

- Lesions usually occur in the lower extremities or in dependent locations. However, urticarial vasculitis is more common on the trunk and proximal extremities.
- The physical examination aims to identify other organ system involvement and should include a musculoskeletal examination looking for arthritis.
  - A neurologic examination is important to identify focal or diffuse weakness that may occur because of mononcuritis multiplex.
  - Palpate for enlarged lymph nodes that may suggest infection or underlying malignancy.
  - Auscultate the heart for murmurs and inspect the nails if endocarditis is suspected.

Diagnostic Criteria

The American College of Rheumatology criteria for hypersensitivity vasculitis are presented in Table 33-2.[6]

Differential Diagnosis

Multiple processes in the skin can result in nonblanching purpura, ulcerations, and urticaria. See Table 33-3 for common nonvasculitic causes of these findings.

Diagnostic Testing

Laboratories
- Investigate renal involvement with **chemistries** and **urinalysis.**
- A **hepatic function panel** can be helpful.
- **Blood cultures** (and cultures from other sites) are mandatory in cases with fever because infections, including endocarditis, can cause vasculitis.
- The **erythrocyte sedimentation rate (ESR)** is often elevated but is nonspecific. Testing for systemic markers of disease is not recommended unless there is clinical suspicion.
- Specific labs to help diagnose systemic causes include but are not limited to antinuclear antibodies (ANA), anti–double-stranded DNA (dsDNA), rheumatoid factor (RF), ANCA, hepatitis serologies, cryoglobulin determination, C3, C4, CH50, SSA, SSB, and urine protein electrophoresis (UPEP).
  - If hypocomplementemic (low C3, C4, C1 esterase inhibitor) with acquired angioedema, consider SLE and B-cell lymphoma.
  - If normocomplementemic, consider IgE-mediated disease.

Imaging
Chest radiographs or computed tomography (CT) scans may be needed to evaluate the lungs and the upper respiratory tract as well as to rule out systemic disease, especially in patients with hypocomplementemia.

TABLE 33-3	MIMICS OF CUTANEOUS VASCULITIS

Hypercoagulable states
Antiphospholipid syndrome
Monoclonal cryoglobulins (Type I): Associated with multiple myeloma and
 Waldenström's macroglobulinemia; may cause hyperviscosity
Warfarin-induced skin necrosis
Protein C and S deficiency
Thrombocytosis

Emboli
Cholesterol, atrial myxoma, endocarditis
Septic vasculitis

Other causes of purpura
Thrombotic thrombocytopenic purpura
Idiopathic thrombocytopenic purpura
Other causes of thrombocytopenia
Other coagulation disorders
Systemic amyloidosis
Scurvy
Pyoderma gangrenosum
Sweet's syndrome
Calciphylaxis

Diagnostic Procedures
- A **skin biopsy** is essential to confirm the diagnosis.
- Indications for biopsy include symptoms of systemic disease or continued formation of new lesions for more than 3 weeks.
- If possible, perform biopsies within 24 to 48 hours after the appearance of a lesion. Biopsies performed before or after this time typically show a nonspecific lymphocytic infiltrate.[7,8]
- Ulcerated sites should be avoided. When it is necessary to biopsy an ulcerated site, the edge should be sampled.
- A punch biopsy provides the appropriate depth for examination, especially for deeper medium-sized vessels.
- Examine specimens under light microscopy and direct immunofluorescence.
- Under light microscopy, the affected blood vessels are characterized by **fibrinoid necrosis** of the vessel wall with an **inflammatory infiltrate within and around the vessel wall.**
  ○ When the infiltrate is only perivascular, the diagnosis of vasculitis cannot be made reliably.
  ○ Hemorrhage and fragments of leukocytes (**leukocytoclasia**) are also seen.
  ○ Cutaneous vasculitic lesions associated with connective tissue diseases often have lymphocytic infiltration.
  ○ Prominence of eosinophils is suggestive of eosinophilic granulomatosis with polyangiitis.
  ○ Urticarial lesions have an LCV histopathology.
- **Direct immunofluorescence** may reveal **Ig and complement deposition** on the vessel wall.
  ○ In particular, IgA deposition is characteristic of HSP. C3 fragments may also be aggregated with IgA.
  ○ **ANCA-associated vasculitides are considered pauci-immune** because few immune reactants are present on immunofluorescence.
  ○ Rheumatoid vasculitis reveals a granular IgM and C3 deposition, suggesting an immune complex–mediated disease.

TREATMENT

- In the absence of other organ involvement and underlying diseases, treatment of cutaneous vasculitis is symptomatic.
    - **Antihistamines and nonsteroidal anti-inflammatory drugs (NSAIDs)** may be helpful.
    - Some severe cases may require **glucocorticoids.**
    - If drug-induced vasculitis is suspected, **stop the offending drug.** Most cases of drug-induced cutaneous vasculitis resolve within 2 to 3 weeks to a few months upon stopping the offending medication.
    - **Colchicine, dapsone,** and **omalizumab** may be considered in normocomplementemic urticarial vasculitis.
- For chronic disease, steroid-sparing agents may be used.
- **The treatment of cutaneous vasculitis, as a manifestation of an underlying disorder, varies according to the type of disorder and other organ involvement.**

MONITORING/FOLLOW-UP

Follow-up is important because cutaneous vasculitis can be the first manifestation of a systemic disease or malignancy.

REFERENCES

1. Russell JP, Gibson LE. Primary cutaneous small vessel vasculitis: approach to diagnosis and treatment. *Int J Dermatol.* 2006;45:3–13.
2. Jennette JC, Falk RJ, Bacon PA, et al. 2012. Revised International Chapel Hill Consensus Conference Nomenclature of Vasculitides. *Arthritis Rheum.* 2013;65:1–11.
3. Loricera J, Blanco R, Ortiz-Sanjuán F, et al. Single-organ cutaneous small-vessel vasculitis according to the 2012 revised International Chapel Hill Consensus Conference Nomenclature of Vasculitides: a study of 60 patients from a series of 766 cutaneous vasculitis cases. *Rheumatology.* 2015;54:77–82.
4. Davis MD, Brewer JD. Urticarial vasculitis and hypocomplementemic urticarial vasculitis syndrome. *Immunol Allergy Clin North Am.* 2004;24:183–213.
5. Gibson LE, el-Azhary RA. Erythema elevatum diutinum. *Clin Dermatol.* 2000;18:295–299.
6. Calabrese LH, Michel BA, Bloch DA, et al. The American College of Rheumatology 1990 criteria for the classification of hypersensitivity vasculitis. *Arthritis Rheum.* 1990;33:1108–1113.
7. Carlson JA. The histological assessment of cutaneous vasculitis. *Histopathology.* 2010;56:3–23.
8. Stone JH, Nousari HC. "Essential" cutaneous vasculitis: What every rheumatologist should know about vasculitis of the skin. *Curr Opin Rheumatol.* 2001;13:23–34.

Behçet's Disease

34

Roseanne F. Zhao and Jonathan J. Miner

GENERAL PRINCIPLES

Definition

- Behçet's disease (BD) is a systemic relapsing and remitting variable vessel vasculitis,[1] affecting both arteries and vein, characterized by **recurrent aphthous oral and genital ulcers as well as uveitis.**
- Skin lesions, joint complaints, vascular disease, gastrointestinal and neurologic manifestations are also associated with BD and may be the presenting symptom.
- BD is relatively unique among the vasculitides in its **ability to affect both venous and arterial vessels of all sizes.**

Epidemiology

- It is most commonly seen along the historic Silk Road extending from **eastern Asia to the Mediterranean basin.**
- **Turkey has the highest prevalence** of BD estimated at 80 to 420 cases per 100,000, whereas the prevalence is much lower in the United States.[2]
- Emigrants from countries with high disease prevalence have a lower incidence of disease compared to their originating countries but higher compared to the local population.
- BD is more common in men in the Mediterranean region but possibly more common in women in East Asia. However, prevalence data may be inaccurate because women in some cultures may not seek medical attention for their symptoms.
- Peak age of onset is in the second to fourth decade. Earlier age of onset is associated with increased severity and mortality.

Risk Factors

- HLA-B51 has been strongly associated with BD in countries with high prevalence rates along the historic Silk Road,[2,3] but the association is much weaker in Caucasian patients. Only about 60% of BD patients carry this risk allele.
- HLA-B15, -B27, -B26, and -B57 are also independent risk factors, whereas HLA-B49 and -A03 may be protective against the development of BD.[2,4]
- Non-HLA associations include variants of endoplasmic reticulum aminopeptidase 1 (ERAP1), interleukin (IL)-23R–IL-12RB2, IL-10, and signal transducer and activator of transcription 4 (STAT4).[2,4]
- Infectious triggers, reduced biodiversity, and other unspecified microbiome signatures may disrupt immune homeostasis and contribute to risk for developing BD.

Pathophysiology

- BD has **features of both autoinflammatory and autoimmune diseases.** The exact cause is unknown but is likely because of a **combination of genetic and environmental factors.**
- Genetic anticipation with symptomatic disease at younger ages in successive generations has been noted in familial clustering of BD.[5]
- Patients with BD may have altered antigen presentation and HLA interaction with receptors on T cells and natural killer cells.[6]

- Cross-reactivity and molecular mimicry between microbial heat shock proteins and self-proteins may contribute to pathogenesis. Herpes simplex virus 1 and streptococcus are possible triggers.
- Evidence points toward a **Th1-mediated disease**, characterized by elevated levels of interferon (IFN)-γ, tumor necrosis factor (TNF)-α, IL-1, IL-6, and IL-2, **with involvement of Th17 cells** and the IL-17/IL-23 pathway, resulting in hyperactivation of neutrophils.
- Neutrophils are the major inflammatory infiltrate in vasculitis of various sized vessels, with endothelial swelling, fibrinoid necrosis, and vascular occlusion. A lymphocytic vasculitis can also be seen.
- Veins are more commonly involved than arteries. Cutaneous thrombophlebitis can result from small- and medium-vessel involvement.
- Larger vessels demonstrate **vasculitis of the vasa vasorum with aneurysmal formation** and superimposed **hypercoagulability,** resulting in thrombosis.
- In Behçet's uveitis, CD8+ T cells are the predominant intraocular infiltrating cells.[7] Neutrophils are predominantly seen in the hypopyon, a layer of pus that can develop in the anterior chamber of the eye.

DIAGNOSIS

BD remains a clinical diagnosis based on characteristic disease manifestations. Diagnostic criteria may be used to help identify and guide diagnosis. However, it should be noted that the emergence of major manifestations of BD may be separated by months to years.

Diagnostic Criteria
- The 1990 International Study Group classification criteria for BD are presented in Table 34-1.[8] A multiethnic study of 300 patients showed an overall sensitivity of 90% and specificity of 95%, but these varied significantly by race.[9]
- The 2013 Revised International Criteria for BD are presented in Table 34-2.[10]
  - A large cohort of Iranian patients demonstrated a sensitivity of 98%, specificity of 95%, and diagnostic accuracy of 97% for the 2006 criteria.[11]
  - Criteria were updated in 2013 to account for geographic variations of BD. These new criteria demonstrate increased sensitivity compared to the previous criteria.

Clinical Presentation
Clinical manifestations of BD may show geographic differences.[12]

History
In most series, the most common symptoms at presentation of BD include oral and genital aphthosis, eye manifestations, and skin lesions.

TABLE 34-1	1990 INTERNATIONAL STUDY GROUP CLASSIFICATION CRITERIA FOR BEHÇET'S DISEASE

Recurrent (≥3 episodes in a 12-month period) oral aphthous ulceration plus two of the following four:
- Genital ulceration
- Skin manifestations (erythema nodosum, pseudofolliculitis, acneiform lesions)
- Eye inflammation (anterior/posterior uveitis, retinal vasculitis)
- Pathergy phenomenon

Adapted from: Criteria for diagnosis of Behçet's disease. International Study Group for Behçet's disease. *Lancet.* 1990;335:1078–1080.

TABLE 34-2	**2013 PROPOSED INTERNATIONAL CRITERIA FOR BEHÇET'S DISEASE (ICBD)**

Patients who present with the following manifestations whose sum of points is four or more are classified as having Behçet's disease:

Oral aphthosis	2 points
Genital aphthosis	2 points
Ocular lesions	2 points
Skin manifestations	1 point
Central nervous system involvement	1 point
Vascular lesions (arterial and venous thrombosis, aneurysm)	1 point
Pathergy test (optional)	1 point

Adapted from: International Team for the Revision of the International Criteria for Behçet's Disease (ITR-ICBD). The International Criteria for Behçet's Disease (ICBD): a collaborative study of 27 countries on the sensitivity and specificity of the new criteria. *J Eur Acad Dermatol Venereol.* 2014;28:338–347.

- **Oral aphthosis** is the most common manifestation and is usually seen in patients throughout the course of the disease.
- **Genital aphthosis** occurs less frequently and may be more common in Caucasians.
- **Ocular symptoms** include changes in visual acuity, pain, photophobia, lacrimation, floaters, and periorbital erythema. It is one of the most frequently diagnosed causes for uveitis in the Far East.
  - Approximately 10% of patients have eye involvement at presentation, whereas approximately 50% develop manifestations during the course of the disease.
  - Ocular manifestations, as the initial symptom, are more common in females, but eye involvement tends to be more severe in males.
  - **Blindness** occurs in approximately 25% of patients with eye involvement.
- **Cutaneous manifestations** of BD include erythema nodosum, pseudofolliculitis, acneiform nodules, and superficial thrombophlebitis. **Erythema nodosum** is observed in approximately 50% of patients in the course of disease and is more common in females.

Physical Examination
- **Oral aphthosis** begins as a raised area of redness that ulcerates, usually occurring in crops of multiple lesions.
  - Lesions are typically round or oval shaped, painful, 2 to 10 mm in size, with a sharp erythematous border, a necrotic white-centered base, and a yellow pseudomembrane.
  - They may occur on the gingiva, tongue, and buccal and labial membranes but rarely on the palate, pharynx, or tonsils. They heal within approximately 10 days but **tend to recur frequently** during the first few years.
- **Ocular findings**, including anterior, posterior, and panuveitis, affects 50% to 90% of BD patients. It is bilateral in 90% of patients, but flares are typically unilateral and alternate between eyes.
  - **Anterior uveitis** tends to be recurrent and self-limited. It causes pain, tearing, eye redness, light sensitivity, or blurry vision.
    - **Hypopyon,** a layer of pus in the anterior ocular chamber, may be visible in up to 20% of patients. This finding is classic for anterior uveitis but has poor prognosis as it is frequently seen with retinal involvement.
    - Repeated attacks can cause iris deformity and glaucoma.

- ○ **Retinal disease** in posterior uveitis is characterized by vasculitis leading to vaso-occlusive disease.
  - ▪ Attacks are recurrent and episodic and result in painless, gradual, bilateral visual loss.
  - ▪ Retinal hemorrhage, exudative lesions, and cellular infiltration of the vitreous humor are visible on examination.
- ○ Patients may develop irreversible visual impairment, loss of visual field, depth and color perception, decreased contrast sensitivity, floaters, glare, and increased light sensitivity.
- • **Cutaneous manifestations** include the following:
  - ○ **Erythema nodosum:** Recurrent and painful subcutaneous nodules that tend to occur on the anterior portion of the lower legs and last for several weeks. Nodules often leave an area of hyperpigmentation and, after spontaneous resolution, they occasionally ulcerate. They occur in 50% of patients.
  - ○ **Pseudofolliculitis and acneiform nodules** occur in about 65% of patients and are more common in men. The lesions are found on the back, face, neck, and along the hairline and are often precipitated by shaving.
  - ○ **Genital ulcers** are rarely the presenting symptoms of BD, but over the course of the disease they appear in approximately 75% of patients.
    - ▪ They are similar in appearance to oral ulcers, but tend to be more painful, larger, last longer, recur less frequently, and often leave scars.
    - ▪ Ulcers commonly form on the scrotum and vulva, and rarely involve the penis, vaginal mucosa, or perianal region.
    - ▪ In young women, the ulcers may be related temporally to the menstrual cycle, occurring in the premenstrual stage, and may be the only manifestation of disease during the early years.
  - ○ The **pathergy test** is performed by using two subcutaneous pricks, to a depth of 5 mm, with blunt 20-gauge sterile needles to one arm and with sharp 20-gauge sterile needles to the other arm.
    - ▪ A test is considered positive if a sterile erythematous papule >2 mm forms at 48 hours.
    - ▪ Blunt needles seem to produce more positive reactions.
    - ▪ The test appears to have high specificity but sensitivity is variable.
    - ▪ Pathergy is less common in European and North American patients and more commonly seen in countries along the historic Silk Road.
- • **Articular manifestations** are common.
  - ○ The inflammatory arthritis of BD is acute, nondeforming, nonerosive, occasionally recurrent, migratory, and rarely chronic.
  - ○ It tends to be monoarticular and asymmetric, commonly affecting the knee, followed by the wrist, ankle, or elbow, but it can also be oligoarticular or polyarticular.
  - ○ It may occasionally present in the distribution and pattern of rheumatoid arthritis.
- • **Venous thrombosis** is a characteristic manifestation.
  - ○ **Superficial thrombophlebitis and deep venous thrombosis** are common after injury to vessels, including cannulation by angiocatheters. Superficial thrombophlebitis is seen in about 25% of patients.
  - ○ The frequency and type (arterial versus venous) of thrombosis may vary by ethnicity and sex.[13–15]
  - ○ Embolic events are rare. Occlusions of major vessels, such as in **Budd–Chiari syndrome**, are associated with high mortality.[16]
- • Arterial disease is less common, seen in <5% of patients, but associated with increased mortality.
  - ○ Thoracic and abdominal aortic aneurysms, as well as aortic root dilation, have been described.

○ **Pulmonary artery and bronchial artery aneurysms with venous thrombosis** occur in Hughes–Stovin syndrome,[17] a subset of BD. It is associated with high morbidity and mortality, with pulmonary hemorrhage being the cause of death in 60% of these patients.

• **Central nervous system (CNS) involvement** in BD occurs in approximately 10% to 20% of patients.

○ It is more common and severe in males, particularly if the disease begins at a young age.

○ Manifestations including **aseptic meningitis, meningoencephalitis, focal neurologic deficits, and personality changes** tend to develop more than 5 years after diagnosis.

○ Focal signs include pyramidal tract disease (e.g., spastic paralysis, Babinski sign, clonus, and speech disturbances), brain stem disease (e.g., dysphagia and fits of laughter alternating with crying), cerebellar ataxia, and pseudobulbar palsy.

○ Sensory deficits are uncommon.

○ **Intracranial venous thrombosis** can lead to intracranial hypertension, seizures, and hemorrhage.[18]

○ CNS BD tends to recur and becomes irreversible. In a study of 200 Turkish patients, 41% have a relapsing–remitting course, 28% a secondary progressive course, 10% a primary progressive course, and 21% silent neurologic involvement.[19]

○ In the terminal stage, approximately 30% of affected BD patients with CNS manifestations may have dementia.

○ Aseptic meningitis or meningoencephalitis, early in the disease course, successfully treated with steroids, carries a good prognosis.

• Other rare manifestations of BD include myocardial infarction, pulmonary embolus, epididymitis, as well as ulcerations along the gastrointestinal tract (esophageal, ileocecal, colonic, etc.).

Differential Diagnosis

• The differential diagnosis depends on the presenting clinical manifestations.

• Erythema nodosum, ileocecal involvement, and ulcerative mouth lesions may suggest Crohn's disease, especially in patients with iron deficiency and an elevated erythrocyte sedimentation rate (ESR) >100.

• **Reactive arthritis** should also be considered if oral and genital ulcers are present in the setting of inflammatory joint symptoms. If ocular manifestations and acneiform nodules are present, **seronegative arthropathies** must be considered in the differential.

• **Malignancies** and **viral infections**, including herpes, human immunodeficiency virus (HIV), and syphilis, may cause ulcers and uveitis that mimic BD.

• **Sweet's syndrome** may cause similar-appearing skin lesions and uveitis.

• **Sarcoidosis** may also produce erythema nodosum and uveitis.

• **SLE** and **systemic vasculitides** should also be considered.

• CNS involvement in BD may mimic **multiple sclerosis** and other neurologic pathologies.

Diagnostic Testing

Laboratories

• No specific test for BD is available. Laboratory findings may include an elevated ESR and C-reactive protein (CRP; do not correlate with disease activity), as well as mild leukocytosis and anemia of chronic disease.

• Cerebrospinal fluid analysis may show elevated protein and immunoglobulin G (IgG), as well as pleocytosis with high numbers of both lymphocytes and neutrophils.

• Joint fluid is inflammatory with increased neutrophils.

Imaging

If neurologic BD is suspected, magnetic resonance imaging (MRI) of the brain and magnetic resonance venography (MRV) can show multiple high-intensity focal lesions in the brain stem, basal ganglia, and white matter.

Diagnostic Procedures
- **A positive pathergy test is often considered diagnostic.**
  - ○ The result may not be consistent throughout the course of the disease, that is, it may appear and then disappear.
  - ○ It is important to note that a positive pathergy test is much less frequently seen in Western countries, including the United States and the United Kingdom, than in Eastern countries along the Silk Road.
- Endoscopy should be performed to confirm gastrointestinal involvement.

TREATMENT

Treatment of BD depends on clinical manifestations, disease severity, and resistance to treatment.[20,21]

Medications

- **Mucocutaneous aphthosis and skin lesions**
  - ○ First-line treatment is **colchicine** at 0.6 mg BID if renal function is not impaired. Side effects are uncommon at this dose.
  - ○ If there is inadequate response, the dose of colchicine may be increased; however, this may be limited by the occurrence of undesirable side effects, usually diarrhea.
  - ○ Second-line therapy includes **levamisole** (150 mg once weekly), **dapsone** (50–150 mg daily), or **thalidomide** (50–150 mg daily; note risk of neuropathy with prolonged use).
  - ○ If no response is noted, consider switching to **methotrexate** (5–20 mg once weekly) or **azathioprine** (2–3 mg/kg daily).
  - ○ **Apremilast** has recently been shown to help mucocutaneous lesions in a subset of BD patients.[22]
  - ○ If these fail, **consider biologic therapy.**
  - ○ In resistant cases of genital aphthosis, **intralesional injection of triamcinolone acetate** may help heal the lesion. Dermatology consultation may be valuable in this setting.
- **Ocular involvement**
  - ○ Ophthalmologic referral is recommended.
  - ○ **Posterior uveitis** is treated with **azathioprine** (2–3 mg/kg daily), cyclosporine A (3–5 mg/kg daily), **IFN-α**, or **TNF-α antagonists** such as infliximab.[23,24] Systemic high-dose glucocorticoids may be used as an adjunct during an acute attack to help suppress inflammation.
    - For severe symptoms, systemic high-dose glucocorticoids, IFN-α, or TNF-α antagonists should be started as first-line therapy. Infliximab has a rapid onset of action with effects within the first 24 hours; other TNF antagonists are also efficacious.
    - Intravitreal glucocorticoids may be used in addition to systemic immunosuppression in severe cases.
  - ○ **Tocilizumab** may be considered in cases of refractory or difficult to manage uveitis associated with BD.[25–28]
  - ○ **Anakinra** and **canakinumab** have also been shown to control ocular inflammation and decrease the frequency of flares.[29–31]
  - ○ **Isolated anterior uveitis** is treated with **topical steroid drops** (e.g., betamethasone, 1–2 drops TID) and mydriatic agents if the symptoms are mild and isolated.
    - Because anterior uveitis is known for recurrent attacks requiring topical steroids that can eventually lead to cataracts and glaucoma, consider switching to cytotoxic agents such as **azathioprine or methotrexate** in these cases.
    - Azathioprine may be considered as first line in patients with hypopyon uveitis; it is not known whether starting systemic treatment is protective against the development of posterior uveitis.
  - ○ Biologic therapy may be considered in frequently recurrent or refractory cases.

- **Neurologic involvement** is treated with **intravenous (IV) cyclophosphamide** or **high-dose systemic steroids** (IV methylprednisolone pulse 1 g daily for 3 to 10 days, followed by prednisone 1 mg/kg daily to be tapered over 6 months).
  - Cyclosporine A should be avoided because it may increase the risk of developing parenchymal neurologic involvement in BD.[32]
  - **TNF-α antagonists**[33,34] and **tocilizumab**[35] may be considered as alternative therapies for parenchymal disease. **Anakinra and canakinumab** have also shown some benefit.[30,31] In patients with **acute cerebral venous thrombosis**, a short course of **anticoagulation may be considered in addition to high-dose steroids**.
- **Vascular involvement**
  - Venous thrombosis (including Budd–Chiari syndrome, deep venous thrombosis, and superficial thrombophlebitis) is treated with immunosuppression, such as glucocorticoids, cyclophosphamide, or azathioprine. Refractory cases may be treated with TNF-α antagonists. **Anticoagulation** may be considered if patients have a low bleeding risk and no concurrent pulmonary artery aneurysms, but it has not shown significant efficacy in reducing the recurrence of thrombosis, though it may reduce the risk of postthrombotic syndrome.
  - **Arterial aneurysms** (including aortic, pulmonary, and peripheral artery aneurysms) should be treated with high-dose glucocorticoids and cyclophosphamide. TNF-α antagonists should be used for refractory cases.[36,37]
    - For stable disease, patients should be treated medically prior to surgical intervention to reduce complications and poor wound healing.
    - Surgery should not be delayed in symptomatic or emergent cases.
- **Arthralgias/arthritis** can usually be treated with colchicine or nonsteroidal anti-inflammatory drugs (NSAIDs) until resolution of symptoms. Intra-articular glucocorticoids may be used in acute monoarticular disease. Methotrexate, azathioprine, and TNF-α antagonists may be considered in chronic or recurrent cases.
- **Gastrointestinal manifestations**
  - Use low-dose **glucocorticoids** and **sulfasalazine** as first-line treatment.
  - Switch to **high-dose steroids and IV cyclophosphamide** if first-line treatment is ineffective.
  - **TNF antagonists** should be considered for severe cases.
- **Treatment with a TNF antagonist** should be considered for patients with **refractory BD** who experience relapsing uveitis, active neurologic manifestations, vascular involvement, refractory gastrointestinal disease, or other symptoms related to BD that are life threatening and/or significantly affecting their quality of life.

Surgical Management

- Surgery is indicated for patients with bowel perforation or recurrent bleeding.
- Arterial aneurysms may require stenting or surgical intervention, including graft insertion, ligation, and bypass.
- Because surgical procedures can result in excessive infiltration of inflammatory cells into treated tissues, intermediate doses of steroids may be used perioperatively to prevent poor wound healing and avoid complications.

MONITORING/FOLLOW-UP

Frequency of follow-up depends on assessment of disease activity and requirements for monitoring drug toxicity.

REFERENCES

1. Jennette JC, Falk RJ, et al. 2012 Revised International Chapel Hill Consensus Conference Nomenclature of Vasculitides. *Arthritis & Rheumatism*. 2013; 65:1–11.
2. Takeuchi M, Kastner DL, Remmers EF. The immunogenetics of Behçet's disease: a comprehensive review. *J Autoimmun*. 2015; 64: 137–148.

3. de Menthon M, Lavalley MP, Maldini C, et al. HLA-B51/B5 and the risk of Behçet's disease: A systematic review and meta-analysis of case-control genetic association studies. *Arthritis Rheum.* 2009;61:1287–1296.

4. Remmers EF, Cosan F, Kirino Y, et al. Genome-wide association study identifies variants in the MHC class I, IL10, and IL23R-IL12RB2 regions associated with Behçet's disease. *Nat Genet.* 2010;42:698–702.

5. Fresko I, Soy M, Hamuryudan V, et al. Genetic anticipation in Behçet's syndrome. *Ann Rheum Dis.* 1998;57:45–48.

6. Giza M, Koftori D, Chen L, et al. Is Behçet's disease a "class 1-opathy"? The role of HLA-B*51 in the pathogenesis of Behçet's disease. *Clin Exp Immunol.* 2018;191:11–18.

7. Park UC, Kim TW, Yu HG. Immunopathogenesis of ocular Behçet's disease. *J Immunol Res.* 2014;2014:653539.

8. Criteria for diagnosis of Behçet's disease. International Study Group for Behçet's disease. *Lancet.* 1990;335:1078–1080.

9. O'Neill TW, Rigby AS, Silman AJ, et al. Validation of the International Study Group criteria for Behçet's disease. *Br J Rheumatol.* 1994;33:115–117.

10. International Team for the Revision of the International Criteria for Behçet's Disease (ITR-ICBD). The International Criteria for Behçet's Disease (ICBD): a collaborative study of 27 countries on the sensitivity and specificity of the new criteria. *J Eur Acad Dermatol Venereol.* 2014;28:338–347.

11. International Team for the Revision of the International Criteria for Behçet's Disease (ITR-ICBD). Revision of the International Criteria for Behçet's Disease (ICBD). *Clin Exp Rheumatol.* 2006; 24:S14–S15.

12. Leonardo NM, McNeil J. Behçet's disease: is there geographical variation? A review far from the Silk Road. *Int J Rheumatol.* 2015;2015:945262.

13. Ames PR, Steuer A, Pap A, et al. Thrombosis in Behçet's disease: a retrospective survey from a single UK centre. *Rheumatology.* 2001;40(6):652–655.

14. Gurler A, Boyvat A, Tursen U. Clinical manifestations of Behçet's disease: an analysis of 2147 patients. *Yonsei Med J.* 1997;38(6):423–427.

15. Koc Y, Gullu I, Akpek G, et al. Vascular involvement in Behçet's disease. *J Rheumatol.* 1992;19(3):402–410.

16. Seyahi E, Caglar E, Ugurlu S, et al. An outcome survey of 43 patients with Budd-Chiari syndrome due to Behçet's syndrome followed up at a single, dedicated center. *Semin Arthritis Rheum.* 2015;44:602–609.

17. Khalid U, Saleem T. Hughes-Stovin syndrome. *Orphanet J Rare Dis.* 2011;6:15.

18. Aguiarr de Sousa D, Mestre T, Ferro JM. Cerebral venous thrombosis in Behçet's disease: a systematic review. *J Neurol.* 2001;258:719–727.

19. Akman-Demir G, Serdaroglu P, Tasçi B. Clinical patterns of neurological involvement in Behçet's disease: evaluation of 200 patients. The Neuro-Behçet study group. *Brain.* 1999;122:2171–2182.

20. Ozguler Y, Leccese P, Christensen R, et al. Management of major organ involvement of Behçet's syndrome: a systematic review for update of the EULAR recommendations. *Rheumatology (Oxford).* 2018;57:2200–2212.

21. Hatemi G, Christensen R, Bang D, et al. 2018 update of the EULAR recommendations for the management of Behçet's syndrome. *Ann Rheum Dis.* 2018;77:808–818.

22. Hatemi G, Melikoglu M, Tunc R, et al. Apremilast for Behçet's syndrome: a phase 2, placebo-controlled study. *N Engl J Med.* 2015; 372:1510–1518.

23. Takeuchi M, Kezuka T, Sugita S, et al. Evaluation of the long-term efficacy and safety of infliximab treatment for uveitis in Behçet's disease: a multicenter study. *Ophthalmology.* 2014;121:1877–1884.

24. Calvo-Río V, Blanco R, Beltrán E, et al. Anti-TNF-α therapy in patients with refractory uveitis due to Behçet's disease: a 1-year follow-up study of 124 patients. *Rheumatology (Oxford).* 2014;53:2223–2231.

25. Atienza-Mateo B, Calvo-Río V, Beltrán E, et al. Anti-interleukin 6 receptor tocilizumab in refractory uveitis associated with Behçet's disease: multicentre retrospective study. *Rheumatology (Oxford).* 2018;57:856–864.

26. Eser Ozturk H, Oray M, Tugal-Tutkun I. Tocilizumab for the treatment of Behçet uveitis that failed interferon alpha and anti-tumor necrosis factor-alpha therapy. *Ocul Immunol Inflamm.* 2018;26:1005–1014.

27. Deroux A, Chiquet C, Bouillet L. Tocilizumab in severe and refractory Behçet's disease: Four cases and literature review. *Semin Arthritis Rheum.* 2016;45:733–737.

28. Calvo-Río V, de la Hera D, Beltrán-Catalán E, et al. Tocilizumab in uveitis refractory to other biologic drugs: a study of 3 cases and a literature review. *Clin Exp Rheumatol.* 2014;32:S54–S57.

29. Fabiani C, Vitale A, Emmi G, et al. Interleukin (IL)-1 inhibition with anakinra and canakinumab in Behçet's disease-related uveitis: a multicenter retrospective observational study. *Clin Rheumatol.* 2017;36:191–197.

30. Emmi G, Talarico R, Lopalco G, et al. Efficacy and safety profile of anti-interleukin-1 treatment in Behçet's disease: a multicenter retrospective study. *Clin Rheumatol.* 2016;35:1281–1286.

31. Cantarini L, Vitale A, Scalini P, et al. Anakinra treatment in drug-resistant Behçet's disease: a case series. *Clin Rheumatol.* 2015;34:1293–1301.

32. Akman-Demir G, Ayranci O, Kurtuncu M, et al. Cyclosporine for Behçet's uveitis: is it associated with an increased risk of neurological involvement? *Clin Exp Rheumatol.* 2008;26:S84–S90.

33. Zeydan B, Uygunoglu U, Saip S, et al. Infliximab is a plausible alternative for neurologic complications of Behçet disease. *Neurol Neuroimmunol Neuroinflamm.* 2016;3:e258.

34. Al-Araji ASA, Saip S. Treatment of NeuroBehçet's disease with infliximab: an international multi-centre case-series of 18 patients. *Clin Exp Rheumatol.* 2010;28:S119.

35. Addimanda O, Pipitone N, Pazzola G, et al. Tocilizumab for severe refractory neuro-Behçet: three cases IL-6 blockade in neuro-Behçet. *Semin Arthritis Rheum.* 2015;44:472–475.

36. Desbois AC, Biard L, Addimanda O, et al. Efficacy of anti-TNF alpha in severe and refractory major vessel involvement of Behçet's disease: a multicenter observational study of 18 patients. *Clin Immunol.* 2018;197:54–59.

37. Hamuryudan V, Seyahi E, Ugurlu S, et al. Pulmonary artery involvement in Behçet's syndrome: effects of anti-TNF treatment. *Semin Arthritis Rheum.* 2015;45:369–373.

VI

Infection-Related Disorders

Infectious Arthritis

35

Colin Diffie and Prabha Ranganathan

GENERAL PRINCIPLES

- Infectious arthritis is caused by **bacteria, fungi, mycobacteria, and viruses.**
- **Prompt joint fluid analysis and culture** is essential to the diagnosis of infectious arthritis as well as tailoring specific antibiotic therapy.
- **Empiric antibiotics** are utilized while awaiting specific culture data.
- Treatment often requires a multidisciplinary approach, involving physical therapy, orthopedic surgery, and infectious disease consultation.

Definition

Infectious arthritis, also referred to as septic arthritis, is an **acute monoarthritis** or oligoarthritis caused by an infectious agent, most often bacteria.

Classification

- Bacterial infectious arthritis is classically divided into gonococcal and nongonococcal arthritis.
- Other etiologies for infectious arthritis include viruses, mycobacteria, and fungi.
- Please see Chapter 36 for discussion on Lyme disease.

Epidemiology

The estimated incidence of infectious arthritis in the United States is approximately 20,000 cases annually, with a rate of 1 in 10,000 per year.

Etiology

- Most cases of bacterial arthritis in adults are caused by *Staphylococcus aureus*, accounting for up to 80% of confirmed cases.[1]
- The second leading pathogen is *Streptococcus pneumoniae*, followed by **gram-negative bacteria**, although any microbial pathogen is capable of causing infectious arthritis.
- The leading cause of bacterial arthritis in young, sexually active adults is *Neisseria gonorrhoeae*, with a male-to-female ratio of 1:4.
- **Viral infections** commonly associated with arthritis include hepatitis, rubella, mumps, Epstein–Barr virus, parvovirus B19, enterovirus, adenovirus, and human immunodeficiency virus (HIV).
- Certain patient characteristics or aspects of a patient's clinical history may suggest certain pathogens. See Table 35-1 for a list of these histories. Note that although these may be suggestive of a pathogen, they are not diagnostic.[2]

Pathophysiology

- **Hematogenous spread** is the most common route by which bacteria reach the joint following inoculation through the skin or mucosa.
- Bacterial colonization usually occurs within the synovial lining, followed by bacterial proliferation in the synovial fluid.

TABLE 35-1	CLINICAL HISTORY SUGGESTIVE OF PATHOGEN	
Clinical History	**Joint Involvement**	**Pathogen**
Cellulitis or skin infection	Mono- or polyarticular	*Staphylococcus aureus, Streptococcus*
Sexually active young women	Polyarticular	*Neisseria gonorrhoeae*
Elderly with skin break-down or UTI	Monoarticular	Gram-negative rods
IV drug use	Sternoclavicular, pubic symphysis, sacroiliac	*Pseudomonas, S. aureus*
Gardening, plant thorn injury	Monoarticular: knee, hand, wrist	*Pantoea agglomerans, Nocardia asteroides, Sporothrix schenckii*
Rheumatoid arthritis	Monoarticular	*S. aureus*
Anti-TNF therapy	Monoarticular	*Salmonella, Listeria*
Unpasteurized dairy products	Sacroiliac, monoarthritis, oligoarthritis of the legs	*Brucella*
Animal bite	Small joints (fingers, toes)	*Pasteurella multocida, oral anaerobes*

IV, intravenous; TNF, tumor necrosis factor; UTI, urinary tract infection.
Adapted from: Sharff KA, Richards EP, Townes JM. Clinical management of septic arthritis. *Curr Rheum Rep.* 2013;15(6):332.

- The presence of bacteria in the joint capsule induces an inflammatory response, recruiting leukocytes that propagate the inflammatory reaction through the release of cytokines.
- Bacterial products, the release of lysosomal enzymes, immune complex deposition, complement activation, metalloproteases, and impairment of chondrocyte function all contribute to articular damage.
- Nongonococcal bacterial arthritis is typically more damaging than gonococcal arthritis.

Risk Factors

- Common risk factors include **inflammatory arthritis** (especially rheumatoid arthritis), **prosthetic joints or heart valves,** **immunosuppression,** diabetes, overlying **skin infection,** and advanced age.
  - Between 1.5% and 2% of prosthetic joints eventually develop septic arthritis.[3]
  - Patients on a tumor necrosis factor (TNF) inhibitor for rheumatoid arthritis have a 0.4% risk per year of a septic joint and 0.2% per year on conventional disease-modifying antirheumatic drug (DMARD) therapy.[4]
- **Immunocompromised patients** are at increased risk for developing opportunistic mycobacterial and fungal infections as well.
- Sepsis and bacteremia can lead to seeding of the joints and increase the risk of infectious arthritis.
- Direct inoculation via arthrocentesis or arthroscopy can occur but is rare; estimated rates vary from 1 in 2,500 to 1 in 15,000.[5]

- **Gonococcal arthritis** should be considered in sexually active young patients and patients engaging in high-risk sexual behavior. Other risk factors for gonococcal arthritis include menstruation, pregnancy, and complement deficiencies.

DIAGNOSIS

Clinical Presentation

- The **acute onset of mono- or oligoarticular arthritis,** especially in the setting of a **fever and constitutional symptoms,** should raise the suspicion of infectious arthritis.
- Delay in diagnosis can lead to rapid and severe joint destruction, causing significant morbidity and increased mortality.

History
- The most common symptoms are joint pain, swelling, and fever.[6]
- Fever occurs in most patients, although up to 20% of patients may be afebrile and patients with other diseases such as gout may also have monoarthritis and fever. Chills and rigors are unusual.
- 50% of cases involve the **knee,** followed by the hip, shoulder, wrist, ankle, elbow, and small joints of the hands and feet. Up to 20% of cases may present with **polyarticular symptoms.**
- **Intravenous drug abusers** tend to develop infectious arthritis in joints of the axial skeleton including the **sternoclavicular and costochondral joints and the pubic symphysis.**
- History should focus on risk factors, recent trauma or procedures, high-risk sexual behavior, and the presence of prosthetic joints.

Physical Examination
- The joint examination should include checking the ability to bear weight, range of motion, and signs of soft-tissue swelling, warmth, erythema, edema, and synovitis within and around the suspected joints.
  - Redness and warmth over a prosthetic joint is highly predictive of a septic joint.
  - Certain indolent organisms, such as mycobacteria, may cause a "cold" arthritis where there is an effusion and pain without warmth or erythema.
- Hematogenous spread to the joint can occur from distant sites. Physical examination should focus on identifying infection in such sites including the oropharynx, skin, respiratory, cardiac, and genitourinary systems.
- The cardiac examination should include evaluation for **new murmurs** or rubs.
- A genitourinary examination is warranted in sexually active patients and should evaluate for **flank pain, urethritis, or cervicitis.**
- A careful skin examination should be performed for signs of cellulitis. **Papules, pustules, bullae, or necrotic lesions** are especially suggestive of gonococcal arthritis.
- **Tenosynovitis, dermatitis, and migratory polyarthritis** are the classic triad for **disseminated gonococcal infections.** Urethritis in men is more likely to be symptomatic than cervicitis in women.

Diagnostic Criteria

The presence of a pathogen in synovial fluid culture is the most specific finding in the diagnosis of septic arthritis. However, timing of antibiotic therapy, arthrocentesis technique, and limitations in microbiologic analysis may affect culture results.

Differential Diagnosis

In addition to infectious arthritis, the differential diagnosis of acute monoarthritis includes trauma, crystalline arthritis (gout and pseudogout), early stages of inflammatory polyarthritis, acute rheumatic fever, infectious bursitis, and Lyme disease. In particular, crystalline arthritis can be a challenging differential and may even coexist with an infectious arthritis.

Diagnostic Testing

Testing should focus on promptly establishing the diagnosis of infectious arthritis and identifying the responsible pathogen.

Laboratories

- **Blood cultures** should be obtained prior to initiation of antibiotics in an effort to isolate the responsible pathogen.
- **Inflammatory markers,** such as white blood cell (WBC) count, erythrocyte sedimentation rate (ESR), and C-reactive protein (CRP), are sensitive but nonspecific. The peripheral WBC count is elevated in approximately half of the affected patients.
- Serum **procalcitonin** elevation above 0.5 ng/mL is more specific but less sensitive than the above markers. It has a specificity and sensitivity of around 90% and 55%, respectively.[7]
- **Culture samples from the cervix, urethra, rectum, pharynx, and skin lesions** may be helpful in isolating a pathogen, especially if gonococcal arthritis is suspected.
- Cultures for unusual organisms should be ordered in cases of suspected tuberculosis, penetrating trauma, animal bites, travel to areas endemic with particular fungal organisms, immunocompromised patients, or monoarthritis refractory to conventional antibiotic therapy.
- In selected cases, synovial biopsy may help demonstrate certain fastidious organisms.
- For Lyme disease, serologies may improve diagnostic yield.

Imaging

- **Plain radiographs** of the suspected joint can be helpful in evaluating joint destruction, bony involvement, effusions, erosions, chondrocalcinosis, and extent of disease but are rarely helpful in the acute setting as radiographic changes of bone and joint destruction may take days to weeks to develop.
- For difficult to access joints, radiographic guidance with ultrasound, fluoroscopy, or computed tomography may be necessary for joint aspiration.
- **Magnetic resonance imaging (MRI)** is useful in assessing whether there is osteomyelitis or adjacent abscess.
- **Echocardiography** can be useful to evaluate for endocarditis as a source of septic emboli, especially in patients with sepsis, bacteremia, known valve disease, or intravenous drug abuse.

Arthrocentesis

- **Prompt synovial fluid analysis is essential** for diagnosing infectious arthritis and guiding appropriate antibiotic therapy. **Arthrocentesis should be performed in any patient presenting with monoarticular joint pain with an effusion.** Entering a joint site with overlying active cellulitis is to be avoided to prevent seeding of infection into the joint.
- Aspiration of purulent drainage is highly suspicious of infectious arthritis.
- The **presence of crystals does not exclude the diagnosis of infectious arthritis.**
- **WBC counts >50,000/μL** with a **predominance of polymorphonuclear neutrophils** is consistent with infectious arthritis. The higher the WBC count, the greater the likelihood ratio (LR) for septic arthritis (>50,000/μL LR 7.7; >100,000/μL LR 28.0).[6]
- Routine **Gram stain** may show bacteria that can guide initial therapy. For nongonococcal infections, these are positive 50% to 75% of the time.
- Chemistries such as synovial lactate dehydrogenase (LDH), glucose, and protein have limited value, although elevated synovial LDH and low glucose are consistent with bacterial infection.

- Special stains and culture, such as acid-fast bacillus stain and fungal cultures, are to be considered for atypical presentation or immunosuppressed patients.
- Microbiologic culture growth of an organism capable of causing infectious arthritis is most helpful in guiding antibiotic therapy. The data may take days to be finalized and may be falsely negative depending on antibiotic timing and arthrocentesis technique.
- For suspected gonococcal infection, conventional Gram stain and routine cultures are less sensitive. Cultures of synovial fluid on **chocolate agar or Thayer–Martin media** may enhance recovery.
- **Polymerase chain reaction (PCR)** of synovial fluid to detect gonococcal DNA may also increase diagnostic yield.

TREATMENT

- The mainstay of treatment of bacterial arthritis includes **intravenous antibiotics and joint drainage.** Antibiotic dosing should be done with consideration of the patient's age, weight, and medical comorbidities, including renal and hepatic function.
- For nongonococcal arthritis, initial antimicrobial therapy should be based on the results of the Gram stain and the clinical setting. **If no organisms are seen on Gram stain, broad-spectrum antibiotic coverage for both gram-positive and gram-negative organisms should be initiated pending culture data.** Recommend coverage for methicillin-resistant *Staphylococcus aureus* (MRSA) based on local community rates, comorbidities, and healthcare exposure.

Medications

- **Nongonococcal arthritis**
  - If MRSA coverage is not required, coverage for gram-positive organisms with anti-staphylococcal penicillin such as **oxacillin or nafcillin** is adequate.
  - For MRSA coverage, start empiric therapy with **vancomycin.**
  - Third-generation cephalosporins, such as **ceftriaxone, ceftazidime, or cefotaxime,** should be started for empiric coverage of gram-negative organisms.
  - If *Pseudomonas aeruginosa* is a possible pathogen, **cefepime** or ceftazidime with an aminoglycoside such as gentamicin should be initiated.
  - When available, culture results and antimicrobial sensitivities should guide treatment.
  - Atypical or resistant organisms may require consultation from infectious diseases to tailor antimicrobial therapy.
  - Most cases of infectious arthritis require **2 to 4 weeks of intravenous antibiotics.** Once a pathogen has been established as causative, this course can often be completed as an outpatient.
- **Gonococcal arthritis**
  - If gonococcal arthritis is suspected, empiric therapy for disseminated gonococcal infection should be initiated.
  - **Ceftriaxone** should be continued for 24 to 48 hours after clinical improvement. This can then be switched to oral cefixime or ofloxacin for 1 week.
- **Nonbacterial arthritis**
  - Arthralgias are common with many acute or chronic viral infections.
  - Viral arthritis tends to present with symmetric polyarthralgias or polyarthritis and may be accompanied by a typical viral exanthem.
  - Supportive treatment with rest and nonsteroidal anti-inflammatory drugs (**NSAIDs**) is usually effective and sufficient.

Surgical Management

- Surgical or arthroscopic drainage is often necessary in cases of septic hip joints, septic arthritis with concurrent osteomyelitis, septic arthritis in a prosthetic joint, persistent infections, complex anatomy, or loculated effusions.

- Most joints can be adequately drained by arthrocentesis. Daily aspiration is generally necessary because certain joints (e.g., the knee) may accumulate fluid for up to 10 days. Serial cell counts and cultures document response to antibiotic therapy.
- Open drainage, arthroscopy, and joint replacement are options for severe and refractory cases.
- Patients with suspected infections involving prosthetic joints warrant prompt orthopedic surgery consultation.

REFERRAL

Complicated joint infections often require a multidisciplinary approach, most often involving orthopedic surgery, infectious diseases, physical therapy, and occupational therapy.

MONITORING/FOLLOW-UP

- Patients should be followed closely, with frequent joint examinations for the first few weeks of treatment with antibiotics.
- Repeated arthrocentesis should confirm sterilization of synovial fluid and decreasing WBC count.
- Failure to improve may warrant alteration in antibiotic regimen or surgical consultation.
- Early rehabilitation should include physical therapy with joint mobilization to prevent loss of joint range of motion.
- Patients should be monitored for side effects from antimicrobials with complete blood counts (CBCs), comprehensive metabolic panels (CMPs), and drug levels, as appropriate.
- ESR and CRP are helpful to follow serially to confirm that inflammation is resolving.

PROGNOSIS

- The **mortality rate** associated with septic arthritis is about 10% and as high as perhaps 50% in polyarticular disease.
- Most patients will recover with prompt medical and surgical management. However, up to a third will go on to have a severe deterioration in joint function, requiring a prosthetic joint, arthrodesis, or even amputation.[8]
- Poor prognostic factors include nongonococcal bacterial arthritis, older age, preexisting joint damage, and infected prosthetic joints.

REFERENCES

1. Matthews CJ, Weston VC, Jones A, et al. Bacterial septic arthritis in adults. *Lancet.* 2010;375:846.
2. Sharff KA, Richards EP, Townes JM. Clinical management of septic arthritis. *Curr Rheum Rep* 2013, 15(6):332.
3. Kurtz SM, Ong KL, Lau E, Bozic KJ, Berry D, Parvizi J. Prosthetic joint infection risk after TKA in the Medicare population. *Clin Orthop Relat Res.* 2010; 468:52–56
4. Galloway JB, Hyrich KL, Mercer LK, et al. Risk of septic arthritis in patients with rheumatoid arthritis and the effect of anti-TNF therapy. *Ann Rheum Dis.* 2011;70:1810–1814
5. Geirsson AJ, Statkevicius S, Víkingsson A. Septic arthritis in Iceland 1990-2002: increasing incidence due to iatrogenic infections. *Ann Rheum Dis.* 2008;67:638–643.
6. Margaretten ME, Kohlwes J, Moore D, et al. Does this adult patient have septic arthritis? *JAMA.* 2007;297:1478–1488.
7. Carpenter CR, Schuur JD, Everett WW, Pines JM. Evidence-based diagnostics: adult septic arthritis. *Acad Emerg Med.* 2011;18:781–796.
8. Kaandorp C, Krijnen P, Moens H, et al. The outcome of bacterial arthritis: a prospective community-based study. *Arthritis Rheum.* 1997;40:884–892

Lyme Disease

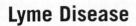

36

Iris Lee and Prabha Ranganathan

GENERAL PRINCIPLES

- Lyme disease is a multisystem illness caused by the spirochete family Borreliaceae. *Borrelia burgdorferi* and, less commonly, *B. mayonii* in the upper Midwest are the only species found in the United States, whereas more species (*B. burgdorferi, B. afzelii,* and *B. garinii*) are found in Europe and Asia. Clinical manifestations and severity of disease may vary with the infecting species. Only *B. burgdorferi* manifestations will be addressed in this chapter.
- **Lyme disease is the most common tickborne illness in the United States** and is transmitted by the *Ixodes* tick (blacklegged tick or deer tick).
- It was initially described in Old Lyme, Connecticut, in 1977 as "Lyme arthritis" in a population of children previously thought to have juvenile rheumatoid arthritis.
- The incidence of Lyme disease in the United States has continued to increase since it was first described. This is thought to be secondary to the **increased deer population and consequent increase in *Ixodes* ticks.**
- According to the Centers for Disease Control and Prevention (CDC), there were over 40,000 confirmed and probable cases of Lyme disease in the United States in 2017.[1]
- Cases of Lyme disease should be reported to the CDC.

Epidemiology

- Lyme disease is transmitted to humans by the *Ixodes* tick. The tick has four developmental stages: egg, larva, nymph, and adult. **Only ticks in nymph and sometimes larva stage transmit Lyme disease to humans.**
- The *Ixodes* tick life cycle
  - Eggs hatch into larvae in the spring. Larvae feed on small rodents (e.g., white-footed mouse), acquiring the spirochete infection from these asymptomatic carriers.
  - In the fall, larvae become dormant for the winter, but molt into nymphs the next spring.
  - Nymphs feed on rodents, rabbits, and humans, transmitting spirochetes to the host during periods of extended attachment.
  - By fall, the nymph matures into an adult. The adult transmits the spirochete less often because it is less likely to go unnoticed during attachment and is not present during peak hiking season.
- Deer are important in the life cycle of the *Ixodes* tick but are not a reservoir for *B. burgdorferi.*

Etiology

- *B. burgdorferi* is a spirochete, a motile corkscrew-shaped bacterium with an outer and inner membrane, and flagella.
- The tick **must be attached for 36 to 48 hours or more** to transmit the spirochete. However, transmission occurs more rapidly in animal models if the spirochete is in the tick salivary gland.[2]

Pathophysiology

- The pathophysiology of Lyme disease is not completely understood, but disease manifestations are thought to be from infection with the spirochete itself as well as the host's immune response to the infection.
- A few pertinent observations include[3]:
  - Patients with HLA-DR4 and HLA-DR2 are more likely to develop a potentially erosive, chronic arthritis.
  - Spirochetes have been isolated from all affected tissues, except peripheral nerves. Containment of the infection requires an intact innate and adaptive immune response.
  - *B. burgdorferi* does not produce toxins or destructive proteases to harm the host.

Risk Factors

- There is a bimodal incidence of infection—ages 5 to 14 and ages 50 and over.[4]
- Males have a slightly higher incidence (53%).[4]
- Residence in the New England, mid-Atlantic states, and northern Midwest states of the United States confers a higher risk.
- Occupation or recreation in fields or woods in endemic areas is a risk factor.[4]
- Location of tick bite on the body on more difficult-to-visualize areas allows for longer tick attachment time and increases the possibility of spirochete transmission.
- The most active season for infection is **May to July**, with the highest infection rate in June. Peak disease manifestations lag 2 to 3 weeks behind inoculation.

Prevention

- Remove ticks promptly.
- Wear insect repellent or long pants and shirts when in endemic areas.
- Reducing tick population when possible may be key to prevention.

DIAGNOSIS

The diagnosis is clinical, manifestations may vary by stage, and laboratory data are only supportive.

Clinical Presentation

History
- Patients may or may not recall a **tick bite** or **erythema migrans** (EM).
- They may complain of constitutional or organ-specific symptoms based on the stage of disease at presentation.
- Constitutional symptoms may include fever, fatigue, myalgias, arthralgias, and headache.

Physical Examination
- EM lesions are usually warm, itchy, and nonpainful. They expand slowly over days to weeks and may reach a diameter of 20 cm or more. The lesion **may develop a central clearing,** classically known as the "bull's-eye" lesion. This is usually only seen in large lesions that have been present for days. However, two-thirds of EM lesions may not present with the classic bull's-eye appearance.
- Lesions are typically found in the intertriginous areas, popliteal fossa, and belt line. In children, head and neck are also common sites.
- In one study of 118 serologically confirmed cases, EM lesions appeared in these patterns[5]:
  - Homogenous erythema (59%)
  - Central erythema (32%)
  - Central clearing (9%)
  - Vesicular or ulcerated (7%)
  - Central purpura (2%)

- Stage I, Early Localized Disease
  - Characterized by the appearance of EM
    - This rash is an expanding annular red macule or papule at the site of the tick bite.
    - This rash occurs within 3 days to 1 month after infection and resolves within 3 to 4 weeks and should be distinguished from irritation from the tick bite itself.
    - **The rash occurs in 60% to 80% of patients** but may go unnoticed.
  - Patients may report malaise, headache, fever, neck stiffness, arthralgias, myalgias, localized lymphadenopathy, and fatigue.
- Stage II, Early Disseminated Disease
  - **Multiple EM lesions** (in locations other than the primary bite) result from hematogenous spread of the spirochete. These lesions are seen days to weeks after the primary infection.
  - **Systemic symptoms** of fever, malaise, headache, arthralgias, and myalgias become more severe. These symptoms may be constant or intermittent.
  - **Cardiac involvement** occurs weeks to months after primary infection and may be the sole manifestation of disseminated disease.
    - Cardiac disease is rare in patients infected with *B. burgdorferi* but occurs more commonly with other species of *Borrelia*.
    - Symptoms include palpitations, light-headedness, syncope, chest pain, and shortness of breath.
    - Most common manifestations are **varying degrees of heart block.**
    - **Myocarditis and pericarditis** are less common, often self-limited and frequently clinically silent. Myocarditis may result in transient cardiomegaly, and pericarditis is associated with mild pericardial effusions.
    - No confirmed cases of valvular damage or chronic cardiomyopathy secondary to Lyme disease have occurred in the United States. It is controversial whether Lyme disease is associated with chronic cardiomyopathy.
  - **Neurologic involvement** occurs weeks to months after primary infection and may affect up to 20% of untreated patients.
    - The most common manifestation is cranial neuropathy, especially unilateral or bilateral **Bell's palsy.**
    - **Meningoencephalitis** may also occur.
  - **Articular involvement** occurs 6 or more months after infection and affects about 60% of untreated patients. In practice, only about 10% of people develop arthritis. This has decreased because of early recognition and treatment of disease.
    - **Arthritis** is oligoarticular with lower extremity predominance, particularly the **knees,** and is associated with large inflammatory effusions.
    - Few patients have persistent arthritis after antibiotic treatment and are classified as having antibiotic-refractory Lyme arthritis.
- Stage III, Late Lyme Disease
  - Occurs months to years after the primary infection and does not have to be preceded by manifestations of stage I or II disease.
  - The most common manifestation is episodic, **lower extremity–predominant oligoarthritis.**
  - **Chronic neurologic sequelae** such as radiculopathy, axonal polyneuropathy, or encephalomyelitis may rarely occur.

Differential Diagnosis

- Cellulitis
- Meningitis
- Dementia
- Multiple sclerosis

- Amyotrophic lateral sclerosis
- Radiculopathy
- Depression
- Ehrlichiosis
- Babesiosis
- Rocky mountain spotted fever
- Reactive arthritis
- Rheumatoid arthritis
- Fibromyalgia

Diagnostic Testing

Laboratory
- Confirmatory laboratory testing is not necessary for diagnosis, especially if the patient has an EM rash. **A seropositive test alone is not adequate to establish the diagnosis.**
- The spirochete is difficult to culture as it grows under microaerophilic or anaerobic conditions. The highest yield for culture is a skin biopsy from the border of the primary EM rash in an untreated patient. Spirochetes may be found in blood and cerebrospinal fluid (CSF) and very rarely in the synovial fluid. Cultures may take up to 12 weeks to reveal the spirochete.
- The CDC recommends two-step serum testing.[6]
  - **Enzyme-linked immunosorbent assay (ELISA) or immunofluorescence assay (IFA)** is the screening test and is more **sensitive** than the western blot. If positive or equivocal, the same serum should be evaluated with western blot. If ELISA or IFA is negative, it is highly unlikely the patient has Lyme disease unless the testing has occurred too early after primary infection (less than 30 days). In the acute phase, patients with disseminated infection have a false-negative rate of about 50%.
  - **Western blot is a more specific** test and only run if the ELISA or IFA is positive.[7] If the immunoglobulin (Ig)M antibody is positive, the patient should be retested in 4 to 6 weeks as they may have early infection. If the IgG antibody is positive, the patient is considered to have infection. If the patient has had symptoms for greater than 30 days, only obtain the IgG western blot.
    - IgM antibodies usually appear 1 to 2 weeks after infection.
    - IgG antibodies usually appear 2 to 6 weeks after infection.
  - **After successful treatment, antibody levels may remain positive, but titers should fall over time.** Titer level and rate of resolution do not correlate with disease severity, chronicity, or treatment.
  - **Seropositivity occurs in less than 40% of patients with early skin disease** but more often in patients with early disseminated extracutaneous disease. Patients with late Lyme disease are almost always IgG positive.
- A lumbar puncture is recommended in patients with neurologic manifestations in an effort to rule out other causes and potentially support the diagnosis.
  - IgG and IgM antibodies in the CSF help confirm the diagnosis but are not mandatory.
  - Polymerase chain reaction (PCR) testing of CSF has low sensitivity.
- Synovial fluid is inflammatory with an average white blood cell (WBC) count of about 25,000/mm^3 and polymorphonuclear leukocytes predominate.
- Mild elevations in transaminases have been observed.
- Although offered by some health departments, testing of ticks removed from a patient is not recommended because presence of the spirochete does not guarantee human infection.

Electrocardiography
- Electrocardiographic abnormalities are only seen in disseminated infection.
- Sustained or intermittent first-, second-, or third-degree **heart block** occurs depending on the location of conduction system dysfunction.

- Variable bundle branch blocks may also be seen.
- Pericarditis can manifest as diffuse ST- and T-wave elevations.

Imaging
- Magnetic resonance imaging (MRI) of the brain may be helpful to rule out other pathology. There are no specific MRI findings in Lyme disease.
- Transthoracic echocardiogram is used to evaluate for the presence of myocarditis and pericarditis.

Diagnostic Procedures
Diagnostic procedures are generally not necessary and often not recommended. If performed, it is frequently in an effort to rule out other diagnoses. Such procedures may include the following:
- Skin biopsy
- Myocardial biopsy
- Lumbar puncture
- Electromyography and nerve conduction studies

TREATMENT

Medications
- **Early lyme disease**
  - Early Lyme disease manifested as only EM may be treated with doxycycline, amoxicillin, or cefuroxime, all of which have equivalent effectiveness.
  - Dosing guidelines in adults are as follows[8,9]:
    - Doxycycline 100 mg PO BID for 10 to 21 days
    - Amoxicillin 500 mg PO TID for 14 to 21 days
    - Cefuroxime axetil 500 mg PO BID for 14 to 21 days
    - Macrolides are not recommended.
  - **Doxycycline is generally preferred** because it has better central nervous system (CNS) penetration.
  - Doxycycline also covers the possibility of coincident *Anaplasma phagocytophilum* infection, which is also transmitted by the *Ixodes* tick.
- **Early disseminated lyme disease**
  - **Intravenous (IV) antibiotics are recommended if there is CNS involvement** (except isolated facial palsy).[8,9]
    - IV ceftriaxone, cefotaxime, or penicillin may be used. Duration of therapy is usually between 10 and 28 days.
    - Isolated Lyme disease with facial palsy can be treated with a 14- to 21-day course of oral doxycycline.
    - Recovery of neurologic symptoms may lag behind clearance of the spirochete and therefore cannot be used to guide length of therapy.
  - **For cardiac involvement, IV ceftriaxone, cefotaxime, or penicillin** is given until resolution of heart block. After this, the patient may be switched to oral therapy to complete a total 21-day course of antibiotics.[8,9] Patients may require a temporary pacemaker.
- **Late lyme disease**
  - Patients usually present with arthritis and are often treated successfully with a 1 month course of oral doxycycline, amoxicillin, or cefuroxime axetil.[8,9]
  - If this fails, another 4-week oral course or 2 to 4 weeks of IV antibiotics may be given.[7,8]
  - The existence of chronic symptomatic *B. burgdorferi* infection after appropriate antibiotic treatment is controversial. The Infectious Disease Society of America does not recommend extended antibiotic treatment for patients with ≥6 months of subjective symptoms.[7–9]

- **Post–lyme disease syndrome**
  - Different from chronic Lyme disease, both are controversial diagnoses.
  - A proposed diagnosis from the Infectious Diseases Society of America (IDSA) is as follows:
    - An adult or a child with a documented episode of early or late Lyme disease fulfilling the case definition of the CDC
    - After treatment with a generally accepted treatment regimen, there is resolution or stabilization of the objective manifestation(s) of Lyme disease
    - Onset of fatigue, widespread musculoskeletal pain or complaints of cognitive difficulties within 6 months of the diagnosis of Lyme disease and persistence of continuous or relapsing symptoms for at least a 6 month period after completion of antibiotic therapy
    - Subjective symptoms cause a substantial reduction in previous levels of occupational, educational, social, or personal activities.
    - However, extensive exclusion criteria exist and include active, untreated coinfection; presence of objective abnormalities on physical examination; prior diagnosis of fibromyalgia, chronic fatigue syndrome, or history of undiagnosed or unexplained somatic complaints; or presence of another condition that may explain the previously mentioned symptoms.
  - There is no evidence for the use of repeated or prolonged antibiotics for this diagnosis.

SPECIAL CONSIDERATIONS

- Must rule out other diseases in the differential diagnosis, because seropositivity is not adequate for diagnosis.
- Pregnant women should not be treated with tetracyclines. Nor should doxycycline be given to young (<8 years old) children.

COMPLICATIONS

Complications depend on the stage of infection and may include the following:
- Acute or chronic arthritis
- Cardiomyopathy, arrhythmia, pericarditis
- Neuropathy, radiculopathy, encephalopathy
- Cognitive dysfunction, dementia
- Conjunctivitis

PATIENT EDUCATION

- Tick Management Handbook from the CDC, available at https://stacks.cdc.gov/view/cdc/11444.[10]
- CDC website: www.cdc.gov/lyme.[11]

MONITORING/FOLLOW-UP

- If seropositive at diagnosis, **repeat testing is not recommended** because titers do not reflect efficacy of treatment.
- The best evaluation of improvement is to monitor the patient's symptoms and resolution of organ dysfunction.

OUTCOME/PROGNOSIS

- Children and patients treated at earlier stages of infection have a better acute and long-term prognosis.
- Infection is rarely fatal.
- Arthritis may take months to resolve and can be chronic.
- Atrioventricular condition abnormalities are usually temporary.
- Cranial nerve palsies usually resolve with or without treatment.

REFERENCES

1. Recent Surveillance Data. Lyme Disease. CDC.gov. https://www.cdc.gov/lyme/datasurveillance/recent-surveillance-data.html. Updated December 21, 2018. Accessed October 10, 2019.
2. Cook, MJ. Lyme borreliosis: a review of data on transmission time after tick attachment. *Int J Gen Med*. 2015;8:1–8.
3. Ilipoulou BP, Huber BT. Infectious arthritis and immune dysregulation: lessons from Lyme disease. *Curr Opin Rheumatol*. 2010;22:451–455.
4. Mead, PS. Epidemiology of Lyme Disease. *Infect Disease Clin North Am*. 2015;29:187–210.
5. Smith RP, Schoen RT, Rahn DW, et al. Clinical characteristics and treatment outcome of early Lyme disease in patients with microbiologically confirmed erythema migrans. *Ann Intern Med*. 2002;136:421–428.
6. Diagnosis and Testing. Lyme Disease. CDC.gov. https://www.cdc.gov/lyme/diagnosistesting/index.html. August 15, 2019. Accessed October 10, 2019.
7. Murray TS, Shapiro ED. Lyme disease. *Clin Lab Med*. 2010;30:311–328.
8. Wormser GP, Dattwyler RJ, Shapiro ED, et al. The clinical assessment, treatment, and prevention of Lyme disease, human granulocytic anaplasmosis, and babesiosis: clinical practice guidelines by the Infectious Diseases Society of America. *Clin Infect Dis*. 2006;43:1089–1134.
9. Lantos PM, Charini WA, Medoff G, et al. Final report of the Lyme disease review panel of the Infectious Diseases Society of America. *Clin Infect Dis*. 2010;51:1–5.
10. Tick management handbook; an integrated guide for homeowners, pest control operators, and public health officials for the prevention of tick-associated disease. CDC.gov. https://stacks.cdc.gov/view/cdc/11444. 2004. Accessed November 10, 2019.
11. Lyme Disease. CDC.gov. https://www.cdc.gov/lyme/. Updated September 12, 2019. Accessed October 10, 2019.

Mosquito-Transmitted Viral Arthritis and Arthralgias

Can M. Sungur and Jonathan J. Miner

GENERAL PRINCIPLES

- Chikungunya virus (CHIKV) and Zika virus (ZIKV) are viruses that can cause joint pain. They are unrelated viruses.
- CHIKV is a mosquito-transmitted alphavirus.
- ZIKV is a mosquito-transmitted flavivirus, related to dengue virus (DENV), West Nile virus (WNV), and yellow fever virus (YFV).
- Whereas CHIKV causes inflammatory arthritis, ZIKV causes arthralgias.
- Both can cause joint pain, but only CHIKV causes chronic arthritis.
- A role for immunosuppressive medications remains undefined. There is concern that immunosuppression could exacerbate the disease.
- Chronic CHIKV arthritis can mimic rheumatoid arthritis and is characterized by profound morning stiffness with a relapsing and remitting course.

Definition

- A variety of viral infections can result in arthritis and arthralgia, which are typically self-limited.
- The initial acute infection is characterized by episodes of fevers, myalgias, rashes, and other constitutional symptoms associated with the particular virus.
- Distribution of joint involvement, symptoms, and chronicity can vary based on viral disease, age of individual, and general variability between individuals.
- CHIKV can manifest as severe arthritis requiring anti-inflammatory treatments.
- ZIKV also can cause severe joint pain.
- Both of these emerging viruses are being studied more extensively because of global spread.

Epidemiology

- CHIKV is endemic to West Africa, with cases seen in Africa, Asia, Europe, Pacific and Indian islands, and recently in the Americas.
  - More cases are seen during the rainy season.
  - The disease is transmitted by *Aedes aegypti* and *Aedes albopictus* mosquitos.
  - In the United States in 2016 there were 4000 cases seen primarily from travelers.[1]
  - Recent outbreak occurred with over 2 million suspected cases in the Western hemisphere.[1]
- ZIKV is prevalent in Africa, Southeast Asia, Americas, the Caribbean, and the Pacific islands.
  - In the United States in 2016 there were 5168 cases of ZIKV, with the majority being travel associated.[2]
  - Transmitted by mosquitos, sexual transmission, blood, nosocomial, and maternal–fetal transmission.

Pathophysiology

- Mosquito-transmitted viral arthritis can manifest with severe joint inflammation with elevated levels of interleukin-6, interferon alpha, and other proinflammatory cytokines.[3]
- The mechanism of development of arthritis in patients is not completely defined at this point, but it is potentially because of persistent low-level viremia in the synovial fluid, antigen mimicry resulting in autoimmunity, or exacerbating preexisting joint disease.[4]
- CD4$^+$ T cells and inflammatory monocytes promote inflammation in mouse models of CHIKV arthritis.[5]

Risk Factors

In patients with CHIKV arthritis, increased risk of development of chronic arthritis can come from preexisting joint disease (osteoarthritis or inflammatory arthritis), metabolic syndromes (hypertension, obesity, diabetes mellitus), and heart failure.[3]

DIAGNOSIS

Clinical Presentation

- CHIKV initially has an incubation period of 2 to 7 days, with ~95% of infected individuals developing high fevers, headaches, rash (which is maculopapular and involves the extremities, trunk, and face), myalgia, and severe arthralgia involving multiple joints. The name means "to walk bent over" because of the severe joint pain. In rare cases, gastrointestinal disease, meningoencephalitis, seizures, cardiovascular disease, hemorrhagic manifestations, and death can occur.[5]
- ZIKV is more frequently asymptomatic, with symptoms developing in only 20% to 25% of patients who were more frequently women and less than 40 years old.
  - Symptoms include low-grade fevers, pruritic rash (maculopapular rash on face, trunk, extremities, palms, and soles), arthralgia (small joints of hands and feet), conjunctivitis, myalgia, headaches, and dysesthesia.
  - Less common symptoms include abdominal pain, nausea, diarrhea, ulcerations in mucous membranes, and petechiae.
  - In rare cases, uveitis, myocarditis, pericarditis, Guillain–Barré syndrome, encephalitis, and myelitis have been reported.[6]

History

- Chikungunya has an acute phase and chronic phase associated with severe arthritis/arthralgia.
  - Acute phase: includes the typical symptoms of fevers, conjunctivitis, rash, headache, and joint and muscle pain. Typically, most patients' disease resolves with no lasting symptoms in days to weeks.
  - Chronic phase: development of chronic arthritis with synovial proliferation; joint stiffness, joint pain, and tenosynovitis occur in up to 40% of patients. Raynaud phenomenon can be seen in the second or third month in 20% of cases as well as cryoglobulinemia. Varying duration of symptoms, with one study showing symptoms in 88% of patients at 1 month, 86% at 3 months, 48% at 6 months, and 4% at 15 months.[7] A different study showed 63% with persistent polyarthralgia and morning stiffness after 18 months.[8]
- ZIKV has an incubation period of 3 to 12 days, and the infection is often asymptomatic in 80% of cases. Symptoms usually resolve within 2 weeks. Persistent or chronic symptoms are rare but can include arthralgia.[6]

Physical Examination

- CHIKV infection: conjunctivitis, periarticular swelling, peripheral lymphadenopathy, maculopapular rash involving face, trunk, and extremities that can be diffuse or patchy.
- ZIKV infection: conjunctivitis, maculopapular rash involving face, trunk, extremities, palms and soles of feet.

Differential Diagnosis

- Viruses with possible associated arthritis and arthralgia include enteroviruses (coxsackie virus and echovirus), hepatitis viruses, parvovirus, rubella, alphaviruses (Ross River, Barmah Forest, chikungunya, Sindbis, Mayaro, O'nyong'nyong, Igbo-ora), flaviviruses (dengue, Zika, mumps), adenovirus, herpesviruses (Epstein–Barr virus, varicella, herpes simplex virus, cytomegalovirus), and human immunodeficiency virus.
- CHIKV and ZIKV infection overlap significantly in their presentations, but CHIKV infection typically presents with higher temperature fevers and symptoms consistent with inflammatory arthritis (e.g., morning stiffness, joint swelling, tenosynovitis).
- Rheumatoid arthritis, reactive arthritis, spondyloarthropathies, and other inflammatory arthritis should also be considered in the differential diagnosis.

Diagnostic Testing

- Immunoglobulin M (IgM) serologies for the particular virus and viral loads by reverse-transcription polymerase chain reaction (RT-PCR) for viral RNA should be obtained. These are done at the Centers for Disease Control and Prevention (CDC) in the United States. IgM testing for ZIKV and DENV can be complicated and have false-positive results because these viruses are closely related and antibodies can cross-react. Plaque reduction neutralization testing (PRNT) may provide more specific results.
- CDC has a single PCR test to evaluate for CHIKV, ZIKV, and DENV.
- Lymphopenia, thrombocytopenia, and elevated transaminases, which are all nonspecific, may be seen in these patients.
- Inflammatory synovial fluid can be seen, but it is rare to see viral load in the synovial fluid, especially in the chronic stage.[4]

TREATMENT

- There are no specific antiviral treatments for either CHIKV or ZIKV. Vaccines are in development.
- Supportive care during acute phase with rest, fluids, acetaminophen, or nonsteroidal anti-inflammatory drugs (NSAIDs) is advised.
- Aspirin should be avoided until DENV infection is excluded. This is because of risk of hemorrhage among DENV-infected patients.
- For the chronic phase with persistent arthralgia or arthritis for more than 3 months, NSAIDs, glucocorticoids for a short course, or disease-modifying antirheumatic drugs (DMARDs) such as methotrexate, leflunomide, or sulfasalazine can be considered, but evidence of safety and efficacy is still very limited.[3]
- Mouse models have studied cytotoxic T-lymphocyte-associated protein 4 (CTLA4)-immunoglobulin (Abatacept) to reduce joint swelling and proinflammatory cytokines in CHIKV.[9]
- **Prevention**
  - Mosquito protection and minimizing exposure is most important.
  - Vaccinations are under development.

○ For ZIKV infection, abstinence or barrier protection is advised during sexual intercourse to avoid sexual transmission. Currently, men are advised to wait at least 3 months after symptom onset or last possible virus exposure if asymptomatic before unprotected sex. Women are currently advised to wait 8 weeks at the minimum.[10]

MONITORING/FOLLOW-UP

• There are no definitive guidelines on long-term management at this time. Management is primarily based on symptom control.
• For chronic CHIKV arthritis, an expert panel has suggested stopping DMARDs after control of symptoms for several months, though this has not been formally studied.[11]

REFERENCES

1. Lindsey NP, Staples JE, Fischer M. Chikungunya virus disease among travelers—United States, 2014-2016. *Am J Trop Med Hyg*. 2018;98:192–197.
2. Hall V, Walker WL, Lindsey NP, et al. Update: Noncongenital Zika virus disease cases—50 U.S. States and the District of Columbia, 2016. *MMWR Morb Mortal Wkly Rep*. 2018;67:265–269.
3. Zaid A, Gerardin P, Taylor A, et al. Chikungunya arthritis: implications of acute and chronic inflammation mechanisms on disease management. *Arthritis Rheumatol*. 2018;70:484–495.
4. Chang AY, Martins KAO, Encinales L, et al. Chikungunya arthritis mechanisms in the Americas: a cross-sectional analysis of chikungunya arthritis patients twenty-two months after infection demonstrating no detectable viral persistence in synovial fluid. *Arthritis Rheumatol*. 2018;70:585–593.
5. Burt FJ, Chen W, Miner JJ, et al. Chikungunya virus: an update on the biology and pathogenesis of this emerging pathogen. *Lancet Infect Dis*. 2017;17:e107–e117.
6. Miner JJ, Diamond MS. Zika virus pathogenesis and tissue tropism. *Cell Host Microbe*. 2017;21:134–142.
7. Simon F, Parola P, Grandadam M, et al. Chikungunya infection: an emerging rheumatism among travelers returned from Indian Ocean islands. Report of 47 cases. *Medicine (Baltimore)*. 2007;86:123–137.
8. Borgherini G, Poubeau P, Staikowsky F, et al. Outbreak of chikungunya on Reunion Island: early clinical and laboratory features in 157 adult patients. *Clin Infect Dis*. 2007;44:1401–1407.
9. Miner JJ, Cook LE, Hong JP, et al. Therapy with CTLA4-Ig and an antiviral monoclonal antibody controls chikungunya virus arthritis. *Sci Transl Med*. 2017;9.
10. Petersen EE, Meaney-Delman D, Neblett-Fanfair R, et al. Update: interim guidance for preconception counseling and prevention of sexual transmission of Zika virus for persons with possible Zika virus exposure. *MMWR Morb Mortal Wkly Rep*. 2016;65:1077–1081.
11. Simon F, Javelle E, Cabie A, et al. French guideline for the management of chikungunya (acute and persistent presentations). *Med Mal Infect*. 2015;45:243–263.

Acute Rheumatic Fever

Philip Chu and Prabha Ranganathan

38

GENERAL PRINCIPLES

- Acute rheumatic fever (ARF) is characterized by arthritis, carditis, chorea, erythema marginatum, and subcutaneous nodules occurring after a group A streptococcal (GAS) pharyngeal infection.
- Early treatment and long-term prophylaxis with antibiotics are important measures to prevent long-term sequelae such as valvular heart disease.

Definition

- ARF is a **delayed reaction to a group A β-hemolytic streptococcal pharyngeal infection,** occurring 2 to 3 weeks after the initial infection.[1]
- Diagnosis is based on the revised Jones criteria (see Table 38-1).[2]

Epidemiology

- The incidence of ARF is highest among children aged 5 to 14 years. ARF is rare in children younger than 5 years or in adults above 30 years. Recurrences can occur but rarely above 40 years.
- Males and females have equal incidence of ARF, but rheumatic heart disease is more common in females.
- ARF was associated with significant morbidity and mortality until the late 1800s. The introduction of antibiotics and improved living conditions in the 20th century significantly reduced the incidence of ARF.
- There are approximately 470,000 new cases of ARF annually, with a mean incidence of 19 per 100,000 school-aged children worldwide; it is lower in the United States (<2 cases per 100,000 school-aged children) and other developed countries.[3]

Pathophysiology

- The pathogenesis of ARF is not clearly understood. GAS pharyngeal infection is necessary for the development of ARF.
- Cellulitis, impetigo, and glomerulonephritis, also caused by GAS, do not cause ARF.
- Some studies suggest that only a few M serotypes of GAS cause ARF, which are referred to as **rheumatogenic strains.**
- **Genetic susceptibility and molecular mimicry,** involving the cross-reaction between GAS antigens and host antigens (e.g., the GAS M protein shares antigenic epitopes with human cardiac myosin and laminin on heart valves) may play a role in pathogenesis.[3]

DIAGNOSIS

Clinical Presentation

- ARF is characterized by a constellation of symptoms that arise **2 to 4 weeks after the pharyngeal infection.**
- The classic manifestations include **arthritis, carditis, neurologic involvement, and rash.**

TABLE 38-1 REVISED JONES CRITERIA (2015)

For all patient populations with evidence of preceding GAS infection[a]

Diagnosis: initial ARF	2 major, or 1 major + 2 minor manifestations
Diagnosis: recurrent ARF	2 major, or 1 major + 2 minor, or 3 minor manifestations

Major criteria

Low-risk populations[b]	Moderate- and high-risk populations
Carditis, clinical or subclinical	Carditis, clinical or subclinical
Arthritis • Polyarthritis only	Arthritis • Monoarthritis or polyarthritis • Polyarthralgia after exclusion of other causes
Chorea	Chorea
Erythema marginatum	Erythema marginatum
Subcutaneous nodules	Subcutaneous nodules

Minor criteria

Low-risk populations[b]	Moderate- and high-risk populations
Polyarthralgia	Monoarthralgia
Fever (≥38.5°C)	Fever (≥38.0°C)
ESR ≥60 mm/h and/or CRP ≥3.0 mg/dL	ESR ≥ 30 mm/h and/or CRP ≥3.0 mg/dL
Prolonged PR interval, after accounting for age variability (unless carditis is a major criterion)	Prolonged PR interval, after accounting for age variability (unless carditis is a major criterion)

[a]Evidence of preceding GAS infection includes any one of the following: rising antistreptolysin O titer or other streptococcal antibodies (anti-DNAse B), a positive throat culture for GAS, a positive rapid GAS antigen test in a child whose clinical presentation suggests a high pretest probability.

[b]Low-risk populations are those with ARF incidence ≤2 per 100,000 school-aged children or all-age rheumatic heart disease prevalence of ≤1 per 1,000 population per year.

ARF, acute rheumatic fever; CRP, C-reactive protein; ESR, erythrocyte sedimentation rate; GAS, group A streptococcal infection.

Adapted from: Gewitz MH, Baltimore RS, Tani LY, et al. Revision of the Jones Criteria for the diagnosis of acute rheumatic fever in the era of Doppler echocardiography: a scientific statement from the American Heart Association. *Circulation.* 2015;131:1806–1818.

- **Arthritis** is usually the first symptom of ARF.
  - It is a migratory polyarthritis usually involving the knees, elbows, ankles, and wrists, which starts in the lower extremity. Typically, 6 to 16 joints are affected.
  - The involved joints become tender without evidence of inflammation.
  - Joints may only be involved for a week before other joints become affected and the initial joint involvement subsides.
  - The synovial fluid is generally inflammatory but sterile.
- **Carditis** is an important manifestation of ARF because it often results in long-term damage.
  - ARF can involve any area of the heart, including the pericardium, epicardium, myocardium, endocardium, and valvular structures.

- Physical examination may show a **new murmur.**
- **Mitral valvulitis** associated with ARF classically causes mitral stenosis and a low-pitched early diastolic murmur at the apex (Carey Coombs murmur). Chronic mitral valve destruction can progress to mitral regurgitation, with a holosystolic apical murmur.
- **Aortic valvulitis** leads to aortic stenosis, with a high-pitched decrescendo murmur along the left sternal border, heard best with the patient leaning forward. Chronic aortic valve destruction can lead to aortic insufficiency, with a late decrescendo systolic murmur and early diastolic murmur at the right upper sternal border.
- **There may be no symptoms despite cardiac involvement,** or patients may experience chest discomfort and dyspnea.
- The 2015 revised Jones criteria account for the increasing use and availability of cardiac ultrasound worldwide, thus allowing for the diagnosis of subclinical carditis. In **subclinical carditis**, classic auscultatory findings of valvular dysfunction may not be present or recognized, but cardiac ultrasound reveals mitral or aortic valvulitis. Thus, echocardiography with Doppler should be performed in all cases of confirmed and suspected ARF.[2]
- The best known neurologic manifestation of ARF is known as **Sydenham's chorea,** also called chorea minor and the St. Vitus' dance.
  - Chorea is characterized by nonrhythmic involuntary abrupt movements and muscle weakness. Usually the movements are more distinct on one side. Muscle weakness is rhythmic, with muscle strength increasing and decreasing on exertion.
  - Frequently, emotional instability (e.g., crying, agitation, and inappropriate behavior) accompanies the chorea.
  - Evidence of a recent GAS infection may be difficult to document because of the latent period between the inciting infection and onset of chorea.
- **Skin manifestations** of ARF include erythema marginatum and subcutaneous nodules.
  - **Erythema marginatum** is a faint, pink, nonpruritic rash that erupts across the trunk, upper arms, and legs; facial involvement does not occur.
    - The lesion begins with a central area of normal skin and extends outward to a distinct border.
    - The rash is transient, coming and going within hours, and worsened by hot conditions (e.g., baths and showers).
    - The rash usually occurs at the onset of disease, but it may recur at any time, including convalescence.
  - **Subcutaneous nodules** are firm, nontender nodules under noninflamed skin that occur on bony prominences and near tendons.
    - They may be solitary or occur in groups. They are symmetric, typically occur on the extensor surfaces, and usually resolve within 4 weeks.
    - The subcutaneous nodules of ARF differ from those of Rheumatoid Arthritis (RA) in that they are smaller and more transient, and are typically found on the olecranon and sometimes on the back.[4]
  - Both erythema marginatum and subcutaneous nodules usually occur only in the presence of carditis.
- Other symptoms may include abdominal pain, malaise, epistaxis, and chest pain.[1]

Diagnostic Criteria

- The diagnosis of ARF is clinical and based on the revised Jones criteria (Table 38-1).[2]
- **Exceptions**
  - **Chorea** may be the only manifestation of rheumatic fever at the time of its presentation.
  - **Indolent rheumatic carditis** may have a slow and insidious onset prior to its realization.

Differential Diagnosis

The differential diagnosis of ARF includes bacterial infections (e.g., septic arthritis, osteomyelitis, and bacterial endocarditis), viral infections (e.g., infectious mononucleosis and coxsackievirus), poststreptococcal reactive arthritis, juvenile idiopathic arthritis, rheumatoid arthritis, systemic lupus erythematosus, Wilson's disease, and malignancies (e.g., lymphoma and leukemia).

Diagnostic Testing
Laboratories
- There may be evidence of recent streptococcal infection, such as:
  - **Increased titers of streptococcal antibodies in the serum** (e.g., antistreptolysin O, DNase B, hyaluronidase, or streptokinase).
  - **Positive throat culture** for group A β-hemolytic streptococci.
- Markers of inflammation, including white blood cell (WBC) count, C-reactive protein (CRP), and erythrocyte sedimentation rate (ESR), may be elevated.

Electrocardiography
- ECG classically shows prolonged PR interval in ARF, but this is a nonspecific finding.
- Other nonspecific ECG changes include T-wave flattening, ST segment and repolarization abnormalities, and P-wave abnormalities.

Imaging
- Echocardiography is useful and should be performed in patients diagnosed or suspected to have ARF because carditis can be subclinical.
- Acute mitral valve changes include annular dilation, chordal elongation, chordal rupture and flail leaflet, anterior leaflet prolapse, and beading of leaflet tips.
- Chronic mitral valve changes include leaflet thickening, chordal thickening, and calcification.
- Aortic valve changes (acute or chronic) include focal leaflet thickening, coaptation defect, restricted leaflet motion, and leaflet prolapse.
- Mitral or aortic valve morphology may be normal on echocardiogram while showing pathologic regurgitation on Doppler.[2]

TREATMENT

Treatment of ARF should include **symptom relief, antibiotic treatment, and prophylaxis.**
- **Antibiotic treatment**
  - **Penicillin** is the treatment of choice for ARF, either IM or PO.[5]
  - **Nonsteroidal anti-inflammatory drugs (NSAIDs), especially aspirin**, are useful for symptomatic relief.
    - Aspirin 4 to 8 g/day for adults
    - NSAIDs can be continued until the patient is asymptomatic and markers of inflammation normalize.
  - Treatment of chorea includes the use of antiepileptic drugs such as phenobarbital, phenytoin, and diazepam.
- **Primary prevention**
  - Primary prevention of ARF consists of recognition of acute GAS pharyngitis and appropriate antibiotic treatment.
  - **Penicillin remains the treatment of choice.**[5,6]
    - Penicillin V 500 mg BID to TID PO for 10 days. For children under 60 lb, the dose is 250 mg.
    - Benzathine penicillin G 1.2 million units IM once. For children under 60 lb, the dose is 600,000 units.
    - Amoxicillin 25 mg/kg (max = 500 mg) BID PO for 10 days is an appropriate alternative to penicillin.
  - For penicillin-allergic patients, appropriate oral alternatives are clindamycin, azithromycin, and clarithromycin.[5,6]

- **Prophylaxis for recurrent ARF** (secondary prevention) is important because symptoms can return, most commonly within 2 years.
  - Penicillin or erythromycin should be started immediately after the initial 10-day antibiotic treatment course: penicillin V 250 mg PO BID or erythromycin 250 mg PO BID if a penicillin allergy is present.
  - Benzathine penicillin G 1.2 million units IM every 4 weeks is the preferred prophylaxis for high-risk individuals.
  - Duration of prophylaxis is controversial. A 5- to 10-year course is usually recommended for patients without residual heart disease, but up to 40 years of age is recommended if there is carditis and residual heart disease.[2,6]

COMPLICATIONS

Cardiac involvement with valvular damage is the most common and serious long-term sequela of ARF.

MONITORING/FOLLOW-UP

- Patients may develop significant valvular abnormalities and heart failure even decades after the initial event.
- ARF requires long-term prophylaxis and sometimes monthly antibiotic injections for years.
- After the planned course for secondary prophylaxis, the risk for GAS reexposure and valvular disease should be assessed.

REFERENCES

1. Guidelines for the diagnosis of rheumatic fever. Jones Criteria, 1992 update. Special Writing Group of the Committee on Rheumatic Fever, Endocarditis, and Kawasaki Disease of the Council on Cardiovascular Disease in the Young of the American Heart Association. *JAMA.* 1992;268:2069–2073.
2. Gewitz MH, Baltimore RS, Tani LY, et al. Revision of the Jones Criteria for the diagnosis of acute rheumatic fever in the era of Doppler echocardiography: a scientific statement from the American Heart Association. *Circulation.* 2015;131:1806–1818.
3. Karthikeyan G, Guilherme L. Acute rheumatic fever. *Lancet.* 2018;392:161–174.
4. Evangelisto A, Werth V, Schumacher HR. What is that nodule? A diagnostic approach to evaluating subcutaneous and cutaneous nodules. *J Clin Rheumat.* 2006;12:230–240.
5. Shulman ST, Bisno AL, Clegg HW, et al. Clinical practice guideline for the diagnosis and management of group A streptococcal pharyngitis: 2012 update by the Infectious Diseases Society of America. *Clin Infect Dis.* 2012;55:e86–e102.
6. Gerber MA, Baltimore RS, Eaton CB, et al. Prevention of rheumatic fever and diagnosis and treatment of acute streptococcal pharyngitis: a scientific statement from the American Heart Association Rheumatic Fever, Endocarditis, and Kawasaki Disease Committee of the Council on Cardiovascular Disease in the Young, the Interdisciplinary Council on Functional Genomics and Translational Biology, and the Interdisciplinary Council on Quality of Care and Outcomes Research: endorsed by the American Academy of Pediatrics. *Circulation.* 2009;119:1541–1551.

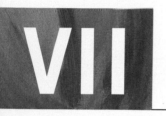

VII

Other Rheumatic Disorders

Mixed Connective Tissue Disease and Undifferentiated Connective Tissue Disease

39

Divya Jayakumar and Richard D. Brasington

MIXED CONNECTIVE TISSUE DISEASE

GENERAL PRINCIPLES

Definition

- Mixed connective tissue disease (MCTD) is a unique connective tissue disease with **overlapping features of systemic sclerosis (SSc), systemic lupus erythematosus (SLE), polymyositis (PM), and rheumatoid arthritis (RA)**, along with the presence of **antibodies to U1-ribonucleoprotein (RNP)**.
- It was first described by Sharp and colleagues in 1972 in a subset of 25 patients with these overlapping features.
- **Overlap syndrome** occurs when a patient possesses characteristics of more than one rheumatologic diagnosis, with distinct autoantibody profiles. MCTD is the prototype of overlap syndrome with high-titer U1-RNP.

Epidemiology and Risk Factors

- Prevalence of MCTD is thought to be approximately 1.9/100,000, but estimates vary widely. Women are affected more often than men.[1]
- It is associated with the HLA-DR4 and -DR2 alleles. Recently, HLA-B*08 and DRB1*04:01 have also been identified as risk alleles.

Pathogenesis

- The sine qua non of MCTD is an antibody against U1-RNP (uridine-rich small nuclear RNP), a spliceosomal complex that splices precursor messenger RNA (pre-mRNA) to form mature mRNA. A high titer of antibodies against U1-RNP, notably against U1-70 kDa and U1-RNA, is present in MCTD patients.
- Posttranslational apoptotic modification of RNP is thought to trigger both innate and adaptive immune responses.
- Innate immune system activation occurs via Toll-like receptor signaling and activation of dendritic cells and lymphocytes.
- T cells appear to have a central role in the pathogenesis of MCTD. CD4 T lymphocytes provide differentiation factors inducing B-cell isotype gene switching and cause tissue injury via cytokines. B lymphocytes serve as antigen-presenting cells and mediate tissue injury via cytokines, immune complex formation, and antibody-dependent cellular cytotoxicity.
- These processes lead to vascular intimal proliferation and medial hypertrophy, which cause disease manifestations, such as Raynaud's phenomenon (RP), puffy hands, sclerodactyly, esophageal dysmotility, pulmonary hypertension, and possibly interstitial lung disease (ILD).[2]

DIAGNOSIS

Clinical Features

- Patients have clinical features of SLE, SSc, PM, and sometimes RA, although the features of each might occur sequentially over the course of the disease.
- **Swollen or puffy fingers,** acrosclerosis, or sclerodactyly are typically seen.
- **Polyarthritis** affects most patients with MCTD and is often a presenting feature. Most have nonerosive disease, resembling Jaccoud's arthropathy, though some may develop erosions many years after disease onset.
- **Myalgias and myositis** range from mild to severe and can be histologically indistinguishable from idiopathic inflammatory myopathies. Often there is no demonstrable weakness, electromyogram (EMG) changes, or elevation in muscle enzymes.
- **RP** is seen in MCTD, with findings of capillary dilatation and drop out on nailfold capillaroscopy, similar to those seen in scleroderma.
- **Pulmonary hypertension is the leading cause of death** in MCTD; hence, periodic screening is encouraged. Blood vessels have intimal hyperplasia (plexiform lesion) and smooth muscle hypertrophy.[3]
- Other pulmonary manifestations of MCTD include **ILD**, pleural effusion, alveolar hemorrhage, diaphragmatic dysfunction, pulmonary vasculitis, and thromboembolic disease.
- **Gastroesophageal reflux disease (GERD)** and **esophageal dysmotility** occur in MCTD, similar to that of scleroderma.
- Severe renal and neurologic disease is rare and should prompt evaluation for another diagnosis.
- Additional features may include fever, malar or discoid rash, hemolytic anemia, leukopenia, thrombocytopenia, secondary Sjögren's syndrome, trigeminal neuralgia, sensorineural hearing loss, membranous glomerulonephritis, renovascular hypertension, and pericarditis.

Diagnostic Criteria

- There are no American College of Rheumatology (ACR) criteria for the diagnosis of MCTD. The diagnosis is made clinically based on the aforementioned characteristics.
- The criteria developed by both Alarcon-Segovia and Kahn have moderate sensitivity and good specificity, though the criteria should not be considered absolute.[4] Their criteria include high-titer U1-RNP antibodies in the appropriate clinical setting, which can be useful to guide the physician toward a diagnosis.
  - Alarcon-Segovia's clinical criteria require three or more of the following clinical features, one of which must be synovitis or myositis: swollen hands, synovitis, myositis, RP, and acrosclerosis.
  - Kahn's clinical criteria require the presence of RP plus at least two of the following: swollen fingers, synovitis, and myositis.
- Thus, the classical clinical presentation of MCTD is puffy or swollen fingers, synovitis, RP, and myositis.

Diagnostic Testing

- Characteristic immunologic findings include speckled pattern fluorescent antinuclear antibody (ANA) in high titers (often $> 1:1,280$) and antibodies to U1-RNP in moderate to high titers.
- Fifty to seventy percent of patients are Rheumatoid factor (RF) positive. Antibodies to Sm, SSA, SSB, dsDNA, and histones may occur as well. A positive Coombs test is often seen, although hemolytic anemia is uncommon. Hypocomplementemia is seen in 25% of patients.

Differential Diagnosis

The differential diagnosis includes SLE, SSc, PM, and RA. MCTD can evolve into one of these diseases over time, so it is essential to reassess these patients periodically. Of note, up to 20% of SLE patients also have anti–U1-RNP antibody positivity, but these are frequently associated with anti-Sm antibodies.

TREATMENT

Treatment should be focused on underlying organ involvement and is based on data extrapolated from treatment of SLE, RA, myositis, or SSc as presented in Table 39-1.[5]

TABLE 39-1	THERAPY OF MIXED CONNECTIVE TISSUE DISEASE BY ORGAN SYSTEM	
Organ System	**Clinical Manifestation**	**Treatment**
Mucocutaneous	Rashes and oral ulcers	Photoprotection, topical steroids, emollients, hydroxychloroquine
Vascular	Raynaud's phenomenon, digital ulcers	Gloves and warm clothing, smoking cessation, calcium channel blockers, digital sympathectomy, topical nitroglycerin, low-dose aspirin, pentoxifylline, phosphodiesterase-5 inhibitors, direct arterial vasodilators (bosentan, prostaglandin infusion therapy)
	Vasculitis	High-dose glucocorticoids, cyclophosphamide
Gastrointestinal	Gastroesophageal reflux, esophageal dysmotility	H2 antagonists, proton pump inhibitors, prokinetics
Respiratory: Arterial	Pulmonary arterial hypertension	Calcium channel blockers, angiotensin-converting enzyme (ACE) inhibitors, phosphodiesterase-5 inhibitors, prostacyclin, treprostinil, bosentan, anticoagulation
Respiratory: Parenchymal	Interstitial lung disease	High-dose glucocorticoids, cyclophosphamide, azathioprine, mycophenolate mofetil
Musculoskeletal	Arthritis	Nonsteroidal anti-inflammatory drugs (NSAIDs), hydroxychloroquine, methotrexate; the use of anti–tumor necrosis factor agents is not recommended
	Myositis	Glucocorticoids, hydroxychloroquine, azathioprine
Cardiovascular	Pericarditis	High doses of NSAIDs and varying doses of steroids; cyclophosphamide for severe cases
Renal	Glomerulonephritis	ACE inhibitors, glucocorticoids, cyclophosphamide, chlorambucil, or mycophenolate mofetil
	Scleroderma renal crisis	ACE inhibitors

(continued)

TABLE 39-1	THERAPY OF MIXED CONNECTIVE TISSUE DISEASE BY ORGAN SYSTEM (*continued*)	
Organ System	**Clinical Manifestation**	**Treatment**
Hematologic	Anemia, leukopenia, thrombocytopenia	Glucocorticoids, danazol, intravenous immunoglobulin, splenectomy
	Thrombotic thrombocytopenic purpura	Plasma exchange, immunosuppressants
Neuropsychiatric	Vascular headaches	Aspirin, NSAIDs, low-dose tricyclic antidepressants
	Transverse myelitis	Pulse glucocorticoids and cyclophosphamide or azathioprine

Adapted from: Kim P, Grossman JM. Treatment of mixed connective tissue disease. *Rheum Dis Clin North Am.* 2005;31:549–565.

PROGNOSIS

The inflammatory features (e.g., arthritis, serositis, myositis) of the disease tend to predominate early in the disease course and fibrotic features (e.g., esophageal dysmotility, pulmonary hypertension, ILD) later. The overall **prognosis is highly variable.**

UNDIFFERENTIATED CONNECTIVE TISSUE DISEASE

GENERAL PRINCIPLES

- A third of patients with undifferentiated connective tissue disease (UCTD) develop a definite connective tissue disease (CTD) within the first 3 to 5 years of diagnosis. The likelihood of transition into a definitive CTD decreases each year from the time of diagnosis.[6]
  - The most common CTD to develop is **SLE.**
  - Patients with predominant skin manifestations, such as discoid lupus, alopecia, and photosensitivity, have a greater chance of evolving into SLE.
- About two-thirds of patients who remain classified as UCTD are considered to have stable UCTD.

Definition

UCTD is a condition in which a patient possesses clinical manifestations and serologic markers suggestive of a CTD but **fails to fulfill enough characteristics for the diagnosis** of a definite CTD.

Epidemiology

Few reliable epidemiologic data are available because of the lack of criteria for diagnosis, but the following have been noted:

- UCTD is significantly more prevalent in females.[7]
- Onset typically occurs between 32 and 44 years of age.[7]

Etiology/Pathophysiology

The cause of UCTD is not well understood, but it is thought to be caused by immune dysregulation by an environmental trigger in a genetically susceptible host.

Risk Factors

Risk factors include female gender and having a family history of autoimmune disease.

DIAGNOSIS

Clinical Presentation

- UCTD physical manifestations are generally mild.
- RP is a typical feature of UCTD and abnormalities on nailfold capillaroscopy may be seen.
- **Inflammatory arthritis** is often a prominent feature but is nonerosive.
- A **nonspecific rash** may be present, and on biopsy, this typically shows interface dermatitis.

History
- Diffuse arthralgia
- RP
- Nonspecific rash with or without photosensitivity
- Oral or nasal ulcerations
- Low-grade fever
- Alopecia
- Sicca symptoms
- Chest pain with reclining or deep inhalation

Physical Examination
- Dry oral and nasal mucosa
- Nonspecific rash
- Hair loss
- Mild inflammatory arthritis
- Digital color changes consistent with RP

Diagnostic Criteria

There are no commonly accepted diagnostic criteria, but the following guidelines are often used to aid in diagnosis:

- **Stable** UCTD manifests signs and symptoms suggestive of a CTD **without fulfilling enough characteristics for the diagnosis of** a definite CTD for at least 3 years, in the setting of **positive** ANAs.[8] Patients with **early** UCTD are those with a shorter follow-up, that is, less than 3 years.
- Proposed exclusion criteria include malar rash, cutaneous lupus, skin sclerosis, heliotrope rash, Gottron's plaques, erosive arthritis, and specific antibodies (anti–double-stranded DNA [dsDNA], anti-Sm, anti–Scl-70, anticentromere, anti-SSA/SSB, anti-Jo1, and anti–Mi-2 antibodies).[9]
- ILD can occur, typically in a nonspecific interstitial pneumonia (NSIP) pattern.
- Stable UCTD is a clinically mild disease often with a single autoantibody profile.
- Neurologic and renal involvement are almost always absent.
- Arthritis is nonerosive and arthralgias are a prominent feature.

Differential Diagnosis

The differential diagnosis of UCTD includes mixed CTD, SLE, Sjögren's syndrome, scleroderma, RA, PM/dermatomyositis, vasculitis, and fibromyalgia.

Diagnostic Testing

Laboratory
- Immunologic[6]
  - **ANA is positive in approximately 90% of patients.**
  - Anti-SSA/SSB and anti-RNP are the other most common autoantibodies.
  - Up to 80% of patients have only a single autoantibody, which persists over time.
  - Patients with ANA in a homogeneous pattern, anti-dsDNA, anti-SSA, anti-Sm, or anticardiolipin antibodies are more likely to develop SLE.
- Hematologic findings are rarely severe enough to warrant treatment. The most common finding is **leukopenia**, but anemia and thrombocytopenia have also been observed.

Imaging
No imaging is specifically required for diagnosis. High-resolution computed tomography (HRCT) can be done if there is suspicion of ILD.

Musculoskeletal imaging may be done to help rule out other diagnoses such as RA.

Diagnostic Procedures
Nailfold capillaroscopy will reveal normal capillaries.

TREATMENT

Medications

Medications are tailored to specific manifestations of the disease. There are no formal studies on medications used for the treatment of UCTD, but the following are often used.

First Line
- **Nonsteroidal anti-inflammatory drugs (NSAIDs)** are the mainstay of therapy. They are used to reduce pain and inflammation and to treat arthralgias.
- **Hydroxychloroquine** is most commonly used to treat patients with myalgias and arthralgias resistant to NSAID monotherapy and to treat mucocutaneous manifestations.
- **Glucocorticoids** may be used for disease resistant to the previously mentioned treatments or for disease flares. Recommended length of glucocorticoid treatment varies. The patient should be treated with the lowest dose for the shortest period possible to minimize glucocorticoid side effects.

Second Line
Immunosuppressive medications other than hydroxychloroquine and glucocorticoids are reserved for severe systemic disease with internal organ involvement.

Nonpharmacologic Therapies

- Physical therapy and exercise
- Decrease sun exposure if photosensitive rash is present.
- Decrease exposure to cold and stress if RP is present.

REFERRAL

Possible referrals depend on the patient's manifestations, but may include rheumatology, dermatology, hematology, pulmonary, and neurology.

FOLLOW-UP

- Review signs and symptoms of CTD at each visit to screen for progression to definite CTD.
- Periodically check complete blood count (CBC), serum chemistries, and urinalysis to monitor for the development of CTD.

PROGNOSIS

About 35% of patients develop definitive CTD and outcomes are then determined by the CTD diagnosis.[6] Others either remain undifferentiated or experience disease remission.

- Many patients only require intermittent symptomatic treatment.
- Internal organ involvement is very rare.

REFERENCES

1. Ungprasert P, Crowson CS, Chowdhary VR, et al. Epidemiology of Mixed Connective Tissue Disease, 1985-2014: A Population-Based Study. *Arthritis Care Res (Hoboken)*. 2016;68:1843.
2. Hoffman RW, Maldonado ME. Immune pathogenesis of mixed connective tissue disease: a short analytical review. *Clin Immunol*. 2008;128:8–17.
3. Bull TM, Fagan KA, Badesh DB. Pulmonary vascular manifestations of mixed connective tissue disease. *Rheum Dis Clin North Am*. 2005;31:451–464.
4. Amiques JM, Cantagrel A, Abbal M, et al. Comparative study of 4 diagnosis criteria sets for mixed connective tissue disease in patients with anti-RNP antibodies. Autoimmunity Group of the Hospitals of Toulouse. *J Rheumatol*. 1998;25:393–394.
5. Kim P, Grossman JM. Treatment of mixed connective tissue disease. *Rheum Dis Clin North Am*. 2005;31:549–565.
6. Bodolay E, Csiki Z, Szekanecz Z, et al. Five-year follow-up of 665 Hungarian patients with undifferentiated connective tissue disease (UCTD). *Clin Exp Rheumatol*. 2003;21(3):313–320.
7. Mosca M, Tani C, Talarico R, et al. Undifferentiated connective tissue diseases (UCTD): simplified systemic autoimmune diseases. *Autoimmun Rev*. 2011;10(5):256–258.
8. Musca M, Neri R, Bombardieri S. Undifferentiated connective tissue diseases (UCTD): a review of the literature and a proposal for preliminary classification criteria. *Clin Exp Rheumatol*. 1999;17:615–620.
9. Doria A, Mosca M, Gambari PF, et al. Defining unclassifiable connective tissue diseases: incomplete, undifferentiated, or both? *J Rheumatol*. 2005;32(2):213–215.

Relapsing Polychondritis

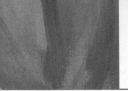

40

Shuang Song and Vladimir Despotovic

GENERAL PRINCIPLES

Definition

Relapsing polychondritis (RPC) is a rare disease characterized by episodic (relapsing–remitting) progressive inflammation of **cartilaginous** structures, most commonly the outer ear, nose, laryngotracheobronchial tree, and peripheral joints. RPC can also affect other **proteoglycan-rich** structures such as the eye, heart, blood vessels, inner ear, and skin.

Epidemiology

- The incidence of RPC is estimated at 3.5 per million per year in the United States.
- RPC occurs mostly in Caucasian patients aged 40 to 60 years but can be found in any race at any age.
- RPC affects both men and women, although there may be a slight female predominance.

Etiology/Pathophysiology

- The etiology of RPC remains unknown, but evidence suggests an autoimmune process. Both humoral and cell-mediated mechanisms are involved.
- The affected tissue is infiltrated by lymphocytes (mainly CD4+ T cells), macrophages, neutrophils, and plasma cells. These inflammatory cells release degradative enzymes and reactive oxygen metabolites that eventually lead to the destruction of cartilage and other proteoglycan-rich tissues.
- A number of proinflammatory cytokines are increased during disease flares, including serum monocyte chemoattractant protein 1 (MCP-1), macrophage inflammatory protein 1β (MIP-1β), and interleukin 8 (IL-8).[1]
- Autoantibodies against collagen (mostly type II, but also types IX and XI), matrilin-1 (an extracellular matrix protein found mainly in tracheal cartilage), and cartilage oligomeric protein (COMP) have been detected in patients with RPC. Some of these autoantigens have induced chondritis in animal models. Serum level of collagen type II autoantibodies seems to correlate with the severity of relapse. Anti–matrilin-1 is elevated during respiratory flares. However, the sensitivity and specificity of these antibodies are poor.[2]
- HLA-DR4 has been associated with RPC. Recently, high-resolution human leukocyte antigen (HLA) typing revealed an association between a specific HLA haplotype (HLA-DRB1*16:02, HLA-B*67:01 and HLA-DQB1*05:02) and RPC, which suggests the importance of HLA class II alleles in RPC susceptibility.[3]

Associated Conditions

- About one-third of cases of RPC are associated with rheumatic, hematologic, or other inflammatory diseases, including myelodysplastic syndrome, Behçet's disease, systemic vasculitis, rheumatoid arthritis, systemic lupus erythematosus, psoriatic arthritis, and inflammatory bowel disease.[1]

DIAGNOSIS

The main manifestations of RPC are otorhinolaryngeal disease, respiratory compromise, arthritis, and ocular inflammation.

Clinical Presentation

- **Auricular chondritis** is the most characteristic manifestation of RPC.
  - Auricular chondritis develops in 80% to 90% of patients with RPC. However, it is the presenting feature in only 40% of patients.
  - Auricular chondritis is characterized by the sudden onset of unilateral or bilateral auricular swelling, pain, warmth, and erythema or violaceous discoloration.
  - The inflammation affects the cartilaginous structures of the outer ear, sparing the lobes that do not contain cartilage.
  - Each episode lasts for days to weeks and usually resolves spontaneously.
  - Recurrent attacks result in a flaccid, nodular, and deformed ear, sometimes referred to as "cauliflower ear."
- **Hearing loss** is found in 30% of patients.
  - Conductive hearing loss is caused by collapse of the auricular cartilage and swelling of the external auditory canal or Eustachian tube. Serous or purulent otitis media can also occur.
  - Sensorineural hearing loss due to cochlear dysfunction is caused by vasculitis of the cochlear branch of the internal auditory artery.
- **Vestibular dysfunction** with symptoms such as vertigo and ataxia is also common.
  - Vasculitis of the vestibular branch of the internal auditory artery can result in vestibular dysfunction manifested by **vertigo, ataxia, nausea, and vomiting**.
  - If acute, these symptoms can mimic a posterior circulation stroke.
- **Nasal chondritis** occurs in approximately 50% of patients.
  - It is characterized by pain at the base of the nose, swelling of the nasal bridge, and tenderness of the distal part of the nasal septum. Patients can have nasal crusting, obstruction, rhinorrhea, or epistaxis.
  - Recurrent attacks may lead to permanent destruction of the septal cartilage with a **saddle nose deformity**.
- **Laryngotracheal and bronchial involvement** occurs in up to 50% of patients.
  - Larynx involvement occurs in more than half of the cases.
  - It is the most common cause of death in RPC.
  - Inflammation of the cartilage in the larynx, trachea, and bronchial tree causes hoarseness, throat pain, dysphonia, aphonia, dyspnea, cough, stridor, wheezing, and choking.
  - Obstruction can occur in varying degrees and at different levels.
    - Total obstruction of the upper airways can occur during attempted bronchoscopy, intubation, or tracheostomy.
    - Involvement of the lower airways is often asymptomatic until detected by imaging, bronchoscopy, or spirometry.
  - Respiratory infections are common and result from impaired drainage of secretions caused by airway collapse and impaired mucociliary function.
  - Parenchymal pulmonary disease is not a common feature of RPC.
- **Arthritis** is the second most common manifestation of RPC. It is a presenting symptom in 30% of patients and occurs in up to 80% of patients during the course of the disease.
  - **Costochondritis, sternoclavicular (SC) arthritis, and manubriosternal arthritis** are typical in RPC.

- ○ Arthritis of other joints is typically asymmetric, episodic, nondeforming, and nonerosive.
- ○ The distribution ranges from monoarthritis to oligoarthritis to polyarthritis. The most commonly affected joints besides the parasternal joints are metacarpophalangeal joints (MCPs), proximal interphalangeal joints (PIPs), wrists, knees, ankles, and metatarsophalangeal joints (MTPs).
- The **eye** is involved in up to 60% of patients.
  - ○ **Scleritis** and **episcleritis** are the most common ocular diseases. **Conjunctivitis** is also relatively common. Uveitis, keratitis, retinal vasculitis, and optic neuritis are rare.
  - ○ All forms of scleritis may occur, ranging from diffuse anterior to nodular or necrotizing. Perforation of the globe is possible yet rare.[1]
- **Systemic vasculitis** is an associated condition in up to one-quarter of patients with RPC. Large, medium, and small vessels may be affected.
  - ○ Associated systemic vasculitis include Behçet's disease, Takayasu's arteritis, polyarteritis nodosa, Henoch–Schönlein purpura, granulomatosis with polyangiitis (GPA), microscopic polyangiitis (MPA), and eosinophilic granulomatosis with polyangiitis (EGPA).
  - ○ The overlap between Behçet's syndrome and RPC is sometime referred to as "MAGIC" syndrome (mouth and genital ulcers with inflamed cartilage).
- Kidney disease is found in approximately 15% of patients and its presence indicates a worse prognosis.
  - ○ The most common histopathologic findings are mild mesangial proliferation and focal segmental necrotizing glomerulonephritis. Tubulointerstitial nephritis and immunoglobulin A (IgA) nephropathy are less common.
  - ○ Deposits of complement and immunoglobulins are found on electron microscopy predominantly in the mesangium.
- **Skin** lesions affect one-third of patients.
  - ○ Palpable purpura, urticaria, aphthous ulcers, limb skin ulceration, distal digital necrosis, erythema nodosum–like nodules, livedo reticularis, Sweet's syndrome, and superficial phlebitis have been reported.
  - ○ The histopathology may show leukocytoclastic vasculitis, neutrophilic infiltrates, or panniculitis.
  - ○ Annular urticaria and erythema annulare centrifugum–like plaques on the upper trunk and shoulders preceding chondritis may be specific for the disorder and more commonly associated with myelodysplastic syndrome.[4]
- **Cardiovascular** disease is the second most common cause of death in RPC and is present in 10% of the patients. Aortic valve disease due to aortic root dilation and ascending thoracic aortic aneurysm are most common. Mitral valvular disease may occur. Aortitis and valvulitis are thought to be contributing factors. Other relatively rare cardiac involvement includes pericarditis, myocarditis, atrioventricular conduction blocks, and extra-aortic large vessel involvement.

Diagnostic Criteria

The diagnosis is based on clinical features, imaging studies, and rarely a biopsy of the cartilage. The first diagnostic criteria for RPC were published by McAdam, and then some modifications were made by Damiani and Levine.[5] Michet's criteria are often used at present and avoid the need for a biopsy (Table 40-1).[6] No new criteria have been published since the 1980s.

Differential Diagnosis

- The differential diagnosis is broad because of the variety of manifestations but is primarily **GPA**.

TABLE 40-1	MICHET'S DIAGNOSTIC CRITERIA FOR RELAPSING POLYCHONDRITIS

Diagnosis requires (1) two major OR (2) one major and two minor criteria. Histologic examination of affected cartilage is not required.

Major criteria	Minor criteria
Auricular chondritis	Ocular inflammation (conjunctivitis, keratitis, episcleritis,
Nasal chondritis	and uveitis)
Laryngotracheal	Hearing loss
chondritis	Vestibular dysfunction
	Seronegative inflammatory arthritis

Adapted from: Michet CJ, McKenna CH, Luthra HS, et al. Relapsing polychondritis. Survival and predictive role of early disease manifestations. *Ann Intern Med.* 1986;104:74–78.

- The manifestations of **auricular chondritis** may resemble redness and swelling of the external ear due to bacterial infectious **cellulitis**. Sparing of the earlobe in RPC is a diagnostic clue, but biopsy is helpful for culture and histology. On the other hand, recurrent "bacterial infections" of the outer ear should raise suspicion for RPC. Another disorder that may locally resemble RPC is chondrodermatitis nodularis helices. Unlike RPC, it tends to be locally limited, most commonly presents in men over age 50 as painful erythematous nodules often with an ulceration in the center.[7]
- **Infectious chondritis** including leprosy and syphilis needs to be excluded.
- **Saddle nose deformity** and **laryngotracheal symptoms** may occur in GPA, although RPC is confined strictly to cartilaginous portions of the airways. GPA is the primary differential diagnosis for RPC. Trauma, lymphoma, and syphilis should also be considered as potential causes of saddle nose deformity.
- Other classes of **systemic vasculitis** should be considered when diagnosing RPC.
- **Aortic root dilation, aortic aneurysms, and valvular diseases** are also found in Marfan syndrome, Ehlers–Danlos syndrome, syphilis, and idiopathic cystic medial necrosis.
- Peripheral inflammatory **arthritis**, especially in conjunction with ocular symptoms, needs to be distinguished from rheumatoid arthritis, seronegative spondyloarthropathies, and sarcoidosis.

Diagnostic Testing

Laboratories
- Laboratory findings of RPC are nonspecific and may demonstrate elevated erythrocyte sedimentation rate (ESR) and/or C-reactive protein (CRP), normochromic normocytic anemia, leukocytosis, thrombocytosis, and hypergammaglobulinemia.
- The diagnostic utility of autoantibodies is poor because of the low sensitivity and specificity.

Imaging
- **Computed tomography (CT)** of the neck and chest should be considered for patients with evidence of laryngeal involvement and for those with abnormal pulmonary function tests, respectively. **Dynamic expiratory CT** imaging appears to have a much greater sensitivity compared to inspiratory CT alone.[8] CT can detect tracheal or bronchial stenosis, excessive dynamic expiratory airway collapsibility and tracheobronchomalacia, smooth airway wall thickening with sparing of the posterior membranous wall, and increased attenuation of the cartilage.

- **F-fluorodeoxyglucose positron emission tomography/CT (FDG PET/CT)** scanning may help to detect tracheobronchial or aortic involvement and occult inflammation in RPC.

Diagnostic Procedures
- Echocardiography should be considered to diagnose aortic and valvular disease.
- Pulmonary function testing is recommended in all suspected cases of RPC. Spirometry may show an obstructive respiratory impairment due to airway collapse and narrowing.
- Bronchoscopy is not routinely performed because of the invasive nature with risks of airway damage and respiratory failure. It may be used if specifically indicated.
- Cartilage biopsy in general is not required but may assist diagnosis in challenging cases. In the early stage, there is inflammatory infiltration of the perichondrium, with CD4+ T cells, macrophages, neutrophils, eosinophils, and plasma cells. These inflammatory cells then invade the cartilage and lead to destruction of the cartilage followed by fibrosis with areas of calcification.
- Biopsy of skin rash may show leukocytoclastic vasculitis, panniculitis, neutrophilic dermatoses, or small-vessel occlusion.

TREATMENT

Treatment is aimed at prevention of flares and managing complications of the disease.

Medications
Anti-inflammatory Agents
- **Nonsteroidal anti-inflammatory drugs (NSAIDs)** may be used for mild episcleritis, costochondritis, arthritis, and minor inflammation of the nose and ear.
- **Dapsone** and **colchicine** have been used for mild chondritis in case reports.

Glucocorticoids
- Glucocorticoids are used in RPC patients with more intense inflammation or those resistant to NSAIDs. RPC is usually steroid responsive.
- Oral prednisone, typically at a dose of 1 mg/kg daily, is often necessary to suppress severe inflammation and induce remission, and then the prednisone dose should be tapered to the lowest maintenance level and eventually discontinued as tolerated. Long-term, low-dose prednisone therapy may be necessary to suppress flares.
- Pulse intravenous (IV) methylprednisolone of 1,000 mg daily for 3 days followed by daily PO prednisone is used for acute airway closure.

Nonbiologic Immunosuppressive Agents
- Disease-modifying treatment is indicated in patients with organ-threatening manifestations and those dependent on higher-dose glucocorticoids.
- There are no randomized controlled trials on RPC treatments.
- **Methotrexate, azathioprine, cyclosporine, cyclophosphamide,** and **mycophenolate mofetil** have shown successful results in some patients with RPC.
- Patients with life-threatening disease should be considered for **pulse IV methylprednisolone** and **cyclophosphamide** therapy.
- **Leflunomide** had mixed outcomes in a couple of case reports.[9,10]
- **Intravenous immunoglobulin (IVIG)** has successfully induced remission in refractory RPC.[1]

Biologics
- Anti–tumor necrosis factor-alpha (anti–TNF-α) agents: Anti–TNF-α agents have had good results in many cases of RPC, including **infliximab, etanercept,**

certolizumab, **adalimumab**, and **golimumab**.[1,2] They are the most commonly used biologics in RPC.
- Interleukin-1 receptor (IL-1R) antagonists: **Anakinra** has been reported to be an effective treatment for RPC refractory to anti–TNF-α therapy.[1]
- Inhibitor of the costimulatory-signaling pathway: **Abatacept** (cytotoxic T-lymphocyte–associated protein 4, CTLA4-Ig) was efficacious for chondritis and inflammatory arthritis from RPC in several patients.[1]
- Anti–IL-6 receptor antibody: **Tocilizumab** has showed therapeutic efficacy in patients with RPC who failed conventional immunosuppressive agents including cyclophosphamide and anti–TNF-α agents. These patients had high serum IL-6 levels despite other medications.[1,11]
- B-cell depletion therapy: The efficacy of **rituximab** in treating RPC is controversial. Further investigation is needed.

Surgical Management

Tracheostomy or bronchial stent placement might be required for symptomatic airway obstruction. Cochlear implantation is useful for patients with sensorineural hearing loss. Heart valve replacement surgery and surgical aortic aneurysm repair may be required. In patients requiring intubation or general anesthesia, difficult airway considerations should be undertaken and awake fiberoptic intubation with surgical airway standby should be considered.

OUTCOME/PROGNOSIS

- Most patients experience intermittent episodes of inflammation and develop some degree of disability (e.g., bilateral deafness, impaired vision, phonation difficulties, or cardiorespiratory problems). Most patients require long-term maintenance therapy.
- In earlier prospective studies, the frequent causes of death included pneumonia, tracheobronchial involvement, vasculitis, and cardiovascular events.
- The survival rate appears to be improving with advances in therapy, and it ranges from 55% at 10 years (1986) to 94% at 8 years (1998).[12]

REFERENCES

1. Mathian A, Miyara M, Cohen-Aubart F, et al. Relapsing polychondritis: a 2016 update on clinical features, diagnostic tools, treatment and biological drug use. *Best Pract Res Clin Rheumatol.* 2016;30:316–333.
2. Lekpa FK, Chevalier X. Refractory relapsing polychondritis: challenges and solutions. *Open Access Rheumatol.* 2018;10:1–11.
3. Terao C, Yoshifuji H, Yamano Y, et al. Genotyping of relapsing polychondritis identified novel susceptibility HLA alleles and distinct genetic characteristics from other rheumatic diseases. *Rheumatology (Oxford).* 2016;55:1686–1692.
4. Watkins S, Magill J, Ramos F. Annular eruption preceding relapsing polychondritis: case report and review of the literature. *Int J Dermatol.* 2009;48:356–362.
5. Damiani JM, Levine HL. Relapsing polychondritis—report of ten cases. *Laryngoscope.* 1979;89:929–946.
6. Michet CJ, McKenna CH, Luthra HS, et al. Relapsing polychondritis. Survival and predictive role of early disease manifestations. *Ann Intern Med.* 1986;104:74–78.
7. Upile T, Patel N, Jerjes W, et al. Advances in the understanding of chondrodermatitis nodularis chronica helicis: the perichondrial vasculitis theory. *Clin Otolaryngol.* 2009;34:147–150.
8. Rafeq S, Trentham D, Ernst A. Pulmonary manifestations of relapsing polychondritis. *Clin Chest Med.* 2010;31:513–518.
9. Handler RP. Leflunomide for relapsing polychondritis: successful long-term treatment. *J Rheumatol.* 2006;33:1916; author reply 1916–1917.

10. Koenig AS, Abruzzo JL. Leflunomide induced fevers, thrombocytosis, and leukocytosis in a patient with relapsing polychondritis. *J Rheumatol*. 2002;29:192–194.
11. Henes JC, Xenitidis T, Horger M. Tocilizumab for refractory relapsing polychondritis–long-term response monitoring by magnetic resonance imaging. *Joint Bone Spine*. 2016;83:365–366.
12. Letko E, Zafirakis P, Baltatzis S, et al. Relapsing polychondritis: a clinical review. *Semin Arthritis Rheum*. 2002;31:384–395.

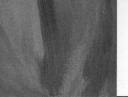

Adult-Onset Still's Disease

41

Michiko Inaba and Richard D. Brasington

GENERAL PRINCIPLES

Definition

Adult-onset Still's disease (AOSD) is a rare autoinflammatory condition, first described by E.G. Bywaters in 1971.[1] It consists of a constellation of clinical and laboratory findings that are similar to those of systemic juvenile arthritis (Still's disease).

AOSD is characterized by quotidian (daily) fevers, arthritis, and an evanescent rash that occurs concurrently with the febrile periods.

Epidemiology

- The incidence of AOSD is estimated to be 0.16 to 0.40 new cases per 100,000 patients per year, depending on the population.[2,3]
- It occurs in a bimodal distribution, most commonly between the ages of 15 and 25 and 36 and 46. However, cases of AOSD have been reported in patients over 60 years.
- There is no gender predilection.

Pathophysiology

- Although the pathogenesis is unknown, immune-mediated mechanisms are clearly involved. A number of viral and bacterial infections have been hypothesized to play a role in its pathophysiology.[4]
- Associations with various human leukocyte antigens (HLAs; HLA B-17, -B18, -B35, -DRB1, -DR2, and -DR5)[5–7] have been reported in different ethnic groups.
- Activation of the innate immune system via neutrophils and macrophages is a hallmark of AOSD. Two proinflammatory cytokines, interleukin (IL)-18 and IL-1β, are thought to be important in causing tumor necrosis factor (TNF)-α, IL-6, IL-8 secretion.[8–10]

DIAGNOSIS

AOSD is a clinical diagnosis and a diagnosis of exclusion.

Clinical Presentation

History

Patients can present with a myriad of symptoms.

- The dominant manifestation is a **spiking fever,** often greater than 39°C. The fever classically follows a **quotidian** (daily) or **double quotidian** (twice a day) pattern of peaks, often with an afebrile period between spikes. The fevers typically occur in the late afternoon or evening and may follow a regular cycle.
- Coincident with fevers is the appearance of a characteristic **transitory salmon-colored rash.**
- Arthralgia involving the knees, wrists, ankles, proximal interphalangeal (PIP) joints, elbows, and shoulders are common manifestations of AOSD.[1,11] Some patients may develop inflammatory arthritis.
- Patients can also present primarily with myalgias.

Physical Examination

- The salmon-colored macular or maculopapular rash may be difficult to identify on routine examination given its transient nature. It is usually found on the trunk or extremities and may be precipitated by stroking the skin in a linear fashion (Koebner phenomenon). The creases in bed sheets may provoke the rash on the back.
- **Oligoarticular joint involvement** is usually gradual in onset and mild in nature but may progress to a more destructive arthritis.
- Additional clinical findings may include **pharyngitis, lymphadenopathy, splenomegaly, hepatomegaly, and cardiopulmonary involvement** (pericarditis, pleural effusions, and pulmonary infiltrates).

Diagnostic Criteria

- The Yamaguchi criteria for AOSD are presented in Table 41-1.[12]
- These criteria carry an estimated sensitivity of 93% when five of the features are present, with at least two from the major criteria.

Differential Diagnosis

The differential diagnosis includes **infection** (viral or bacterial), **granulomatous disorders, vasculitis, connective-tissue diseases** (systemic lupus erythematous, mixed connective tissue disease), **malignancy** (lymphoma, leukemia), and **drug reactions.** The more prolonged the clinical course, in the absence of another definitive diagnosis, the more likely the diagnosis will be AOSD.

Diagnostic Testing

Although laboratory and radiographic abnormalities may lend support to the diagnosis of AOSD, no test alone is specific for the disease.

Laboratory

- A complete blood count (CBC) usually reveals a **leukocytosis** with a predominance of neutrophils, a normocytic normochromic anemia, and thrombocytosis.

TABLE 41-1 **YAMAGUCHI CRITERIA FOR ADULT STILL'S DISEASE[a]**

Definitive diagnosis requires at least two major and three minor criteria.

Major criteria:
- Fever of ≥39°C for ≥1 week
- Arthralgias or arthritis for ≥2 weeks
- Characteristic rash
- Leukocytosis (>10,000 cells/mm^3) with a predominance of neutrophils

Minor criteria:
- Pharyngitis
- Lymphadenopathy
- Hepatomegaly/splenomegaly
- Abnormal liver tests
- Negative ANA and RF

---

[a]Exclusion criteria: current infection, malignancy (especially lymphoma), and other active rheumatologic diseases.

ANA, antinuclear antibody; RF, rheumatoid factor.

Adapted from: Yamaguchi M, Ohta A, Tsunematsu T, et al. Preliminary criteria for classification of adult Still's disease. *J Rheumatol*. 1992;19:424–430.

- **Erythrocyte sedimentation rate (ESR) and C-reactive protein (CRP) are almost always considerably elevated,** which is consistent with an inflammatory process.
- Liver enzymes often demonstrate mild elevations of aminotransferases, alkaline phosphatase, and lactate dehydrogenase (LDH).
- **Serum ferritin levels can be markedly elevated.**
  - Elevated ferritin levels usually correlate with disease activity and have been proposed as markers of treatment response.
  - A threshold of five times the normal value (i.e., 1,000 μg/L) is suggestive of AOSD.[13] Levels between 3,000 and 30,000 are common. However, the specificity for AOSD remains poor (41%–46%) because similar levels may be found during infection, neoplastic conditions, or storage diseases such as Gaucher's disease.
  - The proportion of **glycosylated ferritin is low** and this may also be a clue to diagnosis.[14,15] Hemophagocytic lymphohistiocytosis is also associated with hyperferritinemia and a low percentage of glycosylation.[16]
- Antinuclear antibodies (ANAs) and rheumatoid factor (RF) are usually negative but may be present in low titers. Anti–cyclic citrullinated protein (CCP) antibodies are almost always negative.[17]

Imaging
- Radiographic findings in AOSD are relatively uncommon.
- A nonerosive narrowing of the carpometacarpal joints and the intercarpal spaces within the wrist (with sparing of metacarpophalangeal joints) may be seen, less commonly ankylosis of the wrist.

Diagnostic Procedures
- **Lymph node biopsies** display a large range of nonspecific histologic changes including typical/atypical paracortical hyperplasia, vascular proliferation, histiocyte aggregation, exuberant immunoblastic reaction, and follicular hyperplasia.[18] Clearly, such findings could be confused with lymphoproliferative disorders, but immunohistochemistry can be used to differentiate.
- Skin biopsy reveals a nonspecific mild perivascular inflammation of the superficial dermis with infiltration of lymphocytes and histiocytes.
- Joint fluid aspiration shows a leukocytosis with neutrophil predominance.

TREATMENT

Medications
- **Nonsteroidal anti-inflammatory drugs (NSAIDs)** are effective for mild inflammatory symptoms in 20% of AOSD. Maximal doses (e.g., ibuprofen 800 mg three to four times daily or naproxen 500 mg twice daily) are required. Monitoring for renal, hepatic, and gastrointestinal (GI) toxicity is recommended.[4,11]
- Glucocorticoids are indicated for mild to severe inflammatory manifestations at the onset of therapy. Oral prednisone, dosed at 0.5 to 1 mg/kg daily for mild to moderate inflammatory symptoms, or IV methylprednisolone followed by oral prednisone for severe inflammatory disease with life-threatening organ involvement[19]
- Limited data are available for efficacy of any particular disease-modifying antirheumatic drugs (DMARDs).
- Methotrexate (7.5–17.5 mg/week) remains the most used DMARD in AOSD for its steroid-sparing effects in steroid-dependent patients.[20]
- Other nonbiologic DMARDs previously tried include azathioprine, hydroxychloroquine, cyclophosphamide, and cyclosporine.[21]
- Growing number of studies support the efficacy of several biologic agents including etanercept, infliximab,[22] anakinra,[23] abatacept,[24] tocilizumab,[25] and rituximab in the treatment of AOSD.
- Sulfasalazine has been associated with a high rate of toxicity and should be avoided.[26]

Other Nonpharmacologic Therapies

Local joint injections with steroids may provide symptomatic relief.

COMPLICATIONS

* Patients with AOSD have been noted to develop reactive hemophagocytic syndrome, also known as macrophage activation syndrome (MAS),[27] cardiac tamponade, acute hepatic failure, myocarditis, amyloidosis, disseminated intravascular coagulation (DIC), interstitial lung disease, and pulmonary hypertension.
* MAS can occur in 12% to 19% of AOSD and can occur at any time during the disease course.
* Patients with MAS may have leukopenia and/or thrombocytopenia, very high levels of serum triglyceride, and elevated soluble CD25 (soluble IL-2Rα).

REFERRAL

Patients can benefit from the input of physiotherapists, occupational therapists, psychologists, and/or arthritis support groups.

OUTCOME/PROGNOSIS

* The course of AOSD is variable. Approximately one-third of patients experience a complete resolution within a year of onset. One-third will experience a cyclic relapsing and remitting pattern of the disease. The remaining one-third experiences a chronic active disease, which may evolve into rheumatoid arthritis.[28]
* Factors associated with a poor prognosis include disease refractory to glucocorticoids, polyarthritis, and a persistently elevated ferritin.[29]
* Factors associated with a good prognosis are a prompt resolution of clinical and laboratory abnormalities and lack of a relapse as steroids are reduced (usually over a 2–3 month period).

REFERENCES

1. Bywaters EG. Still's disease in the adult. *Ann Rheum Dis.* 1971:30;121–133.
2. Magadur-Joly G, Billaud E, Barrier JH, et al. Epidemiology of adult Still's disease: estimate of the incidence by a retrospective study in west France. *Ann Rheum Dis.* 1995;54:587–590.
3. Evensen KJ, Nossent HC. Epidemiology and outcome of adult-onset Still's disease in Northern Norway. *Scand J Rheumatol.* 2006;35:48–51.
4. Efthimiou P, Georgy S. Pathogenesis and management of adult-onset Still's disease. *Semin Arthritis Rheum.* 2006;36:144–152.
5. Pouchot J, Sampalis JS, Beaudet F, et al. Adult Still's disease: manifestations, disease course, and outcome in 62 patients. *Medicine (Baltimore).* 1991;70:118–136.
6. Fujii T, Nojima T, Yasuoka H, et al. Cytokine and immunogenetic profiles in Japanese patients with adult Still's disease. Association with chronic articular disease. *Rheumatology.* 2001;40:1398–1404.
7. Joung CL, Lee HS, Lee SW, et al. Association between HLA-DR B1 and clinical features of adult onset Still's disease in Korea. *Clin Exp Rheumatol.* 2003;21:489–492.
8. Kastner DL, Aksentijevich I, Goldbach-Mansky R. Autoinflammatory disease reloaded: a clinical perspective. *Cell.* 2010;140:784–790.
9. Lotito AP, Silva CA, Mello SB. Interleukin-18 in chronic joint diseases. *Autoimmun Rev.* 2007; 6:253–256.
10. Chen DY, Lan JL, Lin FJ, et al. Predominance of Th1 cytokine in peripheral blood and pathological tissues of patients with active untreated adult onset Still's disease. *Ann Rheum Dis.* 2004;63:1300–1306.
11. Efthimiou P, Paik PK, Bielory L. Diagnosis and management of adult onset Still's disease. *Ann Rheum Dis.* 2006;65:564–572.

12. Yamaguchi M, Ohta A, Tsunematsu T, et al. Preliminary criteria for classification of adult Still's disease. *J Rheumatol.* 1992;19:424–430.
13. Coffenils M, Soupart A, Pardier O, et al. Hyperferritinemia in adult onset Still's disease and the hemophagocytic syndrome. *J Rheumatol* 1992;19: 1425–1427.
14. Vignes S, Le Moël G, Fautrel B, et al. Percentage of glycosylated serum ferritin remains low throughout the course of adult onset Still's disease. *Ann Rheum Dis.* 2000;59:347–350.
15. Fautrel B, Le Moël G, Saint-Marcoux B, et al. Diagnostic value of ferritin and glycosylated ferritin in adult onset Still's disease. *J Rheumatol.* 2001;28:322–329.
16. Lambotte O, Cacoub P, Costedoat N, et al. High ferritin and low glycosylated ferritin may also be a marker of excessive macrophage activation. *J Rheumatol.* 2003;30:1027–1028.
17. Riera E, Olivé A, Narváez J, et al. Adult onset Still's disease: review of 41 cases. *Clin Exp Rheumatol.* 2001;29:331–336.
18. Jeon YK, Paik JH, Park SS, et al. Spectrum of lymph node pathology in adult onset Still's disease; analysis of 12 patients with one follow up biopsy. *J Clin Pathol.* 2004;57:1052–1056.
19. Fautrel B. Adult-onset Still disease. *Best Pract Res Clin Rheumatol.* 2008;22:773–792.
20. Manger B, Rech J, Schett G. Use of methotrexate in adult-onset Still's disease. *Clin Exp Rheumatol.* 2010;28:S168–S171.
21. Franchini S, Dagna L, Salvo F, et al. Efficacy of Traditional and biologic agents in different clinical phenotypes of adult-onset Still's disease. *Arthritis Rheum.* 2010;62:2530–2535.
22. Fautrel B, Sibilia J, Mariette X, et al. Tumour necrosis factor alpha blocking agents in refractory adult Still's disease: an observational study of 20 cases. *Ann Rheum Dis.* 2005;64:262–266.
23. Laskari K, Tzioufas AG, Moutsopoulos HM. Efficacy and long-term follow-up of IL-1R inhibitor anakinra in adults with Still's disease: a case-series study. *Arthritis Res Ther.* 2011;13:R91.
24. Quartuccio L, Maset M, De Vita S. Efficacy of abatacept in a refractory case of adult-onset Still's disease. *Clin Exp Rheumatol.* 2010;28:265–267.
25. Perdan-Pirkmajer K, Praprotnik S, Tomšič M. A case of refractory adult-onset Still's disease successfully controlled with tocilizumab and a review of the literature. *Clin Rheumatol.* 2010;29:1465–1467.
26. Jung JH, Jun JB, Yoo DH, et al. High toxicity of sulfasalazine in adult-onset Still's disease. *Clin Exp Rheumatol.* 2000;18:245–248.
27. Hot A, Toh ML, Coppéré B, et al. Reactive hemophagocytic syndrome in adult-onset Still disease: clinical features and long-term outcome: a case-control study of 8 patients. *Medicine (Baltimore).* 2010;89:37–46.
28. Gerfaud-Valentin M, Maucort-Boulch D, Hot A, et al. Adult-onset still disease: manifestations, treatment, outcome, and prognostic factors in 57 patients. *Medicine (Baltimore).* 2014;93:91 99.
29. Ruscitti P, Cipriani P, Masedu F, et al. Adult-onset Still's disease: evaluation of prognostic tools and validation of the systemic score by analysis of 100 cases from three centers. *BMC Med.* 2016;14:194.

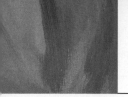

Hereditary Periodic Fever Syndromes

Philip Chu and Richard D. Brasington

42

INTRODUCTION

- Hereditary periodic fever syndromes (also known as familial autoinflammatory syndromes) are rare diseases characterized by recurrent episodes of dramatic inflammation arising from mutations of genes regulating aspects of innate immunity.
- Dysregulation of interleukin-1β (IL-1β) pathway is central to many periodic fever syndromes. As opposed to autoimmune diseases, there is a lack of high-titer autoantibodies or self-reactive T cells. As a result, they are considered a subgroup of autoinflammatory diseases.[1]
- In most hereditary periodic fever syndromes, clinical manifestations usually start during childhood, but diagnosis is often not made until adulthood.
- A trial of IL-1β inhibiting therapy may be helpful for diagnostic and therapeutic purposes.
- The major syndromes are:
  - Familial Mediterranean fever (FMF)
  - Hyperimmunoglobulinemia D with periodic fever syndrome (HIDS)
  - Tumor necrosis factor (TNF) receptor–associated periodic syndrome (TRAPS)
  - Cryopyrin-associated periodic syndrome (CAPS)
  - Periodic fever with aphthous stomatitis, pharyngitis, and adenitis (PFAPA)

FAMILIAL MEDITERRANEAN FEVER

GENERAL PRINCIPLES

Definition

FMF is a hereditary autoinflammatory disease characterized by recurrent attacks of fever and serositis.

Epidemiology

- FMF is the **most common hereditary periodic fever syndrome.**
- FMF is mostly found in people from around the Mediterranean basin (Jewish, Arab, Armenian, Italian, and Turkish populations).
- Prevalence of FMF in Israel is about 1 in 500 but, like the other periodic fever syndromes, is highly variant depending on subgroup and geographical location.[2]

Pathophysiology

- FMF is caused by mutations in the *MEFV* gene, with more than 28 mutations described. The M694V mutation is the most frequent and severe phenotype.[3,4]
- Although FMF is considered an autosomal recessive disease, some patients carry only a single mutation, suggesting a dominant trait with specific mutations.[5]

- *MEFV* encodes the protein pyrin that is involved in regulation of IL-1β processing. *MEFV* is highly expressed in neutrophils, activated monocytes, synovial fibroblasts, and peritoneal fibroblasts.

DIAGNOSIS

Clinical Presentation

- Most patients experience their first clinical episode before the age of 20.
- Patients present with seemingly unprovoked episodes of **fever, serositis, monoarticular arthritis, and rash** of 1 to 3 days duration.
  - Serositis involves peritoneum, pleura, and, less commonly, pericardium. Repeated bouts of serositis can lead to fibrosis and formation of intra-abdominal adhesions.
  - Monoarticular arthritis typically involves the knee, ankle, wrist, or hip. **Arthritis is inflammatory but nonerosive.**
  - The characteristic rash described with FMF is **erysipeloid erythema,** an erythematous, sharply demarcated, tender, swollen area with a predilection for the lower extremity.[6]
  - Other less common symptoms include orchitis, aseptic meningitis, and severe myalgia.[4]
- Episodes spontaneously resolve with return to baseline health between febrile episodes. The time between attacks can range from days to years.

Diagnostic Testing

- During attacks, acute-phase reactant levels like erythrocyte sedimentation rate (ESR), C-reactive protein (CRP), fibrinogen, and serum amyloid A (SAA) are elevated. Proteinuria is suggestive of renal amyloidosis.[3]
- Genetic testing is not required in patients from high-risk groups with typical symptoms who are responsive to colchicine. However, in atypical patients, genetic analysis is recommended. Genetic laboratories usually screen for the most common mutations, and rare mutations can be missed.[3]

TREATMENT

- Lifelong daily **colchicine** (0.6 mg/day to 1.2 to 1.8 mg/day based on age) is the treatment of choice. Colchicine is effective in preventing acute attacks and the development of amyloidosis.[7] Colchicine is safe even when given long term. The most common side effects are gastrointestinal and improve with dose reduction. Less common side effects may include bone marrow suppression and hepatotoxicity.[3]
- IL-1 inhibition with canakinumab or anakinra can be trialed for patients who do not respond to or cannot tolerate colchicine.[8,9]

COMPLICATIONS

- **The most serious adverse effect of FMF is amyloidosis.** Repeated elevated levels of SAA can lead to amyloid deposition in kidneys, lungs, intestine, and adrenal glands. Prior to the use of colchicine, renal failure due to amyloidosis was the leading cause of mortality in FMF patients.
- Risk factors for amyloidosis include a family history of amyloidosis, male gender, and M694V genotype and SAA1 α/α genotype.[2]

HYPERIMMUNOGLOBULINEMIA D SYNDROME

GENERAL PRINCIPLES

Definition

HIDS, also known as mevalonate kinase deficiency (MKD), is an autosomal recessive disorder characterized by recurrent episodes of fever, rash, abdominal pain, polyarticular arthritis, and an elevated immunoglobulin D (IgD) level.

Epidemiology

- Exact prevalence of HIDS is unknown, but it is rare.
- HIDS has been described primarily in Caucasians with origins from Western Europe, notably the Netherlands and France.[7]

Pathophysiology

- HIDS is caused by mutations in *MVK,* a gene encoding **mevalonate kinase,** an enzyme involved in both cholesterol and nonsterol isoprene biosynthesis.
- The exact mechanism of HIDS is unclear. Reduced MVK enzyme activity, possibly related to body temperature, leads to decreased downstream nonsterol isoprenoid products, which leads to a proinflammatory state with elevated IL-1, IL-6, and TNF-α.
- Reduced MVK enzyme activity also leads to elevated mevalonate levels and increased excretion (mevalonic aciduria). However, elevated levels of mevalonate may be protective because treatment with statins (an upstream inhibitor) has worsened disease and addition of downstream products (geraniol, farnesol) attenuates the inflammatory response.[10]

DIAGNOSIS

Clinical Presentation

- The first clinical episode often occurs during infancy.
- Episodes may occur twice a month during childhood but become less frequent and severe during adulthood.
- Likely triggers include **infections, trauma, surgery, stress, and vaccinations.**
- HIDS episodes often start with **headache and chills** followed by **abdominal pain, rash, polyarticular arthritis,** a **palpable tender lymphadenopathy.**
  - Abdominal pain with nausea, vomiting, and diarrhea is a common complaint. Abdominal pain can be severe enough to mimic an acute abdomen.[11]
  - A wide of variety of rashes have been described with HIDS and are nonspecific.
  - Polyarticular arthritis is typically an **inflammatory, symmetric arthritis that involves large joints like the hips and knees.**
  - Although children may get diffuse lymphadenopathy, adults tend to develop only cervical lymphadenopathy.
- Amyloidosis is a rare complication of HIDS.[11]

Diagnostic Testing

- Like other periodic fever syndromes, acute-phase reactants are elevated during attacks.
- **Elevated urinary mevalonic acid** levels during attacks but normal between episodes are suggestive of HIDS.
- Although **elevated serum levels of IgD** (>100 IU/mL) are seen in 85% of patients, levels do not correlate with severity or frequency of attacks.
- Elevated serum levels of IgA are observed in 80% of patients.

- Genetic testing for homozygous or compound heterozygous mutations in the MVK gene in a patient with clinical symptoms establishes the diagnosis. A negative analysis with positive clinical symptoms and laboratory findings may be categorized as variant HIDS because there may be unidentified mutations.[3]

TREATMENT

- Treatment is mainly supportive. Treatment should aim to alleviate current symptoms and avoid unnecessary surgery and unnecessary antibiotics if a patient experiences a typical recurrent episode.
- **Nonsteroidal anti-inflammatory drugs (NSAIDs) or glucocorticoids** can be used from the onset of each episode to reduce the severity and duration but have mixed results.[12–14]
- **IL-1 inhibitors** such as anakinra for on-demand therapy and canakinumab for prophylactic therapy can also be considered for patients who do not respond adequately to NSAIDs.[15,16]
- Colchicine is not effective. Hydroxymethylglutaryl coenzyme A (HMG-CoA) reductase inhibitors show mixed results and may risk exacerbating symptoms.[17]

TNF RECEPTOR–ASSOCIATED PERIODIC SYNDROME

GENERAL PRINCIPLES

Definition

TRAPS, previously known as familial Hibernian fever and benign autosomal dominant familial periodic fever, is an autosomal dominant disease characterized by recurrent episodes of fever, migratory rash, and ocular findings.

Epidemiology

- Prevalence is unknown but is thought to be the second most common hereditary periodic fever syndrome.
- Although TRAPS was initially described in people of Irish and Scottish descent, there is no ethnic predilection.[3]

Pathophysiology

- TRAPS is caused by mutations in *TNFRSF1A,* a gene encoding the p55 receptor for TNF. Currently, over 50 disease-causing mutations have been found.
- Initial studies suggested that pathogenesis occurred by sustained TNF stimulation of target cells by the **impaired shedding of the p55 component.** Recent data suggest that the **intracellular retention of misfolded p55** receptor may be contributing to the inflammatory response.[18]

DIAGNOSIS

Clinical Presentation

- The first clinical episode occurs during childhood or adolescence.
- **Febrile episodes** with a distinctive **migratory rash, myalgia, ocular involvement, and serositis** last anywhere from 1 to 6 weeks.
  ○ The migratory rash associated with TRAPS is distinctive. It is an erythematous macule associated with a significant amount of soft-tissue swelling and myalgias of the muscles underlying the skin. The rash typically starts on the trunk or proximal limbs and migrates distally.

- Ocular involvement seen in TRAPS consists of **periorbital edema and conjunctivitis.** Uveitis is not seen.
- Serositis can involve pleura, peritoneum, and pericardium but is typically less severe than seen in FMF.
- **Amyloidosis** occurs in up to 25% of TRAPS patients, especially patients with ongoing inflammation and frequent episodes. It is unknown whether long-term treatment prevents amyloidosis.[3]

Diagnostic Testing
- Acute-phase reactants are elevated during attacks.
- Diagnosis is confirmed by the presence of a *TNFRSF1A* mutation known to cause disease.
- Proteinuria may suggest secondary amyloidosis affecting the kidney.

TREATMENT
- **NSAIDs** can be used in mild episodes and fever. **Glucocorticoids** are used for aborting more severe attacks.[17]
- Colchicine is not effective.
- **IL-1 receptor inhibitors** such as anakinra or canakinumab for controlling and preventing flares have shown good efficacy.[9,19,20]
- Etanercept can be effective in some patients. However, other TNF inhibitors such as adalimumab and infliximab have shown poor efficacy and even worsening of episodes.[17,21]

CRYOPYRINOPATHIES

GENERAL PRINCIPLES
- CAPS constitutes rare diseases caused by autosomal dominant mutations in *NLRP3*, encoding cryopyrin.
- Cryopyrin is part of a macromolecular complex called an inflammasome, which activates an enzyme that cleaves IL-1β to its active form. Mutations result in a gain of function.
- The mutations in *NLRP3* result in **elevated IL-1β level at baseline or in response to certain triggers.**[7]
- Familial cold autoinflammatory syndrome (FCAS), Muckle–Wells syndrome, and neonatal-onset multisystem inflammatory disease (NOMID; also known as chronic infantile neurologic cutaneous and articular syndrome [CINCA]) are a spectrum of diseases caused by *NLRP3* mutations. NOMID is the most severe, and FCAS is the mildest.[22]

DIAGNOSIS
- **Familial cold autoinflammatory syndrome**
  - Symptoms typically develop in childhood.
  - Attacks occur within 2 hours of cold exposure and last 12 to 48 hours.
  - Symptoms include urticaria followed by fever, arthralgias, and conjunctivitis. Conjunctivitis and cold triggers help to distinguish from other periodic fever syndromes.

- **Muckle–Wells syndrome**
  - Symptoms develop in childhood.
  - Patients develop attacks of fever, urticaria, arthralgia, and abdominal pain. Unlike FCAS, patients do not have attacks reliably after generalized cold exposure, and triggers may not be identifiable.
  - Patients develop progressive sensorineural deafness that can be reversible with treatment.
  - Up to 25% of patients may develop systemic amyloidosis.[6]
- **Neonatal-onset multisystem inflammatory disease**
  - Febrile episodes start during infancy but then start to become more chronic than recurrent acute episodes.
  - Along with fevers, rash, and sensorineural hearing loss, patients also develop uveitis, disabling arthropathy because of overgrowth of the patella and epiphyses of long bones, chronic meningitis, and mental retardation.
  - Patients also display dysmorphic facies, such as prominent forehead, saddleback nose, and midface hypoplasia.[7]
  - Twenty percent of patients die within the first two decades.[6]
  - Patients may develop systemic amyloidosis.

TREATMENT

All the three cryopyrinopathies show a dramatic clinical and laboratory response to treatment with **IL-1 inhibitors** including anakinra (IL-1 receptor antagonist), rilonacept (IL-1 Trap, a fusion protein of the extracellular domain of the IL-1 receptor and the Fc region of IgG), and canakinumab (monoclonal antibody against IL-1β).[23–25]

PERIODIC FEVER WITH APHTHOUS STOMATITIS, PHARYNGITIS, AND ADENITIS

GENERAL PRINCIPLES

Definition

PFAPA syndrome is a recurrent fever syndrome characterized by seemingly unprovoked inflammation. The etiology is related to defects in the innate immune system. However, unlike the autoinflammatory syndromes earlier, **PFAPA does not have a known single genetic cause.**

Epidemiology

- PFAPA is considered the most common periodic fever syndrome of childhood.
- The onset of episodes typically begins **prior to age 5**, with a slight male predominance and no predilection for ethnic groups.[26]

Pathophysiology

- PFAPA is likely a complex disease of polygenic inheritance or a group of Mendelian diseases with a common phenotype. Some cohorts may suggest familial clustering, and some pedigrees suggest an autosomal dominant pattern with variable penetrance. Genetic screening has revealed several candidate genes with variants, but none predicted to be causal.[27]

- Inflammation involves the innate immune system. IL-1β, IL-6, TNF-α, and interferon gamma (IFNγ) are elevated in patients with PFAPA.[28]
- The efficacy of tonsillectomy draws attention to the role of the tonsils in immune pathogenesis. PFAPA tonsils have higher polyclonal T lymphocyte and lower B lymphocyte populations. PFAPA tonsil microbiome also shows relative differences in flora, but no common microbe to suggest an infectious cause. It is unclear whether the differences in tonsil microbiome play a causal role or are because of repeated inflammation.[26]

DIAGNOSIS

Clinical Presentation

Proposed diagnostic criteria include[29]:

- Regularly recurring fevers with an onset <5 years of age. Fevers begin abruptly with a prodrome of malaise, headache, vomiting, and last 4 days on average. The interval between febrile episodes among different patients can range from 14 to 50 days with a mean interval of 30 days, the **predictability of the interval between febrile episodes is a hallmark of the syndrome.**[30]
- Constitutional symptoms in the absence of upper respiratory infection with **aphthous stomatitis, cervical lymphadenitis, or pharyngitis**.
  - Aphthous ulcers may be limited to one to four aphthae, small, and therefore easy to miss.
  - Pharyngitis ranges from tonsillar erythema to exudative, ulcerated palatine tonsils.[30]
- Exclusion of cyclic neutropenia
- Asymptomatic intervals between episodes
- Normal growth and development

Diagnostic Testing

It is crucial that an appropriate evaluation for infection, malignancy, chronic inflammatory conditions, and malabsorption syndromes has been performed.

- There is no diagnostic test for PFAPA.
- Leukocytosis and elevated inflammatory markers (ESR, CRP) are present during attacks but normalize between episodes.
- CBC, Ig levels, rheumatoid factor, and antinuclear antibody (ANA) can be checked for assessing other potential etiologies, such as neutropenia, immunodeficiency, and autoimmune diseases.[30]

TREATMENT

- Treatment is primarily for symptom management because PFAPA is generally a self-limited disease that improves over time.
- **Prednisone** 1 to 2 mg/kg can be given for flares and resolve fever within hours. However, glucocorticoids can potentially increase the frequency of attacks.[30]
- **Cimetidine** or **colchicine** can be given as prophylaxis to decrease the frequency and severity of attacks.[30]
- **Tonsillectomy** has shown to be efficacious for patients who do not respond to medical management.[31]

REFERENCES

1. Masters SL, Simon A, Aksentijevich I, et al. Horror autoinflammaticus: the molecular pathophysiology of autoinflammatory disease. *Annu Rev Immunol.* 2009;27:621–668.
2. Ben-Chetrit E, Levy M. Familial Mediterranean fever. *Lancet.* 1998;351:659–664.
3. Drenth JP, van der Meer JW. Hereditary periodic fever. *N Engl J Med.* 2001;345:1748–1757.
4. Brasington R. How to recognize, diagnose periodic fever syndromes in adults. *The Rheumatologist* 2017. https://www.the-rheumatologist.org/article/recognize-diagnose-periodic-fever-syndromes-adults. Accessed September 1, 2018.
5. Booty MG, Chae JJ, Masters SL, et al. Familial Mediterranean fever with a single MEFV mutation: where is the second hit? *Arthritis Rheum.* 2009;60:1851–1861.
6. Goldfinger S. The inherited autoinflammatory syndrome: a decade of discovery. *Trans Am Clin Climatol Assoc.* 2009;120:413–418.
7. Rigante D, Frediani B, Cantarini L. A comprehensive overview of the hereditary periodic fever syndromes. *Clin Rev Allergy Immunol.* 2018;54:446–453.
8. van der Hilst J, Moutschen M, Messiaen PE, et al. Efficacy of anti-IL-1 treatment in familial Mediterranean fever: a systematic review of the literature. *Biologics.* 2016;10:75–80.
9. De Benedetti F, Gattorno M, Anton J, et al. Canakinumab for the treatment of autoinflammatory recurrent fever syndromes. *N Engl J Med.* 2018;378:1908–1919.
10. Houten SM, Schneiders MS, Wanders RJ, et al. Regulation of isoprenoid/cholesterol biosynthesis in cells from mevalonate kinase-deficient patients. *J Biol Chem.* 2003;278:5736–5743.
11. van der Hilst JC, Bodar EJ, Barron KS, et al. Long-term follow-up, clinical features, and quality of life in a series of 103 patients with hyperimmunoglobulinemia D syndrome. *Medicine (Baltimore).* 2008;87:301–310.
12. Picco P, Gattorno M, Di Rocco M, et al. Non-steroidal anti-inflammatory drugs in the treatment of hyper-IgD syndrome. *Ann Rheum Dis.* 2001;60:904.
13. de Dios Garcia-Diaz J, Alvarez-Blanco MJ. Glucocorticoids but not NSAID abort attacks in hyper-IgD and periodic fever syndrome. *J Rheumatol.* 2001;28:925–926.
14. Drenth JP, Haagsma CJ, van der Meer JW. Hyperimmunoglobulinemia D and periodic fever syndrome. The clinical spectrum in a series of 50 patients. International Hyper-IgD Study Group. *Medicine (Baltimore).* 1994;73:133–144.
15. Ter Haar N, Lachmann H, Ozen S, et al. Treatment of autoinflammatory diseases: results from the Eurofever Registry and a literature review. *Ann Rheum Dis.* 2013;72:678–685.
16. Galeotti C, Meinzer U, Quartier P, et al. Efficacy of interleukin-1-targeting drugs in mevalonate kinase deficiency. *Rheumatology (Oxford).* 2012;51:1855–1859.
17. ter Haar NM, Oswald M, Jeyaratnam J, et al. Recommendations for the management of autoinflammatory diseases. *Ann Rheum Dis.* 2015;74:1636–1644.
18. Kimberley FC, Lobito AA, Siegel RM, et al. Falling into TRAPS—receptor misfolding in the TNF receptor 1-associated periodic fever syndrome. *Arthritis Res Ther.* 2007;9:217.
19. Grimwood C, Despert V, Jeru I, et al. On-demand treatment with anakinra: a treatment option for selected TRAPS patients. *Rheumatology (Oxford).* 2015;54:1749–1751.
20. Gattorno M, Pelagatti MA, Meini A, et al. Persistent efficacy of anakinra in patients with tumor necrosis factor receptor-associated periodic syndrome. *Arthritis Rheum.* 2008;58:1516–1520.
21. Jacobelli S, Andre M, Alexandra JF, et al. Failure of anti-TNF therapy in TNF Receptor 1-Associated Periodic Syndrome (TRAPS). *Rheumatology (Oxford).* 2007;46:1211–1212.
22. Hoffman HM, Wanderer AA. Inflammasome and IL-1beta-mediated disorders. *Curr Allergy Asthma Rep.* 2010;10:229–235.
23. Hawkins PN, Lachmann HJ, Aganna E, et al. Spectrum of clinical features in Muckle-Wells syndrome and response to anakinra. *Arthritis Rheum.* 2004;50:607–612.
24. Lachmann HJ, Kone-Paut I, Kuemmerle-Deschner JB, et al. Use of canakinumab in the cryopyrin-associated periodic syndrome. *N Engl J Med.* 2009;360:2416–2425.
25. Hoffman HM, Throne ML, Amar NJ, et al. Efficacy and safety of rilonacept (interleukin-1 Trap) in patients with cryopyrin-associated periodic syndromes: results from two sequential placebo-controlled studies. *Arthritis Rheum.* 2008;58:2443–2452.
26. Manthiram K, Lapidus S, Edwards K. Unraveling the pathogenesis of periodic fever, aphthous stomatitis, pharyngitis, and cervical adenitis through genetic, immunologic, and microbiologic discoveries: an update. *Curr Opin Rheumatol.* 2017;29:493–499.

27. Di Gioia SA, Bedoni N, von Scheven-Gete A, et al. Analysis of the genetic basis of periodic fever with aphthous stomatitis, pharyngitis, and cervical adenitis (PFAPA) syndrome. *Sci Rep.* 2015;5:10200.

28. Stojanov S, Hoffmann F, Kery A, et al. Cytokine profile in PFAPA syndrome suggests continuous inflammation and reduced anti-inflammatory response. *Eur Cytokine Netw.* 2006;17:90–97.

29. Thomas KT, Feder HM, Jr., Lawton AR, Edwards KM. Periodic fever syndrome in children. *J Pediatr.* 1999;135:15–21.

30. Feder HM, Salazar JC. A clinical review of 105 patients with PFAPA (a periodic fever syndrome). *Acta Paediatr.* 2010;99:178–184.

31. Burton MJ, Glasziou PP, Chong LY, Venekamp RP. Tonsillectomy or adenotonsillectomy versus non-surgical treatment for chronic/recurrent acute tonsillitis. *Cochrane Database Syst Rev.* 2014:Cd001802.

IgG4-Related Disease

43

Kelvin J. Lee and Deborah L. Parks

GENERAL PRINCIPLES

Definition

- Immunoglobulin (Ig)G4-related disease is an increasingly recognized fibroinflammatory condition comprising a collection of disorders that share common histopathologic features. The multiorgan nature of this disease entity did not appear in medical literature until 2003.[1] It now links many conditions once regarded as isolated, single-organ diseases (e.g., Mikulicz's syndrome, Küttner's tumor, and Riedel's thyroiditis) as part of the systemic disease spectrum.
- The disease is characterized by tumefactive lesions, a dense lymphoplasmacytic infiltrate rich in IgG4-positive plasma cells, storiform fibrosis, and often, but not always, elevated serum IgG4 concentrations.[2]
- IgG4-related disease has been described in virtually every organ system. Often, more than one organ is affected. Major presentations include type 1 autoimmune pancreatitis, salivary gland disease, orbital disease, and retroperitoneal fibrosis.

Epidemiology

- IgG4-related disease generally has a slight predominance for middle-aged and older males. The predilection for older males has been reported for disease involving the pancreas,[3] kidney,[4] and retroperitoneum.[5] This male predominance contrasts starkly with other autoimmune diseases that mimic IgG4-related disease, such as Sjögren's syndrome and primary biliary cirrhosis, which have markedly female predominance.
- Similar male predilection was not seen in disease involving organs of the head and neck, however. The reasons for this difference are unclear.[6]
- Overall, the disease epidemiology is not well understood. The prevalence of organ manifestations is also unclear. Study of the various conditions was initially hampered by lack of knowledge about IgG4-related disease.

Pathophysiology

- The pathogenesis of IgG4-related disease is poorly understood; findings consistent with both an autoimmune disorder and an allergic disorder are present. The physiologic role of IgG4 is also not well understood. A specific autoantigenic target has not been identified, and it is not clear that the IgG4 antibodies are pathogenic. Moreover, elevations in serum and tissue IgG4 concentrations are not specific to IgG4-related disease.[7]
- An emerging hypothesis suggests CD4+ cytotoxic T cells as the main orchestrators of disease.[8] These cells elaborate interleukin (IL)-1, transforming growth factor beta (TGF-β), and interferon-γ—important mediators of the fibrosis characteristic of IgG4-related disease. It is believed that these cells are sustained by continuous antigen presentation by B cells and plasmablasts. A separate T-follicular helper cell response is thought to be responsible for the development of germinal centers and the production of cytokines (e.g., IL-4) that drive the IgG4 class switch, culminating in the creation of IgG4-secreting plasmablasts and long-lived plasma cells. This would explain why current B-cell depletion therapy often doesn't lead to complete normalization of serum IgG4 concentrations even after clinical remission.[9]

DIAGNOSIS

Clinical Presentation

- IgG4-related disease usually presents subacutely, and most patients are not constitutionally ill. Involvement of virtually every organ system has been described.[10] Multiple organs are affected in 60% to 90% of patients, and the disease can often cause major tissue damage. The disorder is often recognized incidentally through a radiologic finding or histopathologic examination of a tissue specimen.
- Two common findings in IgG4-related disease are tumefactive lesions and allergic disease.[10] Symptoms of asthma or allergy are present in approximately 40% of patients.
- The major organ manifestations are summarized as follows:
- **Lymphadenopathy**
  - Asymptomatic lymphadenopathy is common in IgG4-related disease. It is usually observed together with other clinical or laboratory manifestations of the syndrome but may be the initial or only manifestation.
  - Multiple groups of lymph nodes are usually involved—mediastinal, hilar, intraabdominal, and axillary being the most common.
  - Individual nodes are typically no more than a few centimeters in diameter, and symptoms occasionally occur due to mass effect of the enlarging nodes. The lymphadenopathy is generally rubbery and nontender.
- **Autoimmune pancreatitis**
  - Type 1 autoimmune pancreatitis, also denoted as lymphoplasmacytic sclerosing pancreatitis, was the first manifestation recognized to be associated with high serum IgG4 concentrations. It often presents as a pancreatic mass or as a painless obstructive jaundice that can be mistaken for pancreatic cancer.
  - Most patients have another concomitant IgG4-related condition, such as lymphadenopathy or salivary/lacrimal gland involvement.
- **Sclerosing cholangitis**
  - IgG4-related sclerosing cholangitis commonly accompanies type 1 autoimmune pancreatitis.[11] It rarely occurs in the absence of pancreatitis. It is thought to be clinically distinct from primary sclerosing cholangitis, which carries a drastically different prognosis.
  - Patients may present with obstructive jaundice, pancreatic enlargement, and lymphadenopathy.
- **Salivary and lacrimal gland involvement**
  - Major salivary gland (parotid and submandibular) involvement is a common feature of IgG4-related disease.
  - Patients may present with prominent parotid and lacrimal gland enlargement, which was historically called Mikulicz's disease. Patients may also present with submandibular gland enlargement, which was previously called Küttner's tumor or sclerosing sialadenitis.[12] Bilateral involvement is typical, even though the two glands may be clinically asynchronous at disease onset.
  - Despite marked lacrimal and salivary gland enlargement, these patients experience relatively mild dryness of the eyes and of the mouth, a feature that may help differentiate from Sjögren's syndrome.
- **Retroperitoneal fibrosis** is one of the most commonly encountered manifestations of IgG4-related disease. Chronic inflammatory and fibrotic change can involve regional tissues, such as the ureters (leading to obstructive uropathy), infrarenal aorta, and iliac arteries.[13]
- **Aortitis and periaortitis:** Inflammation affecting the thoracic and/or abdominal aortic wall is a well-recognized manifestation of IgG4-related disease. Patients may present with aneurysms and aortic dissections; those with abdominal aortitis can have associated retroperitoneal fibrosis.[13]

- **Ophthalmic disease:** The typical ophthalmic presentation of IgG4-related disease involves swelling within the ocular region or frank proptosis. These patients develop orbital inflammation/pseudotumors or orbital myositis.[14]
- **Renal disease**
  - Patients with renal disease often have involvement of other organs. The most common renal abnormality is tubulointerstitial nephritis; IgG4-related membranous nephropathy is much less common.
  - Clinically, patients may present with urinary abnormalities (proteinuria), renal dysfunction, and/or imaging abnormalities, including nodular parenchymal lesions mimicking renal cell carcinoma.[15]
- **Thyroid disease:** IgG4-related thyroid involvement is infiltrative. Two forms have been described and pathologically linked: Riedel's thyroiditis[16] and the fibrous variant of Hashimoto thyroiditis.[17]
- **Others**
  - IgG4-related disease rarely affects the brain parenchyma but is one of the most common causes of hypertrophic pachymeningitis.[18]
  - Lung involvement has the greatest diversity of clinical and radiologic presentations and includes thickening of the bronchovascular bundle, pulmonary nodules, ground-glass opacities, pleural thickening, and interstitial lung disease.[19]

Diagnostic Criteria

- Tissue biopsy and histopathologic analysis remain the cornerstone in the diagnosis of IgG4-related disease. Elevated concentrations of IgG4 in tissue and serum are helpful but are neither specific nor diagnostic for this disease.
- Key morphologic features include a dense lymphoplasmacytic tissue infiltration of mainly IgG4-positive plasma cells and lymphocytes, accompanied by fibrosis that is organized in a storiform pattern, with obliterative phlebitis and a modest tissue eosinophilia. These histopathologic and immunohistochemical staining features are strikingly similar across different tissues, regardless of the organ or tissue involved.[10]
- The number of IgG4-positive plasma cells per high-power field (HPF) that is regarded as consistent with or suggestive of IgG4-related disease varies somewhat from tissue to tissue. Tissue IgG4-positive cell counts and the ratios of IgG4- to IgG-positive cells are considered secondary in importance to the histopathologic appearance of the tissue and should be correlated carefully.

Differential Diagnosis

The differential diagnosis for IgG4-related disease is broad and depends on the specific site of involvement and clinical presentation.

Diagnostic Testing

The diagnosis of IgG4-related disease requires characteristic findings upon biopsy of affected tissue, but additional organ involvement may be possible to identify through a comprehensive history, physical examination, routine laboratory testing, and selected imaging studies.

Laboratories

- Complete blood count (CBC) with differential, comprehensive metabolic panel (CMP), erythrocyte sedimentation rate (ESR), C-reactive protein (CRP), and urinalysis (UA) provide useful information and should be obtained in patients being considered for IgG4-related disease.
- Serum IgG4 levels should also be measured but the degree of elevation correlates imperfectly with disease activity. Serum levels tend to increase with the number of organs involved and usually decreases after treatment with glucocorticoids. Again, it should

be emphasized that increased serum levels are insufficient to establish a diagnosis of IgG4-related disease.

- Complement (C3 and C4) levels can be beneficial in patients with renal disease because those with IgG4-related tubulointerstitial nephritis are likely to be profoundly hypocomplementemic.[15]
- Markers of allergic disease such as serum IgE concentrations and the peripheral eosinophil count should be tested at baseline and monitored if abnormal.[10]
- Blood plasmablast concentration measurements, particularly those for IgG4+ plasmablasts,[20] are not widely available.

Imaging
- Computed tomography (CT) scan of the chest, abdomen, and pelvis performed at baseline is helpful for establishing the extent of disease as well as subclinical disease.
- Positron emission tomographic (PET) scanning is also useful for determining the extent of disease.
- Selected patients require additional imaging studies depending on their symptom complex.
- Characteristic imaging findings of IgG4-related disease are generally nonspecific and do not reliably distinguish from other conditions but include diffuse and focal organ infiltration and encasement by inflammatory and fibrotic tissue.

Diagnostic Procedures
As mentioned, tissue biopsy should be performed to confirm diagnosis, especially when a discrete mass is present. A core needle biopsy is preferred over fine-needle aspirates (FNAs) because FNAs do not provide adequate tissue.

TREATMENT

- The optimal treatment for IgG4-related disease has not been established. No randomized treatment trials have been conducted, but there are observational data and open-label trials to help guide therapy.
- Not all manifestations of the disease require immediate treatment. For example, IgG4-related lymphadenopathy is often asymptomatic and indolent; watchful waiting is appropriate in this case. In contrast, patients who are symptomatic from their organ involvement often benefit from treatment. Also, when vital organs are involved, aggressive treatment is needed because the disease can lead to serious organ dysfunction and failure.
- Most patients respond to glucocorticoids and this is typically the first-line agent for remission induction, usually at a dose ≥ 0.6 mg/kg/day.[10] A response is frequently seen within several weeks and it is reasonable to initiate tapering once a significant response is established. There is, however, disagreement among experts on using combination therapy (glucocorticoids and a steroid-sparing immunosuppressive agent) at the start of treatment, plus most patients experience disease flares during or after steroid tapering.
- A growing number of reports support the efficacy of B-cell depletion with rituximab (1 g intravenously [IV] every 15 days for a total of two doses). It has been shown to be effective as both induction and maintenance treatment, as well as in patients with disease refractory to glucocorticoids and other medications.[21]
- XmAb5871 is a novel anti-CD19 agent that is being investigated in IgG4-related disease.[22]
- There is one case report of successful treatment with abatacept.[23]
- Azathioprine, mycophenolate mofetil, and methotrexate have also been used, but rigorous assessment of these treatments is needed.[10]

MONITORING

- The serum IgG4 concentration usually decreases after treatment with glucocorticoids. B-cell depletion also often leads to swift, targeted reduction of serum IgG4 concentrations relative to other subclasses.
- The utility of PET in monitoring disease activity and response to treatment is not clear.
- In patients with tubulointerstitial nephritis secondary to IgG4-related disease, following serum complement levels can be useful in gauging response to treatment.

PROGNOSIS

- The natural history and prognosis of IgG4-related disease have not been well-defined. Spontaneous improvement can be seen, but the disease often recurs without treatment. Significant organ dysfunction may arise from uncontrolled and progressive inflammatory and fibrotic changes in affected tissues.
- Patients with advanced fibrotic changes may respond poorly to treatment.
- A possible increased risk of malignancy associated with IgG4-related disease is controversial and requires further study.

REFERENCES

1. Kamisawa T, Funata N, Hayashi Y, et al. A new clinicopathological entity of IgG4-related autoimmune disease. *J Gastroenterol.* 2003;38:982–984.
2. Stone JH, Zen Y, Deshpande V. IgG4-related disease. *N Engl J Med.* 2012;366:539–551.
3. Kanno A, Masamune A, Okazaki K, et al. Nationwide epidemiological survey of autoimmune pancreatitis in Japan in 2011. *Pancreas.* 2015;44:535–539.
4. Raissian Y, Nasr SH, Larsen CP, et al. Diagnosis of IgG4-related tubulointerstitial nephritis. *J Am Soc Nephrol.* 2011;22:1343–1352.
5. Zen Y, Onodera M, Inoue D, et al. Retroperitoneal fibrosis: a clinicopathologic study with respect to immunoglobulin G4. *Am J Surg Pathol.* 2009;33:1833–1839.
6. Zen Y, Nakanuma Y. IgG4-related disease: a cross-sectional study of 114 cases. *Am J Surg Pathol.* 2010;34:1812–1819.
7. Strehl JD, Hartmann A, Agaimy A. Numerous IgG4-positive plasma cells are ubiquitous in diverse localized non-specific chronic inflammatory conditions and need to be distinguished from IgG4-related systemic disorders. *J Clin Pathol.* 2011;64:237–243.
8. Mattoo H, Mahajan VS, Maehara T, et al. Clonal expansion of CD4(+) cytotoxic T lymphocytes in patients with IgG4-related disease. *J Allergy Clin Immunol.* 2016;138:825–838.
9. Perugino CA, Mattoo H, Mahajan VS, et al. Emerging treatment models in rheumatology: IgG4-related disease: insights into human immunology and targeted therapies. *Arthritis Rheumatol.* 2017;69(9):1722–1732.
10. Kamisawa T, Zen Y, Pillai S, et al. IgG4-related disease. *Lancet.* 2015;385:1460–1471.
11. Hamano H, Arakura N, Muraki T, et al. Prevalence and distribution of extrapancreatic lesions complicating autoimmune pancreatitis. *J Gastroenterol.* 2006;41:1197–1205.
12. Geyer JT, Deshpande V. IgG4-associated sialadenitis. *Curr Opin Rheumatol.* 2011;23:95–101.
13. Stone JR. Aortitis, periaortitis, and retroperitoneal fibrosis, as manifestations of IgG4-related systemic disease. *Curr Opin Rheumatol.* 2011;23:88–94.
14. Wallace ZS, Deshpande V, Stone JH. Ophthalmic manifestations of IgG4-related disease: single-center experience and literature review. *Semin Arthritis Rheum.* 2013;43:806–817.
15. Saeki T, Nishi S, Imai N, et al. Clinicopathological characteristics of patients with IgG4-related tubulointerstitial nephritis. *Kidney Int.* 2010;78:1016–1023.
16. Dahlgren M, Khosroshahi A, Nielsen GP, et al. Riedel's thyroiditis and multifocal fibrosclerosis are part of the IgG4-related systemic disease spectrum. *Arthritis Care Res (Hoboken).* 2010;62:1312–1318.
17. Deshpande V, Huck A, Ooi E, et al. Fibrosing variant of Hashimoto thyroiditis is an IgG4-related disease. *J Clin Pathol.* 2012;65:725–728.

18. Wallace ZS, Carruthers MN, Khosroshahi A, et al. IgG4-related disease and hypertrophic pachymeningitis. *Medicine (Baltimore)*. 2013;92:206–216.

19. Inoue D, Zen Y, Gabata T, et al. Immunoglobulin G4-related lung disease: CT findings and pathologic correlations. *Radiology*. 2009;251:260–270.

20. Wallace ZS, Mattoo H, Carruthers M, et al. Plasmablasts as a biomarker for IgG4-related disease, independent of serum IgG4 concentrations. *Ann Rheum Dis*. 2015;74:190–195.

21. Carruthers MN, Topazian MD, Khosroshahi A, et al. Rituximab for IgG4-related disease: a prospective, open-label trial. *Ann Rheum Dis*. 2015;74:1171–1177.

22. Stone JH, Wallace ZS, Perugino CA, et al. A trial of XmAbVR 5871, a reversible inhibitor of CD191 cells, in IgG4-related disease [abstract]. *Arthritis Rheumatol*. 2016;68 Suppl 10. http://acrabstracts.org/abstract/a-trial-of-xmab5871-a-reversible-inhibitor-of-cd19-cellsin-igg4-related-disease/.

23. Yamamoto M, Takahashi H, Takano K, et al. Efficacy of abatacept for IgG4-related disease over 8 months. *Ann Rheum Dis*. 2016;75:1576–1578.

Antiphospholipid Syndrome

44

Iris Lee and Deepali Sen

GENERAL PRINCIPLES

Definition

Antiphospholipid syndrome (APS) is a **hypercoagulable disorder** manifested by recurrent arterial and venous thromboses and adverse outcomes in pregnancy that is associated with antiphospholipid (aPL) antibodies.

Classification

- APS may occur as a primary autoimmune condition or in association with another systemic disease (e.g., systemic lupus erythematosus [SLE]).
- **Catastrophic APS** is a variant of APS characterized by widespread thrombotic disease resulting in multiorgan failure and has a high mortality rate.

Epidemiology

- Although aPLs occur in 1% to 5% of the general population, the prevalence of primary APS is thought to be 40 to 50 cases per 100,000 individuals.[1]
- In patients with SLE, 10% to 44% will develop aPLs, and of those, about half will eventually develop secondary APS. Among patients with APS, 37% have SLE.[2] Catastrophic APS occurs in less than 1% of patients with APS.
- Cardiovascular risk factors such as smoking and estrogen use increase the risk of thrombosis in APS.
- About 13% of individuals with stroke, ~11% of individuals with myocardial infarction and ~9.5% of individuals with deep vein thrombosis are positive for aPL antibodies.[1]

Pathophysiology

- The pathophysiology of APS is poorly understood, although aPLs are implicated in the disorder.
- aPLs are not by themselves sufficient to incite thrombosis but require a trigger to tip the hemostatic balance toward thrombosis (infection, inflammation, trauma, etc.)—the two-hit hypothesis.
- There may be associations with HLA-DR4 and HLA-DRw53.
- aPLs affect coagulation and thrombosis through a variety of mechanisms.[3–5]
  - These antibodies may bind platelets, upregulating production of thromboxane A2 and expression of glycoprotein IIb/IIIa; endothelial cells and monocytes, increasing production of tissue factors; or endothelial cells, increasing expression of adhesion molecules. These interactions favor thrombosis.
  - aPLs also activate complement, which can initiate an inflammatory cascade, resulting in thrombosis. Complement activation has also been linked to fetal loss in APS.
  - Some authors propose that coagulation may result from disruption of proteins that regulate thrombosis, such as protein C, by aPL. Also, antibodies against β2-glycoprotein I (β2-gpI), a naturally occurring anticoagulant, may induce a prothrombotic state.[1,4]

- The mechanism of pregnancy complications is different in early and late pregnancy. aPLs in early pregnancy are thought to have a direct inhibitory effect on the proliferation of trophoblast cells. Late complications are caused by impaired remodeling of the spiral arteries, reduced proliferation and invasion of the extravillous trophoblasts, and inflammation at the maternal–fetal interface.

Associated Conditions

- Secondary APS has been associated with various rheumatologic conditions, most commonly SLE, but also Sjögren's syndrome, rheumatoid arthritis, scleroderma, and systemic vasculitis.
- aPL in the absence of APS can be induced by infections, neoplasms, medications, and other diseases. These aPL are usually immunoglobulin (Ig)M antibodies at low titers and are usually transient and rarely associated with thrombosis.

DIAGNOSIS

- APS should be suspected in patients presenting with **venous or arterial thromboembolism** (deep venous thrombosis or pulmonary embolism, stroke, myocardial infarction, etc.) or **pregnancy complications** (miscarriage, preeclampsia, or placental insufficiency).
- Consider APS when a patient has unexplained or recurrent thromboses or thrombotic events at **unusual sites** (e.g., adrenal veins), when thrombosis occurs in **young patients,** and when recurrent pregnancy losses occur in the **second and third trimesters.**

Clinical Presentation

- Clinical presentation of APS varies on the basis of the affected blood vessel. Patients typically present in one of three ways:
  - Venous thrombosis
  - Arterial thrombosis
  - Pregnancy loss
- Other manifestations commonly include livedo reticularis (20%), thrombocytopenia (22%), and transient ischemic attack/stroke (13%), but many organs can be affected (Table 44-1).
- Definitive **catastrophic APS presents** with (1) involvement of **more than three organs** (2) within **1 week** as a result of multiple-vessel occlusion; (3) histopathology confirms small-vessel occlusion in at least one organ or tissue; and (4) laboratory tests show presence of aPL. The mortality rate is high (30%–50%).

Diagnostic Criteria

- The updated International Consensus Statement on classification criteria for definite APS states that the diagnosis of APS should be considered when at least one clinical criterion and one lab criterion are met (Table 44-2).[6]
- The clinical criteria include vascular thrombosis and pregnancy morbidity, and the laboratory criteria include the presence of anticardiolipin antibody (aCL), anti–β2-gpI antibody, or lupus anticoagulant (LA).

Differential Diagnosis

- Diagnoses of **other prothrombotic conditions** must be entertained: protein C or S deficiency, antithrombin III deficiency, factor V Leiden mutation, dysfibrinogenemias, hyperhomocysteinuria, malignancies, thrombotic thrombocytopenic purpura, heparin-induced thrombocytopenia, nephrotic syndrome, severe diabetes, paroxysmal nocturnal hemoglobinuria, pregnancy, smoking, estrogen therapy, and immobility.

TABLE 44-1	CLINICAL MANIFESTATIONS OF ANTIPHOSPHOLIPID SYNDROME

Cardiovascular: Myocardial infarction, angina, premature atherosclerotic valvular lesions, pseudoinfective endocarditis, intracardiac thrombosis
Dermatologic: Livedo reticularis, splinter hemorrhages, skin infarcts, leg ulcers, superficial thrombophlebitis, blue toe syndrome, Raynaud's phenomenon, necrotizing purpura
Endocrine: Adrenal insufficiency
Gastrointestinal: Hepatic infarction, Budd–Chiari syndrome
Hematologic: Thrombocytopenia, leukopenia, hemolytic anemia, positive Coombs test
Musculoskeletal: Deep venous thrombosis, avascular necrosis
Neurologic: Cerebrovascular accidents, transient ischemic attacks, migraines, chorea, multi-infarct dementia, pseudotumor cerebri, peripheral neuropathy, myasthenia gravis, seizures, transverse myelopathy
Obstetric: Eclampsia/preeclampsia; intrauterine growth retardation; hemolysis, elevated liver enzymes, and low platelet count (HELLP) syndrome; oligohydramnios; chorea gravidarum; postpartum syndrome
Pulmonary: Pulmonary embolus, nonthromboembolic pulmonary hypertension
Renal: Renal artery/vein thrombosis, hypertension, glomerular thrombosis, renal insufficiency

- aPLs can also be found in the general population, those with lymphoproliferative disorders, viral infections (e.g., human immunodeficiency virus [HIV]), or malignancies. These individuals may not necessarily have APS.

Diagnostic Testing
- Three types of assays are available to detect aPL.
  - LA is a misnomer; it was characterized by in vitro prolongation of clotting, but it confers a hypercoagulable state in vivo. It is not a specific analyte but a lab phenomenon, which may be found in conditions other than SLE (see Chapter 5). Assays for LA include the **dilute Russell viper venom time, activated partial thromboplastin time (aPTT), kaolin clotting time, and tissue thromboplastin inhibition;** none has a >70% sensitivity to detect all LA antibodies. Mixing normal platelet-poor plasma with the patient's plasma will not correct an LA-associated prolonged aPTT, but addition of excess phospholipids will.
  - aCL and anti–β2-gpI are measured by enzyme-linked immunosorbent assay (ELISA) and reported by isotypes (IgG, IgA, IgM) and titers. IgG and IgM antibodies are clinically significant at high titer (>99th percentile) and have high specificity for the diagnosis of APS.
- The diagnostic criteria require the presence of LA or medium- to high-titer aCL antibodies or high-titer anti–β2-gpI antibodies to be present on at least two occasions, at least 12 weeks apart.
- aPLs can cause **false-positive syphilis serology.**
- Although aPLs can be found in healthy individuals, **triple positivity** of these antibodies is associated with recurrence of thrombosis as well as first thrombosis.
- Other lab tests to consider in the evaluation of the patient include complete blood count (CBC) and blood chemistries, to evaluate for renal and liver dysfunction. Radiologic studies (computed tomography [CT]/magnetic resonance imaging [MRI]) are helpful to assess damage and guide management.

TABLE 44-2	REVISED CLASSIFICATION CRITERIA FOR DIAGNOSIS OF ANTIPHOSPHOLIPID SYNDROME

Definite antiphospholipid syndrome is considered to be present if at least one of the following clinical criteria and one of the laboratory criteria are met.[a]

Clinical criteria:
- **Vascular thrombosis:** ≥1 clinical episodes of venous, arterial, or small-vessel thrombosis (except superficial venous thrombosis) in any tissue or organ, which must be confirmed by imaging or by histopathology. For histopathologic confirmation, thrombosis should be present without significant evidence of inflammation in the vessel wall.

Pregnancy morbidity:
- ≥1 unexplained deaths of a morphologically normal fetus at or beyond the 10th week of gestation, with normal fetal morphology documented by ultrasound or by direct examination of the fetus, or
- ≥1 premature births of a morphologically normal neonate at or before the 34th week of gestation because of severe preeclampsia or eclampsia or severe placental insufficiency, or
- ≥3 unexplained consecutive spontaneous abortions before the 10th week of gestation, with maternal anatomic or hormonal abnormalities and paternal and maternal chromosomal causes excluded.

Laboratory criteria:
- **Lupus anticoagulant** present in plasma, on ≥2 occasions at least 12 weeks apart, detected according to the guidelines of the International Society on Thrombosis and Haemostasis.
- **Anticardiolipin antibody** (IgG and/or IgM) in blood, present in medium or high titer, on ≥2 occasions, at least 12 weeks apart, measured by a standardized enzyme-linked immunosorbent assay.
- **Anti–β2-glycoprotein I antibody** (IgG and/or IgM) in blood, present in titer >99th percentile, on ≥2 occasions, at least 12 weeks apart, measured by a standardized enzyme-linked immunosorbent assay.

[a]Classification of APS should be avoided if the positive aPL test and clinical manifestation are separated by less than 12 weeks or more than 5 months.

aPL, antiphospholipid; APS, antiphospholipid syndrome; Ig, immunoglobulin.

Adapted from: Miyakis S, Lockshin MD, Atsumi T, et al. International consensus statement on an update of the classification criteria for definite antiphospholipid syndrome (APS). *J Thromb Haemost.* 2006;4:295–306.

TREATMENT

Prevention of thrombosis is a major goal of therapy in patients with aPL antibodies. Therapy is divided into two clinical settings: primary prophylaxis (aPL carriers without previous thrombosis) and secondary prophylaxis (patients with APS who have already had a thrombotic event).

Medications
- **Primary prophylaxis**
  - Primary prophylaxis can be considered in purely asymptomatic individuals (who had testing done for unclear reasons), patients with SLE, or women with obstetric APS.

- ○ Healthy patients with high aPL titers but no manifestation of thromboses may be advised to take low-dose aspirin (LDA) as prophylaxis based on cardiac risk factors and risk of thrombosis (i.e., immobility). Lifestyle modification is important, as discussed later.
- ○ Current European League Against Rheumatism (EULAR) guidelines recommend LDA in patients with SLE and aPLs because it has a protective effect in this population.[7,8]
- ○ On the basis of data from animal models and indirect evidence from human studies, hydroxychloroquine has been found to be protective against future thrombosis in SLE; more studies are needed to determine whether this should be recommended for healthy patients with aPLs.
- **Secondary prophylaxis**
  - ○ For patients with documented thrombotic events, long-term intensive anticoagulation is recommended on the basis of the type of thrombotic event.
  - ○ **Venous event: Heparin (unfractionated [UFH] or low-molecular-weight [LMWH]) followed by warfarin** with a goal international normalized ratio (INR) of 2.5 (range 2.0–3.0) is the treatment of choice for patients presenting with a first venous event.[2,3]
    - ▪ The optimal duration of anticoagulation for prevention of recurrent thrombosis is unknown, but the risk of recurrence appears to be highest in the 6-month period after discontinuing anticoagulant drugs. To date, **the general consensus is to treat indefinitely with anticoagulation.**[3] However, if the thrombosis was clearly provoked, the risks and benefits of stopping after 3 to 6 months can be discussed with the patient.
    - ▪ **Recurrent venous thrombosis** has been reported from 3% to 24% per year. If recurrent thrombosis occurs despite adequate anticoagulation, high-intensity anticoagulation with INR goal range 3.0 to 4.0 or switching to LMWH may be recommended. Some experts recommend the addition of LDA, hydroxychloroquine, and/or statin.[10]
    - ▪ **Direct oral anticoagulants are currently not standard of care;** however, current studies are ongoing. In addition to their anticoagulant effect, they appear to decrease complement activation.
  - ○ **Arterial events** most commonly involve the cerebral circulation (i.e., transient ischemic attack, stroke) and less commonly myocardial infarction or other arterial thrombosis. Evidence for treatment of these groups is controversial and lacks prospective randomized controlled trials. Current therapy includes warfarin therapy at moderate dose (goal INR 2.0–3.0) with LDA or high (goal INR 3.0–4.0) dose.[1,3] In older adults with low aPL titers, LDA may be appropriate.
  - ○ **Pregnancy morbidity prevention:** The optimal treatment of pregnant women with aPL and recurrent fetal loss without thrombosis is controversial. Treatment depends on the clinical manifestations of obstetric APS and includes LDA with or without heparin.[9]
    - ▪ **LDA** should be started when attempting conception.
    - ▪ **UFH or LMWH** can be administered as prophylactic (if no prior history of thrombosis) or therapeutic (if history of thrombosis) doses.
    - ▪ **All postpartum women should receive LMWH prophylaxis** for 1 to 6 weeks postpartum with transition to warfarin in women who have thrombotic APS.
    - ▪ Historically, pregnant patients were treated with prednisone, but because of significant side effects of hyperglycemia, preeclampsia, diabetes, and infection, as well as lack of compelling benefit, this is no longer recommended.
  - ○ **Catastrophic APS:** This requires early diagnosis and treatment. Combination therapy includes the following[10,11]:
    - ▪ Treatment of precipitating factors (e.g., infection, underlying SLE flare).
    - ▪ Effective anticoagulation with intravenous (IV) **heparin** followed by oral anticoagulation.

- **High-dose steroids** (methylprednisolone 500–1,000 mg IV daily) for 3 or more days followed by oral or parenteral therapy at 1 mg/kg prednisone equivalents.
- **Plasma exchange** and/or **IV immunoglobulin** (400 mg/kg body weight daily for 4–5 days). Of note, thrombosis with intravenous immunoglobulin use has been reported, so it needs to be cautiously given, especially when delivered rapidly or when anticoagulation needs to be interrupted.
- If ineffective, alternative therapies for catastrophic APS with reported success include cyclophosphamide (in patients with SLE, not patients with primary APS), rituximab (in patients with thrombocytopenia or autoimmune hemolytic anemia), and eculizumab.

Lifestyle/Risk Modification

Lifestyle modifications are recommended in both patients with APS and patients with asymptomatic aPL. This includes **smoking cessation, avoidance of supplemental estrogens, and controlling hypertension and diabetes.**

REFERENCES

1. Schreiber K, Sciascia S, de Groot PG, et al. Antiphospholipid syndrome. *Nat Rev Dis Primers.* 2018. 4:1–19.
2. Cohen D, Berger SP, Steup-Beekman GM, et al. Diagnosis and management of the antiphospholipid syndrome. *BMJ.* 2010;340:1125–1132.
3. Ruiz-Irastorza G, Crowther M, Branch W, et al. Antiphospholipid syndrome. *Lancet.* 2010;376:1498–1509.
4. Matsuura E, Shen L, Matsunami Y, et al. Pathophysiology of B2-glycoprotein I in antiphospholipid syndrome. *Lupus.* 2010;19:379–384.
5. Chen PP, Giles I. Antibodies to serine proteases in the antiphospholipid syndrome. *Curr Rheumatol Rep.* 2010;12:45–52.
6. Miyakis S, Lockshin MD, Atsumi T, et al. International consensus statement on an update of the classification criteria for definite antiphospholipid syndrome (APS). *J Thromb Haemost.* 2006;4:295–306.
7. Hereng T, Lambert M, Hachulla E, et al. Influence of aspirin on the clinical outcomes of 103 anti-phospholipid antibodies-positive patients. *Lupus.* 2008;17:11–15.
8. Erkan D, Harrison MJ, Levy R, et al. Aspirin for primary thrombosis prevention in the antiphospholipid syndrome: a randomized double-blind, placebo-controlled trial in asymptomatic antiphospholipid antibody-positive individuals. *Arthritis Rheum.* 2007;56:2382–2391.
9. Schreiber K, Hunt BJ. Pregnancy and antiphospholipid syndrome. *Semin Thromb Hemost.* 2016;42(7):780–788.
10. Cervera R. Update on the diagnosis, treatment, and prognosis of the catastrophic antiphospholipid syndrome. *Curr Rheumatol Rep.* 2010;12:70–76.
11. Kazzaz NM, McCune WJ, Knight JS. Treatment of catastrophic antiphospholipid syndrome. *Curr Opin Rheumatol.* 2016;28(3):218–227.

Thromboangiitis Obliterans

45

Roseanne F. Zhao and Jonathan J. Miner

GENERAL PRINCIPLES

- **Thromboangiitis obliterans** (TAO), or **Buerger's disease**, is a chronic, recurring inflammatory occlusive disease of medium- and small-sized vessels in the upper and lower extremities, **associated with tobacco use.**
- It was first described by Hans von Winiwarter[1] in 1879 and subsequently described histologically by Leo Buerger[2] in 1908.
- It is characterized by **segmental, nonatherosclerotic, thrombotic vessel stenosis and occlusion** with **subsequent limb ischemia and necrosis or thrombophlebitis.**

Epidemiology

- TAO tends to affect **male smokers younger than 40 years of age.**
- Incidence in women (previously thought to be <2%) has increased to 11% to 30%.[3,4]
- Prevalence is difficult to determine accurately because of a lack of uniform diagnostic criteria.
- It is seen with **higher frequencies in Middle East and Asian countries**, including Israel, Nepal, India, and Japan.
- The prevalence of TAO in the United States has decreased, in part because of a decline in smoking.[5] Rates documented at Mayo Clinic decreased from 104 cases per 100,000 in 1947 to approximately 12.6 cases per 100,000 in 1986.
- TAO constitutes a higher proportion of peripheral arterial disease (PAD) in countries where atherosclerosis is less common.[6]
- The prevalence of PAD is as low as 0.5% to 5.6% in Western Europe and the United States.
  - Approximately 16% to 66% in Japan and Korea, and 45% to 63% in India
  - Highest in Jews of Ashkenazi descent, representing 80% of all cases of PAD
- Recent observations cast suspicion on arsenic, suggesting a closer correlation between disease prevalence and the risk of arsenic poisoning.[7]

Pathophysiology

- The exact etiology of TAO is unknown but is strongly associated with tobacco use. Disease exacerbation is seen in patients who resume use, even years later.
- Histopathology reveals **cellular, inflammatory thrombus occluding the lumen, with initial sparing of the blood vessel wall.** This is distinct from other common vasculitides that show inflammatory changes starting in the adventitia of the vessel wall and progressing inward toward the lumen. TAO may be pathologically divided into three phases:
  - **Acute:** Occlusive highly cellular inflammatory thrombi with fibrovascular granulation tissue in distal limb arteries or veins composed of polymorphonuclear leukocytes, microabscesses, mononuclear cells, and multinucleated giant cells. The internal elastic lamina is intact but may be infiltrated by macrophages, T cells, and few B cells.[8] The media is structurally normal. Dendritic cells are found in the intima, along with media and adventitia to a lesser extent.

- ○ **Subacute:** Progressive organization of thrombus with relative preservation of the vessel wall
- ○ **Chronic:** Organized thrombus and vascular fibrosis are now prominent, without inflammatory infiltrate. At this stage, the histopathology is nonspecific and resembles other types of vascular occlusive disease.
- The inflammatory disease process is not well understood.[9,10]
- Nicotine and other components of tobacco (including known carcinogens and toxins such as arsenic) alter innate and adaptive immunity, and can cause direct toxicity to endothelium.
- TAO patients have increased cellular and humoral immunity to Type I and III collagens (constituents of blood vessels), as well as Type IV collagen, elastin, and laminin.[11,12]
- Autoantibodies against endothelial cells, collagen, and elastin[13,14] may form immune complexes, fix complement, and deposit in vessels.[15]
- Endothelial injury and activation promote the recruitment of inflammatory cells. Vascular dysfunction, including impaired endothelium-dependent vasodilation,[16] is thought to be an initiating factor in pathogenesis.
- Increased production of various proinflammatory cytokines is seen.[10,17,18]
- Prothrombotic factors, such as the prothrombin gene mutation G20210A and anticardiolipin antibodies, are associated with increased risk[19] in the setting of an inflammatory trigger, such as tobacco use.

Risk Factors

- **Smoking,** especially heavy smokers (>1.5 packs per day) and those who use raw tobacco
- Can also be seen in patients who use smokeless tobacco, snuff, cigars, cannabis, or cocaine
- Chronic arsenic poisoning

Prevention

Abstinence of tobacco use is the only known preventative measure.

DIAGNOSIS

- **Definitive diagnosis is by biopsy** of the affected limb revealing pathology consistent with an acute phase vascular lesion in the appropriate clinical setting.
- Other causes of distal extremity ischemia must be ruled out.

Diagnostic Criteria

- The American College of Rheumatology does not have diagnostic or classification criteria for TAO. However, several authors, including Shionoya, Papa et al., Mills and Porter, and Olin et al., have suggested criteria, and most propose a combination of clinical, angiographic, and histopathologic, as well as exclusionary findings.
- Commonly used criteria of Olin and colleagues are presented in Table 45-1.[6]

Clinical Presentation

- Typically seen in **male smokers,** younger than 40 years of age
- Ischemia usually starts at distal fingertips or toes and progresses proximally.
- **Ischemic findings and symptoms** are common (e.g., claudication or ulcerations). Ulcerations are a common initial symptom because TAO has the tendency to affect smaller arteries first.
- **Pain at rest and sensory deficits** are very common and are usually secondary to ischemic neuritis.
- **Migratory superficial thrombophlebitis** and **Raynaud's phenomenon** are present in about 40% of patients.[6]

TABLE 45-1	CRITERIA FOR THROMBOANGIITIS OBLITERANS

Age of onset <45 years
- Current or recent tobacco use
- Distal extremity ischemia manifested as claudication, pain at rest, ulceration, or gangrene plus consistent noninvasive vascular testing
- Consistent angiographic findings
- Exclusion of proximal sources of emboli (by echocardiography and arteriography)
- Exclusion of autoimmune diseases, hypercoagulable states, diabetes mellitus

Adapted from: Olin JW. Thromboangiitis obliterans (Buerger's disease). *N Engl J Med. 2000*; 343:864–869.

- Signs of peripheral vascular disease (e.g., extremity poikilothermia, pallor, pulselessness, and paresthesia) are present in the affected as well as unaffected limbs.
- TAO rarely affects the cerebral, coronary, pulmonary, mesenteric, iliac or renal arteries, or the aorta. However, if these arteries are affected, ischemic symptoms in the affected organ may be seen.

History
- Digital pain, ulceration, or color changes from blood vessel obstruction and eventual tissue necrosis are presenting complaints in a third of patients.
- Claudication of upper or lower extremities with use.
- Superficial thrombophlebitis may occur before digital ischemia.
- Symptoms and color changes consistent with Raynaud's phenomenon.
- Nonspecific, episodic, joint pains in the extremities may be observed months to years before the occlusive phase of the disease. Most commonly affected joints are wrists and knees.

Physical Examination
- Digital ulcerations and necrosis that are usually bilateral
- Claudication with exercise of the extremity in question
- Raynaud's phenomenon
- Superficial thrombophlebitis
- Altered Allen's test (used to evaluate radial and ulnar perfusion of the hand)[6]

Differential Diagnosis
- Thrombotic or embolic disease (cholesterol, atrial myxoma, etc.)
- Peripheral vascular disease
- Chilblains
- Hypercoagulable states and hyperviscosity syndrome (myeloproliferative diseases)
- Raynaud's disease
- Scleroderma or CREST syndrome
- Small vessel vasculitis
- Systemic lupus erythematosus
- Mixed connective tissue disease
- Trauma
- Infection

Diagnostic Testing
There is no definitive laboratory or radiographic test to diagnose TAO. However, disease mimics must be ruled out.

Laboratory
- Test for systemic vasculitis or other autoimmune disorders associated with vasculitis. Consider checking antinuclear antibodies (ANAs), extractable nuclear antigen (ENA) panel, antineutrophil cytoplasmic antibodies (ANCAs), rheumatoid factor (RF), anti–cyclic citrullinated protein (CCP) antibodies, complement levels, Scl-70 antibodies, and antiphospholipid antibodies. Autoimmune serologies should be negative. However, a few patients with TAO may have a low titer positive antiphospholipid screen.
- Evaluate for possible hypercoagulable states.
- Unlike some other vasculitides, TAO does not have laboratory signs of systemic inflammation (e.g., elevated erythrocyte sedimentation rate [ESR] and C-reactive protein [CRP], thrombocytosis, normochromic normocytic anemia).
- Ensure patients are screened for diabetes mellitus.

Imaging
- Arteriography
  - Perform angiography of **all four limbs,** even those without clinical evidence of occlusive disease.
  - Arteriogram should reveal normal proximal arteries with **distal segmental occlusive disease of small- and medium-sized vessels** (e.g., palmar, plantar, tibial, peroneal, radial, ulnar, or digital arteries), with severe distal disease and collateralization around the occlusion ("corkscrew" collaterals).
  - These findings are not pathognomonic because they may be seen in hypercoagulable states, autoimmune diseases, and vasculitis.
- Transthoracic echocardiography (TTE) with follow-up transesophageal echocardiography (TEE) if there is suspicion of intracardiac thrombus

COMPLICATIONS

- Gangrene that may become progressive, especially if the patient continues to use tobacco products
- Infection of necrotic tissue
- Amputation in about 25% at 5 years and more than 50% in patients who continue to smoke
- Rare involvement of coronary, mesenteric, renal, and splenic arteries

TREATMENT

- Crucial to the treatment of TAO is **complete cessation of tobacco use and avoidance of nicotine replacement products.**
- It is inconclusive whether second-hand smoke causes disease exacerbation or progression.
- With complete tobacco cessation, patients can largely avoid amputation but may still have claudication or Raynaud's phenomenon.
- Nicotine replacement therapy may perpetuate disease activity.[6]
- Many medications are under investigation for treatment, but none have been proven to be as beneficial as smoking cessation.
- Different medical and surgical treatments have been tried, with varying degrees of success, in patients with critical limb ischemia.[20] None have shown particular efficacy in preventing major amputation.

Medications
- Smoking cessation aids
  - Do not use nicotine replacement therapy because this may trigger disease activity.

- ○ Consider Food and Drug Administration (FDA)-approved non–nicotine-containing medications such as **bupropion or varenicline.**
- **Foot care**: moisturize, Lamb's wool between toes, avoid trauma. Trial of **cilostazol** for ischemic ulcers
- The following medications are investigational. Most have been tried in the acute and chronic phases of the disease.
  - ○ There is no study showing overwhelming support for the use of aspirin or anticoagulation during acute or chronic phases of TAO.
  - ○ Thrombolytic therapy may be beneficial in a limited number of patients in the acute phase but remains investigational.
  - ○ **Prostacyclin (prostaglandin I2 [PGI2]) analogs: Iloprost** is considered the most effective and may improve ulcer healing, decrease pain, and reduce the need for amputation.[21,22] These results have only been seen with intravenous (IV) but not oral administration. Continuation or reinitiation of smoking may completely blunt these potentially beneficial effects.
    - ▪ **Bosentan**: Treatment with this oral dual endothelin-1 receptor antagonist may result in clinical and angiographic improvement, even in smokers or those with disease refractory to smoking cessation.[23,24] This treatment shows promise, but more studies are needed.
    - ▪ **Calcium channel blockers**, β-blockers, and **sildenafil** may be of benefit but have not been studied in clinical trials and do not have clear-cut evidence for efficacy.
- **Other nonpharmacologic investigative therapies**
  - ○ Epidural spinal cord stimulators are under investigation.
  - ○ **Stem cell therapy for angiogenesis induction**: Studies evaluating the effect of autologous bone marrow mononuclear cell implantation for critical limb ischemia show promising results in the short term.[25,26] However, more studies are needed because the long-term efficacy, safety, and complications are not well defined.
  - ○ **Angiogenesis growth factors**: Intramuscular injections of vascular endothelial growth factor (VEGF) recombinant protein[27] and DNA plasmid for gene therapy[28] may decrease ischemic pain and improve ulcer healing. Promising results have also been reported with injections of hepatocyte growth factor gene therapy.[29] These therapies are currently undergoing further evaluation.
  - ○ **Immunoadsorption** clears plasma immunoglobulins and immune complexes and is approved for the treatment of several autoimmune diseases. Preliminary studies suggest significant improvement in physiologic and functional measures, as well as pain at 6 months.[30] Further investigation is needed.

Surgical Management

- Ischemic digits or limbs may require amputation.
- **Arterial bypass** is usually not an option or recommended because of the mostly distal and intermittent occlusive nature of the disease. However, in other countries, there are reports of successful surgical bypass with autologous vein or omental transfers.
- **Sympathectomy** may be tried in patients with resistant disease, but results are mixed and controversial.

REFERRAL

Consider referral to a vascular surgeon.

PATIENT EDUCATION

Educate the patient about the need to stop smoking!

OUTCOME/PROGNOSIS

- Resolution may occur with discontinuation of tobacco products. However, even if digital ischemia resolves, some patients may have persistent Raynaud's phenomenon, claudication, or rest pain.
- If the patient continues to smoke, they are much more likely to require major amputations; 43% of patients who continued smoking required at least one amputation, whereas 94% of those who quit smoking prior to developing gangrene avoided amputations.[6]

REFERENCES

1. von Winiwarter F. Ueber eine eigenthumliche Form von Endarteriitis und Endophlebitis mit Gangran des Fusses. *Arch Klin Chir.* 1879;23:202–226.
2. Buerger L. Thrombo-angiitis obliterans: a study of the vascular lesions leading to presenile spontaneous gangrene. *Am J Med Sci.* 1908;136:567–580.
3. Sasaki S, Sakuma M, Kunihara T, et al. Current trends in thromboangiitis obliterans (Buerger's disease) in women. *Am J Surg.* 1999;177:316–320.
4. Mills JL, Taylor LM Jr, Porter JM. Buerger's disease in the modern era. *Am J Surg.* 1987;154:123–129.
5. Lie, JT. The rise and fall and resurgence of thromboangiitis obliterans (Buerger's disease). *Acta Pathol Jpn.* 1989;39:153–158.
6. Olin JW. Thromboangiitis obliterans (Buerger's disease). *N Engl J Med.* 2000;343:864–869.
7. Noël B. Buerger disease or arsenic intoxication? *Arch Intern Med.* 2001;161:1016.
8. Kobayashi M, Ito M, Nakagawa A, et al. Immunohistochemical analysis of arterial wall cellular infiltration in Buerger's disease (endarteritis obliterans). *J Vasc Surg.* 1999;29:451–458.
9. Ketha SS, Cooper LT. The role of autoimmunity in thromboangiitis obliterans (Buerger's disease). *Ann N Y Acad Sci.* 2013;1285:15–25.
10. Sun XL, Law BY, de Seabra Rodrigues Dias IR, et al. Pathogenesis of thromboangiitis obliterans: Gene polymorphism and immunoregulation of human vascular endothelial cells. *Atherosclerosis.* 2017;265:258–265.
11. Adar R, Papa MZ, Halpern Z, et al. Cellular sensitivity to collagen in thromboangiitis obliterans. *N Engl J Med.* 1983;308:1113–1116.
12. Hada M, Sakihama T, Kamiya K, et al. Cellular and humoral immune responses to vascular components in thromboangiitis obliterans. *Angiology.* 1993;44:533–540.
13. Berlit P, Kessler C, Reuther R, et al. New aspects of thromboangiitis obliterans (von Winiwarter-Buerger's disease). *Eur Neurol.* 1984;23:394–399.
14. Eichhorn J, Sima D, Lindschau C, et al. Antiendothelial cell antibodies in thromboangiitis obliterans. *Am J Med Sci.* 1998;315:17–23.
15. Gulati SM, Madhra K, Thusoo TK, et al. Autoantibodies in thromboangiitis obliterans (Buerger's disease). *Angiology.* 1982;33:642–651.
16. Makita S, Nakamura M, Murakami H, et al. Impaired endothelium-dependent vasorelaxation in peripheral vasculature of patients with thromboangiitis obliterans (Buerger's disease). *Circulation.* 1996;94:II211–II215.
17. Slavov ES, Stanilova SA, Petkov DP, et al. Cytokine production in thromboangiitis obliterans patients: new evidence for an immune-mediated inflammatory disorder. *Clin Exp Rheumatol.* 2005;23:219–226.
18. Dellalibera-Joviliano R, Joviliano EE, Silva JS, et al. Activation of cytokines corroborate with development of inflammation and autoimmunity in thromboangiitis obliterans patients. *Clin Exp Immunol.* 2012;170:28–35.
19. Avcu F, Akar E, Demirkiliç U, et al. The role of prothrombotic mutations in patients with Buerger's disease. *Thromb Res.* 2000;100:14–17.
20. Fazeli B, Dadgar MM, Niroumand S. How to treat a patient with thromboangiitis obliterans: a systematic review. *Ann Vasc Surg.* 2018;49:219–228.
21. Fiessinger JN, Schafer N. Trial of iloprost versus aspirin treatment for critical limb ischaemia of thromboangiitis obliterans. The TAO Study. *Lancet.* 1990;335:555–557.
22. The European TAO Study Group. Oral iloprost in the treatment of thromboangiitis obliterans (Buerger's disease): a double-blind, randomised, placebo-controlled trial. The European TAO Study Group. *Eur J Vasc Endovasc Surg.* 1998;15:300–307.

23. De Haro J, Acin F, Bleda S, et al. Treatment of thromboangiitis obliterans (Buerger's disease) with bosentan. *BMC Cardiovasc Disord.* 2012;12:5.
24. Narváez J, García-Gómez C, Álvarez L, et al. Efficacy of bosentan in patients with refractory thromboangiitis obliterans (Buerger disease): A case series and review of the literature. *Medicine (Baltimore).* 2016;95:e5511.
25. Motukuru V, Suresh KR, Vivekanand V, et al. Therapeutic angiogenesis in Buerger's disease (thromboangiitis obliterans) patients with critical limb ischemia by autologous transplantation of bone marrow mononuclear cells. *J Vasc Surg.* 2008;48:53S–60S.
26. Matoba S, Tatsumi T, Murohara T, et al. Long-term clinical outcome after intramuscular implantation of bone marrow mononuclear cells (Therapeutic Angiogenesis by Cell Transplantation [TACT] trial) in patients with chronic limb ischemia. *Am Heart J.* 2008;156:1010–1018.
27. Isner JM, Baumgartner I, Rauh G, et al. Treatment of thromboangiitis obliterans (Buerger's disease) by intramuscular gene transfer of vascular endothelial growth factor: preliminary clinical results. *J Vasc Surg.* 1998;28:964–973; discussion 73–75.
28. Kim HJ, Jang SY, Park JI, et al. Vascular endothelial growth factor-induced angiogenic gene therapy in patients with peripheral artery disease. *Exp Mol Med.* 2004;36:336–344.
29. Makino H, Aoki M, Hashiya N, et al. Long-term follow-up evaluation of results from clinical trial using hepatocyte growth factor gene to treat severe peripheral arterial disease. *Arterioscler Thromb Vasc Biol.* 2012;32:2503–2509.
30. Baumann G, Stangl V, Klein-Weigel P, et al. Successful treatment of thromboangiitis obliterans (Buerger's disease) with immunoadsorption: results of a pilot study. *Clin Res Cardiol.* 2011; 100:683–690.

Avascular Necrosis

46

Shuang Song and Deepali Sen

GENERAL PRINCIPLES

Definition

Avascular necrosis (AVN), also known as **osteonecrosis, ischemic necrosis, and aseptic necrosis,** is caused by compromise of the bone vasculature with subsequent bone death and joint destruction.

Epidemiology

- It is estimated that 10,000 to 30,000 new cases of AVN are diagnosed every year in the United States.
- AVN accounts for about 10% of the 500,000 joint replacements performed annually in the United States.[1]
- AVN is more commonly seen in males (male–female ratio of 7:3), with the exception of AVN in systemic lupus erythematosus (SLE). The age of AVN onset is relatively young, with 75% of patients between 30 and 60 years.[2] A recent study, however, suggested greater heterogeneity of the epidemiologic characteristics of AVN.[3]
- **Osteonecrosis of the femoral head the most common and has the most severe morbidity.** In addition, osteonecrosis can affect humeral heads, femoral condyles, tibial plateaus, wrists, ankles, shoulders, bones of the hands and feet, vertebrae, jaws, and bony structures of the face.
- About half of patients with femoral head AVN develop bilateral disease.[2]
- Osteonecrosis of the jaw occurs predominantly with the use of intravenous bisphosphates (88%), and about 90% of patients have an underlying malignancy.[4]

Pathophysiology

- The pathogenesis of AVN is multifactorial and not fully understood. The **disruption of blood supply** to the bone is the final common pathway and is believed to be precipitated by several mechanisms, such as vasculature disruption through mechanical injury, inflammation, thrombotic or embolic intravascular obstruction and extravascular compression by increased marrow fat, and intraosseous pressure.[2,5] Recent studies have revealed more specific mechanisms leading to nontraumatic AVN, including:
  - Osteoblast/osteoclast imbalance leading to inhibited osteogenesis
  - Apoptosis of osteoblasts, osteoclasts, and osteocytes
  - Adipogenesis and fatty infiltration of bone marrow
  - Oxidative stress
  - Endothelial nitric oxide synthase (eNOS) defects
  - Hypercoagulation, hypofibrinolysis, and thrombophilia[5,6]
- After infarction in the femoral head, subchondral fractures occur if the necrotic lesion is weight bearing. The femoral head eventually collapses, which causes loss of cartilage and degenerative changes of the joint.

Risk Factors

- The most common risk factor for developing AVN is **glucocorticoid use, followed by alcoholism.** The AVN risk associated with glucocorticoid therapy depends on both the maximum daily dose and the cumulative dose. There is no consensus on a "safe" dose but studies reported that an equivalent of prednisone dose of 20 mg or more, especially if 40 mg or more, and a cumulative prednisone dose of 12 g or more per year are associated with a higher risk of development of AVN.[7]
- **Other risk factors** include cigarette smoking, SLE, anti–phospholipid antibody syndrome, rheumatoid arthritis (RA), vasculitis, trauma, organ transplantation, hematologic malignancies, chemotherapy, radiation exposure, sickle cell disease, HIV infection, severe acute respiratory syndrome (SARS), Gaucher's disease, Fabry's disease, hyperlipidemia, pregnancy, dysbaric conditions (caisson disease), and bisphosphonate use especially in malignancies.
- AVN may be idiopathic in approximately 12% of patients, where no clear cause is identified.[2]
- Genetic associations of AVN include polymorphisms in alcohol-metabolizing enzyme genes, eNOS genes, plasminogen activator inhibitor-1 (PAI-1) genes, vascular endothelial growth factor (VEGF) genes, and sterol regulatory element-binding factor (SREBP-2) genes involved in lipid metabolism. Mutations in the type II collagen gene (COL2A1) were identified in some families, demonstrating autosomal dominant inheritance of AVN.[8]

DIAGNOSIS

Clinical Presentation

History
- Many patients may be asymptomatic in the early phases of the disease.
- AVN commonly presents as vague, mild **joint pain** with gradual progression. It less commonly presents with acute and severe pain.
- Early in the course of the disease, pain is increased with activity, but over time it progresses to pain with rest.
- More severe pain can occur with larger infarcts (most often associated with Gaucher's disease, dysbarism, and hemoglobinopathies).
- Some patients remain relatively asymptomatic despite advanced radiographic changes.
- Early and small lesions generally progress slowly. It often takes more than 5 years for a small AVN to progress from a very early stage to a stage where there are clinical symptoms and radiographic changes; progression accelerates as the disease becomes more advanced.[2]

Physical Examination
- The physical examination is nonspecific but may reveal tenderness to palpation over the bone, mild joint swelling, and decreased range of motion of the affected joint.
- Joint effusions are sometimes seen when large joints like the knee are involved.

Differential Diagnosis

Other diagnoses to consider include infections, fractures, sickle cell disease, osteoporosis, tumors, soft-tissue injuries, and exacerbation of existing joint disease.

Diagnostic Testing

Laboratories
Laboratory tests are useful only for evaluating an underlying cause of AVN or excluding other diagnoses.

Imaging

- **Imaging plays a key role in confirming the diagnosis of AVN.** Evaluation may begin with plain radiographs, but early in the disease course these can be normal. The earliest radiographic finding is the "crescent sign" as a result of subchondral collapse. Later, radiographs will show sclerosis, further collapse, and degenerative joint changes.
- Bone scans (i.e., Technetium-99m scintigraphy) are useful for early diagnosis of AVN. Typical findings in early AVN show a dead central area surrounded by increased activity described as the **"doughnut sign."** As disease progresses, it shows only a uniformly high level of activity. Bone scans are less sensitive than MRI for evaluation of AVN.
- Although there is no definitive role of F-18 fluoride positron emission tomography–computed tomography (PET/CT) in the diagnosis of AVN, some studies have shown good agreement of PET/CT with MRI in the diagnosis of femoral head AVN and even higher sensitivity in early disease than MRI.[9]
- CT scanning is not commonly used for diagnosing AVN but can be helpful because it allows more detailed evaluation than plain radiographs.
- **MRI is the gold standard for imaging of osteonecrosis** because of the specificity and sensitivity of 99% or more demonstrated by multiple studies. The earliest sign is marrow edema that is nonspecific. As disease progresses, the border of the subchondral necrotic lesion shows a high-intensity signal on T2-weighted images, and the surrounding band-like lesion shows a low-intensity signal on T1-weighted images, producing the **"double-line sign"** that is usually pathognomonic for AVN.
- **Staging of AVN:** AVN of the femoral head is generally staged based on imaging findings. The staging system is used to guide treatment strategies and to bring uniformity to clinical trials. Different staging systems are shown in Table 46-1.[10]

TREATMENT

The goal of therapy is to prevent collapse in early disease and to preserve the native joint for as long as possible in late, irreversible disease.

Medications

- Treatment varies according to the site of AVN, the underlying cause, and the stage of progression. **Cessation of the offending agent** may be beneficial.
- Pharmacologic measures are intended to allow **revascularization and bone growth.** They include the following[11]:
  - Vasodilators—a prostacyclin (prostaglandin I2 [PGI2]) iloprost has shown significant improvement in both clinical and radiologic outcomes in early stages.[12]
  - Bisphosphonates—alendronate has been shown to reduce the incidence of collapse of the femoral head in Steinberg stages 2 and 3 AVN.
  - Statins may provide protective effects on the osteonecrosis risk for patients receiving glucocorticoid, according to retrospective analyses.
  - Anticoagulants such as warfarin or enoxaparin have been shown to reduce progression of early AVN. They are primarily beneficial in patients with risk factors of hypercoagulation, thrombophilia, or hypofibrinolysis.

Other Nonpharmacologic Therapies

- Conservative treatment modalities including assisted weight bearing with canes or crutches, analgesics, anti-inflammatory medications, and physiotherapy are effective for symptomatic relief, but do not seem to alter the natural course of the disease.
- Several other biophysical treatment modalities are under study, including hyperbaric oxygen treatment, extracorporeal shock wave therapy, and pulsed electromagnetic therapy.[11]

TABLE 46-1	RADIOGRAPHIC CLASSIFICATION OF OSTEONECROSIS OF THE FEMORAL HEAD

Stage   Description

Ficat and Arlet

I	Normal (only evident on MRI)
II	Sclerotic or cystic lesions, without subchondral fracture
III	Crescent sign (subchondral collapse)
IV	Osteoarthritis with decreased articular cartilage, osteophytes

University of Pennsylvania System of Staging

I, II	First two stages are the same as Ficat and Arlet
III	Crescent sign only
IV	Flattening of articular surface
V	Joint narrowing or acetabular changes
VI	Advanced degenerative changes

Each stage is divided into A, B, and C subclasses based on the extent of femoral head involvement (small, moderate, and large).

ARCO (Association Research Circulation Osseous)

0	Negative imaging findings but with risk factors
1	X-ray and CT normal; at least one of bone scintigraphy and MRI is positive
2	Sclerosis, osteolysis, focal porosis
3	Crescent sign and/or flattening of articular surface
4	Osteoarthritis, acetabular changes, joint destruction

Japanese Investigation Committee

1	Demarcation line, subdivided by relationship to weight-bearing area (from medial to lateral): 1A, 1B, 1C
2	Early flattening without demarcation line around necrotic area
3	Cystic lesions, subdivided by site in the femoral head: 3A (medial), 3B (lateral)

Adapted from: Mont MA, Marulanda GA, Jones LC, et al. Systemic analysis of classification systems of osteonecrosis of the femoral head. *J Bone Joint Surg Am.* 2006;88(suppl 3):16–26.

Surgical Management

Surgical modalities include the following:

- Core decompression decreases the intraosseous and intramedullary pressure.
- Osteotomy helps redistribute forces to healthy bone by moving necrotic tissues away from the weight-bearing region.
- Nonvascularized bone grafting provides structural support.
- Vascularized bone grafting provides mesenchymal stem cells, vascular supply, and structural support to the subchondral bone and cartilage.

- For younger patients with later-stage AVN, resurfacing arthroplasty showed comparable success rates to total hip arthroplasty [THA].
- In hemiarthroplasty, the femoral head alone is replaced with prosthesis.
- THA is the most common surgical procedure for advanced cases. It is reserved for patients with late-stage disease, older age, and more severe arthritis. About 17% of patients require revision after 10 years.[13]
- Young or active patients should be candidates for procedures that delay total joint arthroplasty, such as bone grafts or bone-preserving operations like resurfacing arthroplasty.

COMPLICATIONS

Complications include incomplete fractures and superimposed degenerative arthritis.

REFERENCES

1. Mankin HJ. Nontraumatic necrosis of bone (osteonecrosis). *N Engl J Med.* 1992;326:1473–1479.
2. Assouline-Dayan Y, Chang C, Greenspan A, et al. Pathogenesis and natural history of osteonecrosis. *Semin Arthritis Rheum.* 2002;32:94–124.
3. Cooper C, Steinbuch M, Stevenson R, et al. The epidemiology of osteonecrosis: findings from the GPRD and THIN databases in the UK. *Osteoporos Int.* 2010;21:569–577.
4. Reid IR, Cornish J. Epidemiology and pathogenesis of osteonecrosis of the jaw. *Nat Rev Rheumatol.* 2011;8:90–96.
5. Seamon J, Keller T, Saleh J, et al. The pathogenesis of nontraumatic osteonecrosis. *Arthritis.* 2012;2012:601763.
6. Shah KN, Racine J, Jones LC, et al. Pathophysiology and risk factors for osteonecrosis. *Curr Rev Musculoskelet Med.* 2015;8:201–209.
7. Powell C, Chang C, Naguwa SM, et al. Steroid induced osteonecrosis: an analysis of steroid dosing risk. *Autoimmun Rev.* 2010;9:721–743.
8. Pouya F, Kerachian MA. Avascular necrosis of the femoral head: are any genes involved? *Arch Bone Jt Surg.* 2015;3:149–155.
9. Pierce TP, Jauregui JJ, Cherian JJ, et al. Imaging evaluation of patients with osteonecrosis of the femoral head. *Curr Rev Musculoskelet Med.* 2015;8:221–227.
10. Mont MA, Marulanda GA, Jones LC, et al. Systematic analysis of classification systems for osteonecrosis of the femoral head. *J Bone Joint Surg Am.* 2006;88 Suppl 3:16–26.
11. Klumpp R, Trevisan C. Aseptic osteonecrosis of the hip in the adult: current evidence on conservative treatment. *Clin Cases Miner Bone Metab.* 2015;12:39–42.
12. Claßen T, Becker A, Landgraeber S, et al. Long-term clinical results after iloprost treatment for bone marrow edema and avascular necrosis. *Orthop Rev (Pavia).* 2016;8:6150.
13. Fyda TM, Callaghan JJ, Olejniczak J, et al. Minimum ten-year follow-up of cemented total hip replacement in patients with osteonecrosis of the femoral head. *Iowa Orthop J.* 2002;22:8–19.

Deposition and Storage Arthropathies

47

Kelvin J. Lee and María C. González-Mayda

INTRODUCTION

- A number of unusual arthropathies result from cellular deposition of normal metal ions (e.g., hemochromatosis) *or* cellular storage of abnormal lipids (e.g., Gaucher's disease).
- Because of storage and deposition arthropathies being relatively rare, they are often mistaken for more common diseases like osteoarthritis (OA) and rheumatoid arthritis (RA).
- Given the systemic nature of these arthropathies, an accurate diagnosis is important to guide appropriate therapy.

HEMOCHROMATOSIS

GENERAL PRINCIPLES

Definition

Hemochromatosis is a disease characterized by **iron overload** and visceral **deposition of hemosiderin** in susceptible organs such as the liver, heart, pancreas, bones, and joints.

Classification

- **Hereditary hemochromatosis** (HH) is an **autosomal recessive** disorder. A **C282Y mutation in the HFE gene** is found in 80% to 90% of patients.[1] Individuals who are heterozygous for the mutation are generally asymptomatic carriers.
- **Secondary hemochromatosis** occurs in the setting of excessive iron ingestion or repeated blood transfusions in patients with chronic hypoproliferative anemia, sickle cell anemia, and thalassemia. End-organ damage because of secondary hemochromatosis tends to be milder than that of HH.

Epidemiology

- HH is seen more commonly in populations of Northern European ancestry, approximately 1 in 250 individuals.[1]
- Owing to several factors such as physiologic blood loss in women and higher iron intake in men, HH is approximately 10 times more common in men than in women, and men tend to have symptom onset at an earlier age.

Pathophysiology

- HFE gene mutation leads to **increased intestinal iron absorption** *and* **decreased hepatic expression of hepcidin**, resulting in iron deposition in hepatocytes and other viscera.
- The pathogenesis of HH arthropathy is unclear, but there is speculation that iron deposition within joints may trigger free radical generation and promote calcium pyrophosphate crystal deposition.[2]

Associated Conditions

Patients with HH also have increased susceptibility to infection from siderophilic microorganisms such as *Vibrio, Yersinia, Listeria*, and *Escherichia coli*.

DIAGNOSIS

Clinical Presentation

- Patients with HH can present with **cirrhosis, hypogonadism, heart failure, diabetes, or polyarthropathy.**
- **Chronic progressive arthritis,** mechanical in nature, is a frequent complaint (about 50%) and often predates other symptoms of iron overload.
  - **Second and third metacarpophalangeal (MCP)** joints are the most common joints affected (about 50%), with the **dominant hand** either solely or more severely involved.
  - On examination, joint inflammation is typically minimal, with mild tenderness and slightly decreased range of motion.
  - The arthritis may then progress to involve the larger joints such as shoulders, hips, and knees. The wrists can also be affected.
  - HH can manifest as an acute episode of monoarticular arthritis. Chondrocalcinosis is a late but characteristic feature of HH arthropathy.[3]

Diagnostic Testing

Laboratories

Diagnosis is based on detection of HFE genotype in the setting of elevated ferritin (>300 µg/L in men, >200 µg/L in women) and transferrin saturation greater than 45%.

Imaging

- Radiologic changes resemble OA with **irregular joint space narrowing and sclerotic cyst formation.** HH arthropathy has less osteophytosis and no involvement of carpometacarpal (CMC) joints as classically seen in OA. Disease-specific changes include subchondral radiolucency of the femoral head, hook-like osteophytes on the metacarpal heads, and a degenerative predilection for the MCP joint rather than the scapholunate.
- **Chondrocalcinosis** can be seen in up to 49% of patients with HH arthropathy.[3]

TREATMENT

- Treatment is aimed at reduction of iron load using **phlebotomy and iron chelators.** However, **reduction in body iron stores has little effect on HH arthropathy.**
- Symptoms are managed much like OA, with **acetaminophen, nonsteroidal anti-inflammatory drugs (NSAIDs), physical therapy, and local steroid injections.**
- Limiting alcohol and red meat intake while increasing consumption of substances that inhibit iron absorption, such as high-tannin teas, may be of benefit.

WILSON'S DISEASE

GENERAL PRINCIPLES

Definition

Wilson's disease, also known as **hepatolenticular degeneration,** is an autosomal recessive disorder resulting in **excess copper accumulation.**

Epidemiology

- Incidence is one in 30,000 to 40,000.[4]
- The majority present between ages 5 and 35.

Pathophysiology

- Wilson's disease is caused by mutations in the **ATP7B gene,** which is translated into a **membrane-bound copper-transporting adenosine triphosphatase (ATPase).**
- Membrane-bound copper-transporting ATPase deficiency leads to **excess copper accumulation, affecting the liver, kidney, brain, cornea, and joints.**
- The pathogenesis of arthropathy is unclear but its severity does not correlate with neurologic, hepatic, or renal disease. By elemental analysis, copper has been found in the synovium of Wilson's disease patients and is thought to contribute to the development of arthropathy.

DIAGNOSIS

Clinical Presentation

- Patients presenting before the age of 20 usually have **progressive hepatic failure.** Patients presenting after their 20s tend to have more **psychiatric or neurologic manifestations.**
- Arthropathy tends to be mild and is common with other manifestations of Wilson's disease.[5]
  - Joint manifestations are **similar to those of OA** with mechanical pain and crepitus.
  - Commonly affected joints include knees and spine, but hips, feet/ankles, and wrists can also be involved. MCP involvement seems rare.[5]
- **Kayser–Fleischer rings** are present in more than 99% of patients if neurologic or psychiatric symptoms are present. The presence of Kayser–Fleischer rings on slit-lamp examination supports the diagnosis of Wilson's disease.

Diagnostic Testing

Laboratories

- Approximately 90% of Wilson's patients have low **serum ceruloplasmin** levels. It is the cheapest test, but it can also be low in patients without the disease and may be normal or elevated in patients with the disease.
- **24-hour urine copper** (>100 mg/day) has greater than 98% sensitivity but can easily be contaminated or collected improperly.
- The "gold standard" for diagnosis is a **liver biopsy** with quantitative copper assays.
- Genetic testing is useful when the diagnosis remains unclear despite liver biopsy.

Imaging

- Radiographic changes seen resemble OA with **irregular joint space narrowing** and **marked osteophyte formation.** Calcified loose bodies have also been seen in the wrist.[5]
- Generalized osteoporosis is seen in the majority of patients.

TREATMENT

- Treatment is aimed at reduction of copper load using **chelation therapy.** Penicillamine was previously the chelator of choice but because of its toxicity, it has been supplanted by **zinc and trientine (triethylenetetramine).**
- Avoidance of high-copper food items including mushrooms, nuts, chocolate, shellfish, and liver is recommended.

- Arthropathy is managed with local therapy because symptoms are mild. **Acetaminophen and NSAIDs should be used with great caution in patients with liver and possible renal tubular acidosis.**

OCHRONOSIS (ALKAPTONURIA)

GENERAL PRINCIPLES

Definition
Alkaptonuria (AKU) is a rare autosomal recessive disorder resulting from a **deficiency of homogentisate 1,2-dioxygenase (HGD).**

Epidemiology
Incidence is 1 in 250,000.[6]

Pathophysiology
- A loss-of-function mutation leading to a complete deficiency of HGD leads to **accumulation of homogentisic acid (HGA)**, a normal intermediate in tyrosine metabolism.
- Oxidative conversion of HGA leads to production of a pigmented polymer, a process termed ochronosis.
- The ochronotic tissue becomes stiff and brittle; this change in mechanical properties of the connective tissue results in multisystem disease dominated by spinal involvement.

DIAGNOSIS

Clinical Manifestation
- Suspect AKU in a young patient who complains of passing dark urine with progressive arthritic pain affecting weight-bearing joints such as the spinal column, hips, and knees.
- Patients usually present with **progressive degenerative arthropathy** (noninflammatory and nonerosive in nature) beginning in their late 30s or early 40s. There are few symptoms or signs before the late 20s or early 30s, apart from constant dark urine.
- Symptoms worsen from the 4th decade onward, including progressive kyphoscoliosis and impaired spinal and thoracic mobility.
- Other systemic features include stones (renal, prostatic, salivary, gallbladder), renal damage/failure, osteopenia/fractures, ruptures of tendons/muscle/ligaments, respiratory compromise, hearing loss, and aortic valve disease.

Diagnostic Testing
Laboratories
- The presence of HGA in urine is the gold standard for confirmation of the diagnosis. This can be quantitatively measured. Urine color change upon alkalinization is unpredictable and nonspecific.
- Genetic testing is available but usually not necessary for diagnosis.

Imaging
- Lumbosacral radiographs show premature degenerative changes along with prominent vacuum discs and intervertebral disc calcification. Sacroiliac (SI) joints are spared.
- The radiographic changes of large peripheral joints (knees, hips, shoulders) in ochronotic arthritis are virtually indistinguishable from that in primary OA.[7]

TREATMENT

- Current available therapy includes joint protection, physical/occupational therapy, analgesia, and dietary restriction of phenylalanine and tyrosine. **Total joint arthroplasty** is reserved for severe cases.
- Nitisinone (Orfadin), an agent blocking an earlier step in tyrosine metabolism, has been studied in AKU as this medication has shown to decrease levels of HGA. Suitability Of Nitisinone In Alkaptonuria 1 (SONIA 1) showed that 2 mg of nitisinone per day decreased HGA by 95% or more.[8] Ranganath and colleagues showed nitisinone reduced the rate of progression of AKU in 39 patients over a 3-year period.[9] The Suitability of Nitisinone in Alkaptonuria 2 (SONIA 2) is a Phase 3 trial currently underway evaluating nitisinone's efficacy in AKU.[10]

MULTICENTRIC RETICULOHISTIOCYTOSIS

GENERAL PRINCIPLES

Definition

Multicentric reticulohistiocytosis (MRH) is a rare dermatoarthritis primarily affecting middle-aged women and is characterized by cellular accumulation of **glycolipid-laden histiocytes in joints and in skin.**

Pathophysiology

- Etiology is unknown but is thought to involve an often self-limited inflammatory reaction triggered by autoimmunity, malignancy, and infections.[11,12]
- Studies have shown increased levels of tumor necrosis factor (TNF)-α, interleukin (IL)-1B, IL-2, IL-6, and IL-12 in blood and tissue. Osteoclastic activity may also play a role in pathogenesis.[11]
- MRH is **associated with autoimmune diseases** like scleroderma, Sjögren's syndrome, and dermatomyositis in about 10% to 15% of cases.[11,12]
- At diagnosis, up to 30% of patients were found to have a **concomitant malignancy.**[11,12]

DIAGNOSIS

Clinical Manifestation

- About two-thirds of patients present with **arthritis as their initial sign of disease.**[11] The arthritis of MRH is inflammatory, usually chronic, symmetric, and polyarticular. **It characteristically affects the hands and is destructive.**[11,12]
- Active synovitis is seen on examination and hence is most often mistaken for aggressive seronegative RA. However, MRH tends to destroy **both the distal interphalangeals (DIPs) and proximal interphalangeals (PIPs) prior to significant destruction of the MCPs.**
- **Cutaneous manifestations** comprise **papulonodular lesions** ranging from a few millimeters to a centimeter in diameter. The lesions are scattered and isolated well-circumscribed, round, yellow-brown nodules preferentially affecting fingers, nailfolds, as well as oral and nasal mucosa.

Diagnostic Testing

- Diagnosis is made by skin or synovial biopsy demonstrating the presence of numerous multinucleated giant cells and histiocytes with an abundant eosinophilic, finely granular cytoplasm (glycolipids).

- Hand radiographs may show articular punched-out lesions like gouty tophi, but these will rapidly progress to severe joint destruction and even arthritis mutilans.

TREATMENT

- When not associated with a malignancy, MRH often **spontaneously resolves** within 10 years. However, by that time, many patients have already developed an irreversible deforming arthritis.
- Because of the rarity of MRH, treatment has been mostly empirical. NSAIDs and glucocorticoids are generally utilized as first-line agents. Various disease-modifying antirheumatic drugs (DMARDs) have also been used with some success. These include methotrexate, leflunomide, hydroxychloroquine, and azathioprine. Cyclophosphamide and cyclosporine have also been used to treat this condition.[13]
- There is also evidence supporting the use of TNF-α inhibitors and bisphosphonates, with efficacy for both skin lesions and arthritis.[13] This is based on the observed levels of proinflammatory cytokines in MRH tissues and association with osteoclastic activity as previously mentioned.

LYSOSOMAL STORAGE DISEASES

GENERAL PRINCIPLES

- There are almost 50 lysosomal storage diseases (LSDs), which are generally classified by the nature of the primary stored material involved.
- LSDs affect mostly children; however, those with a mild or attenuated form may look "normal" and present later in life with rheumatic symptoms.
- Gaucher's disease and Fabry's disease are two of the more common LSDs with musculoskeletal manifestations. They will be briefly reviewed, but further details are beyond the scope of this manual.

GAUCHER'S DISEASE

GENERAL PRINCIPLES

Definition

Gaucher's disease is an **autosomal recessive** disease of **glucocerebrosidase deficiency**.

Epidemiology

It is difficult to assess the incidence of Gaucher's worldwide as only certain countries have reported their numbers. The incidence also varies significantly by country. For example, Australia has reported their incidence to be 1:57,000,[14] whereas the Netherlands has reported their incidence to be 1:86,000.[15] All agree, however, Gaucher's is more commonly seen in the Ashkenazi Jewish population.[16]

Pathophysiology

Mutations in the glucocerebrosidase gene located on chromosome 1q21 cause glucocerebrosidase deficiency.[17] This leads to accumulation of glucocerebroside within the lysosomes of macrophages that circulate through the reticuloendothelial system depositing in liver, spleen, lymph nodes, bone marrow, and other organs.

DIAGNOSIS

Clinical Manifestations

- Presentation can be variable and because of this, patients have been classified into three different variants:
  - Type 1: (non-neuropathic variant) is the most common form and is characterized by hepatomegaly, splenomegaly, anemia, and thrombocytopenia.
  - Type 2: The most severe variant. Symptoms present within the first year of life with oculomotor dysfunction, seizures, and rigidity. Some may also develop ichthyosis.[18]
  - Type 3: Presents in childhood, typically later than Type 2. Can manifest with neurologic, hematologic, cardiac, and skeletal abnormalities along with hepatosplenomegaly.
- Patients have infiltration of bone marrow by lipid-laden macrophages (Gaucher cells), which lead to long bone pain from **osteonecrosis**, as well as **osteopenia, osteoporosis, and fractures**. Patients can also develop acute "bone crises" because of sudden ischemia of infiltrated bone.[19]

Diagnostic Testing

- Diagnosis is confirmed by measuring enzyme activity in circulating lymphocytes. It is suspected when Gaucher cells are seen on bone marrow biopsy.
- Radiographic findings are commonly seen in Gaucher's. In the Gaucher registry that evaluated almost 1,700 patients, the most common radiographic bone manifestations were Erlenmeyer flask deformity (46%), osteopenia (42%), marrow infiltration (40%), infarction (25%), avascular necrosis (25%), and multiple manifestations (59%).[18]

TREATMENT

Treatment is with enzyme replacement therapy with modified glucocerebrosidases. Enzyme replacement is effective in diminishing hematologic findings. Bone pain and disease decrease with enzyme replacement.[20]

FABRY'S DISEASE

GENERAL PRINCIPLES

Definition

Fabry's disease is an X-linked lipid storage disease caused by deficiency of lysosomal hydrolase α-galactosidase A (αGalA).

Pathophysiology

Mutations in the *Gal* gene at Xq22 lead to deficiency of the lysosomal hydrolase αGalA.[21] This leads to accumulation of glycosphingolipids, specifically globotriaosylceramide (Gb3), in nerves, viscera, skin, cornea, and cardiac and renal tissues.

DIAGNOSIS

Clinical Manifestations

- Disease manifestations include cornea verticillata, angiokeratomas, abdominal pain as well as progressive cardiac, cerebrovascular, and renal disease.
- A significant portion of patients with Fabry's also experience acroparesthesia, which is burning limb pain, often affecting peripheral joints. Fever can also accompany the pain

and can be mistaken for Juvenile Idiopathic Arthritis (JIA), RA, or rheumatic fever. The symptoms are often brought on by physical exertion, stress, or extremes in temperature.[21,22]

Diagnostic Testing

Diagnosis of Fabry's is confirmed in males by measuring αGalA activity in circulating leukocytes. By contrast, female carriers must be tested for genetic mutational analysis of the GLA gene because their levels of αGalA can vary and in some cases can be near normal.

TREATMENT

Early diagnosis is important because enzyme replacement therapy with recombinant agalsidase α or β can provide benefit when initiated prior to the development of end-organ damage.[23,24]

REFERENCES

1. Bacon BR, Adams PC, Kowdley KV, et al. Diagnosis and management of hemochromatosis: 2011 practice guideline by the American Association for the Study of Liver Diseases. *Hepatology.* 2011;54:328–343.
2. Richette P, Bardin T, Doherty M. An update on the epidemiology of calcium pyrophosphate dehydrate crystal deposition disease. *Rheumatology (Oxford).* 2009;48:711–715.
3. Carroll GJ, Breidahl WH, Olynyk JK. Characteristics of the arthropathy described in hereditary hemochromatosis. *Arthritis Care Res (Hoboken).* 2012;64:9–14.
4. European Association for Study of Liver. EASL clinical practice guidelines: Wilson's disease. *J Hepatol.* 2012;56:671–685.
5. Golding DN, Walshe JM. Arthropathy of Wilson's disease. Study of clinical and radiological features in 32 patients. *Ann Rheum Dis.* 1977;36:99–111.
6. Phornphutkul C, Introne WJ, Perry MB, et al. Natural history of alkaptonuria. *N Engl J Med.* 2002;347:2111–2121.
7. Monnoni A, Selvi E, Lorenzini S, et al. Alkaptonuria, ochronosis, and ochronotic arthropathy. *Semin Arthritis Rheum.* 2004;33:239–248.
8. Ranganath LR, Milan AM, Hughes AT, et al. Suitability Of Nitisinone In Alkaptonuria 1 (SONIA 1): an international, multicentre, randomised, open-label, no-treatment controlled, parallel-group, dose-response study to investigate the effect of once daily nitisinone on 24-h urinary homogentisic acid excretion in patients with alkaptonuria after 4 weeks of treatment. *Ann Rheum Dis.* 2016;75:362–367.
9. Ranganath LR, Khedr M, Milan AM, et al. Nitisinone arrests ochronosis and decreases rate of progression of Alkaptonuria: Evaluation of the effect of nitisinone in the United Kingdom National Alkaptonuria Centre. *Mol Genet Metab.* 2018;125(1–2):127–134.
10. https://clinicaltrials.gov/ct2/show/NCT01916382. Accessed February 13, 2019.
11. Islam AD, Naguwa SM, Cheema GS, et al. Multicentric reticulohistiocytosis: a rare yet challenging disease. *Clin Rev Allergy Immunol.* 2013;45(2):281–289
12. Trotta F, Colina M. Multicentric reticulohistiocytosis and fibroblastic rheumatism. *Best Pract Res Clin Rheumatol.* 2012;26:543–557.
13. Selmi C, Greenspan A, Huntley A, et al. Multicentric reticulohistiocytosis: a critical review. *Curr Rheumatol Rep.* 2015;17(6):511.
14. Meikle PJ, Hopwood JJ, Clague AE, et al. Prevalence of lysosomal storage disorders. *JAMA.* 1999;281(3):249–254.
15. Poorthuis BJ, Wevers RA, Kleijer WJ, et al. The frequency of lysosomal storage diseases in The Netherlands. *Hum Genet.*1999;105(1–2):151–156.
16. Meikle PJ, Fuller M, Hopwood JJ. Gaucher disease: epidemiology and screening policy. In: Futerman AH, Zimran A eds. *Gaucher Disease.* CRC Press, Boca Raton, FL, 2007:321.
17. Zimran A, Elstein D. Gaucher disease and related lysosomal storage diseases. In: Kaushansky K, Lichtman M, Prchal J, eds. *Williams Hematology.* 9th ed. New York, NY: McGraw-Hill; 2016.

18. Gupta N, Oppenheim IM, Kauvar EF, et al. Type 2 Gaucher disease: phenotypic variation and genotypic heterogeneity. *Blood Cells Mol Dis.* 2011;46(1):75.
19. Charrow J, Andersson HC, Kaplan P, et al. The Gaucher registry: demographics and disease characteristics of 1698 patients with Gaucher disease. *Arch Intern Med.* 2000;160:2835–2843.
20. Weinreb NJ, Goldblatt J, Villalobos J, et al. Long-term clinical outcomes in type 1 Gaucher disease following 10 years of imiglucerase treatment. *J Inherit Metab Dis.* 2013;36:543–553.
21. Masson C, Cissé I, Simon V, Insalaco P, Audran M. Fabry disease: a review. *Joint Bone Spine.* 2004;71(5):381–383.
22. Manger B, Mengel E, Schaefer RM. Rheumatologic aspects of lysosomal storage diseases. *Clin Rheumatol.* 2007;26(3):335–341.
23. Germain DP, Charrow J, Desnick RJ, et al. Ten-year outcome of enzyme replacement therapy with agalsidase beta in patients with Fabry disease. *J Med Genet.* 2015;52:353–358.
24. Rombach SM, Smid BE, Bouwman MG, et al. Long term enzyme replacement therapy for Fabry disease: effectiveness on kidney, heart and brain. *Orphanet J Rare Dis.* 2013;8:47.

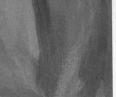

Amyloidosis and Amyloid Arthropathy

48

Colin Diffie and Vladimir Despotovic

GENERAL PRINCIPLES

- Amyloidosis is a heterogeneous disorder characterized by deposition of various protein subunits in extracellular tissue.
- Amyloidosis is an occasional cause of musculoskeletal complaints and a serious complication of rheumatologic disease.
- Currently, 36 different proteins have been identified as causes of amyloidosis. Amyloid can be found in a systemic disease, which is the focus of this chapter. It may also be **localized amyloidosis**, such as neurofibrillary tangles isolated to the central nervous system (CNS) in Alzheimer's disease.[1]
- There are four major classes of **systemic amyloidosis.** However, only amyloid light chain (AL [primary]) and amyloid A (AA [secondary]) systemic amyloidosis will be discussed in detail here. Hereditary amyloidosis and dialysis-related amyloid β-2-microglobulin (AB2M) are the remaining two types.
- **Amyloid arthropathy** is rare but occurs in up to 5% of patients with AL amyloidosis.

Definition/Classification

- Amyloid fibrils are extracellular insoluble polymers comprising various low-molecular-weight protein subunits. These undergo a conformational change into insoluble antiparallel β-pleated sheets that deposit in tissues.
- **AL amyloidosis**
  - Also known as **immunoglobulin light chain** or **primary** amyloidosis
  - This group includes all forms of systemic amyloidosis in which the fibrils are derived from **monoclonal light chains.** Causal conditions include monoclonal gammopathy of undetermined significance (**MGUS**), multiple myeloma (**MM**), and Waldenström's macroglobulinemia (WM).
  - It may be distinguished from a similar disorder, **light chain deposition disease** (LCDD), by the fact that fibril formation of monoclonal light chains does not occur in LCDD.
- **AA amyloidosis** also known as **serum amyloid A (SAA)** or **secondary** amyloidosis
- It is characterized by extracellular tissue deposition of fragments of SAA. SAA is an **acute-phase reactant** that can pathologically accumulate in uncontrolled inflammatory diseases.

Epidemiology

- AL amyloidosis is more common in developed countries and AA amyloidosis is more common in developing countries, where chronic infections are more prevalent and where treatment of chronic inflammatory diseases is more challenging.
- AL amyloidosis has a prevalence of around 10 per 1,000,000.

Pathophysiology

- Except in Alzheimer's disease, where direct cell cytotoxicity from amyloid is observed, other systemic manifestations and organ dysfunction from amyloidosis are thought to be secondary to mechanical disruption by the amyloid plaques.

- Disease manifestations depend on the tissue distribution, concentration of deposits, and specific precursor protein leading to fibril formation.
- **Primary amyloidosis is a clonal plasma cell proliferative disorder** that results in monoclonal **light chain** fibril deposition in multiple organs. Seventy-five percent are derived from the λ light chain variable region, and the remaining 25% are derived from the κ light chain variable region.
- **Secondary amyloidosis** is characterized by extracellular tissue deposition of fragments of an acute-phase reactant protein, SAA.
- **Hemodialysis-related amyloidosis** is a result of β-2-microglobulin deposition.

Risk Factors

- AA and AL amyloidosis are both related to conditions discussed below.
- Hereditary amyloid
  - Most familial mutations are autosomal dominant missense mutations that alter the precursor proteins.
  - Almost all hereditary mutations cause kidney, nervous system, and cardiac disease.
  - A significantly higher prevalence of these diseases is seen in patients of Turkish descent.
- Dialysis-related amyloid
  - The result of β-2-microglobulin deposition
  - This is more common with patients using low-flux or bioincompatible dialysis membranes. It is much less common with modern dialysis machines. It is therefore seen more often in developing nations.[2]
- The longer a patient has been on dialysis, the higher the risk.

Associated Conditions

- AL amyloid is often associated with **plasma cell dyscrasias.** Most classically, MM t(11;14) (q13;32) translocation is frequently found in MM or MGUS patients.
- Secondary amyloid is associated with **systemic inflammatory conditions.** One large UK-based study[3] identified the following etiologies:
  - It was associated with inflammatory arthritis in 60% of patients. This is most commonly rheumatoid arthritis but also includes juvenile idiopathic arthritis and seronegative spondyloarthropathies.
  - Chronic infections, such as bronchiectasis, tuberculosis (TB), or osteomyelitis, were associated in 15%.
  - Periodic fevers were associated in 10%, especially Familial Mediterranean Fever.
- It is less commonly seen as a complication of Crohn's disease (5%), non-Hodgkin's lymphoma, Castleman's disease, and injection drug abuse.

DIAGNOSIS

Amyloidosis may be diagnosed in the appropriate clinical setting, but definitive diagnosis requires tissue biopsy.

Clinical Presentation

- Primary amyloidosis most classically presents with **nephrotic range proteinuria** (from deposition of fibrils in the glomerulus), **edema, hepatosplenomegaly, heart failure, and carpal tunnel syndrome.**
  - CNS disease is almost never seen, but peripheral neuropathy and autonomic instability may occur.
  - **Cardiac involvement** is insidious and often advanced at the time of diagnoses. It may result in **restrictive cardiomyopathy.**
  - The most common **gastrointestinal (GI) manifestations** are stomach and small intestinal bleeding from ulcers, polyps, or hematomas, and motility disorders such as dysphagia, gastroparesis, constipation, or pseudo-obstruction.

- AA amyloid most classically presents with nephrotic range proteinuria.[3]
  - Ninety-seven percent will have renal involvement; 11% have end-stage renal disease (ESRD).
  - Cardiac involvement is rare, occurring in 1% of amyloid patients.
  - Hepatic involvement occurs in a quarter and results in hepatomegaly in 9%.
- Hemodialysis-related amyloid (AB2M) most commonly presents with musculoskeletal complaints such as shoulder pain, tendonitis, and nerve entrapment syndromes such as carpal tunnel syndrome. Less commonly, it may present with GI-predominant symptoms.
- **Amyloid arthropathy is most commonly seen in patients with primary amyloidosis** and usually does not occur in patients with inflammatory arthritis.[4]
  - Patients will typically describe symmetric **noninflammatory arthralgias** affecting the metacarpophalangeal joints (MCPs), proximal interphalangeal joints (PIPs), wrists, shoulders, and knees without morning stiffness.
  - Case reports exist of erosive disease but are rare.
  - Muscular deposition may lead to pseudohypertrophy, causing classic **macroglossia** (23%) or a positive **shoulder pad sign** (2%).

History

The clinical presentation is highly variable, depending on the type of amyloidosis and the systems involved. Symptoms may include:

- Constitutional symptoms of fatigue, weight loss, anorexia, and early satiety.
- Cardiovascular symptoms such as palpitations, dyspnea, or lower extremity edema are prominent in AL amyloidosis. Edema can occur from nephrotic syndrome in AL or AA amyloid.
- Syncope can be a symptom of autonomic instability or of cardiac involvement. It is a very poor prognostic factor if it is because of cardiac disease.
- GI involvement in AL amyloid can cause hematemesis, melena, or bloody stool.
- Enlarged muscles, especially the deltoids or tongue.
- Neurologic manifestations including decreased fine touch sensation and nerve entrapment syndromes, most classically **carpal tunnel syndrome.**
- Cutaneous manifestations including waxy skin papules and easy bruising, especially of the face.

Physical Examination

Similarly, the physical findings vary with the organ system involved and may include:

- **Macroglossia** and visible indentations on the tongue where it abuts the teeth.
- Patients may have visible swelling around the glenohumeral joint, giving a positive **shoulder pad sign** reflecting amyloid deposition. This is rare but specific for AL amyloidosis.
- Abnormal heart rate or rhythm, S3, elevated jugular venous distention (JVD), or holosystolic murmur (tricuspid or mitral regurgitation).
- Palpable hepatomegaly occurs in both AL and AA amyloid. Splenomegaly or ascites can occur. Lower extremity edema can occur from renal or cardiac failure.
- Decreased peripheral sensation, with or without focal weakness.
- Waxy papules most commonly located on the face, neck, groin, armpits, perianal area, tongue, external auditory canals; hair loss.

Diagnostic Criteria

- **Primary amyloidosis** should be suspected when classic history and physical examination findings occur along with typical organ involvement in the setting of a serum or urine monoclonal protein or free light chains (FLCs).[5]
- Diagnostic criteria for systemic AL amyloidosis are presented in Table 48-1.[6]
- **Secondary amyloidosis:** Biopsy staining positive by immunohistochemical methods and electron microscopy with anti-AA serum and absence of AL amyloid. Laboratory testing is of no confirmatory utility but is useful in ruling out AL amyloid and related disorders. The vast majority of patients have renal disease.

TABLE 48-1	**DIAGNOSTIC CRITERIA FOR PRIMARY SYSTEMIC AMYLOIDOSIS**

All of the following four criteria are required:

- Presence of amyloid-related systemic syndrome (e.g., renal, heart, liver, or peripheral nerve)
- Positive amyloid staining by Congo red from any biopsied tissue (under polarized light amyloid protein glows green after staining with Congo red)
- Immunohistochemical staining for light chain amyloid
- Evidence of monoclonal plasma cell proliferative disorder: serum or urine electrophoresis with a monoclonal protein, disproportionate light chain ratio (normal total serum κ to λ ratio is approximately 2, normal free serum κ to λ ratio 0.26–1.65), or clonal plasma cells on bone marrow biopsy

Adapted from: Rajkumar SV, Dispenzieri A, Kyle RA. Monoclonal gammopathy of undetermined significance, Waldenström macroglobulinemia, AL amyloidosis, and related plasma cell disorders: diagnosis and treatment. *Mayo Clin Proc.* 2006;81:693–703.

Diagnostic Testing

Laboratories
- Primary amyloidosis
  - **Immunofixation** will identify 90% of patients.
  - **Serum protein electrophoresis (SPEP)** will reveal a **monoclonal paraprotein**.
  - **Urine protein electrophoresis (UPEP)** will reveal **monoclonal light chains**.
  - **Serum FLC analysis** may identify monoclonal FLC in patients who fail to have a positive SPEP or UPEP.[5]
- Synovial fluid from patients with amyloid arthropathy shows a mononuclear predominance with a mean white cell count of 2,000 to 3,000.
- Secondary amyloidosis has no specific serum or urine laboratory testing that will reveal the diagnosis.

Electrocardiography
There are changes seen in patients with cardiac amyloidosis.
- Most common abnormality is decreased voltage in limb leads.
- Conduction abnormalities (e.g., first-, second-, or third-degree heart block), nonspecific intraventricular conduction delay, atrial fibrillation or flutter, ventricular tachycardia, or pseudoinfarct patterns.[7]

Imaging
- **Radiography** in amyloid arthropathy
  - Preservation or widening of joint space without periarticular erosions or bone cysts. Amyloid bone erosions are generally extra-articular.[8]
  - Soft-tissue swelling and bone demineralization.
  - Lytic lesions may be seen if arthropathy is associated with MM.
- Transthoracic **echocardiography**[7]:
  - Amyloid infiltration into the myocardium causes increased echogenicity, giving a "**granular sparkling**" appearance to the myocardium under echocardiography.
  - **Left ventricular wall thickening with diastolic dysfunction** is the most commonly observed abnormality. With advanced disease, restrictive cardiomyopathy may be seen with a normal to small left ventricle, biatrial enlargement, and right ventricular dilation. Mitral and aortic valve thickening may also occur.
- Nuclear scintigraphy with radiolabeled serum amyloid P can measure the extent of amyloid deposition but is not available in most countries.[9]

Diagnostic Procedures
- **Tissue biopsy** is required for the diagnosis of primary or secondary amyloidosis.
- **Abdominal fat pad biopsy** has a relatively high sensitivity (up to 80%) and specificity (up to 99%) for identifying primary and secondary amyloidosis in patients with multi-organ involvement.[6]
- Kidney and liver biopsy will be positive in about 90% of patients but is invasive and, therefore, not recommended as first line.
- If the above sites are negative and the diagnosis is still in question, **a rectal, bone marrow, or skin biopsy** may be considered.
- Amyloid fibers stained with **Congo red** will produce **green birefringence** under polarized light. Fibers stained with thioflavin T will produce yellow-green fluorescence.
- **Immunohistochemical staining and immunofluorescence** microscopy will reveal κ or λ light chains in AL amyloidosis.

TREATMENT

Regardless of the type of amyloid, the goal of treatment is to decrease fibril production and extracellular deposition as well as target the specific disease etiology. Novel therapies targeting removal of the amyloid deposits from the affected tissues are in development.

Medications
- **Primary amyloidosis**
  ○ Treatment should be directed by an experienced hematologist. Generally, patients are considered for **hematopoietic stem cell transplantation** (HSCT) to eliminate the pathologic clonal cells. Decision-making regarding this therapy is complex, and most amyloidosis patients are not candidates because of advanced age and advanced disease at the time of diagnosis.
  ○ In patients who are not candidates for HSCT, patients can be treated with a regimen of melphalan, bortezomib, and dexamethasone or with a regimen of cyclophosphamide, bortezomib, and dexamethasone.[10]
- **Amyloid arthropathy** is managed by treating the underlying amyloidosis. For patients with refractory symptoms, nonsteroidal anti-inflammatory drugs (NSAIDs) or steroids can be used, either intra-articular or systemic.
- **Secondary amyloidosis:**
  ○ **Control of the primary inflammatory disease** to stabilize and possibly reduce amyloid burden is important. In general, attaining adequate control of the primary disease is the most important prognostic factor. Depending on the inflammatory disease, this may be done with immunosuppressive, cytotoxic, or biologic medications.
  ○ **Tocilizumab**, a humanized anti-interleukin (IL)-6 receptor antibody, quickly normalizes serum C-reactive protein (CRP) and SAA levels. In one study of Rheumatoid Arthritis (RA) patients with amyloid, tocilizumab was better than tumor necrosis factor (TNF) inhibitors at normalizing SAA levels and at improving glomerular filtration rate (GFR).[11]
  ○ **Colchicine** is commonly used in Familial Mediterranean Fever (FMF), with only 2% of compliant patients developing amyloidosis after 10 years of therapy compared to 50% of noncompliant patients. Use of colchicine for amyloidosis secondary to other etiologies is questionable.[12]
  ○ Disease-specific treatment is recommended in other **autoinflammatory syndromes**.
  ○ **Dimethyl sulfoxide (DMSO)** has been investigated as an alternative therapy, but studies are limited to animal models and small case series.
  ○ For infectious etiologies, antibiotics and removal of infected tissue are helpful.

Other Nonpharmacologic Therapies

Physical therapy and occupational therapy are useful in amyloid arthropathy.

Surgical Management

- Organ transplantation for failure or complications (kidney, heart, liver)
- Surgical resection of enlarged tissue (e.g., tongue)
- Carpal tunnel and other peripheral nerve releases
- Joint replacement

PATIENT EDUCATION

Amyloidosis Foundation (www.amyloidosis.org)

OUTCOME/PROGNOSIS

- Survival in **AL amyloidosis** may be months or years depending on the organs affected, bone marrow involvement, and circulating plasma cell percentages.
  - The main causes of death are **cardiac dysfunction, infection, and hepatic failure.**
  - Primary amyloidosis is often diagnosed after identification of the blood cell dyscrasias. Progression to MM after the diagnosis of primary amyloidosis is rare.
- Treatment of the underlying disorder can lead to favorable outcomes in **AA amyloidosis.**[3]
  - Serum GFR may improve in chronic kidney disease (CKD), but most patients with ESRD will still require dialysis.
  - On serial scintigraphy of treated patients, 12% had progressive SAA deposition, 48% had stable disease burden, and 39% had improved SAA deposition. Lower serum SAA concentrations correlated with less tissue-level deposition.

REFERENCES

1. Sipe JD, Benson MD, Buxbaum JN, et al. Nomenclature 2014: Amyloid fibril proteins and clinical classification of the amyloidosis. *Amyloid.* 2014;21:221–224.
2. Jadoul M, Drueke TB. beta2 microglobulin amyloidosis: an update 30 years later. *Nephrol Dial Transplant.* 2016;31:507–509.
3. Lachmann HJ, Goodman HJ, Gilbertson JA, et al. Natural history and outcome in systemic AA amyloidosis. *N Engl J Med.* 2007;356:2361–2371.
4. Prokaeva T, Spencer B, Kaut M, et al. Soft tissue, joint, and bone manifestations of AL amyloidosis: Clinical presentation, molecular features, and survival. *Arthritis Rheum.* 2007;56:3858–3868.
5. Katzmann JA, Clark RJ, Abraham RS, et al. Serum reference intervals and diagnostic ranges for free kappa and free lambda immunoglobulin light chains: relative sensitivity for detection of monoclonal light chains. *Clin Chem.* 2002;48:1437–1444.
6. Rajkumar SV, Dispenzieri A, Kyle RA. Monoclonal gammopathy of undetermined significance, Waldenström macroglobulinemia, AL amyloidosis, and related plasma cell disorders: diagnosis and treatment. *Mayo Clin Proc.* 2006;81:693–703.
7. Grogan M, Dispenzieri A. Natural history and therapy of AL cardiac amyloidosis. *Heart Fail Rev.* 2015;20:155–162.
8. Elsaman AM, Radwan AR, Akmatov MK, et al. Amyloid arthropathy associated with multiple myeloma: a systematic analysis of 101 reported cases. *Semin Arthritis Rheum.* 2013;43:405–412.
9. Hazenberg BP, van Rijswijk MH, Piers DA, et al. Diagnostic performance of 123I-labeled serum amyloid P component scintigraphy in patients with amyloidosis. *Am J Med.* 2006;119:355.
10. Wechalekar AD, Hawkins PN, Gillmore JD. Perspectives in treatment of AL amyloidosis. *Br J Haematol.* 2008;140:365–377.
11. Okuda Y, Ohnishi M, Matoba K, et al. Comparison of the clinical utility of tocilizumab and anti-TNF therapy in AA amyloidosis complicating rheumatic diseases. *Mod. Rheumatol.* 2014;24:137–143.
12. Zemer D, Pras M, Sohar E, et al. Colchicine in the prevention and treatment of the amyloidosis of familial Mediterranean fever. *N Engl J Med.* 1986;314:1001–1005.

Sarcoid Arthropathy

Michiko Inaba and Vladimir Despotovic

49

GENERAL PRINCIPLES

Definition

- Sarcoidosis is a **granulomatous inflammatory disease** of unknown etiology that can involve any organ, most commonly the lung, skin, eye, and joints.
- The **lung is the most commonly involved organ,** with pulmonary involvement occurring in over 80% of patients. Patients usually present with fatigue and pulmonary symptoms (e.g., cough, dyspnea, and chest pain).
- Extrapulmonary involvement frequently accompanies the pulmonary symptoms. Lymph nodes, liver, and spleen are frequently involved. Heart, kidney, and pancreas are less commonly involved.[1]
- The disease remits within 3 years in most patients and about 10% to 30% of patients develop a chronic form of the disease and require ongoing treatment.
- This chapter will focus mainly on the musculoskeletal manifestations of sarcoidosis, which occur in 15% to 25% of patients.[2]

Classification

- Arthritic syndromes of sarcoidosis may involve the joints, muscles, and bones, causing a variety of musculoskeletal complaints through different mechanisms and can be categorized as acute or chronic.[3]
- **Acute sarcoid arthritis** occurs most commonly as a polyarthritis of the ankles, knees, elbows, and wrists, and often occurs concomitantly with bilateral hilar lymphadenopathy, uveitis, and erythema nodosum as a part of Löfgren's syndrome.
- Involvement is usually **symmetrical,** and **periarticular swelling,** rather than joint effusions, is common. Acute arthritis usually lasts several weeks to months and often does not recur.
- **Löfgren's syndrome** is the triad of acute arthritis, erythema nodosum, and bilateral hilar adenopathy. It is usually self-limiting and has a good prognosis.
- **Chronic sarcoid arthritis** is rare, presenting several months after the onset of disease.
  - It commonly involves the knees but also can involve the ankles, wrists, proximal interphalangeal (PIP) and metacarpophalangeal (MCP) joints. This form of arthritis is not associated with erythema nodosum.
  - In contrast to acute arthritis, chronic arthritis in sarcoidosis usually occurs in the setting of more diffuse organ involvement and occurs at an older age.
  - It can mimic rheumatoid arthritis in clinical presentation.
  - Rarely, chronic arthritis can present as Jaccoud's arthropathy, sarcoid dactylitis, as well as arthritis because of granulomatous synovitis or adjacent sarcoid bony lesions.[4]
  - Joint destruction can occur very rarely with shortening and deformity of the phalanges.
- **Muscle and bone involvement** is relatively common in sarcoidosis.
- Osseous sarcoidosis occurs in 3% to 13% of patients with sarcoidosis. The hands and feet are the most frequent sites of involvement, whereas the spine is less commonly affected. Only about half of patients with bony lesions have pain and stiffness, whereas the other half remain asymptomatic.

- Sarcoidosis affects muscle (less than 5% of sarcoidosis cases) in the form of **myopathy, atrophy, myositis, or palpable nodules.** Asymptomatic granulomatous involvement of the muscles is documented frequently at autopsy.
- Sarcoidosis causes **lytic and sclerotic lesions in the bone,** both of which can be painful. Along with bone resorption, the lesions contribute to a high risk of fracture in sarcoid patients.

Epidemiology

- The prevalence of sarcoidosis is 10 to 20 cases/100,000 population.
- The incidence is higher among blacks than other races.
- The disease also varies by geographic region and may have a genetic component.
- Sarcoidosis occurs most commonly in patients aged 20 to 40 years.

Etiology

The underlying etiology of sarcoidosis is not known. Evidence exists for genetic, environmental, and infectious associations.[5]

Pathophysiology

- Sarcoidosis is characterized pathologically by the presence of **noncaseating granulomas.** This process has been best characterized in the lung.
- Granulomas consist of a dense collection of epithelioid macrophages and CD4+ T cells, with fewer CD8+ T cells restricted to the periphery.
- Over time, the granulomas can heal without sequelae or undergo fibrosis, leading to organ dysfunction.

Associated Conditions

Sarcoidosis has been described in association with other autoimmune disorders, including rheumatoid arthritis, systemic lupus erythematosus, Sjögren's syndrome, and psoriatic arthritis.

DIAGNOSIS

Clinical Presentation

- Clinical manifestations of sarcoidosis vary depending on which organ systems are involved. It may be easy to diagnose sarcoidosis in a patient with bilateral hilar adenopathy, pulmonary infiltrates, or characteristic skin and eye involvement but more difficult if arthritis is the only manifestation.
- A thorough history and physical examination is important to identify any extra-articular manifestations that can lead to the proper diagnosis.
- Bone involvement in chronic arthritis is commonly asymptomatic, but pain and soft-tissue swelling over affected areas (joints or bones) can occur.
- Skin lesions may be the first manifestation to occur. They most commonly present as papules around the eyelids and nasolabial folds or in old scars. Larger subcutaneous nodules, plaques, or indurated purplish facial lesions (**lupus pernio**) may also occur.

Differential Diagnosis

- The differential diagnosis will vary depending on the symptoms manifested by individual patients.
- Patients with Löfgren's syndrome have primarily a lower extremity–predominant inflammatory arthritis, which may also be seen in reactive arthritis or infectious arthritides (viral, gonococcal). Septic arthritis should always be considered if monoarticular or acute in nature.

- In patients with significant lymphadenopathy, **infections and malignancy** should be excluded.
- Sarcoidosis can also manifest with pulmonary infiltrates, myositis, and vasculitis and rheumatologic causes of those symptoms should be considered as well.

Diagnostic Testing

Laboratories
- Erythrocyte sedimentation rate (ESR) and C-reactive protein (CRP) can be elevated but are not specific for sarcoidosis.
- Serum **angiotensin-converting enzyme (ACE) levels** are high in up to three-fourths of untreated patients, including in 15% of acute sarcoid arthritis and up to 50% of chronic sarcoid arthritis; however, false positives occur frequently and **limit diagnostic utility.**
- **Hypercalcemia** and more often **hypercalciuria** occur because of dysregulated calcitriol (1,25-dihydroxyvitamin D) metabolism and its production in the granulomatous tissue.
- Serum 1,25-dihydroxyvitamin D levels may also be elevated.

Imaging
- Chest radiograph findings in sarcoidosis include **bilateral hilar lymphadenopathy, diffuse parenchymal changes,** or a combination of both. Computed tomography (CT) or magnetic resonance imaging (MRI) may be required to better characterize the lung and mediastinum, especially in a patient with suspected Löfgren's syndrome and a normal chest radiograph.[6]
- Joint radiographs in acute arthritis can be normal or show soft-tissue swelling. In patients with chronic arthritis or bone involvement, radiographs can be striking.
  - Characteristic bone involvement involves bilateral metacarpals, metatarsals, and phalanges, although any bone can be affected, even vertebrae.
  - Radiographs of affected hands show **subchondral lesions or cysts** that sometimes can extend into joint spaces. The bone itself can have a lacy reticulated appearance from granulomatous involvement.
  - MRI may be more sensitive to detect bony lesions from sarcoidosis; however, it can be difficult to distinguish from bony metastasis.
  - MRI of affected muscles shows nonspecific muscle edema or fatty atrophy and is not diagnostic.
  - Gallium-67 scanning and positron emission tomography (PET) scanning are useful in identifying muscles affected by granulomatous infiltration. PET scanning is useful in monitoring response to therapy.

Diagnostic Procedures
- **Biopsy** of the affected organ(s) is the most effective way to demonstrate the noncaseating granulomas.
  - Biopsy of lymph nodes, skin, and lacrimal glands often yields diagnostic histology.
  - Biopsy of lung tissue requires fiberoptic bronchoscopy with transbronchial lung biopsy. Open lung biopsy is usually not required.
  - When vertebral sarcoidosis is suspected without other features of sarcoidosis, a histopathologic confirmation is mandatory to exclude other possible causes, especially malignancy or tuberculosis.
  - Synovial biopsy occasionally reveals granulomas or nonspecific mononuclear infiltrates and synovial hypertrophy but is not often performed.[7]
- **Arthrocentesis** of an involved joint can be performed and is characterized by noninflammatory or only mildly inflammatory synovial fluid in both acute and chronic forms of arthritis.

TREATMENT

- The decision to start medications in patients with sarcoidosis should be based on clinical assessment of disease activity.
- For the acute arthritis seen in Löfgren's syndrome, nonsteroidal anti-inflammatory drugs (NSAIDs) are the first-line therapy and may be sufficient. In acute arthritis, there is a high likelihood of complete remission within weeks to months. Low-dose glucocorticoids are sometimes needed if the symptoms are not adequately controlled with NSAIDs.
- The decision to use glucocorticoids is typically guided by persistence of symptoms for greater than 2 to 3 months, and the type and severity of extra-articular disease (e.g., ocular involvement, significant cardiac involvement, neurologic impairment, or severe constitutional symptoms such as fevers, fatigue, and weight loss).
- Chronic arthritis may or may not be controlled with glucocorticoids alone and may require second-line agents.

Medications

There are no Food and Drug Administration (FDA)-approved treatments for extrapulmonary sarcoidosis. Large randomized clinical trials have not been performed and treatments are based on case reports and unblinded case series.

First Line

- Mild joint symptoms often can be controlled with NSAIDs.
- **Glucocorticoids** are effective for patients with moderate to severe symptoms, including musculoskeletal symptoms. Although glucocorticoid therapy clearly reduces inflammation and symptoms attributable to disease, there is a paucity of data regarding the optimal dose and duration of treatment.
  - For severe vital organ dysfunction, initial doses of prednisone 1 mg/kg/day PO for 4 to 6 weeks are used, followed by slow tapering.
  - Löfgren's syndrome can be treated with observation alone, NSAIDs, or low doses of prednisone (10–20 mg/day) depending on the severity of symptoms.
  - Disease can recur after withdrawal of steroids, requiring reinitiation of therapy.
  - In patients who have relapse of disease off prednisone or are unable to taper prednisone to a tolerable dose (5–10 mg/day), second-line agents should be considered.

Second Line

- **Methotrexate** has been successfully used to treat pulmonary and extrapulmonary manifestations of sarcoidosis at doses similar to those used in rheumatoid arthritis.
- **Antimalarials** (hydroxychloroquine and chloroquine) have also been used to treat extrapulmonary manifestations successfully.
- There may be a role for other medications such as leflunomide, sulfasalazine, and minocycline.
- **Anti–tumor necrosis factor (TNF) medications** are used as therapy in patients who have contraindications to or have not responded well to other treatments, although high-quality data for their use are lacking. Preliminary evidence suggests that infliximab and adalimumab may be efficacious in pulmonary and extrapulmonary sarcoidosis.[8,9] However, there are also case reports and series that demonstrate sarcoidosis (pulmonary and extrapulmonary) can develop in patients treated with these medications for other indications.

OUTCOME/PROGNOSIS

- Sarcoidosis **clears spontaneously** in approximately 50% to 90% of patients. Relapse is rare, and most (90%) of the patients have remission with few sequelae.

• Overall sarcoidosis-related mortality is less than 5%. Mortality is usually from the sequelae of long-term steroid use for progressive pulmonary or cardiac involvement.

REFERENCES

1. Rao DA, Dellaripa PF. Extrapulmonary manifestations of sarcoidosis. *Rheum Dis Clin North Am.* 2013;39(2):277–297.
2. Visser H, Vos K, Zanelli E, et al. Sarcoid arthritis: clinical characteristics, diagnostic aspects, and risk factors. *Ann Rheum Dis.* 2002;61(6):499–504.
3. Sweiss N, Patterson K, Sawaqued R, et al. Rheumatologic manifestations of sarcoidosis. *Semin Respir Crit Care Med.* 2010;31:463–473.
4. Lima I, Ribeiro DS, Cesare A, et al. Typical Jaccoud's arthropathy in a patient with sarcoidosis. *Rheumatol Int.* 2013;33(6):1615–1617.
5. Ungprasert P, Crowson CS, Maeson EL. Epidemiology and clinical characteristics of sarcoidosis: an update from a population-based cohort study from Olmsted County, Minnesota. *Rheumatism.* 2017;69:16–22.
6. Pitt P, Hamilton EB, Innes EH, et al. Sarcoid dactylitis. *Ann Rheum Dis.* 1983;42(6):634–639.
7. Keijsers RG, van den Heuvel DA, Grutters JC. Imaging the inflammatory activity of sarcoidosis. *Eur Respir J.* 2013;41:743–751.
8. Baughman RP, Drent M, Kavuru M, et al. Infliximab therapy in patients with chronic sarcoidosis and pulmonary involvement. *Am J Respir Crit Care Med.* 2006;174:795–802.
9. Clementine RR, Lyman J, Zakem J, et al. Tumor necrosis factor-alpha antagonist-induced sarcoidosis. *J Clin Rheumatol.* 2010;16:274–279.

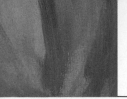

Cutaneous Conditions Associated with Rheumatic Disease

Christine N. Schafer and Heather A. Jones

INTRODUCTION

The skin is often a target organ in autoimmune disease and for that reason, a careful skin examination may yield the first clinical clue to the diagnosis of an internal, systemic inflammatory disorder.

PALPABLE PURPURA

GENERAL PRINCIPLES

Definition

Purpura is defined as visible hemorrhage into the skin or mucous membranes.

Classification

- There are many different types of purpura, with an extensive differential diagnosis largely based on morphology.
- Six major subsets include petechiae (<4 mm), macular purpura (5–9 mm), macular ecchymoses (>1 cm), palpable purpura, noninflammatory retiform purpura, and inflammatory retiform purpura. This section will focus on **palpable purpura**.[1]

Pathophysiology

Most cases of palpable purpura are caused by **leukocytoclastic vasculitis** (LCV), which is a **histologic term** referring to a specific pattern of inflammation that can involve both medium- and small-sized blood vessels (see Diagnostic Testing section, Pathology).

DIAGNOSIS

Clinical Presentation

- Palpable purpura presents with **raised, nonblanching violaceous papules and plaques** that can have prominent early erythema, which is because of underlying inflammatory cell infiltrate and extravasation of red cells from damaged vessels.
- Lesions are usually asymptomatic; however, burning, pain, or pruritus can be present.
- Associated clinical features are related to the underlying cause.

Differential Diagnosis

- LCV because of immune complex disease
  - **Infection:** Infective endocarditis, septic emboli, beta-hemolytic streptococci, *Neisseria* infections, *Rickettsia* infections (e.g., Rocky Mountain spotted fever, typhus), acute

viral infections (e.g., human immunodeficiency virus [HIV], hepatitis B and C, herpes simplex virus [HSV], and Epstein–Barr virus [EBV])
- ○ **Drug exposure:** Allopurinol, cephalosporins, hydralazine, minocycline, nonsteroidal anti-inflammatory drugs (NSAIDs), oral contraceptives, propylthiouracil, penicillins, phenytoin, and sulfonamides (including loop and thiazide diuretics)[2-4]
- ○ **Idiopathic immunoglobulin A (IgA) complex vasculitis**
  - Most commonly occurs in children in the setting of preceding respiratory infection, also referred to as Henoch–Schönlein purpura (Chapter 31)
  - Characterized **by IgA-dominant immune deposits** in walls of small blood vessels
  - IgA small vessel vasculitis in adults is uniquely associated with **solid-organ malignancy.** Although other forms of small vessel vasculitis are most commonly linked to hematologic malignancy, 60% to 90% of adults with neoplasm-associated IgA vasculitis will have cancer of a solid organ, particularly the lung.[5,6]
  - Adults with IgA vasculitis are also more likely to develop **chronic renal disease;** therefore, IgA staining on **direct immunofluorescence** (DIF) is important to guide prognosis and should prompt close monitoring of kidney function.[7]
- ○ **Hypergammaglobulinemic purpura of Waldenström**
- ○ **Urticarial vasculitis**
- ○ **Mixed cryoglobulinemia**
- ○ **Systemic lupus erythematosus (SLE), rheumatoid arthritis (RA), Sjögren's syndrome**
- **Pauci-immune LCV** (vessel damage is mediated by neutrophils rather than by immune complex deposition)
  - ○ **Mixed small- and medium-sized vessel vasculitis**
  - ○ **Antineutrophil cytoplasmic autoantibody (ANCA) associated**
    - Granulomatosis with polyangiitis (Chapter 28)
    - Microscopic polyangiitis (Chapter 30)
    - Eosinophilic granulomatosis with polyangiitis (Chapter 29)

Diagnostic Testing

- **With skin biopsy,** the classic histopathologic features of palpable purpura are LCV, which consists of a perivascular neutrophilic infiltrate, leukocytoclasis (nuclear dust), fibrin deposition within vessel walls, and red cell extravasation.
- Biopsy for DIF is helpful because **the presence of IgA** may provide prognostic information.
- **Special Note:** Leukemic vasculitis is a specific form of vasculitis mediated by a perivascular infiltrate of leukemic blast cells, as opposed to inflammatory cells. This is a rare manifestation of leukemia cutis and portends a poor prognosis.[8]

TREATMENT

Management of the underlying cause

LIVEDOID VASCULOPATHY

GENERAL PRINCIPLES

Definition

Livedoid vasculopathy, also known as **atrophie blanche,** is a chronic vascular occlusive disease of unclear etiology that results from the formation of microthrombi within superficial dermal blood vessels.[1]

Classification

There is a primary (idiopathic) form and a secondary form.

Associated Conditions

The secondary form has been associated **with chronic venous hypertension** and **hypercoagulable states,** such as factor V Leiden, deficiency of protein C or S, hyperhomocysteinemia, essential cryoglobulinemia, and antiphospholipid antibodies.[9–11]

DIAGNOSIS

Clinical Presentation

Livedoid vasculopathy presents with **painful, recurrent punched-out ulcers** favoring the lower extremities, especially the medial malleolus of the ankle and dorsum of the feet. Ulcers often heal with **white, atrophic circular scars** with peripheral telangiectasias. The disease has a predilection for **middle-aged females.**

Differential Diagnosis

Livedoid vasculopathy must first be distinguished from inflammatory vasculitis. History of ulceration should be used to distinguish this disorder from other conditions that can lead to atrophic scarring, such as venous stasis with varicosities.

Diagnostic Testing

With skin biopsy, histology shows hyaline thrombi in the lumen of small vessels with extravasated red cells in the upper and mid-dermis. A sparse perivascular lymphocytic infiltrate may be present, but there is **no vasculitis.**[10,11]

TREATMENT

No treatment has been shown to be consistently effective. One proposed therapeutic strategy is a step-wise approach that includes **smoking cessation**, low-dose **aspirin**, oral **pentoxifylline**, and oral **dipyridamole**. Management should otherwise be tailored to treat an underlying coagulopathy if indicated.[12]

ERYTHEMA NODOSUM

GENERAL PRINCIPLES

Definition

Erythema nodosum (EN) is the most common **panniculitis.**

Pathophysiology

- It is considered a delayed hypersensitivity response to a variety of antigenic stimuli, including bacteria, viruses, and chemical agents.[1,13,14]
- Majority of cases are idiopathic.

Associated Conditions

- **Infections** (e.g., *Streptococcus* most common; coccidioidomycosis, bacterial gastroenteritis)
- **Medications** (e.g., estrogens and oral contraceptives most common; sulfonamides, penicillin, rarely tumor necrosis factor [TNF] inhibitors)

- **Sarcoidosis** (Löfgren's syndrome is the triad of bilateral hilar lymphadenopathy, EN, and polyarthritis seen in acute sarcoidosis)
- **Inflammatory bowel disease** (IBD) (Crohn's disease has a stronger association than ulcerative colitis; EN may precede or accompany IBD flare)[15]
- **Spondyloarthropathies**
- **Malignancy** (most often acute myelogenous leukemia [AML])
- Interestingly, can be a **prognostic indicator** in certain disorders: associated with a more **self-limited form of sarcoidosis** and has a **protective effect** against disseminated disease in patients with **coccidioidomycosis**[1,13]

DIAGNOSIS

Clinical Presentation

EN presents with **tender, erythematous subcutaneous nodules** most commonly over the **bilateral tibial areas**. Rarely, the thighs and forearms are involved.[16] In later stages, lesions can have a bruise-like appearance. Unlike other forms of panniculitis, **EN does not ulcerate**. Systemic symptoms may occur, including **arthralgia, fever, and malaise**.

Differential Diagnosis

When lesions are few or present in atypical locations, EN may resemble other forms of panniculitis, such as pancreatic panniculitis and erythema induratum (nodular vasculitis).

Diagnostic Testing

Skin biopsy: EN is the prototype of a "septal" panniculitis with widened septa and little to no necrosis of the fat lobule. A neutrophilic septal infiltrate predominates in the acute phase, whereas mononuclear cells and granulomatous inflammation are seen in the chronic phase. Small collections of macrophages, called **Miescher's microgranulomas**, can be found within septa and are considered a pathognomonic feature of EN.[17]

TREATMENT

Identification and treatment of the underlying etiology is of primary importance. Symptomatic treatment includes **NSAIDs, salicylates** and **intralesional steroid injections**. Severe and unresponsive cases may require **oral glucocorticoids**. Oral **potassium iodide** may also be useful.[18]

CHOLESTEROL MICROEMBOLIZATION SYNDROME

GENERAL PRINCIPLES

Definition

Cholesterol microembolization syndrome (CES), also known as cholesterol emboli or warfarin blue toe syndrome, is caused by **embolization of lipid debris from an ulcerated atherosclerotic plaque**, generally from a large artery to smaller arterioles or end arteries.

Pathophysiology

Three clinical scenarios are known to prompt embolization

- **Arterial or coronary catheterization** or intervention including bypass surgery and intra-aortic balloon pump therapy. **Embolization occurs within hours to days of catheterization.**

- **Prolonged anticoagulation** may precipitate cholesterol emboli by dissolving protective thrombi coating a friable atheromatous plaque, permitting the release of cholesterol. **Cholesterol embolism typically occurs after 1 to 2 months of anticoagulant therapy.** Note that "Warfarin blue toe syndrome" is not restricted to anticoagulation with warfarin.[19]
- Acute thrombolytic therapy given for treatment of myocardial infarction or stroke may also result in cholesterol embolism. Typically, **embolism occurs within hours to days of lytic therapy.**

DIAGNOSIS

Clinical Presentation

- **Systemic features** are related to **ischemia** of organ(s) distal to the occlusion. Common symptoms include **fever, myalgia, altered mental status, affected limb pain**, and sudden-onset **arterial hypertension.**[1]
  - Frequently involved sites are the lower extremities (toes), intestine, pancreas, central nervous system (CNS), kidneys, spleen, liver, and bone marrow.
  - Up to 40% of patients have **acute renal failure** (ARF) at onset, as a direct result of preglomerular renal emboli, as well as an indirect inflammatory response to the emboli.
- **Cutaneous findings** are reported in 35% of patients with cholesterol embolism.[20]
  - The most common presentation is the **abrupt onset of distal livedo reticularis.**
  - Other findings include multiple sites of **peripheral gangrene, cyanosis, and** ulceration.
- Both cutaneous and systemic disease may be progressive because of repeated showers of emboli or secondary vascular inflammation induced by the emboli.

Differential Diagnosis

- Differential diagnosis includes all causes of retiform purpura or livedo reticularis including oxalate embolus, small or medium vessel vasculitis, thromboangiitis obliterans, cocaine-induced ischemia, disorders of cryoagglutination, septic vasculitis, and gangrene.
- A high threshold of suspicion is needed for making the diagnosis.

Diagnostic Testing

Laboratories
Laboratory findings include elevated erythrocyte sedimentation rate (ESR), C-reactive protein (CRP), serum creatinine, leukocytosis, and **peripheral blood eosinophilia**, which occur in up to 80% of cases.[21] Urine should be examined for eosinophils, proteinuria, and hyaline and granular casts.

Diagnostic Procedures
Skin biopsy: Histopathology is the gold standard for diagnosis. Routine staining reveals **biconvex, needle-shaped clefts** indicating the site of cholesterol crystals in arterioles and small arteries in the lower dermis or subcutis.[22]

TREATMENT

Medications

- Medical treatment is mainly supportive.
- Although no therapeutic standard exists, some advocate for the use of **aspirin** and other **antiplatelet agents, pentoxifylline**, and the discontinuation of anticoagulation.[19]
- Systemic glucocorticoids have a variable rate of response.
- Although some advocate for the initiation of anticoagulation in patients with severe renal failure, in other studies it has been shown to worsen outcomes.[19]

Surgical Management
- Surgical treatment includes bypass or endarterectomy to eliminate the source of embolism, as well as amputation or resection of gangrenous tissues to prevent infection.
- Angiographic confirmation of the embolic source is needed prior to removal of atheromatous lesions by endarterectomy, stenting, or bypass.

COMPLICATIONS

Prognosis remains guarded with significant mortality rates, limb-threatening consequences, and chronic renal failure.

PYODERMA GANGRENOSUM

GENERAL PRINCIPLES
Definition
Pyoderma gangrenosum (PG) is an uncommon, chronic **ulcerative, neutrophilic dermatosis.**

Classification
There are four major clinical variants: **ulcerative, bullous, pustular, and superficial granulomatous/vegetative.** Clinical variants have also been described based on location, such as **peristomal** and **genital.**

Pathophysiology
Although PG is idiopathic in 25% to 30% of patients, it is suspected to have an autoimmune pathogenesis given its **frequent association with systemic autoimmune diseases.**[23]

Associated Conditions
IBD, seronegative RA, pyogenic arthritis with PG and acne (PAPA syndrome), and hematologic disorders (IgA monoclonal gammopathy, AML, myelodysplasia)

DIAGNOSIS
Clinical Presentation
- The characteristic initial lesion is an inflammatory pustule or nodule that ulcerates and enlarges. The ulcers are **painful**, appear necrotic with **violaceous, undermined borders**, and may be as large as 20 cm. Cutaneous lesions occur most frequently on the **lower extremities.**
- Pathergy, in which trivial trauma initiates or aggravates existing lesions, is an important characteristic of PG. **Debridement may therefore worsen PG.**

Differential Diagnosis
- Differential diagnosis is broad and depends on the stage of the lesion. Other causes of ulceration must be excluded, namely, infection, vasculitis, and vasculopathy.
- Although PG remains a "diagnosis of exclusion," **diagnostic criteria** were recently created following a Delphi consensus of international experts.
- This Delphi exercise produced **one major criterion** and **eight minor criteria** for the diagnosis of ulcerative PG. Receiver operating characteristic analysis revealed that four of

eight minor criteria maximized discrimination, yielding sensitivity and specificity of 86% and 90%, respectively.[24]
- ○ **Major criterion:** Biopsy of ulcer edge demonstrating neutrophilic infiltrate
- ○ **Minor criteria**
  - Exclusion of infection
  - Pathergy
  - History of IBD or inflammatory arthritis
  - History of papule, pustule, or vesicle ulcerating within 4 days of appearing
  - Peripheral erythema, undermining border, and tenderness at ulceration site
  - Multiple ulcerations, at least one on an anterior lower leg
  - Cribriform or "wrinkled paper" scar(s) at healed ulcer sites
  - Decreased ulcer size within 1 month of initiating immunosuppressive medication(s)

Diagnostic Testing
- It is recommended that patients undergo skin biopsy as clinicopathologic correlation can aid in the diagnosis and exclude other etiologies.
- Histopathology can be nonspecific; however, biopsy of an ulcer edge showing **neutrophilic infiltrate** is highly suggestive of PG.

TREATMENT
- There is no consensus on gold-standard therapy for PG.
- If there is an underlying systemic disorder, then management of the associated disorder may result in improvement of PG.
- The current mainstay of treatment is **local** or **combined local and systemic glucocorticoid therapy** with or without **adjuvant systemic therapy**.[25]
- One recent randomized control trial demonstrated similar healing times with **cyclosporine** compared to prednisolone, making cyclosporine a promising treatment option.[26,27]
- Additionally, several studies suggest that there may be a potential role for **intravenous immunoglobulin** (IVIG) as adjuvant therapy for refractory PG. Prospective clinical trials are needed to further validate these findings.[28]
- Patients with **concurrent IBD** may specifically benefit from **TNF α inhibitors** (e.g., infliximab, adalimumab).[27,29]
- Other steroid-sparing agents include **dapsone, methotrexate, and azathioprine**.[25]

SWEET'S SYNDROME

GENERAL PRINCIPLES
Definition
Sweet's syndrome, also known as **acute febrile neutrophilic dermatosis**, is a rare **neutrophilic dermatosis** that may **occur in the setting of various systemic conditions.**

Classification
Sweet's syndrome can be divided into three subtypes based upon etiology:
- **Classical Sweet's syndrome** (idiopathic; can be associated with infections, IBD, pregnancy)
- **Malignancy-associated Sweet's syndrome** (accounts for 20% of cases; most commonly associated with hematologic disease)[30]
- **Drug-induced Sweet's syndrome**

Pathophysiology

The pathogenesis of Sweet's syndrome is not well understood. The association with under-lying systemic disease suggests that hypersensitivity reactions, cytokine dysregulation, and genetic susceptibility may contribute to the development of the disease.[31]

Associated Conditions

Malignancy (especially AML), infections (upper respiratory and gastrointestinal (GI) infections most common), IBD, medications (e.g., furosemide, oral contraceptives, tri-methoprim–sulfamethoxazole, minocycline, granulocyte colony–stimulating factor), RA, sarcoidosis, Behçet's syndrome, and pregnancy.

DIAGNOSIS

Clinical Presentation

- Sweet's syndrome presents with an **abrupt onset of tender, erythematous or violaceous, edematous papules, plaques, or nodules** favoring the **head, neck, upper extremities, and dorsal hands.** Marked edema can result in a **pseudovesicular** or **bullous** appearance. Like in PG, lesions in Sweet's syndrome demonstrate **pathergy.**
- Cutaneous manifestations are usually accompanied by **fever** and **malaise.**
- Less common systemic manifestations include arthralgias, arthritis, ocular, pulmonary, and renal involvement.
  - **Pulmonary Sweet's syndrome** or neutrophilic alveolitis is a rare systemic manifestation of Sweet's syndrome presenting with cough, dyspnea, and pleuritic chest pain. Chest radiograph may show interstitial infiltrates, nodules, and pleural effusions.
  - **Multifocal sterile osteomyelitis** or **SAPHO syndrome** (synovitis, acne, pustulosis, hyperostosis, osteitis) has also rarely been seen in association with Sweet's syndrome.[1]

Differential Diagnosis

- Bullous PG, EN, erythema multiforme, urticarial vasculitis, small vessel vasculitis, and exaggerated arthropod bites
- Papulonodules of Sweet's syndrome involving the lower legs may mimic EN. In fact, **EN and PG can occur concomitantly** in some patients with Sweet's syndrome.[1]

Diagnostic Testing

Laboratories
Laboratory findings include leukocytosis, elevated ESR, and CRP

Diagnostic Procedures
With skin biopsy, histopathology shows a dense, nodular and perivascular **neutrophilic infiltrate with leukocytoclasia** but with **no evidence of vasculitis.**

TREATMENT

- The most effective therapy for Sweet's syndrome is **oral prednisone** (0.5 to 1.0 mg/kg/day) for 4 to 6 weeks, which provides prompt **relief of cutaneous and systemic manifestations.**
- Some patients may require a prolonged course of low-dose prednisone over several months to prevent recurrence.
- The major steroid-sparing agents include **dapsone, colchicine, and potassium iodide.**[1]
- Treatment of the underlying condition is essential.

CALCIPHYLAXIS

GENERAL PRINCIPLES

Definition

Calciphylaxis is a rare disease characterized by **progressive calcification** of **small- and medium-sized vessels** in the dermis and subcutis, leading to ischemic necrosis of the skin and soft tissues.

Pathophysiology

The pathogenesis of this disorder is poorly understood.

Associated Conditions

Calciphylaxis is most often associated with **end-stage renal disease** with **secondary hyperparathyroidism**,[32,33] but it can also be seen in other systemic conditions including:
- **Endocrine:** primary hyperparathyroidism, diabetes, obesity, and excess vitamin D
- **Renal:** uremia, calcium–phosphate product greater than 70 mg^2/dL^2, serum aluminum greater than 25 ng/mL.[34]
- **Autoimmune:** RA, SLE, sarcoidosis, Sjögren's syndrome, Crohn's disease, and antiphospholipid syndrome
- **Other conditions:** paraneoplastic, deficiency of protein C or S, alcoholic liver disease

DIAGNOSIS

Clinical Presentation

Calciphylaxis presents with **painful, violaceous reticulated patches and tender erythematous plaques and nodules** that may **become necrotic, ulcerate, or form eschars.** Lesions favor the **lower extremities** and **areas of adiposity** such as the breasts, abdomen, buttocks, and thighs.

Differential Diagnosis

- **Vasculitis:** granulomatosis with polyangiitis, pancreatic panniculitis, polyarteritis nodosa (PAN), hypersensitivity vasculitis, bullous SLE
- **Vasculitis mimics:** cholesterol emboli syndrome, cryoglobulinemia, PG, livedoid vasculopathy, warfarin skin necrosis, antiphospholipid syndrome, deficiency of protein C or S
- **Infections:** cellulitis, necrotizing fasciitis, brown recluse spider bite, *Vibrio vulnificus* infection, fungal and atypical mycobacterial infections

Diagnostic Testing

The clinical diagnosis is confirmed by biopsy. Histopathology shows **epidermal ulceration, focal dermal necrosis, and calcified small vessels,** particularly in the subcutis. **Fibrin thrombi in capillaries**, a **mixed inflammatory infiltrate**, and acute and chronic **calcifying panniculitis** are also common findings.

TREATMENT

- First-line treatment includes medical management to normalize the calcium–phosphate product by **low calcium dialysis** and use of **phosphate binders**. If medical management of hypercalcemia fails, surgical treatment with **parathyroidectomy** may be required.[1]
- **Aggressive wound care** is essential. In fact, a multivariate analysis demonstrated that overall survival is improved by **surgical debridement** and aggressive management of wound infections.[35]

- Other proposed treatment modalities, based on small case series of patients:
  - **Sodium thiosulfate** has shown benefit in some patients, usually at a dose of 25 g after each dialysis.[36]
  - **Cinacalcet** (a calcimimetic) may be beneficial by controlling secondary hyperparathyroidism.[37]
  - **Hyperbaric oxygen**[38]
  - **Bisphosphonates** have proven to be helpful by increasing osteoprotegerin production and inhibiting arterial calcification.[39]
  - **Anticoagulation** can be beneficial in cases of underlying hypercoagulable states.[40]

COMPLICATIONS

Complications include mesenteric ischemia, GI hemorrhage, ischemic myopathy. Mortality is most often because of **gangrene** and **sepsis**.[1]

ERYTHROMELALGIA

GENERAL PRINCIPLES

Definition

Erythromelalgia is a rare condition characterized by episodic **painful burning** and **erythema of acral sites**, which may be **idiopathic, familial,** or can occur as a **secondary phenomenon.**

Classification

- The **familial form** is the result of a disease-specific **autosomal dominant mutation** in **voltage-gated sodium channels,** resulting in overexcitability in nociceptive fibers.[41]
- **Secondary erythromelalgia** is most closely associated with **essential thrombocythemia.** This form of secondary erythromelalgia is caused by platelet-mediated acral vasodilation, inflammation, and microvascular occlusion.[1]

Associated Conditions

- **Essential thrombocythemia**
- **Myeloproliferative disorders:** polycythemia vera, pernicious anemia, myelodysplastic syndrome
- **Drug induced:** cyclosporine, calcium channel blockers, norepinephrine, bromocriptine
- **Infections:** HIV, hepatitis B, EBV
- **Other conditions:** SLE, RA, diabetic neuropathy, multiple sclerosis

DIAGNOSIS

Clinical Presentation

- Erythromelalgia presents **with paroxysmal intense burning, erythema, and warmth** of **acral sites.** The feet are involved in the majority of patients, while the hands are affected less commonly. Rarely, there is also involvement of the head and neck.
- Classically, symptoms are precipitated by heat and relieved by cooling.

Differential Diagnosis

Differential includes complex regional pain syndrome and peripheral neuropathy. Clinically, erythromelalgia can be distinguished by its close relationship to temperature and episodic nature. Peripheral neuropathy can also be differentiated by nerve conduction studies. It is important to always consider erythromelalgia because it may be the first sign of an underlying myeloproliferative disorder.

Diagnostic Testing

Erythromelalgia is a **clinical diagnosis**. In general, biopsies are nonspecific and not recommended. If biopsies are taken from areas of erythromelalgia associated with thrombocythemia, there is fibromuscular intimal proliferation involving arterioles and small arteries.[42]

TREATMENT

- No single therapy is consistently effective for the treatment of erythromelalgia.
- Topical therapies that may aid in analgesia include **10% capsaicin cream** and **lidocaine patches.**
- Oral medications to consider include **selective serotonin reuptake inhibitors (SSRIs)** (venlafaxine, fluoxetine), **tricyclic antidepressants** (amitriptyline), **anticonvulsants** (gabapentin, carbamazepine), **calcium channel blockers** (diltiazem), and the prostaglandin analogue **misoprostol.**[1]
- In **familial erythromelalgia, sodium channel blocking agents** (mexiletine, flecainide) can be effective.[43]
- **Low-dose aspirin** administration is very effective in treating **thrombocythemic erythromelalgia**, whereas idiopathic or other secondary forms typically show minimal to no improvement with aspirin.[44]
- Supportive measures:
  - **Avoidance of triggers** that induce vasodilation, such as strenuous exercises, warm climate, or hot baths
  - **Cooling the limbs** during attacks using fans, wet dressings, ice packs, leg elevation
- Treatment of underlying conditions, in particular myeloproliferative disorders, is essential.

LEVAMISOLE-CONTAMINATED COCAINE VASCULOPATHY

GENERAL PRINCIPLES

Definition

- **Cutaneous vasculopathy** associated with levamisole-contaminated cocaine is an emerging syndrome characterized by **retiform purpura involving the ears, ANCA positivity, and bone marrow suppression.**[45,46]
- Levamisole is an antihelminthic and immune-modulating medication for use in animals that is also a common additive to cocaine.[47]

Pathophysiology

The mechanism of levamisole-contaminated cocaine vasculopathy is unknown; however, the syndrome is believed to be driven by **immune dysfunction.**[45,46]

DIAGNOSIS

Clinical Presentation

- **Cutaneous features** include characteristic **tender, retiform purpura** frequently involving **the external ear** and **malar region of the cheek.** The purpura may progress to **bullae,** which can be followed by **necrosis.** Lesions appear days after using levamisole-contaminated cocaine and resolve over several weeks with cessation of the drug.
- **Systemic features** are common and include **arthralgias** affecting the large joints, **rhinorrhea, sinusitis,** and **fever.** Pulmonary hemorrhage and ARF have also been reported.[47]

Differential Diagnosis

Differential is broad and includes other causes of vasculitis, including cryoglobulinemia, PAN, granulomatosis with polyangiitis, and idiopathic thrombocytopenic purpura.[45]

Diagnostic Testing

Laboratories

Laboratory abnormalities include **leukopenia, neutropenia, and agranulocytosis.** Serology is often positive with high-titer **ANCA**, as well as positive antinuclear antibodies (ANA), lupus anticoagulant, anti–myeloperoxidase antibodies, anti–proteinase 3 and antiphospholipid antibodies.[46]

Diagnostic Testing

Histopathology demonstrates a nonspecific pattern of vasculopathy, including **LCV, fibrin thrombi,** and, most commonly, **bland vascular occlusive disease** without a true vasculitis. DIF studies are nonspecific, but support an immunocomplex-mediated process. Skin biopsy is helpful to rule out other diseases but will not implicate cocaine or levamisole directly.[46]

TREATMENT

Treatment includes abstinence from levamisole-contaminated cocaine, as well as supportive wound care. The role of steroids and anticoagulation is yet to be determined.

COMPLICATIONS

Complications include infection and autoamputation of affected tissue.

CLINICAL CLUES TO SEPARATE COMMON MIMICKING DISEASES IN CUTANEOUS RHEUMATOLOGY

ACUTE CUTANEOUS LUPUS ERYTHEMATOSUS (ACLE), ROSACEA, AND SEBORRHEIC DERMATITIS

- ACLE, rosacea, and seborrheic dermatitis can present similarly with prominent erythematous patches and plaques involving the malar region of the cheek.
- In ACLE, the rash tends to **spare the nasolabial folds.** There is often a clearly demonstrable **photodistribution.** Systemic signs such as fever, weight loss, fatigue, and myalgias should also raise your suspicion of SLE in patients presenting with malar rash.
- There are several forms of rosacea. In erythematotelangiectatic rosacea, in addition to centrofacial erythema, patients often present with distinguishing features of **flushing, telangiectasias, and skin sensitivity. Papulopustular rosacea** is characterized by a centrofacial eruption of multiple small erythematous papules and pustules. Importantly, both ACLE and seborrheic dermatitis **lack the pustules** seen in rosacea.
- In contrast to ACLE, seborrheic dermatitis of the face presents with **distinct greasy, yellow scale involving the nasolabial folds and eyebrows.** Of note, seborrheic dermatitis and rosacea often can coexist.

ACLE AND DERMATOMYOSITIS

- Although ACLE and dermatomyositis can both present with a **photodistributed, erythematous rash** involving the face, chest, and hands, subtle cutaneous clues and systemic symptoms can help distinguish the two diseases.

- In ACLE, the rash typically **spares the nasolabial folds,** whereas the facial rash of dermatomyositis involves them. Additionally, the rash of dermatomyositis has a distinct **violaceous hue.**
- On the hands, the rash of ACLE spares the knuckles, whereas dermatomyositis characteristically presents with pink, scaly papules overlying the metacarpophalangeal joints, which are known as **Gottron's papules.** Dermatomyositis also has a predilection for **extensor surfaces,** particularly the elbows and knees.
- Other informative clues that suggest a diagnosis of dermatomyositis **include prominent nail fold telangiectasias,** as well as symptoms of **pruritus** and **proximal muscle weakness.**

SYSTEMIC SCLEROSIS, MORPHEA, AND EOSINOPHILIC FASCIITIS

- Systemic sclerosis (SSc), morphea, and eosinophilic fasciitis are distinct inflammatory diseases that ultimately lead to **scar-like sclerosis of the skin.**
- Although generalized morphea may resemble early diffuse SSc, the presence of **digital sclerosis, nail fold abnormalities, Raynaud's phenomenon,** and **involvement of the GI tract and lungs** help to make the diagnosis of SSc. Unlike SSc and eosinophilic fasciitis, **morphea does not lead to involvement of internal organs.**
- Deep morphea can often be difficult to distinguish from eosinophilic fasciitis. In both processes, there is deep inflammation and fibrosis of the deep dermis and subcutis, resulting in a **"pseudo-cellulite"** rippled appearance of the involved skin. The **"groove sign"** is fairly specific to eosinophilic fasciitis, where veins appear as sunken, linear depressions within the indurated skin. Although SSc and eosinophilic fasciitis characteristically present with symmetric induration of the skin, **morphea lacks symmetric distribution.**
- Laboratory findings and **autoantibody profiles** can also help to distinguish these conditions. Patients with SSc often have high-titer positive ANA, anti–centromere antibodies, and anti–topoisomerase I (Scl-70) antibodies. As the name suggests, patients with eosinophilic fasciitis have a striking **peripheral eosinophilia** and negative ANA.

REFERENCES

1. Bolognia J, Jorizzo J, Schaffer J, eds. *Dermatology.* 3rd ed. Philadelphia, PA: Elsevier Saunders, 2012.
2. Pendergraft WF 3rd, Niles JL. Trojan horses: drug culprits associated with antineutrophil cytoplasmic autoantibody (ANCA) vasculitis. *Curr Opin Rheumatol.* 2014;26(1):42–49.
3. Martinez-Taboada VM, Blanco R, Garcia-Fuentes M, Rodriguez-Valverde V. Clinical features and outcome of 95 patients with hypersensitivity vasculitis. *Am J Med.* 1997;102(2):186.
4. Calabrese LH, Duna GF. Drug-induced vasculitis. *Curr Opin Rheumatol.* 1996;8(1):34.
5. Zurada JM, Ward KM, Grossman ME. Henoch-Schönlein purpura associated with malignancy in adults. *J Am Acad Dermatol.* 2006;55:s65–s70.
6. Uppal SS, Hussain MA, Al-Raqum HA, et al. Henoch-Schönlein's purpura in adults versus children/adolescents: a comparative study. *Clin Exp Rheumatol.* 2006;24(2 Suppl 41):s26–s30.
7. Pillebout E, Thervet E, Hill G, et al. Henoch-Schönlein purpura in adults: outcome and prognostic factors. *J Am Soc Nephrol.* 2002;13:1271–1278.
8. Jones D, Dorfman DM, Barnhill RL, Granter SR. Leukemic vasculitis. A feature of leukemia cutis in some patients. *Am J Clin Pathol.* 1997;107:637–642.
9. Maessen-Visch MB, Koedam M, Hamulyak K, Neumann HA. Atrophie blanche. *Int J Dermatol.* 1999;38:161–172.
10. Hairston BR, Davis MDP, Pittelkow MR, Ahmed I. Livedoid vasculopathy. Further evidence for procoagulant pathogenesis. *Arch Dermatol.* 2006;142:1413–1418.
11. Milstone LM, Braverman IM, Lucky P, Fleckman P. Classification and therapy of atrophie blanche. *Arch Dermatol.* 1983;119:963–969.
12. Callen JP. Livedoid vasculopathy. What it is and how the patient should be evaluated and treated. *Arch Dermatol.* 2006;142:1481–1482.
13. Braverman IM. Protective effects of erythema nodosum in coccidioidomycosis. *Lancet.* 1999;353:168.

14. Honma T, Bang D, Lee S, et al. Ultrastructure of endothelial cell necrosis in classical erythema nodosum. *Hum Pathol.* 1992;24:384–390.
15. Hanauer SB. How do I treat erythema nodosum, aphthous ulcerations, and pyoderma gangrenosum? *Inflamm Bowel Dis.* 1998;4:70.
16. Cribier B, Caille A, Heid E, et al. Erythema nodosum and associated diseases. A study of 129 cases. *Int J Dermatol.* 1998;37:667–672.
17. White WL, Hitchcock MG. Diagnosis: erythema nodosum or not? *Semin Cutan Med Surg.* 1999;18:47–55.
18. Gilchrist H, Patterson JW. Erythema nodosum and erythema induratum (nodular vasculitis): diagnosis and management. *Dermatol Ther.* 2010;23:320–327.
19. Kronzon I, Saric M. Cholesterol embolization syndrome. *Circulation.* 2010;122:631–641
20. Falanga V, Fine MJ, Kapoor WN. The cutaneous manifestations of cholesterol crystal embolization. *Arch Dermatol.* 1986;122:1194–1198.
21. Lawson JM. Cholesterol crystal embolization: more common than we thought? *Am J Gastroenterol.* 2001;96:3230–3232.
22. Manganoni AM, Venturini M, Scolari F et al. The importance of skin biopsy in the diverse clinical manifestations of cholesterol embolism. *Br J Dermatol.* 2004;150:1230–1232.
23. Powell FC, Su WPD, Perry HO. Pyoderma gangrenosum: classification and management. *J Am Acad Dermatol.* 1996;34:395–409.
24. Maverakis E, Ma C, Shinkai K, et al. Diagnostic criteria of ulcerative pyoderma gangrenosum: a Delphi consensus of international experts. *JAMA Dermatol.* 2018;154(4):461–466.
25. Miller J, Yentzer BA, Clark A, et al. Pyoderma gangrenosum: a review and update on new therapies. *J Am Acad Dermatol.* 2010;62:646–654.
26. Ormerod AD, Thomas KS, Craig FE, et al. Comparison of the two most commonly used treatments for pyoderma gangrenosum: results of the STOP GAP randomised controlled trial. *BMJ.* 2015;350:h2958.
27. Patridge ACR, Bai JW, Rosen CF, et al. Effectiveness of systemic treatments for pyoderma gangrenosum: a systematic review of observational studies & clinical trials. *Br J Dermatol.* 2018;179(2):290–295.
28. Song H, Lahood N, Mostaghimi A. Intravenous immunoglobulin as adjunct therapy for refractory pyoderma gangrenosum: systematic review of cases and case series. *Br J Dermatol.* 2018;178(2):363–368.
29. Juillerat P, Christen-Zäch S, Troillet FX, et al. Infliximab for the treatment of disseminated pyoderma gangrenosum associated with ulcerative colitis. Case report and literature review. *Dermatology.* 2007;215:245–251.
30. Raza S, Kirkland RS, Patel AA, et al. Insight into Sweet's syndrome and associated-malignancy: a review of the current literature. *Int J Oncol.* 2013;42(5):1516–1522.
31. Giasuddin AS, El-Orfi AH, Ziu MM, et al. Sweet's syndrome: is the pathogenesis mediated by helper T cell type 1 cytokines? *J Am Acad Dermatol.* 1998;39:940–943.
32. Cockerell CJ, Dolan ET. Widespread cutaneous and systemic calcification (calciphylaxis) in patients with the acquired immunodeficiency syndrome and renal disease. *J Am Acad Dermatol.* 1992;26:559–562.
33. Ivker RA, Woosley J, Briggaman RA. Calciphylaxis in three patients with end-stage renal disease. *Arch Dermatol.* 1995;131:63–68.
34. Weenig RH, Sewell LD, David MD, et al. Calciphylaxis: natural history, risk factor analysis, and outcome. *J Am Acad Dermatol.* 2007;56:569–579.
35. Lal G, Nowell AG, Liao J, et al. Determinants of survival in patients with calciphylaxis: a multivariate analysis. *Surgery.* 2009;146:1028–1034.
36. Noureddine L, Landis M, Patel N, et al. Efficacy of sodium thiosulfate for the treatment for calciphylaxis. *Clin Nephrol.* 2011;75:485–490.
37. Robinson MR, Augustine JJ, Korman NJ. Cinacalcet for the treatment of calciphylaxis. *Arch Dermatol.* 2007;143:152–154.
38. Basile C, Montanaro A, Masi M, et al. Hyperbaric oxygen therapy for calcific uremic arteriolopathy: a case series. *J Nephrol.* 2002;15:676–680.
39. Shiraishi N, Kitamura K, Miyoshi T, et al. Successful treatment of a patient with severe calcific uremic arteriolopathy (calciphylaxis) by etidronate disodium. *Am J Kidney Dis.* 2006;48:151–154.
40. Harris RJ, Cropley TG. Possible role of hypercoagulability in calciphylaxis: review of the literature. *J Am Acad Dermatol.* 2011;64:405–412.
41. Yang Y, Wang Y, Li S, et al. Mutations in SCN9A, encoding a sodium channel alpha subunit, in patients with primary erythermalgia. *J Med Genet.* 2004;41:171–174.

42. Drenth JPH, Vuzevski V, Van Joost T, et al. Cutaneous pathology in primary erythermalgia. *Am J Dermatopathol*. 1996;18:30–34.
43. Iqbal J, Bhat MI, Charoo BA, et al. Experience with oral mexiletine in primary erythromelalgia in children. *Ann Saudi Med*. 2009;29:316–318.
44. Michiels JJ, Berneman Z, Schroyens W, et al. Platelet-mediated thrombotic complications in patients with ET: Reversal by aspirin, platelet reduction, and not by coumadin. *Blood Cells Mol Dis*. 2006;36(2):199–205.
45. Chung C, Tumeh PC, Birnbaum R, et al. Characteristic purpura of the ears, vasculitis, and neutropenia--a potential public health epidemic associated with levamisole-adulterated cocaine. *J Am Acad Dermatol*. 2011;65(4):722–725.
46. Gross RL, Brucker J, Bahce-Altuntas A, et al. A novel cutaneous vasculitis syndrome induced by levamisole-contaminated cocaine. *Clin Rheumatol*. 2011;30:1385–1392.
47. Lee KC, Ladizinski B, Nutan FN. Systemic complications of levamisole toxicity. *J Am Acad Dermatol*. 2012;67(4):791–792.

Interstitial Lung Disease

51

Yuka Furuya and Adrian Shifren

GENERAL PRINCIPLES

- Pulmonary disease is an important cause of morbidity and mortality in patients with connective tissue diseases (CTDs). **Interstitial lung disease (ILD) is a well-known manifestation of CTDs**, although airways, pulmonary vessels, and the pleura can also be affected to varying degrees.
- Pulmonary involvement is especially common in systemic sclerosis (SSc), rheumatoid arthritis (RA), inflammatory myopathies (IMs), Sjögren's syndrome, and systemic lupus erythematosus (SLE), all of which will be reviewed in this chapter.
- **Drug-induced ILD must be considered in the differential diagnosis** of any lung disease occurring in the context of disease-modifying antirheumatic drug (DMARD) therapy because many DMARDs are associated with the development of pulmonary toxicity. However, in many cases, it is difficult to distinguish drug-induced ILD from pulmonary manifestations of the underlying CTD. Drug-induced ILD will be discussed separately.
- Some individuals with ILD have clinical features or serologic markers suggestive of an underlying CTD but do not meet the established criteria for defined CTDs. In 2015, the term **"interstitial pneumonia with autoimmune features" (IPAF)** was proposed to further characterize these patients.[1] Table 51-1 summarizes the current diagnostic criteria for IPAF.[1]
- A **multidisciplinary approach** involving pulmonology, rheumatology, radiology, and pathology has become increasingly important in the diagnosis and management of these complex multiorgan diseases.

Definition

- ILD, also known as diffuse parenchymal lung disease (DPLD), is a heterogeneous group of diseases with variable involvement of the **pulmonary interstitium, airways, pleura, and pulmonary vessels**.
- In some cases, lung disease may be the **first manifestation** of a CTD that may become apparent at a later time.

Classification

- There is no established classification system for ILD associated with CTDs. The histologic and radiographic classification for idiopathic interstitial pneumonia (IIP) has been used historically to describe patterns of disease in CTD-ILD.[2,3]
- Common histologic/radiographic patterns observed in CTDs include nonspecific interstitial pneumonia (NSIP), usual interstitial pneumonia (UIP), organizing pneumonia (OP), and lymphoid interstitial pneumonia (LIP).
- Other manifestations may include pleural effusions, pleural inflammation (pleuritis), bronchiolar inflammation (bronchiolitis), pulmonary nodules (with or without cavitation), and diffuse alveolar hemorrhage (DAH).

TABLE 51-1   DIAGNOSTIC CRITERIA FOR IPAF

1. Presence of an interstitial pneumonia (by HRCT or surgical lung biopsy) *and,*
2. Exclusion of alternative etiologies *and,*
3. Does not meet criteria of a defined connective tissue disease *and,*
4. At least one feature from at least two of these domains:
   - A. Clinical domain
   - B. Serologic domain
   - C. Morphologic domain

A. Clinical domain
   1. Distal digital fissuring (i.e., "mechanic hands")
   2. Distal digital tip ulceration
   3. Inflammatory arthritis *or* polyarticular morning joint stiffness ≥60 min
   4. Palmar telangiectasia
   5. Raynaud's phenomenon
   6. Unexplained digital edema
   7. Unexplained fixed rash on the digital extensor surfaces (Gottron's sign)
B. Serologic domain
   1. ANA ≥1:320 titer, diffuse, speckled, homogeneous patterns *or*
      a. ANA nucleolar pattern (any titer) *or*
      b. ANA centromere pattern (any titer)
   2. Rheumatoid factor ≥2× upper limit of normal
   3. Anti-CCP
   4. Anti-dsDNA
   5. Anti-Ro (SS-A)
   6. Anti-La (SS-B)
   7. Anti-ribonucleoprotein (RNP)
   8. Anti-Smith
   9. Anti–topoisomerase I (Scl-70)
   10. Anti-tRNA synthetase (e.g., Jo-1, PL-7, PL-12, EJ, OJ, KS, Zo, tRS)
   11. Anti-PM-Scl
   12. Anti-MDA-5
C. Morphologic domain
   1. Suggestive radiology patterns by HRCT:
      a. NSIP
      b. OP
      c. NSIP with OP overlap
      d. LIP
   2. Histopathology patterns or features by surgical lung biopsy:
      a. NSIP
      b. OP
      c. NSIP with OP overlap
      d. LIP
      e. Interstitial lymphoid aggregates with germinal centers
      f. Diffuse lymphoplasmacytic infiltrates (with or without lymphoid follicles)
   3. Multicompartment involvement (in addition to interstitial pneumonia):
      a. Unexplained pleural effusion or thickening
      b. Unexplained pericardial effusion or thickening
      c. Unexplained intrinsic airway disease (by PFT, imaging, or pathology)
      d. Unexplained pulmonary vasculopathy

ANA, antinuclear antibody; HRCT, high-resolution computed tomography; NSIP, nonspecific interstitial pneumonia; OP, organizing pneumonia; PFT, pulmonary function tests.

Pathophysiology

- CTD-ILDs are a heterogeneous group of diseases with **varied clinical presentations and natural histories**. Much remains unknown regarding the pathogenesis of ILD in this patient population.
- The exact mechanism of injury, inflammation, and fibrosis is poorly understood and is likely specific to the underlying CTD.

DIAGNOSIS

- Diagnosis of ILD is suggested by abnormal pulmonary function tests (PFTs), chest x-rays, and high-resolution computed tomography (HRCT).
- **Complete PFTs** (spirometry, lung volumes, and diffusion capacity) along with **arterial blood gases** (ABGs) are obtained on the initial visit for all patients with suspected ILD.

Clinical Presentation

- In addition to ILD, some CTDs commonly present with airway and pleural complications, and these are summarized in Table 51-2.
- Gradual onset **dyspnea** and a persistent nonproductive **cough** are the most common presenting symptoms.
- In patients with airway involvement, a history of wheezing, productive cough, and episodes of exacerbation can be present.
- Patients with pleural involvement may complain of pleuritic pain—sharp chest pain that worsens with inspiration.
- Patients with DAH may manifest with hemoptysis. However, lack of cough productive of bloody sputum does not exclude the presence of DAH.

History

- **Smoking history** is particularly important to obtain because some IIPs such as desquamative interstitial pneumonia (DIP) or respiratory bronchiolitis–associated ILD (RB-ILD) are strongly associated with cigarette smoking and typically respond to smoking cessation.
- **Occupational and environmental exposures** can explain some ILDs such as hypersensitivity pneumonitis (HP) or heavy metal pneumoconiosis.
- Some ILDs have a strong hereditary pattern, and **family history** can aid in diagnosis.
- Lastly, knowledge of prior **medication** use is vital for evaluation of CTD-ILD because many therapeutic agents used in the treatment of CTD are associated with pulmonary toxicity.

Physical Examination

- Physical examination can be fairly nonspecific, including **inspiratory crackles**, squeaks, and wheezes.
- Digital clubbing can be appreciated in pulmonary fibrosis.
- Airway involvement should be suspected in patients with wheezing.
- Signs of **underlying systemic disease** such as mechanic's hands, Gottron's papules, specific skin rashes, Raynaud's phenomenon, or digital edema can aid in the diagnosis.

Diagnostic Testing

Laboratories

- As lung disease can be the first manifestation of an underlying CTD, we recommend **serologic testing** in newly diagnosed ILD patients without a previous workup, especially if high-risk features are present (NSIP or OP pattern, clinical features of CTD, patulous esophagus on CT).

TABLE 51-2	AFFECTED ANATOMIC COMPARTMENT AND CHARACTERISTICS IN DIFFERENT CTDs					
		SSc	RA	IM	pSS	SLE	Drug induced

		SSc	RA	IM	pSS	SLE	Drug induced
Pleura	Pleural effusion, pleuritis		+			++	
Airway	Bronchiectasis	+	+		++		
	Follicular bronchiolitis		+				
Parenchyma	NSIP	++	+	++	++	+	
	UIP	+	++	+	+	+	
	OP	+	+	+		+	++
	LIP				+		
	DAD					+	+
	Pulmonary nodules		+				
Vasculature	PAH	++	+	+	+	+	
	DAH					+	

CTDs, connective tissue diseases; DAD, diffuse alveolar damage; DAH, diffuse alveolar hemorrhage; IM, inflammatory myopathies; LIP, lymphoid interstitial pneumonia; NSIP, nonspecific interstitial pneumonia; OP, organizing pneumonia; PAH, pulmonary arterial hypertension; pSS, primary Sjögren's syndrome; RA, rheumatoid arthritis; SLE, systemic lupus erythematosus; SSc, systemic sclerosis; UIP, usual interstitial pneumonia.

- Typically, serologies for antinuclear antibody (ANA), anti–rheumatoid factor (RF), anti–cyclic citrullinated peptide (CCP), anti–double-stranded DNA (dsDNA), anti–topoisomerase I (Scl-70), anti-Smith (Sm), anti-SSA, anti-SSB, anti-ribonucleoprotein (RNP) are sent.
- Creatine kinase (CK) and aldolase are checked when screening for IM.
- Myositis-specific antibodies can also be tested if proximal muscle weakness is present, if muscle enzymes are elevated, or in cases where there is clinical suspicion for clinically amyopathic dermatomyositis (CADM).

Imaging
- **HRCT is the standard for diagnosis of ILD.** By using a thin (1–2 mm) slice thickness, HRCT optimizes spatial resolution. Many protocols include imaging during the expiratory phase of respiration, which aids in diagnosing air trapping. Images obtained in the prone position can minimize the distortion created by atelectasis in the dependent lung regions.
- **NSIP on HRCT is characterized by relatively symmetric bilateral reticulations (alveolar septal thickening), ground-glass opacities (GGO), and traction bronchiectasis** (Fig. 51-1). These findings are frequently lower lobe predominant. **Subpleural sparing** of the lung parenchyma, when present, is considered specific for NSIP and can help

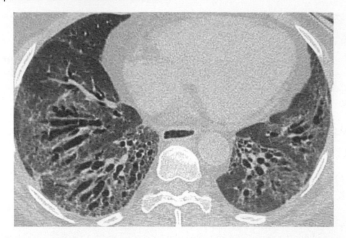

FIGURE 51-1. High-resolution computed tomography pattern of nonspecific interstitial pneumonia.

distinguish NSIP from early UIP. Histologically, NSIP is characterized by either diffuse homogeneous interstitial inflammation and infiltrating lymphocytes (cellular NSIP) or homogeneous interstitial fibrosis (fibrotic NSIP).

- UIP on HRCT manifests as **lower lung and subpleural predominant bilateral reticulation in the presence of honeycombing, with/without traction bronchiectasis** (Fig. 51-2). Histologically, UIP is characterized by temporal and spatial heterogeneity of lung involvement with areas of interstitial inflammation and fibrosis alternating with spared regions. Additional features include architectural distortion, frequently with microscopic honeycombing, and the presence of pathognomonic fibroblastic foci.
- OP, in contrast, exhibits **patchy consolidation and GGO in a peripheral and peribronchovascular pattern** (Fig. 51-3). Pulmonary nodules can be seen, at times with a central clearing or GGO, which is termed the "reverse halo sign."

Diagnostic Procedures
- Pulmonary function testing
  - Spirometry and lung volumes often show a **restrictive ventilatory defect (RVD)**, defined by a **decrease in total lung capacity (TLC)**. A symmetric reduction in both Forced Expiratory Volume in the first second (FEV1) and Forced vital capacity (FVC) with a preserved FEV_1:FVC ratio (>80%) may suggest underlying restriction when lung volume measurement is not performed.
  - **Airway involvement**, not uncommon in RA, is suggested when an **obstructive ventilatory defect** is detected. Obstruction is characterized by a decreased FEV_1:FVC ratio (<70%).
  - In addition, air trapping, characterized by increase in residual volumes (RVs), may suggest small airway disease.
  - **Diffusing capacity for carbon monoxide (DL_{CO})** evaluates alveolar gas exchange by measuring the amount of carbon monoxide (CO) transferred from alveolar gas to the red blood cells in the pulmonary capillaries. An isolated decrease in DL_{CO} in the setting of normal PFTs can be a sign of underlying pulmonary hypertension (PH).

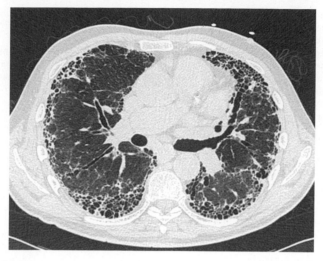

FIGURE 51-2. High-resolution computed tomography pattern of usual interstitial pneumonia.

- Bronchoscopy
  - There is a **limited role for bronchoscopy and transbronchial biopsy** in the diagnosis of diffuse lung disease given the low yield because of random sampling error, the patchy disease process, and small biopsy size.
  - However, **bronchoscopy and bronchoalveolar lavage (BAL) can be useful in ruling out pulmonary infection**, particularly in cases that warrant high-dose immunosuppression.

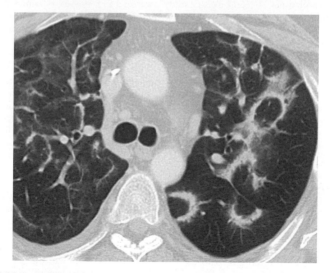

FIGURE 51-3. High-resolution computed tomography pattern of organizing pneumonia.

- Surgical lung biopsy
  - Surgical lung biopsies, typically via video-assisted thoracoscopic surgery (VATS), yield adequate sample sizes for evaluation of lung architecture.
  - **In general, lung biopsies are not performed in CTD-ILD**, as it is uncommon that the histopathologic pattern dictates treatment in this population. In addition, many patients with limited lung function and impaired oxygenation will not tolerate a surgical lung biopsy.

TREATMENT

Medications

- In most cases, the **decision to initiate therapy should be individualized** depending on symptoms, severity of physiologic dysfunction on PFTs, rate of disease progression, and patient preference.
- Treatment varies depending on the underlying etiology.
- In general, **systemic glucocorticoids** are initiated for more severe disease or acute exacerbations of disease, along with a scheduled taper.
- Regardless of the etiology, patients with OP are often most responsive to glucocorticoid therapy, followed by NSIP and then UIP, which is almost always very poorly responsive to therapy of any kind.
- Other immunosuppressive agents used for treating CTD-ILD include **mycophenolate mofetil (MMF), cyclophosphamide, rituximab, azathioprine, and calcineurin inhibitors (CNIs)**.
- For **drug-induced ILD, withdrawal of the offending agent** is the first-line treatment.

Other Nonpharmacologic Therapies

- Many patients are significantly physically deconditioned as a result of their underlying disease and benefit from **pulmonary rehabilitation**.
- **Lung transplantation** is a viable option for end-stage CTD-ILD patients without significant comorbidities. A recent registry study compared 275 nonscleroderma CTD-ILD patients undergoing lung transplantation with patients transplanted for idiopathic pulmonary fibrosis (IPF). There was no difference in survival (adjusted for demographic data), episodes of acute rejection, or development of chronic rejection.[4]
- As for scleroderma, posttransplant survival rates reported for SSc-ILD patients were similar to survival rates observed in recipients without SSc.[5] However, given the association between chronic rejection and gastroesophageal reflux, some centers consider significant esophageal disease (often seen in SSc) to be a relative contraindication for lung transplantation.
- Although patients with single organ disease are generally thought to be ideal transplant candidates, determination of transplant candidacy varies widely between transplant centers. Some centers may consider patients with multiorgan involvement (e.g., renal disease) to be a transplant candidate.

OUTCOME/PROGNOSIS

- **Prognosis and outcome vary widely depending on the underlying disease and histologic pattern.** In general, CTD-ILD patients have a more favorable prognosis compared to those with comparable histology of an idiopathic nature such as IPF.
- In a retrospective analysis of 422 patients with undifferentiated CTD or IIP, 144 of whom met IPAF criteria, patients with defined CTD-ILD had the best prognosis, compared to IPAF or IPF. IPAF patients with UIP pattern and IPF patients had

a similar survival and fared worse compared to those with non-UIP pattern IPAF or CTD-ILD.[6]

- In another study, survival was better for CTD-UIP patients compared to patients with IPF even after controlling for age, sex, and baseline lung function.[7]

SCLERODERMA

GENERAL PRINCIPLES

- The prevalence of RVDs on PFT in SSc patients is approximately 40%.[8] Subtle fibrosis may be found in up to 90% of patients on HRCT.[9] **Along with pulmonary vascular disease, ILD accounts for about 60% of all SSc-related deaths.**[10,11]
- Group 1 PH, or pulmonary arterial hypertension (PAH) based on the World Health Organization (WHO) classification, manifests in 10% to 15% of SSc patients and can occur with or without concomitant ILD.
- In addition to PAH, group 2 (pulmonary venous hypertension) PH can occur with cardiac involvement in SSc, and group 3 (lung disease and/or hypoxia) PH can be seen in cases of severe underlying ILD and resultant hypoxemia.

DIAGNOSIS

- **All SSc patients should be screened for the presence of ILD with a full PFT and HRCT.**
- PFTs typically show RVD with reduced FEV1, FVC, and TLC. Although uncommon, airway involvement should be suspected when an obstructive pattern with reduced FEV1 and reduced FEV1/FVC ratio is seen.
- NSIP, and in particular the fibrotic form, **is the most commonly seen HRCT pattern** in SSc. Bronchiectasis can be pronounced, especially in the lower lobes owing to both traction bronchiectasis from the underlying fibrosis and chronic aspiration. A patulous esophagus is often seen on CT scan supporting the diagnosis.
- UIP is the next most commonly noted ILD pattern.

TREATMENT

- In the Scleroderma Lung Study (SLS) II,[12] 142 SSc-ILD patients were randomized to MMF (target dose 1,500 mg twice daily) for 24 months or oral cyclophosphamide for 12 months followed by placebo for 12 months. Improvement in %FVC was seen in both groups; however, **MMF was better tolerated with fewer withdrawals** and had less episodes of leukopenia and thrombocytopenia. The role of adjuvant glucocorticoids was unclear based on the results of this study.
- Based on the above findings, we recommend initial therapy with MMF over cyclophosphamide.

MONITORING/FOLLOW-UP

- We recommend **yearly screening with full PFTs** in all asymptomatic SSc patients.
- Yearly HRCT in this population is not currently recommended because of concern for cumulative radiation dose.
- Because of the risk of development of PH, **yearly screening echocardiogram with estimation of pulmonary arterial pressure** is recommended.

- In patients with confirmed SSc-ILD, we recommend pulmonary consultation and co-management.

OUTCOME/PROGNOSIS

- In a systematic review of SSc-ILD patients, lower % predicted DLCO, older age, and lower FVC predicted mortality in more than one study. However, the **extent of disease on HRCT** was the only variable that independently predicted both mortality and progression of ILD.[13]
- In a cohort study of 215 patients with SSc who had HRCT, the overall 10-year survival was 59%.[14]

RHEUMATOID ARTHRITIS

GENERAL PRINCIPLES

- **RA-ILD is the most common cause of CTD-ILD.**
- Up to 81% of asymptomatic patients with RA may exhibit abnormal PFTs or an abnormal chest CT.
- One study estimated the lifetime risk of developing RA-ILD at 7.7%. However, the study almost certainly underestimates the true prevalence of RA-ILD because no screening protocol was implemented, and diagnostic tests such as CT and PFTs were conducted only as clinically indicated.[15]
- **RA can affect all pulmonary compartments**, including the parenchyma, airways, pleura, and vasculature to various degrees.
- Risk factors for the development of ILD include **older age, male sex, smoking history, and seropositivity for RF or anti-CCP antibodies.**
- High titers for RF and anti-CCP antibodies are predictive of the development of RA-ILD.
- It is postulated that smoking may lead to production of anti-CCP antibodies that cross-react to citrullinated proteins. The production of anti-CCP antibody in the lung parenchyma and the observation that ILD may precede extrapulmonary disease in RA support this hypothesis.

DIAGNOSIS

- Diagnosis of RA-ILD is made through a combination of PFT, HRCT, and clinical presentation.
- Clinical presentation may vary depending on the affected component.
- With **upper airway involvement**, patients may present with hoarseness, dysphagia, odynophagia, or coughing. **Lower airway and parenchymal involvement** may manifest with coughing, dyspnea, decreased exercise tolerance, and wheezing.
- Unlike most other CTD-ILD, **UIP is the most common (56%) HRCT finding** in RA-ILD, followed by NSIP (33%) and OP (11%).[16]
- Other pulmonary manifestations include pulmonary nodules, pleural effusions, follicular bronchiolitis, bronchiectasis, and bronchiolitis obliterans.[17]
- Follicular bronchiolitis can manifest as small centrilobular nodules with or without peribronchial nodules and GGO. Mosaic attenuation, signifying air trapping, can be seen on expiratory scans.
- Given its variable presentation and high prevalence of DMARD use in this population, it may be difficult to distinguish RA-ILD from drug-induced ILD.

TREATMENT

- Asymptomatic patients with mild radiographic disease and/or mild impairment in PFT may be monitored carefully with serial imaging and PFTs.
- **Responsiveness to glucocorticoid varies based on the histopathology/HRCT findings,** with OP being the most responsive and UIP least responsive.
- In a retrospective study of 125 CTD-ILD patients, 18 of whom had RA-ILD, MMF was well tolerated with a discontinuation rate of 10%. The % predicted FVC (%FVC) improved after initiation of MMF compared to pretreatment, although the difference did not reach statistical significance.
- The **improvement in %FVC and %DLCO was greater** in CTD-ILD patients with a **non-UIP pattern**, compared with those with UIP.[18]
- Other immunosuppressive drugs such as azathioprine or cyclophosphamide are used in patients who fail to respond to glucocorticoids or as steroid-sparing agents.
- Given its similarity in morphology and disease course with IPF, the role of antifibrotics (e.g., pirfenidone and nintedanib) in the treatment of RA-ILD manifesting with a UIP pattern is currently under investigation.

OUTCOME/PROGNOSIS

Those with **UIP pattern of disease** have more progressive decline in DLCO[19] and **worse 5-year survival compared to** those with **NSIP or OP** pattern on CT scan.[20]

INFLAMMATORY MYOPATHIES

GENERAL PRINCIPLES

The prevalence of ILD in PM/dermatomyositis (DM) patients ranges from 23.1% to 65%, depending on the method of diagnosis.[21,22] However, in select populations such as in CADM and those with antisynthetase syndrome, the prevalence and the extent of pulmonary involvement can be much higher.

DIAGNOSIS

- Clinical presentation can vary significantly, from **asymptomatic disease to rapidly progressive and often fatal ILD** seen in those with anti-melanoma differentiation-associated gene 5 (MDA-5) antibody.
- In addition to the classic presentation of IM (symmetrical proximal muscle weakness, heliotrope rash, Gottron's papules, or shawl sign), patients should be carefully questioned and examined for features consistent with antisynthetase syndrome (nonerosive polyarthritis, fever, **mechanic's hands**, Raynaud's phenomenon).
- The presence of myositis-specific antibodies, in particular, anti-tRNA synthetase (antisynthetase) antibodies, in conjunction with supporting history and imaging can be helpful in the diagnosis and, in some cases, prognostication.
- Muscle enzymes (**CK and aldolase**) can be helpful in monitoring disease activity.
- Room air ABG should be checked periodically as restrictive lung disease and **hypercapnic respiratory failure can result from involvement of the diaphragm and other chest wall muscles.**
- HRCT in antisynthetase syndrome typically shows NSIP, often with superimposed areas of OP.
- In one study of 33 patients with antisynthetase syndrome, GGO (100%) and reticulations (87%) were the most common finding, followed by traction bronchiectasis (76%)

and consolidations (45%). **NSIP (45%) was the most commonly observed pattern, followed by OP (21%), then NSIP-OP overlap (24%).**

- Esophageal dysmotility should be suspected in patients with dysphagia and those with HRCT findings suggestive of **chronic aspiration.** These include a patulous esophagus and infiltrates in dependent lung regions including GGO, tree-in-bud infiltrates suggesting bronchiolitis, and bronchiolectasis/bronchiectasis. These findings should prompt additional diagnostic testing.

TREATMENT

- It is reasonable to initiate early therapy in individuals with high-risk antibodies such as anti-MDA-5.
- **Systemic glucocorticoids** are the initial treatment for IM-related ILD at a dose of 1 mg/kg/day with a gradual taper over months, for a total duration of therapy for 6 to 12 months.
- Approximately 50% of patients may be steroid refractory[23] and require additional therapy. Although no randomized controlled trials (RCTs) have been conducted, there have been reports of successful treatment with **azathioprine, MMF, CNIs, rituximab, and methotrexate (MTX).**
- **Tacrolimus** has been used to treat myositis-associated ILD refractory to other therapies with favorable outcome.[24]
- A retrospective study from Japan comparing 25 previously untreated patients who were treated with tacrolimus plus conventional therapy (prednisolone, intravenous [IV] cyclophosphamide, and/or cyclosporine) with 24 propensity-matched patients treated with conventional therapy only showed a longer event-free survival in the tacrolimus group compared to the conventional therapy group (adjusted hazard ratio [HR] 0.32 [95% confidence interval (CI) 0.14–0.75]; p = 0.0008).
- **Rituximab** has also been used mostly in cases with positive antisynthetase antibodies. Although a standardized dosing regimen has not been established, 1,000 mg given on day 0 and days 7–14 is commonly used.[25] Doses can then be repeated every 6 months as needed.

OUTCOME/PROGNOSIS

- A large retrospective study of 107 IM-ILD patients identified three distinct patterns of disease course: 32.7% responded to immunosuppression with complete radiographic and functional resolution, 51.4% showed improvement without complete resolution, and 15.9% showed radiographic and functional deterioration. Histologic patterns of **OP and NSIP were more frequent in patients that had resolution or improvement,** and **UIP was associated with deterioration.** Overall mortality rate was 7.5%.[26]
- **Anti-MDA-5 positivity** has been associated with a high incidence (50%) of ILD, a rapidly **progressive course of ILD,** and **worse survival** compared to DM and CADM patients without the antibody.[27]

SJÖGREN'S SYNDROME

GENERAL PRINCIPLES

- Primary Sjögren's syndrome (pSS) is the second most common CTD after RA.
- Pulmonary involvement occurs in about 9% to 20% of patients[28,29] and most **commonly affects the airways.**
- Involvement of the airway epithelial glands can lead to xerotrachea, or dryness of the airway epithelium, and can present as nonproductive cough.

- Airway disease can involve the central and peripheral bronchi/bronchioles and result in bronchiectasis and bronchial wall thickening.

DIAGNOSIS

- ILD in pSS most commonly manifests as **NSIP, followed by UIP, LIP, and OP. Anti-SSA positivity is a risk factor for the development of ILD.**
- LIP and follicular bronchiolitis both fall within the spectrum of lymphoproliferative **disorders and are considered benign.**
- PFT typically shows RVD in the majority of cases, but in cases of airway involvement obstructive patterns can be seen.
- HRCT findings in **LIP** include scattered GGO, centrilobular nodules, bronchial wall thickening, and reticulation. In some cases, it presents as a predominantly **cystic disease with thin-walled cysts that are randomly distributed.** Mosaic attenuation on expiratory images suggests air trapping and small airway involvement.

TREATMENT

- Asymptomatic patients may be monitored closely without ILD-specific therapy.
- As with other CTD-ILD, NSIP and OP are frequently responsive to **systemic glucocorticoids** and other immunosuppressive agents. Although there are reports of successful treatment with **azathioprine, MMF, and rituximab**, no RCTs exist to date.
- LIP may be responsive to systemic glucocorticoids, although the cystic component usually persists despite treatment.

COMPLICATIONS

- Patients with pSS are **at risk for non-Hodgkin's lymphoma (NHL).** In a pooled analysis that included 12 case–control studies, the **odds ratio** of pSS patients having NHL was **4.8**, compared to 2.7 in SLE and 1.06 in RA.[30]
- **Mucosa-associated lymphoid tissue (MALT) lymphoma**, a form of marginal zone B-cell lymphoma, is the most common NHL identified.
- Although NHL occurs most frequently in the salivary glands, primary pulmonary lymphoma occurs in 1% to 2% of the patients, and any **focal pulmonary nodules noted on CT warrant close follow-up.**

SYSTEMIC LUPUS ERYTHEMATOSUS

GENERAL PRINCIPLES

- SLE commonly involves the pleura, and pleuritis and/or pleural effusions can be detected in >90% of SLE patients at autopsy.
- Other pulmonary manifestations of SLE include **acute lupus pneumonitis, DAH, chronic ILD, and shrinking lung syndrome.**
- Chronic ILD in SLE is not as prevalent as in other CTD-ILDs, with a reported prevalence of around 3%.[31]

DIAGNOSIS

- SLE primarily involves the pleura and less commonly the airways, interstitium, and pulmonary vasculature.
- Clinical presentation varies depending on the location of disease.

- Patients with pleural disease can present with **pleuritic chest pain** or dyspnea when significant effusion is present. Pleural effusion can be unilateral or bilateral.
- **Pleural effusions in lupus are exudative** and characteristically but not inevitably have **low glucose concentration and a low pH**. Positive ANA $\geq$ **1:160 in the pleural fluid** may aid in diagnosis.
- **Acute lupus pneumonitis** is similar to acute interstitial pneumonia (AIP), also known as Hamman–Rich syndrome. Patients may have a mild prodromal period lasting 1 to 2 weeks prior to presentation. Symptoms include **fever, cough, and dyspnea that can be rapidly progressive, resulting in hypoxemia frequently requiring invasive mechanical ventilation**. AIP is clinically indistinguishable from adult respiratory distress syndrome (ARDS), and an underlying etiology for ARDS (sepsis, toxic inhalation, drugs) must be sought before AIP/acute lupus pneumonitis can be considered.
- Acute lupus pneumonitis will show diffuse bilateral airspace opacities and interstitial thickening on imaging. HRCT typically demonstrates **diffuse symmetric GGO, patchy consolidations, and septal thickening**. These findings are similar to those seen in AIP or ARDS. Histologic findings in acute lupus pneumonitis show diffuse alveolar damage (DAD), which is the typical histologic finding in ARDS. Vasculitic changes are uncommon.
- **DAH** typically presents with cough, dyspnea, and hemoptysis, with or without fevers. It should be noted that **hemoptysis may be absent** on presentation, and the lack of hemoptysis does not rule out DAH.
- In chronic ILD, symptoms can include exertional dyspnea, nonproductive cough, and pleuritic chest pain. Chronic ILD in SLE can manifest in any form including OP, NSIP, UIP, bronchiolitis, or LIP.
- **Shrinking lung syndrome** manifests as an insidious onset of **dyspnea, episodic pleuritic chest pain, progressive lung volume loss on imaging** in the absence of pulmonary or pleural disease, and **RVD on PFTs**. The etiology of this syndrome is unknown.
- When there is **diffuse parenchymal involvement, bronchoscopy and BAL should be performed** to rule out etiologies such as infection or pulmonary hemorrhage. Sequential BAL can be diagnostic of DAH. BAL fluid should be sent for microbiologic studies and cytology. BAL cytology may reveal hemosiderin-laden macrophages in DAH.

TREATMENT

- Lupus pleuritis, in mild cases, responds well to **nonsteroidal anti-inflammatory drug (NSAID) monotherapy**. In refractory cases, systemic glucocorticoids can be used.
- For acute lupus pneumonitis, the mainstay of treatment is supportive care. Moderate-dose **systemic glucocorticoids** (1 to 1.5 mg/kg/day) should be initiated if there is suspicion for AIP. In refractory or severe cases, high-dose glucocorticoid (1 g methylprednisolone for 3 days) is often administered in an attempt to control the disease.
- Broad-spectrum antibiotics should be initiated and continued until an infectious etiology is ruled out.

OUTCOME/PROGNOSIS

- **Acute lupus pneumonitis has a high mortality rate** (33% to 100%). In a case series of 12 patients with SLE and "acute pneumonitis," the mortality rate was 50%.[32]
- In a longitudinal study of 14 patients with SLE-ILD with a mean follow-up of 7.3 years, the mortality because of respiratory involvement was 21%. Two patients died of pulmonary fibrosis, and one died of a bacterial pneumonia.[31]

DRUG-INDUCED ILD

GENERAL PRINCIPLES

- Methotrexate
  - **Acute pulmonary toxicity** following MTX exposure has been well documented. The incidence of acute pulmonary toxicity is thought to be between 0.3% and 8%.
  - It is clinically manifested by dyspnea, nonproductive cough, and fever.
  - Several risk factors including **age >60 years, DM, hypoalbuminemia, rheumatoid pleuropulmonary involvement, and previous DMARD use** have been recognized.
  - HRCT typically shows interstitial opacity, poorly defined micronodules, and GGO. Chest x-ray, especially in the initial stages, may appear normal.
  - The presentation may be indistinguishable from an acute respiratory infection and exclusion of an infectious process, usually through **bronchoscopy, is essential**.
  - Although it has been reported sporadically, chronic fibrosing ILD as a result of MTX use has not been demonstrated to occur in longitudinal studies.[33] Although chronic fibrosing lung disease that develops in the context of MTX does exist, this is difficult **to differentiate retrospectively from RA-ILD**.
- Leflunomide
  - Cases of pulmonary complications have been reported with leflunomide (LEF) use, including **DAD, acute eosinophilic pneumonia, and OP**.
  - Most cases are reported from Japan, and LEF **pulmonary complications seem to be higher in Asian populations** (0.5%–1%) than in the West (<0.1%). This may be because of a genetic susceptibility or increased awareness leading to a higher rate of diagnosis.
  - In a partially industry-sponsored large-scale cohort study of 62,734 RA patients prescribed DMARDs, the increased risk of ILD with LEF was restricted to those with a prior history of ILD or to those who had previously taken MTX (relative risk [RR] 2.6; 95% CI [1.2–5.6]), suggesting the possibility of channeling bias.[34] In 2016, a **meta-analysis of RCTs did not demonstrate any increased respiratory adverse events in patients who received LEF** versus placebo or other DMARDs.[35]
- Tumor necrosis factor (TNF)-α inhibitors
  - TNF-α has been shown to play both pro- and antifibrotic roles in animal models.
  - There have been published case reports, case series, and postmarketing surveys reporting new-onset ILD in patients treated with the TNF inhibitors infliximab, etanercept, adalimumab, and certolizumab. However, several confounding factors such as infection, previous or concomitant treatment with other DMARDs (particularly MTX), and underlying disease severity were not accounted for. As such, **causality has not been clearly established**.
- Other drug toxicities: Table 51-3 summarizes pulmonary toxicities associated with therapies used in the treatment of CTD-ILD.

TREATMENT

In mild cases, **removal of the offending agent** alone may suffice. In severe cases, the equivalent of **prednisone** 1 mg/kg/day may be given, although definitive data for mortality benefit are lacking.

TABLE 51-3   PULMONARY DRUG TOXICITY

	GLD	DAD	Pneumonitis	Fibrosis	Infection Risk	OP	OB	EP	DAH
Cyclophosphamide		x	x	x	x	x			x
Methotrexate	x (HP pattern)	x		?	small	x			
Leflunomide			x	?	x				
TNF-α inhibitors	x (infection)				Mycobacterial	x			
Mycophenolate			x	?	x	x			
Azathioprine		x	x	x	x	x		x	
Rituximab			x		x	x			
Gold			x			x	x		
Sulfasalazine	x			x	x	x	x	x	
Penicillamine				x	x		?		x

DAD, diffuse alveolar damage; DAH, diffuse alveolar hemorrhage; EP, eosinophilic pneumonia; GLD, granulomatous lung disease; HP, hypersensitivity pneumonitis; OB, obliterative bronchiolitis; OP, organizing pneumonia.

? reported but relation between drug and effect uncertain.

REFERENCES

1. Fischer A, Antoniou KM, Brown KK, et al. An official European Respiratory Society/American Thoracic Society research statement: interstitial pneumonia with autoimmune features. *Eur Respir J.* 2015;46:976–987.
2. American Thoracic S and European Respiratory S. American Thoracic Society/European Respiratory Society International Multidisciplinary Consensus Classification of the Idiopathic Interstitial Pneumonias. This joint statement of the American Thoracic Society (ATS), and the European Respiratory Society (ERS) was adopted by the ATS board of directors, June 2001 and by the ERS Executive Committee, June 2001. *Am J Respir Crit Care Med.* 2002;165:277–304.
3. Travis WD, Costabel U, Hansell DM, et al. An official American Thoracic Society/European Respiratory Society statement: update of the international multidisciplinary classification of the idiopathic interstitial pneumonias. *Am J Respir Crit Care Med.* 2013;188:733–748.
4. Courtwright AM, El-Chemaly S, Dellaripa PF, et al. Survival and outcomes after lung transplantation for non-scleroderma connective tissue-related interstitial lung disease. *J Heart Lung Transplant.* 2017;36:763–769.
5. Pradere P, Tudorache I, Magnusson J, et al. Lung transplantation for scleroderma lung disease: An international, multicenter, observational cohort study. *J Heart Lung Transplant.* 2018;37:903–911.
6. Oldham JM, Adegunsoye A, Valenzi E, et al. Characterisation of patients with interstitial pneumonia with autoimmune features. *Eur Respir J.* 2016;47:1767–1775.
7. Strand MJ, Sprunger D, Cosgrove GP, et al. Pulmonary function and survival in idiopathic vs secondary usual interstitial pneumonia. *Chest.* 2014;146:775–785.
8. Chang B, Wigley FM, White B, et al. Scleroderma patients with combined pulmonary hypertension and interstitial lung disease. *J Rheumatol.* 2003;30:2398–2405.
9. White B. Interstitial lung disease in scleroderma. *Rheum Dis Clin North Am.* 2003;29:371–390.
10. Steen VD, Medsger TA. Changes in causes of death in systemic sclerosis, 1972-2002. *Ann Rheum Dis.* 2007;66:940–944.
11. Tyndall AJ, Bannert B, Vonk M, et al. Causes and risk factors for death in systemic sclerosis: a study from the EULAR Scleroderma Trials and Research (EUSTAR) database. *Ann Rheum Dis.* 2010;69:1809–1815.
12. Tashkin DP, Roth MD, Clements PJ, et al. Mycophenolate mofetil versus oral cyclophosphamide in scleroderma-related interstitial lung disease (SLS II): a randomised controlled, double-blind, parallel group trial. *Lancet Respir Med.* 2016;4:708–719.
13. Winstone TA, Assayag D, Wilcox PG, et al. Predictors of mortality and progression in scleroderma-associated interstitial lung disease: a systematic review. *Chest.* 2014;146:422–436.
14. Goh NS, Desai SR, Veeraraghavan S, et al. Interstitial lung disease in systemic sclerosis: a simple staging system. *Am J Respir Crit Care Med.* 2008;177:1248–1254.
15. Bongartz T, Nannini C, Medina-Velasquez YF, et al. Incidence and mortality of interstitial lung disease in rheumatoid arthritis: a population-based study. *Arthritis Rheum.* 2010;62:1583–1591.
16. Lee HK, Kim DS, Yoo B, et al. Histopathologic pattern and clinical features of rheumatoid arthritis-associated interstitial lung disease. *Chest.* 2005;127:2019–2027.
17. Jokerst CA, Azok J, Cummings W, et al. High-resolution CT imaging findings of collagen vascular disease-associated interstitial lung disease. *Curr Respir Med Rev.* 2015;11:73–82.
18. Fischer A, Brown KK, Du Bois RM, et al. Mycophenolate mofetil improves lung function in connective tissue disease-associated interstitial lung disease. *J Rheumatol.* 2013;40:640–646.
19. Zamora-Legoff JA, Krause ML, Crowson CS, et al. Progressive decline of lung function in rheumatoid arthritis-associated interstitial lung disease. *Arthritis Rheumatol.* 2017;69:542–549.
20. Tsuchiya Y, Takayanagi N, Sugiura H, et al Lung diseases directly associated with rheumatoid arthritis and their relationship to outcome. *Eur Respir J.* 2011;37:1411–1417.
21. Marie I, Hachulla E, Cherin P, et al. Interstitial lung disease in polymyositis and dermatomyositis. *Arthritis Rheum.* 2002;47:614–622.
22. Fathi M, Dastmalchi M, Rasmussen E, et al. Interstitial lung disease, a common manifestation of newly diagnosed polymyositis and dermatomyositis. *Ann Rheum Dis.* 2004;63:297–301.
23. Dickey BF, Myers AR. Pulmonary disease in polymyositis/dermatomyositis. *Semin Arthritis Rheum.* 1984;14:60–76.
24. Ando M, Miyazaki E, Yamasue M, et al. Successful treatment with tacrolimus of progressive interstitial pneumonia associated with amyopathic dermatomyositis refractory to cyclosporine. *Clin Rheumatol.* 2010;29:443–445.

25. Andersson H, Sem M, Lund MB, et al. Long-term experience with rituximab in anti-synthetase syndrome-related interstitial lung disease. *Rheumatology (Oxford)*. 2015;54:1420–1428.

26. Marie I, Hatron PY, Dominique S, et al. Short-term and long-term outcomes of interstitial lung disease in polymyositis and dermatomyositis: a series of 107 patients. *Arthritis Rheum*. 2011;63:3439–3447.

27. Moghadam-Kia S, Oddis CV, Sato S, et al. Anti-melanoma differentiation-associated gene 5 is associated with rapidly progressive lung disease and poor survival in US patients with amyopathic and myopathic dermatomyositis. *Arthritis Care Res (Hoboken)*. 2016;68:689–694.

28. Nannini C, Jebakumar AJ, Crowson CS, et al. Primary Sjogren's syndrome 1976-2005 and associated interstitial lung disease: a population-based study of incidence and mortality. *BMJ Open*. 2013;3:e003569.

29. Strimlan CV, Rosenow EC, III, Divertie MB, et al. Pulmonary manifestations of Sjogren's syndrome. *Chest*. 1976;70:354–361.

30. Ekstrom Smedby K, Vajdic CM, Falster M, et al. Autoimmune disorders and risk of non-Hodgkin lymphoma subtypes: a pooled analysis within the InterLymph Consortium. *Blood*. 2008;111:4029–4038.

31. Weinrib L, Sharma OP, Quismorio FP, Jr. A long-term study of interstitial lung disease in systemic lupus erythematosus. *Semin Arthritis Rheum*. 1990;20:48–56.

32. Matthay RA, Schwarz MI, Petty TL, et al. Pulmonary manifestations of systemic lupus erythematosus: review of twelve cases of acute lupus pneumonitis. *Medicine (Baltimore)*. 1975;54:397–409.

33. Dawson JK, Graham DR, Desmond J, et al. Investigation of the chronic pulmonary effects of low-dose oral methotrexate in patients with rheumatoid arthritis: a prospective study incorporating HRCT scanning and pulmonary function tests. *Rheumatology (Oxford)*. 2002;41:262–267.

34. Suissa S, Hudson M, Ernst P. Leflunomide use and the risk of interstitial lung disease in rheumatoid arthritis. *Arthritis Rheum*. 2006;54:1435–1439.

35. Conway R, Low C, Coughlan RJ, et al. Leflunomide use and risk of lung disease in rheumatoid arthritis: a systematic literature review and metaanalysis of randomized controlled trials. *J Rheumatol*. 2016;43:855–860.

Osteoporosis

52

Kelvin J. Lee and Deborah L. Parks

GENERAL PRINCIPLES

Definition

- Osteoporosis is a skeletal disorder characterized by poor bone mass and quality, resulting in decreased bone strength and increased risk of fracture.
- Conceptually, low bone strength relates to low bone mineral density (BMD) and poor bone quality.
  - **BMD** refers to the number of grams of mineral per area (or volume) of bone. This information is easily obtained through dual-energy x-ray absorptiometry (DEXA) and is expressed as two values:
    - **Z-score:** Number of standard deviations (SDs) a patient's BMD differs from the mean BMD of an age-matched population.
    - **T-score:** Number of SDs a patient's BMD differs from the mean BMD of a young-adult reference population.
  - **Bone quality** refers to the architectural characteristics of bone (e.g., rate of bone remodeling, trabecular connectivity, degree of mineralization, and damage accumulation). A bone biopsy is the best way to obtain information on bone quality, which makes it difficult to routinely assess.

Classification

- Osteoporosis can be classified as primary or secondary on the basis of causality.
- In **primary osteoporosis,** the deterioration of bone mass is related to aging or decreased gonadal function. It is typically seen in postmenopausal women and older men, usually over age 70.
- **Secondary osteoporosis** results from chronic conditions or medications, like glucocorticoids, that accelerate bone loss.

Epidemiology

- Osteoporosis is generally asymptomatic until complications develop. Approximately 1.5 million osteoporosis-related fractures occur each year in the United States.[1]
- Postmenopausal women comprise the vast majority of fragility fractures. **White and Mexican American postmenopausal women are especially at high risk for osteoporosis and related fractures.** The age-adjusted prevalence of osteoporosis is lowest in men and black adults.[2,3]
- Osteoporosis is a **common comorbidity in patients with rheumatologic diseases** because of the increased use of glucocorticoids, decreased physical activity, systemic inflammation, and alteration of the normal balance of bone resorption/formation.

Pathophysiology

- Osteoporosis is characterized by **either low bone density or poor bone quality.**
- Loss of bone mass occurs during bone remodeling when bone resorption (a result of osteoclast activity) occurs more quickly than bone formation (a consequence of osteoblast activity).

- ○ Crucial regulators of osteoclastic bone resorption include **RANK ligand** (RANKL; a member of the tumor necrosis factor [TNF] ligand family) and **its two receptors, RANK and osteoprotegerin (OPG).**
- ○ RANKL is expressed by osteoblasts. It interacts with its corresponding receptor, RANK, which is expressed by osteoclasts.
- ○ This interaction promotes osteoclast differentiation, activation, and prolonged survival.
- ○ OPG, which is secreted by osteoblasts and stromal cells, blocks the interaction of RANKL with RANK, thereby regulating bone turnover (see Fig. 52-1).
- After age 40, cortical bone is lost at a rate of 0.3% to 0.5% per year.
  - ○ Trabecular bone loss may begin at an even younger age. This loss of cortical and trabecular bone accelerates after menopause because **estrogen deficiency results in increased bone turnover and a remodeling imbalance.**
  - ○ The enhanced activity and function of osteoclasts during this period appear to be because of the increased expression of **osteoclastogenic proinflammatory cytokines like interleukin (IL)-1 and TNF,** which are negatively regulated by estrogen.
- Histologically, the bone has decreased cortical thickness and a decreased number and size of trabeculae.
  - ○ Although trabecular or cancellous bone found mainly in the axial skeleton comprises only 20% of bone, and cortical bone found primarily in the diaphyses of long bones comprises 80% of bone, **trabecular bone is the site of the greatest bone turnover** as a result of its greater surface area.
  - ○ Thus, it is more susceptible to imbalances in remodeling and more frequently associated with osteoporotic fractures.
  - ○ **The most frequent sites of osteoporotic fractures are the spine, hip, and distal radius.**

Risk Factors

- Low BMD correlates with an increased risk of primary osteoporosis. **Predictors of low BMD** include female gender, increased age, estrogen deficiency, white or Asian race, low weight and body mass index, family history of osteoporosis, smoking, history of fracture, late menarche, and early menopause.
- Secondary causes of osteoporosis are extensive.

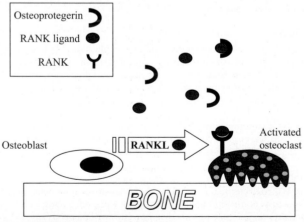

FIGURE 52-1. Pathophysiology of osteoporosis.

○ They involve **diseases of hormone dysregulation** including Cushing's syndrome, primary or secondary amenorrhea, hypogonadism, hyperthyroidism, diabetes mellitus type I, and hyperparathyroidism.

○ Malnutrition, malabsorption syndromes, pernicious anemia, parenteral nutrition, and gastrectomy are predisposing factors.

○ Severe liver and renal diseases, chronic obstructive pulmonary disease, hemochromatosis, and mastocytosis also place patients at a higher risk for osteoporosis.

○ **Rheumatologic diseases** such as rheumatoid arthritis and ankylosing spondylitis also predispose to osteoporosis even after excluding patients on glucocorticoids.[4]

○ **Certain drugs and toxins** (e.g., glucocorticoids, anticonvulsants, heparin, lithium, thyroxine, cytotoxic drugs, ethanol use, and tobacco) have also been implicated.

DIAGNOSIS

Clinical Presentation

History

- Osteoporosis is commonly asymptomatic until fractures occur.
- **Vertebral compression fractures** most commonly occur in the T-11 to L-2 region and may present as loss of height rather than back pain.
- Other common fracture sites are the **distal wrist (Colles fracture), hip, and pelvis.**

Physical Examination

- Physical examination may reveal tenderness along the spine, scoliosis, kyphosis, or dowager's hump.
- Signs and symptoms of secondary causes can be elicited during the history and physical examination (e.g., hypogonadism, evidence of thyroid disease, and cushingoid features).

Diagnostic Criteria

- Osteoporosis should be diagnosed in **any patient who sustains a fragility fracture regardless of BMD.**
- **Current World Health Organization (WHO) criteria for patients greater than 50 years are as follows:**
  ○ **Normal:** BMD within 1 SD of the reference mean (T ≥ −1.0)
  ○ **Osteopenia:** BMD between 1 and 2.5 SDs below the reference mean (−2.5 < T < −1.0)
  ○ **Osteoporosis:** BMD 2.5 SDs or more below the reference mean (T ≤ −2.5)
- **In premenopausal women or men under age 50, the diagnosis cannot be made based on BMD score alone** because the relationship between BMD and fracture risk is not the same in younger women and men. Also, Z-scores, not T-scores, should be used. A change in T- or Z-score of 1 SD roughly corresponds to a 10% change in BMD.
- BMD is an excellent predictor of fracture risk but when it is combined with clinical risk factors, it is a better predictor than either alone. **The Fracture Risk Assessment Tool (FRAX)** estimates the 10-year probability of fracture on the basis of clinical risk factors and BMD at the femoral neck. FRAX is an electronic clinical tool (www.shef.ac.uk/FRAX) and is only helpful in making treatment decisions in patients with osteopenia.
- The American College of Rheumatology and National Osteoporosis Foundation currently recommend **screening all women over age 65 and men over age 70, along with any adult with a condition or taking medication-associated low bone mass or bone loss.**
- Patients with rheumatic diseases at higher risk of osteoporosis should be screened when **glucocorticoids are initiated at doses of 10 mg or more and length of treatment is anticipated for more than 3 month for consideration of prophylactic treatment to prevent bone loss.**

Differential Diagnosis

The differential diagnosis of osteoporosis includes osteomalacia, metastatic malignancy to bone, multiple myeloma, hyperthyroidism, hyperparathyroidism, renal osteodystrophy, malabsorption syndromes, vitamin deficiencies, and Paget's disease.

Diagnostic Testing

Laboratories
- Limited laboratory testing as suggested by history and physical examination (e.g., serum and urine calcium, serum phosphorus, alkaline phosphatase, thyroid hormone levels, serum protein electrophoresis, parathyroid hormones [PTHs], vitamin D level, serum testosterone in men, cortisol, and renal and liver functions) can be helpful in diagnosing secondary causes.
- Markers of bone turnover are not useful in making the diagnosis of osteoporosis.

Imaging
- **Plain radiography** can demonstrate osteopenia and vertebral compression fractures but is a generally unreliable marker of bone mass because 20% to 50% of bone must be lost before changes are evident on radiographs.
- BMD testing techniques include **DEXA**, single-energy x-ray absorptiometry, peripheral DEXA, quantitative computed tomography (CT), and ultrasound densitometry.
  - **Central DEXA is the gold standard and recommended for adults who have had osteoporotic fractures or who are undergoing general screening.**
  - DEXA imaging results in a low level of radiation exposure (one-tenth of a traditional radiograph) and has excellent reproducibility and precision.
  - Bone density testing should be obtained at both the spine and the hip. **In women younger than 65 years, spine imaging may be more helpful** because bone is apt to be lost more rapidly in the spine, and vertebral fractures are the most common fracture in this age group. **In women older than 65 years, bone density at the hip is more clinically useful** as hip fractures are more of a concern and the spine bone density has a higher chance of false elevations because of vascular calcifications or osteoarthritis of the spine.
  - DEXA can also be used to measure the wrist, but measurements at that site are of limited clinical significance because of lower predictive values and less reproducibility.
- **Quantitative CT** has a similar ability to predict fractures as central DEXA. Quantitative CT is less affected by superimposed osteoarthritis. However, quantitative CT scans are more expensive and require a larger dose of radiation, so clinically they are not frequently used.
- **Peripheral bone density** performed with either DEXA or single-energy x-ray absorptiometry can measure forearm, finger, or heel BMD, whereas peripheral ultrasonography most commonly measures bone mass of the heel. The advantages of peripheral bone density testing and ultrasonography are the portability and the ability of these tests to be performed in primary care offices. However, there are no universally agreed upon diagnostic criteria for the different machines available. In addition, the precision of the machines does not allow for their use in monitoring response to therapy. **Peripheral testing has not been endorsed for use in the diagnosis of osteoporosis,** but if it is performed, abnormal results should be followed up with central DEXA to establish or confirm the diagnosis.

TREATMENT

- The National Osteoporosis Foundation has issued clinical practice guidelines for treating osteoporosis and addresses postmenopausal women and men over the age of 50 for all ethnic groups in the United States. It is intended for use by clinicians in making decisions in the care of individual patients.

- **The main goal in treatment of osteoporosis is the prevention of fractures.** On average, risk of fracture approximately doubles for each 1 SD decrease in T-score. The following are indications to initiate specific therapy for osteoporosis. It is important to be aware that the prospective randomized controlled pharmacologic trials for the treatment of osteoporosis have taken place mainly in the population of white women, so limited data are available on therapeutic benefit of pharmacologic agents in men or minority groups.
  - All adults with osteoporotic fractures of the hip or spine
  - Adults with a T-score lesser than or equal to -2 SD who do not have specific risk factors for osteoporosis
  - Adults with a T-score lesser than or equal to -1.5 SD who have risk factors for osteoporosis
  - Women more than 70 years old with multiple risk factors are at high enough risk to begin treatment without BMD testing.
- Adequate intake of **calcium and vitamin D is recommended for all patients.**
  - Daily intake of elemental **calcium** should be at least **1,200 mg.** Calcium supplements are mostly available as calcium carbonate or calcium citrate. Foods rich in calcium include dairy products, sardines, and fortified juices.
  - All adults should receive at least **800 to 1,000 IU of vitamin D** per day. Foods rich in vitamin D include fortified milk and cereals, egg yolks, and liver.
- Regular **weight-bearing exercise** is also recommended for all patients.
- **Fall prevention:** Most osteoporotic fractures involve falling or low-impact trauma. Patients should be assessed for reversible causes of falls like overmedication, neurologic or vision problems, and poor footwear.
- Smoking cessation and avoidance of excessive alcohol intake should also be encouraged.

Medications

Pharmacologic agents for the treatment of osteoporosis can be classified as either antiresorptive or anabolic. Drugs of each type have been shown to improve BMD and reduce the risk of fractures.

- **Bisphosphonates**
  - **Bisphosphonates:** Alendronate, risedronate, ibandronate, and zoledronic acid are commonly used as first-line treatment in women who do not have contraindications.
  - Bisphosphonates bind avidly to hydroxyapatite crystals in bone and are resistant to metabolic degradation. They **reduce the ability of osteoclasts to resorb bone and accelerate osteoclast apoptosis.**
  - Oral bisphosphonates are now used in weekly doses (alendronate and risedronate) or monthly doses (ibandronate and risedronate). In clinical practice, **esophageal and gastric side effects** are the most commonly reported, and oral bisphosphonates should not be prescribed for patients with clinically significant esophageal disease.
  - Intravenous bisphosphonates (ibandronate [every 3 months] and zoledronic acid [annually]) are alternatives that do not require frequent patient use. Intravenous administration of bisphosphonates can cause an **acute-phase reaction (flu-like symptoms).** An increased risk of atrial fibrillation has been reported in some trials of zoledronic acid but not in others.
  - Two rare but more serious adverse effects have been observed in bisphosphonates: **osteonecrosis of the jaw (ONJ)** and **atypical femoral fractures (AFF).**
    - Most cases of ONJ have been associated with the use of intravenous bisphosphonates in patients with metastatic bone disease.
    - The incidence of AFF increases with duration of bisphosphonate exposure, approximately 1 per 1,000 patient-years after 10 years of exposure.[5]
  - Long-term data with alendronate and risedronate have demonstrated efficacy and safety for 10 and 7 years, respectively.

○ Stopping therapy after 5 years or a "drug holiday" of a year or two may be reasonable because there appears to be residual BMD and fracture benefit.[6]

• **Denosumab**
  ○ **Denosumab** is a humanized monoclonal antibody that specifically binds RANKL and blocks the binding of RANKL to RANK. It thereby decreases the differentiation of osteoclasts and reduces fractures. It is administered as 60 mg subcutaneously every 6 months.
  ○ Unlike bisphosphonates, it is not cleared by the kidney; thus, there is no restriction of its use in chronic kidney disease.
  ○ Also in contrast to bisphosphonates, discontinuation of denosumab results in immediate bone loss and is associated with increased risk of fracture. It has also been shown through monitoring of bone turnover markers that the effect on bone remodeling is reversible within a short time of discontinuation. Consideration for alternative therapy following cessation should be given.
  ○ As with bisphosphonates, rare cases of AFF and ONJ have been observed with denosumab. Skin reaction is also a potential side effect.

• **Synthetic PTH: Teriparatide** is a recombinant formation of the active 34 N-terminal peptide portion of PTH.
  ○ The skeletal effects of PTH depend upon the pattern of systemic exposure. Continuous exposure to PTH (as in patients with primary hyperparathyroidism) leads to increased bone resorption, whereas intermittent exposure increases bone formation.
  ○ Teriparatide is an anabolic agent that works by preferentially stimulating osteoblastic activity over osteoclastic activity. It is administered by daily self-injection and is approved for up to 2 years of use.
  ○ **BMD improvement seen with teriparatide is greater than other available agents for osteoporosis.** However, because of its significant cost, the medication would be best served for patients with severe osteoporosis (i.e., T-score below −3) or those who fail antiresorptive therapy.
  ○ There is a black-box warning about risk of osteosarcoma based on studies of long-term, high-dose use in rodents. It should therefore not be prescribed for patients with metastatic bone disease and those at increased baseline risk for osteosarcoma, such as Paget's disease and prior radiation therapy involving the skeleton.

• **Selective Estrogen Receptor Modulators: Raloxifene is a selective estrogen receptor modulator (SERM)** that exhibits proestrogen effects on some tissues and antiestrogen effects on other tissues. It has been shown in trials to decrease the rate of new vertebral fractures by 40% to 50% and improve BMD at the spine and hip. It has not been found to have a significant effect on hip or total nonvertebral fractures. The ideal candidate for raloxifene is a woman who cannot tolerate a bisphosphonate. Typical dose is 60 mg PO daily. On raloxifene, there is an increased risk of stroke or deep vein thrombosis and pulmonary embolism.

• **Others**
  ○ **Hormone replacement therapy** has been shown to prevent bone loss but it is not used in the treatment of osteoporosis because of an **unfavorable risk–benefit ratio**, especially cardiovascular disease and thromboembolic events.
  ○ **Calcitonin** is an endogenous peptide that enhances BMD by inhibiting osteoclast activity. It is available in both subcutaneous and intranasal forms. Evidence of its effect on osteoporosis is limited compared to the aforementioned agents. Of note, intranasal calcitonin has been found to be **beneficial in treating the pain of acute vertebral compression fractures.**
  ○ **Strontium ranelate** is an agent approved in Europe but not approved by the Food and Drug Administration (FDA). It increases calcium uptake and bone formation, and inhibits bone resorption.

- ○ **Romosozumab** is a humanized monoclonal antibody that binds to sclerostin, an osteocyte-derived inhibitor of osteoblast activity. It results in increased bone formation. The medication is not currently FDA-approved, but results from the pivotal ARCH trial showed that it outperformed alendronate.[7]
- **Combination therapy** with two antiresorptive medicines has not demonstrated a reduction in the fracture risk above what would be found with a single agent. Starting antiresorptive therapy after completing anabolic therapy makes conceptual sense and is especially supported by results of the DATA-Switch study[8]; however, more studies are needed to validate this. Bone loss occurred in patients switching from denosumab to teriparatide, further illustrating the importance of treatment sequence.

SPECIAL CONSIDERATIONS

- **Glucocorticoid therapy** causes bone loss through a number of different mechanisms, including impaired intestinal calcium absorption, increased urinary calcium excretion, decreased bone formation, increased bone resorption through the stimulation of osteoclast activity by macrophage colony–stimulating factor, and suppression of endogenous gonadal steroid production.[9]
- Therapy with glucocorticoids leads to an early and sometimes dramatic loss of trabecular bone with less effect on cortical bone.
- Glucocorticoid use is **the most common form of drug-related osteoporosis** and is often seen in patients with rheumatic diseases.
  - ○ Glucocorticoids should be prescribed at the **lowest effective dose for the shortest duration possible.**
  - ○ Patients who receive glucocorticoids (e.g., prednisone at >5 mg PO/day) for more than 2 months are considered at high risk for excessive bone loss, but there has been some controversy regarding the dose at which an increased risk of fracture occurs.
  - ○ To diagnose and prevent glucocorticoid-induced osteoporosis, **obtain a baseline assessment of BMD of the hip or spine before initiating any long-term (>3 months) therapy.**
- For steroid-induced osteoporosis, randomized controlled studies demonstrate calcium carbonate 1,000 mg PO daily and vitamin D 500 IU PO daily to be an effective preventive therapy for some patients receiving prednisone.
- The American College of Rheumatology updated guidelines for the prevention and treatment of glucocorticoid-induced osteoporosis in 2017.[10]
  - ○ Postmenopausal women and men over age 50 with an estimated steroid course of at least 3 months were stratified into low-, moderate-, and high-risk groups on the basis of their FRAX and BMD testing with consideration of other risk factors.
  - ○ Low-risk patients should require no further treatment and clinically monitored annually with BMD testing every 2 to 3 years. Moderate- and high-risk groups should be on a bisphosphonate for any dose of steroid.
  - ○ For premenopausal women and men less than age 50, the data are inadequate to make a recommendation. Individual circumstances and childbearing potential in women need to be considered.

COMPLICATIONS

- Possible consequences of fracture because of osteoporosis are acute and chronic pain, depression, deconditioning, dependency, and changes in appearance including loss of height and kyphosis.
- Hip fractures are associated with an up to 20% mortality rate in women and a 30% mortality rate in men within the first year of fracture, most often because of comorbidities.

Twenty percent of patients with hospitalization because of a hip fracture require nursing home care, and 50% of survivors are unable to ambulate independently or have some other permanent disability.

MONITORING/FOLLOW-UP

- Follow-up of patients includes monitoring for complications, side effects, and response to treatment. Continued assessment for modifiable risk factors and fall risk is necessary. Height should be followed to screen for asymptomatic vertebral fractures.
- **BMD should be reevaluated every 1 to 2 years to assess response to therapy.** Repeat measurements made sooner than that can be difficult to interpret because the expected change in BMD over a short period of time may be similar to the precision of the machine. **BMD changes need to be 3% or more to be considered significant.** Repeat measurements need to be made on the same DEXA machine to allow results to be accurately compared. Patients who are being screened for osteoporosis but are not on treatment should wait 2 years before undergoing repeat BMD testing.
- Monitoring with markers of bone turnover is another option. Fasting urinary N-telopeptide (NTX) or serum carboxy-terminal collagen cross-links (CTX) can be measured before and then 3 to 6 months after initiating therapy. A decrease of greater than 50% in urinary NTX excretion or 30% in serum CTX provides evidence of compliance and drug efficacy. A decrease in markers of less than this amount may not necessarily indicate treatment failure, and noncompliance or poor absorption should be considered.[11]

REFERENCES

1. Black DM, Rosen CJ. Postmenopausal osteoporosis. *N Engl J Med.* 2016;374:254–262.
2. Wright NC, Looker AC, Saag KG, et al. The recent prevalence of osteoporosis and low bone mass in the United States based on bone mineral density at the femoral neck or lumbar spine. *J Bone Miner Res* 2014;29:2520–2526.
3. Looker AC, Borrud LG, Dawson-Hughes B, et al. Osteoporosis or low bone mass at the femur neck or lumbar spine in older adults: United States, 2005-2008. *NCHS Data Brief.* 2012;1–8.
4. Roux C. Osteoporosis in inflammatory joint diseases. *Osteoporos Int.* 2011;22:421–433.
5. Dell RM, Adams AL, Greene DF, et al. Incidence of atypical nontraumatic diaphyseal fractures of the femur. *JBMR.* 2012;27:2544–2550.
6. Black DM, Schwartz AV, Ensrud KE, et al. Effects of continuing or stopping alendronate after 5 years of treatment: the Fracture Intervention Trial Long Term Extension (FLEX), a randomized trial. *JAMA.* 2006;296:2927–2938.
7. Saag KG, Peterson J, Brandi ML, et al. Romosozumab or alendronate for fracture prevention in women with osteoporosis. *N Engl J Med.* 2017;377:1417–1427.
8. Leder BZ, Tsai JN, Uihlein AV, et al. Denosumab and teriparatide transitions in postmenopausal osteoporosis (the DATA-Switch study): extension of a randomised controlled trial. *Lancet.* 2015;386:1147–1155.
9. Weinstein RS. Clinical practice. Glucocorticoid-induced bone disease. *N Engl J Med.* 2011;365:62–70.
10. Buckley L, Guyatt G, Fink HA, et al. 2017 American College of Rheumatology Guideline for the prevention and treatment of glucocorticoid-induced osteoporosis. *Arthritis Rheumatol.* 2017;69:1521–1537.
11. Naylor K, Eastell R. Bone turnover markers: use in osteoporosis. *Nat Rev Rheumatol.* 2012;8:379–389.

Fibromyalgia Syndrome

53

Divya Jayakumar and Amy M. Joseph

GENERAL PRINCIPLES

Definition

- Fibromyalgia syndrome (FMS) is a chronic pain syndrome of unknown etiology that is characterized by altered central afferent pain processing associated with unexplained diffuse pain as well as fatigue, cognitive impairment, and sleep disturbance.
- This disorder is not considered to be autoimmune or inflammatory, and whether this is a rheumatologic condition is controversial. However, it is a condition seen by rheumatologists because patients present with musculoskeletal pain.

Epidemiology

- Estimated prevalence of fibromyalgia is 2% to 5%, with a female-to-male ratio of 2:1 based on the 2010 American College of Rheumatology criteria that do not require a tender point examination.[1]
- FMS may present at any age.
- Psychiatric disorders, including depression, posttraumatic stress disorder (PTSD), and anxiety disorder, are seen significantly more frequently in patients with FMS than in the general population.

Pathophysiology

- The pathophysiology of fibromyalgia is poorly understood.
- FMS is a disorder of **heightened pain response,** characterized by both hyperalgesia, defined as increased pain sensitivity, and allodynia, defined as pain experienced in response to nonpainful stimuli.
- FMS may be a result of neuroendocrine axis alterations with subsequent **disturbances in mood, sleep, and pain perception.**
- Abnormalities of the joint, muscle, or soft tissue have not been identified in FMS patients, although musculoskeletal conditions can coexist with FMS.
- Studies show that patients often have low serum serotonin, growth hormone, and cortisol levels as well as elevated cerebrospinal fluid (CSF) substance P concentrations. Substance P, regulated by serotonin, can cause exaggerated perception of normal sensory stimuli.
- Functional MRI studies have demonstrated that the pain centers in the brains of FMS patients are activated by low-level stimuli and show expanded receptive fields for central pain perception in a very similar way to patients with other chronic pain disorders.[2]
- FMS patients have sleep disturbances, with decreased sleep efficiency, increased arousals, and decreased deep sleep, resulting in nonrestorative sleep and daytime somnolence. It is unknown whether pain disturbs sleep, the disturbed sleep causes pain, or both.[3]

Associated Conditions

- Patients with FMS often have other symptom-based conditions such as irritable bowel syndrome, migraine headache, interstitial cystitis/bladder pain syndrome, chronic fatigue syndrome, and temporomandibular syndrome.
- Primary fibromyalgia occurs alone, whereas secondary fibromyalgia may coexist with other disease conditions. Patients with rheumatologic disorders, such as rheumatoid

arthritis (RA), Sjögren's syndrome (SS), and systemic lupus erythematosus (SLE), have concomitant FMS at a higher prevalence than in the general population.

DIAGNOSIS

Clinical Presentation

- **The cardinal feature of FMS is diffuse musculoskeletal pain,** which is often described as burning, tingling, or gnawing. The pain may be located in the neck, back, chest, or limbs. Usually patients have pain on both sides of the body as well as above and below the waist.
- In addition, patients may complain of **morning stiffness, fatigue, sleep disturbances, or headaches.** The symptoms of pain and fatigue are worsened by inactivity but also after seemingly minor activity.
- **The physical examination is normal except for the presence of tenderness.** It is important to perform a complete joint examination to look for synovitis to avoid missing a concomitant inflammatory arthritis.

Diagnostic Criteria

The American College of Rheumatology published preliminary criteria for the diagnosis and measurement of symptom severity of FMS in 2010.[4] These criteria are outlined in Table 53-1.

Differential Diagnosis

Other diagnoses to consider include hypothyroidism, drug-induced myopathies (e.g., 3-hydroxy-3-methyl-glutaryl-coenzyme A (HMG-CoA) reductase inhibitor induced), polymyalgia rheumatica (PMR), myofascial pain syndrome, Lyme disease, sciatica, multiple sclerosis, metabolic myopathy, depression, temporomandibular joint syndrome, sleep apnea, and rheumatologic disorders (e.g., RA, SLE, SS, ankylosing spondylitis [AS]).

Diagnostic Testing

- The diagnosis of FMS is made clinically.
- Lab tests and radiologic studies often are unrevealing but are helpful in excluding other diseases.
- Perform a careful sleep history and consider **sleep studies,** especially in obese patients and in males with fibromyalgia.
- **Screen patients for coexistent depression,** which commonly occurs in patients with chronic pain regardless of the source.

Laboratories
- Initial tests should include a complete blood count (CBC), an erythrocyte sedimentation rate (ESR), standard chemistries, creatine phosphokinase, and thyroid function studies.
- Because of the number of false positives, reserve testing for rheumatoid factor (RF), antinuclear antibodies (ANAs), and Lyme antibodies for patients in whom clinical suspicion is high based on history and physical examination.

Imaging
Radiologic studies may be ordered for patients with evidence of arthritis or radiculopathy.

TREATMENT

Both pharmacologic and nonpharmacologic therapies should be included when tailoring a treatment plan to an individual patient.

TABLE 53-1	**THE AMERICAN COLLEGE OF RHEUMATOLOGY 2010 FIBROMYALGIA DIAGNOSTIC CRITERIA**

A patient satisfies diagnostic criteria for fibromyalgia if the following three conditions are met:

- Widespread pain index (WPI) ≥7 and symptom severity (SS) scale score ≥5 OR WPI 3–6 and SS scale score ≥9.
- Symptoms have been present at a similar level for at least 3 months.
- The patient does not have a disorder that would otherwise explain the pain.

WPI: Quantify the number of areas in which the patient has had pain over the last week. Score will be between 0 and 19.

Shoulder girdle, left	Hip (buttock, trochanter), left	Jaw, left	Upper back
Shoulder girdle, right	Hip (buttock, trochanter), right	Jaw, right	Lower back
Upper arm, left	Upper leg, left	Chest	Neck
Upper arm, right	Upper leg, right	Abdomen	
Lower arm, left	Lower leg, left		
Lower arm, right	Lower leg, right		

SS Scale Score: The sum of the severity of the three symptoms (fatigue, waking unrefreshed, and cognitive symptoms) plus the extent (severity) of somatic symptoms in general. The final score is between 0 and 12.

For each of the three symptoms below, indicate the level of severity over the past week using the following scale:

Fatigue
Waking unrefreshed
Cognitive symptoms

0 = no problem
1 = slight or mild problems, generally mild or intermittent
2 = moderate, considerable problems, often present and/or at a moderate level
3 = severe, pervasive, continuous, life-disturbing problems

Considering somatic symptoms in general, indicate whether the patient has[a]:

0 = no symptoms
1 = few symptoms
2 = a moderate number of symptoms
3 = a great deal of symptoms

[a]Somatic symptoms to consider: fatigue, muscle pain/weakness, irritable bowel syndrome, abdominal pain/cramps, nausea, vomiting, constipation, diarrhea, dry mouth, heartburn, oral ulcers, loss of/change in taste, loss of appetite, thinking problems, memory problems, headache, numbness/tingling, dizziness, blurred vision, hearing problems, tinnitus, seizures, insomnia, depression, nervousness, shortness of breath, wheezing, chest pain, urinary frequency, dysuria and bladder spasms, itching, Raynaud's phenomenon, hives, dry eyes, rash, sun sensitivity, easy bruising, hair loss.

Adapted from: Wolfe F, Clauw DJ, Fitzcharles M, et al. The American College of Rheumatology preliminary diagnostic criteria for fibromyalgia and measurement of symptom severity. *Arth Care Res.* 2010;62:600–610.

Nonpharmacologic Therapies

- There is strong evidence to support the use of exercise and cognitive-behavioral psychotherapy (CBT) in the treatment of FMS.[5]

- Physical activity helps maintain function in patients. Aerobic activity (e.g., swimming, water aerobics, bicycling, brisk walking) should be performed for at least 20 minutes daily, at a moderate intensity. It can be split into two 10-minute periods. Long intervals between workouts may require the patient to start over on their exercise regimen. Strength training should be performed 2 to 3 times per week with 8 to 12 repetitions per exercise.
- Behavioral therapy, CBT, and biofeedback combined with relaxation and movement therapy have been proven effective.
- Some patients find relief from tai chi and yoga. Acupuncture and balneotherapy can also be of benefit.
- Treatment of sleep disorders, including education regarding sleep hygiene principles, is important in FMS.
- Psychiatric disorders such as depression, PTSD, and anxiety disorder can amplify pain perception in FMS and so should be treated.
- Patient education is an important component of therapy for FMS. Patients often find it somewhat reassuring that the pain of FMS does not signify tissue damage, but rather is thought to be from a disorder in processing pain signals to the brain. Support groups are also available for FMS patients.
- Establishing a close patient–physician relationship with frequent visits often helps patients cope with their disease.

Medications

- Pharmacologic therapies with proven effectiveness include antidepressants, antiepileptics, and analgesics.
- Antidepressants, including tricyclic antidepressants (TCAs), monoamine oxidase inhibitors (MAOIs), selective serotonin reuptake inhibitors (SSRIs), along with serotonin and norepinephrine reuptake inhibitors (SNRIs), have been shown to be effective in decreasing symptoms of fibromyalgia.[6]
- Two SNRI antidepressants, **duloxetine and milnacipran,** have been approved by the Food and Drug Administration (FDA) for FMS. They affect pain and sleep disturbance in FMS, but this is thought to be independent of their effect on mood.[7,8]
  - Duloxetine is usually started at 30 mg daily and increased to 60 mg daily.
  - Milnacipran is started at 12.5 mg daily and titrated slowly to 50 mg twice daily (maximum 200 mg daily).
- The SNRI venlafaxine is another option that benefits some patients. The MAOIs and SSRIs have been shown to diminish pain in FMS patients.
- Antiepileptic medications such as **pregabalin and gabapentin** have been studied in fibromyalgia, and pregabalin has been approved by the FDA for treatment of FMS after being shown to significantly reduce pain and fatigue and to improve sleep and health-related quality of life.[9,10]
  - Pregabalin is initiated at 150 mg daily and titrated to 300 to 450 mg/day in divided doses.
  - Gabapentin is dosed at 300 to 2,400 mg daily in divided doses.
- **Medications that target sleep patterns** by promoting stage 4 sleep and providing analgesic effects include the TCAs such as amitriptyline, which is dosed at 10 to 50 mg PO at bedtime. Amitriptyline has been shown to reduce pain, sleep disturbance, and fatigue in FMS patients.[11]
- The centrally acting muscle relaxant **cyclobenzaprine** has been shown to be beneficial in FMS (global assessment, sleep, and pain). It is usually dosed at 10 to 20 mg daily in divided doses.[12] The actual mechanism of action is unclear, but its structure is related to TCAs and cyproheptadine.
- Trials have shown improvement in pain and mood with low-dose naltrexone in 30% of patients.[13]

- Analgesics are generally not beneficial in FMS.
  - There is some evidence that tramadol can be effective, however, in doses of 50 to 400 mg daily.[14,15]
  - Topical agents (e.g., capsaicin cream and topical lidocaine) may be used as adjunctive therapies.
  - **Opioids should not be prescribed for FMS** because FMS patients have worse outcomes with opioids than without them.[13]

REFERENCES

1. Wolfe F, Ross K, Anderson J, et al. The prevalence and characteristics of fibromyalgia in the general population. *Arthritis Rheum.* 1995;38(1):19–28.
2. Gracely RH, Petzke F, Wolf JM, et al. Functional magnetic resonance imaging evidence of augmented pain processing in fibromyalgia. *Arthritis Rheum.* 2002;46(5):1333–1343.
3. Abad VC, Sarinas PS, Guilleminault C. Sleep and rheumatologic disorders. *Sleep Med Rev.* 2008;12(3):211–228.
4. Wolfe F, Clauw DJ, Fitzcharles MA, et al. The American College of Rheumatology preliminary diagnostic criteria for fibromyalgia and measurement of symptom severity. *Arthritis Care Res (Hoboken).* 2010;62(5):600–610.
5. Busch AJ, Barber KA, Overend TJ, et al. Exercise for treating fibromyalgia syndrome. *Cochrane Database Syst Rev.* 2007;(4):Cd003786.
6. Hauser W, Bernardy K, Uceyler N, et al. Treatment of fibromyalgia syndrome with antidepressants: a meta-analysis. *JAMA.* 2009;301(2):198–209.
7. Mease PJ, Clauw DJ, Gendreau RM, et al. The efficacy and safety of milnacipran for treatment of fibromyalgia. a randomized, double-blind, placebo-controlled trial. *J Rheumatol.* 2009;36(2):398–409.
8. Mease PJ, Russell IJ, Arnold LM, et al. A randomized, double-blind, placebo-controlled, phase III trial of pregabalin in the treatment of patients with fibromyalgia. *J Rheumatol.* 2008;35(3):502–514.
9. Arnold LM, Goldenberg DL, Stanford SB, et al. Gabapentin in the treatment of fibromyalgia: a randomized, double-blind, placebo-controlled, multicenter trial. *Arthritis Rheum.* 2007;56(4):1336–1344.
10. Russell IJ, Crofford LJ, Leon T, et al. The effects of pregabalin on sleep disturbance symptoms among individuals with fibromyalgia syndrome. *Sleep Med.* 2009;10(6):604–610.
11. Hauser W, Petzke F, Uceyler N, et al. Comparative efficacy and acceptability of amitriptyline, duloxetine and milnacipran in fibromyalgia syndrome: a systematic review with meta-analysis. *Rheumatology (Oxford).* 2011;50(3):532–543.
12. Harris RE, Clauw DJ, Scott DJ, et al. Decreased central mu-opioid receptor availability in fibromyalgia. *J Neurosci.* 2007;27(37):10000–10006.
13. Younger J, Noor N, McCue R, et al. Low-dose naltrexone for the treatment of fibromyalgia: findings of a small, randomized, double-blind, placebo-controlled, counterbalanced, crossover trial assessing daily pain levels. *Arthritis Rheum.* 2013;65(2):529–538.
14. Tofferi JK, Jackson JL, O'Malley PG. Treatment of fibromyalgia with cyclobenzaprine: a meta-analysis. *Arthritis Rheum.* 2004;51(1):9–13.
15. Bennett RM, Kamin M, Karim R, et al. Tramadol and acetaminophen combination tablets in the treatment of fibromyalgia pain: a double-blind, randomized, placebo-controlled study. *Am J Med.* 2003;114(7):537–545.

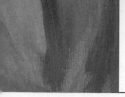

Cutting-Edge Technologies in Rheumatology

54

Michael A. Paley and Wayne M. Yokoyama

GENETIC MANIPULATION

Scientific manipulation of the genome has evolved from random mutagenesis to targeted deletion or insertion of desired genetic material, allowing for detailed analysis of phenotypes attributable to the altered genome.

Homologous Recombination

- Deletion or insertion of genetic material into research animals was initially based on the process of homologous recombination in mouse embryonic stem cells, a development that was awarded the Nobel Prize in Physiology or Medicine (2007).[1]
- Although effective and specific, this process is labor-intensive and inefficient.
- "Knocking out" a gene of interest with homologous recombination might require more than 12 months of cloning, cell culture, *in vitro* fertilization, and screening to generate a specific mouse strain.

Clustered Regularly Interspaced Short Palindromic Repeats (CRISPR)

- The most recent revolution of genetic engineering is based on **CRISPR** and **Cas nucleases**, such as Cas9.[2,3]
- Cas9 is directed by guide RNA sequences to selectively alter genomic DNA targets based on sequence homology.
- The Cas9 nuclease and guide RNA can be directly introduced into eukaryotic cells, including the fertilized egg.[4] This allows for development of new genetically altered embryos, without need for development of embryonic stem cells. By serial targeting of mice and their progeny, this strategy can also generate new mutant strains carrying multiple mutations.
- This process is **highly specific** with off-target effects ranging from 1 to 0.01%.[5,6]
- Because the mutagenesis occurs directly in the embryo, the time to develop a new gene-targeted mouse strain has **decreased to 6 weeks,** expediting testing of new hypotheses in vivo and accelerating the rate of scientific advancement.[7]

Knock Out or Knock In

- The Cas9 nuclease creates a DNA break at the target gene, which often leads to a frameshift mutation during DNA repair, thus "knocking out" the target gene.
- Disease-causing point mutations or other genetic material can be introduced on DNA constructs for faithful "knock-in" mutations. The donor DNA sequences are incorporated into the genomic DNA at the site of the DNA break.

Repression/Activation

Researchers have removed the enzymatic activity of the Cas9 protein and attached either transcriptional activators or repressors to specifically activate or repress target genes, respectively.

CYTOMETRY-BASED MEASUREMENTS: MASS CYTOMETRY

Flow cytometry has helped form the bedrock of today's understanding of immunology and inflammatory or autoimmune diseases.

Traditional Flow Cytometry

- Developed in the 1960s[8]
- Cells are tagged with fluorescent dyes and then passed through lasers that cause the tags to fluoresce.
- The most common method of tagging cells is specific monoclonal antibodies that target a unique molecule.
- By measuring the number of photons emitted from each cell, the relative abundance of the target molecule can be quantified.
- Using different color fluorochromes and their associated optics (e.g., lasers, mirrors, filters, and detectors), multiple parameters can be determined for each cell.
- The cytometer employs advanced fluidics or acoustics to pass cells in a single stream in front of the laser beam at a rate of thousands to tens of thousands of cells per second, allowing for high-throughput analysis at the single-cell level.
- One major **limitation** of this technique, however, is that spectral overlap of different fluorescent tags leads to one dye bleeding over into the detector of another dye. This limits the number of parameters in an individual experiment.
- A second **limitation** is baseline "autofluorescence," in that laser-excited cells will fluoresce even if unlabeled, increasing background.

Mass Cytometry: Cytometry by Time-of-Flight

Cytometry by Time-of-Flight (CyTOF) measures cells labeled with heavy metal tags instead of fluorescent dyes, by high-throughput mass cytometry.[9]

Advantages of CyTOF

- CyTOF markedly increases the number of parameters per cell assessed over traditional flow cytometry.
- By using heavy metal tags that are not naturally found in organic materials, CyTOF is not affected by background signals.
- There is minimal "spectral overlap" between channels as seen by traditional flow cytometry.
- The power to measure so many parameters at once has led to the discovery of new pathogenic mechanisms in rheumatologic disease.

Examples of rheumatologic discoveries based on CyTOF

- CyTOF demonstrated the similarities between viral arthritis and rheumatoid arthritis.[10]
- CyTOF allowed for the identification of a novel type of CD4 helper T cells in seropositive rheumatoid arthritis patients.[11] These CD4 T cells directly interact with B cells within the synovium, promoting adaptive B-cell responses that had previously thought to mainly occur in the spleen or lymph node.
- CyTOF has been used to identify aberrant production of proinflammatory cytokines in the synovium of spondyloarthritis patients.[12]

RNA EXPRESSION MEASUREMENTS: SINGLE-CELL RNA SEQUENCING

- The ability to measure the expression of each gene in the entire genome has led to new understanding in terms of gene regulation, immune cell development, and autoimmunity.

- **Microarray analysis** is accomplished by reverse-transcribing messenger RNA into a complementary DNA (cDNA) library, which is then hybridized to a microarray chip containing probes for each gene of interest.
- **RNA sequencing** uses next-generation, high-throughput sequencers to directly sequence the cDNA library.
- Both of these techniques, however, use large pools of cells that average the expression of each gene in the entire population.
- Rare cell behavior, small populations, and cell-to-cell variation in gene expression are lost by the pooling process.

Single-Cell RNA Sequencing

- Single-cell RNA sequencing (scRNAseq) has provided an opportunity for the rapid accumulation of scientific discoveries.[13]
- scRNAseq uses cell sorting or microfluidics to isolate a single cell in a single well or chamber, or a water micro droplet within an oil immersion.[14,15]
- Inside the chamber or droplet, the cell is lysed, and the RNA is exposed to reagents for synthesis of cDNA.
- Each droplet or chamber is uniquely barcoded, allowing for high-throughput sequencing and discrimination of each cell.
- Commercial products of scRNAseq allow for the high-throughput processing of tens of thousands of cells, creating millions of data points for a single sample.

Advantages of scRNAseq
- scRNAseq facilitates for the discovery of **rare cell types** within a much larger and heterogeneous pool, even if there is no tag or marker previously identified for them.
- scRNAseq allows for analysis of gene expression from single cells in a **mixed cell population**, rather than older methods that would require isolation of the cell of interest before mRNA expression analysis.
- Translational studies no longer have to choose which cell type is believed to be important in disease pathology but rather can identify appropriate cases and controls and allow the biology and bioinformatics to identify the important processes.
- 3D-printed, low-cost droplet microfluidic instruments may be able to bring single-cell transcriptome profiling to the clinical setting.[16]

TISSUE SAMPLING: SYNOVIAL BIOPSIES

- With some exceptions, our understanding of human rheumatologic disease has been largely based on analysis of circulating immune cells in the blood. However, these cells may not completely reflect pathologic changes at the site of inflammation and tissue destruction.
- Tissue-specific injury may be more relevant in understanding the disease process, which could affect medical decision-making.
- A renewed focus on synovial biopsies has thus been developed.

Technique

- **Arthroscopic biopsies** utilize an arthroscope to directly visualize the synovium for biopsy. This technique is most commonly performed in either an operating room or a dedicated procedure room and requires irrigation of the joint for proper visualization. Local anesthesia can be sufficient; however, sedation is often required.[17] This technique is largely limited to large joints.
- **Ultrasound-guided biopsies** use ultrasonography to visualize the placement of the biopsy needle.

- **Blind needle biopsy** uses anatomic landmarks to obtain appropriate synovial tissue. This technique is less reliable for sampling synovial tissue compared to arthroscopic or ultrasound-guided biopsies.[18]
- Both ultrasound-guided and blind needle biopsies can be performed in the outpatient setting, commonly in a dedicated procedure room. Local anesthesia is sufficient, and sedation is not often needed. This technique is less invasive than arthroscopy and is suitable for sampling of both large and small joints.[18,19]

Personalized Medicine

- At the present time, there is little clinical or laboratory data that help rheumatologists select conventional or targeted disease-modifying antirheumatic drugs (DMARDs).
- Current targeted therapies may only be effective in a fraction of patients depending on the rheumatologic disease, such as rheumatoid arthritis.[20]
- Integration of histologic scores and RNA sequencing has revealed three distinct subtypes of synovial inflammation.[21]
- Tissue sampling such as synovial biopsies may provide opportunities to tailor treatment choices to individual patients and improve patient outcomes.[20–22]

REFERENCES

1. The Nobel Prize in Physiology or Medicine 2007. NobelPrize.org. https://www.nobelprize.org/prizes/medicine/2007/summary/. Accessed October 11, 2019.
2. Hsu PD, Lander ES, Zhang F. Development and applications of CRISPR-Cas9 for genome engineering. *Cell.* 2014;157(6):1262–1278.
3. Adli M. The CRISPR tool kit for genome editing and beyond. *Nat Commun.* 2018;9(1):1911.
4. Parikh BA, Beckman DL, Patel SJ, et al. Detailed phenotypic and molecular analyses of genetically modified mice generated by CRISPR-Cas9-mediated editing. *PLoS One.* 2015;10(1):e0116484.
5. Gori JL, Hsu PD, Maeder ML, et al. Delivery and specificity of CRISPR-Cas9 genome editing technologies for human gene therapy. *Hum Gene Ther.* 2015;26(7):443–451.
6. Tycko J, Barrera LA, Huston NC, et al. Pairwise library screen systematically interrogates Staphylococcus aureus Cas9 specificity in human cells. *Nat Commun.* 2018;9(1):2962.
7. Shalem O, Sanjana NE, Zhang F. High-throughput functional genomics using CRISPR-Cas9. *Nat Rev Genet.* 2015;16(5):299–311.
8. Picot J, Guerin CL, Le Van Kim C, et al. Flow cytometry: retrospective, fundamentals and recent instrumentation. *Cytotechnology.* 2012;64(2):109–130.
9. Spitzer MH, Nolan GP. Mass cytometry: single cells, many features. *Cell.* 2016;165(4):780–791.
10. Miner JJ, Aw-Yeang HX, Fox JM, et al. Chikungunya viral arthritis in the United States: a mimic of seronegative rheumatoid arthritis. *Arthritis Rheumatol.* 2015;67(5):1214–1220.
11. Rao DA, Gurish MF, Marshall JL, et al. Pathologically expanded peripheral T helper cell subset drives B cells in rheumatoid arthritis. *Nature.* 2017;542(7639):110–114.
12. Al-Mossawi MH, Chen L, Fang H, et al. Unique transcriptome signatures and GM-CSF expression in lymphocytes from patients with spondyloarthritis. *Nat Commun.* 2017;8(1):1510.
13. Stubbington MJT, Rozenblatt-Rosen O, Regev A, et al. Single-cell transcriptomics to explore the immune system in health and disease. *Science.* 2017;358(6359):58–63.
14. Kolodziejczyk AA, Kim JK, Svensson V, et al. The technology and biology of single-cell RNA sequencing. *Mol Cell.* 2015;58(4):610–620.
15. Baran-Gale J, Chandra T, Kirschner K. Experimental design for single-cell RNA sequencing. *Brief Funct Genomics.* 2018;17(4):233–239.
16. Stephenson W, Donlin LT, Butler A, et al. Single-cell RNA-seq of rheumatoid arthritis synovial tissue using low-cost microfluidic instrumentation. *Nat Commun.* 2018;9(1):791.
17. Kane D, Veale DJ, FitzGerald O, et al. Survey of arthroscopy performed by rheumatologists. *Rheumatology (Oxford).* 2002;41(2):210–215.
18. Humby F, Romao VC, Manzo A, et al. A multicenter retrospective analysis evaluating performance of synovial biopsy techniques in patients with inflammatory arthritis: arthroscopic versus ultrasound-guided versus blind needle biopsy. *Arthritis Rheumatol.* 2018;70(5):702–710.

19. Kelly S, Humby F, Filer A, et al. Ultrasound-guided synovial biopsy: a safe, well-tolerated and reliable technique for obtaining high-quality synovial tissue from both large and small joints in early arthritis patients. *Ann Rheum Dis.* 2015;74(3):611–617.

20. Romao VC, Vital EM, Fonseca JE, et al. Right drug, right patient, right time: aspiration or future promise for biologics in rheumatoid arthritis? *Arthritis Res Ther.* 2017;19(1):239.

21. Orange DE, Agius P, DiCarlo EF, et al. Identification of three rheumatoid arthritis disease subtypes by machine learning integration of synovial histologic features and RNA sequencing data. *Arthritis Rheumatol.* 2018;70(5):690–701.

22. Mandelin AM, II, Homan PJ, Shaffer AM, et al. Transcriptional profiling of synovial macrophages using minimally invasive ultrasound-guided synovial biopsies in rheumatoid arthritis. *Arthritis Rheumatol.* 2018;70(6):841–854.

Index

Note: Page locators followed by *f* and *t* indicates figure and table respectively.